STATISTICS
for
HEALTH
PROFESSIONALS

SUSAN SHOTT, Ph.D.

Assistant Professor
Section of Epidemiology and Biostatistics
Department of Preventive Medicine
Rush-Presbyterian-St. Luke's Medical Center
Chicago, Illinois

W. B. SAUNDERS COMPANY

Harcourt Brace Jovanovich, Inc.

Philadelphia, London, Toronto, Montreal, Sydney, Tokyo

W. B. SAUNDERS COMPANY
Harcourt Brace Jovanovich, Inc.

The Curtis Center
Independence Square West
Philadelphia, PA 19106

Library of Congress Cataloging-in-Publication Data

Shott, Susan, 1954–
    Statistics for health professionals.

    Includes bibliographical references.
    1. Medical
statistics.   I. Title.   [DNLM: 1. Biometry.
2. Statistics.   WA 950 5559s]
RA407.s56   1990   610'.21   89-70016
ISBN 0-7216-8254-5

Cover design by Miriam Recio

Sponsoring Editor: Thomas Eoyang

STATISTICS FOR HEALTH PROFESSIONALS   ISBN   0-7216-8254-5

Printed in the United States of America

Last digit is the print number: 9   8   7   6   5   4   3

This book is dedicated to three health professionals
who exemplify the best in their fields:

U. Yun Ryo, M.D., Ph.D.

Joan A. Uebele, M.S., R.N.

Susan E. Yohn, D.V.M.

PREFACE

The importance of correct statistical analyses in medical and health care research cannot be overemphasized. Decisions about treatment methods are often made on the basis of research articles. If these articles rest on faulty statistics, a great deal of harm may result. Unfortunately, incorrect statistical analyses are not uncommon in the medical and health care literature.[1-8]

Traditionally taught statistics courses can do little to reduce the number of statistical errors. Students in such courses spend so much time memorizing formulas, studying proofs, and calculating numbers that they often fail to learn the basic principles of sound statistical analysis. All too often, statisticians assume that what is obvious to them must be obvious to nonstatisticians. The result is statistics courses and textbooks that gloss over the application and interpretation of statistical methods. But these are the areas that cause students and researchers the greatest difficulty. Most statistical errors in the classroom and in the medical and health care literature involve misapplications or misinterpretations of statistical procedures.

This text emphasizes *understanding* of statistical procedures rather than memorization or calculation. The assumptions required by statistical methods are discussed in detail, and numerous examples illustrating common violations of assumptions are presented. Correct interpretations of statistical results are emphasized, again through the use of examples. The problems do not ask for rote applications of statistical formulas. Instead, they ask the student to choose correct statistical procedures, identify violations of statistical assumptions, and interpret statistical results.

Because some knowledge of formulas is necessary to understand statistics, statistical formulas are presented and discussed. Proofs are omitted, however, and notation is kept to a minimum. Some calculation is also required. Although computers are commonly used to carry out statistical analyses, the methods used to generate statistical output should not be a mystery. Whenever possible, calculations are simplified to eliminate excessive number crunching.

The sequence of topics in this text differs slightly from the usual sequence. I have found that students grasp analysis of variance more easily if it is taught immediately after hypothesis testing. A more common sequence places the analysis of frequency data immediately after hypothesis testing. In addition, the McNemar test for comparing proportions is discussed in the chapter on analysis of frequency data (Chapter 10) rather than the chapter on nonparametric statistics (Chapter 11). I believe that this test is best discussed with the chi-square test of association. All too often, the chi-square test of association is mistakenly applied to data that should be analyzed with the McNemar test.

Preferences vary, and the sequence of topics here can be changed to suit different tastes. Statistical inference, confidence intervals, and hypothesis testing are described in Chapters 4–7, which require Chapters 2 and 3. Once these six chapters have been covered, the topics discussed in Chapters 8–13 may be taken up in any order, with the exception of the three chapters on analysis of variance. Familiarity with Chapter 8 (one-way analysis of variance) is needed before beginning Chapter 13 (two-way analysis of variance) or Chapter 9 (one-factor repeated-measures analysis of variance). An optional chapter on experimental design is also included. Since experimental designs warrant an entire book, only a brief discussion of basic principles is given.

The text contains more material than can be covered in a single course, and several topics that are not usually covered in a first statistics course have been included. One-factor repeated-measures analysis of variance, two-way analysis of variance, and regression and correlation (Chapters 9, 13, and 12) have been discussed because they are so commonly used in medical and health care research. Their inclusion should make this text more useful as a reference. In addition, instructors who prefer to cover these topics can use this text to do so. Instructors who prefer not to cover these topics can omit them.

Although the text requires almost no mathematical sophistication, a certain amount of clinical knowledge is assumed. The text will be most useful to students and professionals with some knowledge of medicine and health care. Graduate students and advanced undergraduate students are most likely to be comfortable with the clinical level of the text. The text is also appropriate for highly motivated beginning undergraduates with a strong interest in medicine or health care.

Because the text is aimed at diverse health professionals, a variety of data is used. Most of the examples and problems are based on data from the medical, health care, and veterinary literature. Although examples that please everyone do not exist, the large number of diverse examples should provide most readers with something of interest. An excess of problems is given, allowing selective assignment of problems to suit various tastes.

I have attempted to make this book complete enough to serve as a reference as well as a text. It is also designed for self-study. To this end, answers to half of the problems are given in Appendix D.

The goal of this text is to foster the kind of statistical understanding that leads to sound research. If this text can guide health professionals past the statistical pitfalls that trap so many, it will serve its purpose.

A few words about pronouns: In the interest of fairness and readability, I have alternated the use of "she" and "he." This convention avoids the awkward "he/she" phrase while providing equal time for both sexes. It may also have the unintended consequence of infuriating everyone half of the time. If anyone has a better solution to the pronoun problem, please let me know.

Acknowledgments: Numerous people have been kind enough to read various drafts of this text, and their comments have greatly improved the book. I am especially indebted to Judith Brown, Sandra Gaynor, Douglas Hammer, Sharon Handelsman, Marija Norusis, Glen Richardson, Wendy Tuzik, Joan Uebele, June Valient, Paul Zorn, and several anonymous reviewers. I also wish to acknowledge Jessie, Granger, Scout, Trig, Saunders, and Mugsy for making me learn about medicine.

References

1. Schor S, Karten I: Statistical evaluation of medical journal manuscripts. J Am Med Assoc *195*:1123–1128, 1966.

2. Lionel NDW, Herxheimer A: Assessing reports of therapeutic trials. Br Med J *3*:637–640, 1970.
3. Hoffman JIE: The incorrect use of Chi-square analysis for paired data. Clin Exper Immunol *24*:227–229, 1976.
4. Gore SM, Jones IG, Rytter EC: Misuse of statistical methods: Critical assessment of articles in BMJ from January to March 1976. Br Med J *1*:85–87, 1977.
5. White SJ: Statistical errors in papers in the British Journal of Psychiatry. Br J Psychiatry *135*:336–342, 1979.
6. Glantz SA: Biostatistics: How to detect, correct and prevent errors in the medical literature. Circulation *61*:1–7, 1980.
7. Gore SM, Altman DG: Statistics in Practice. London: British Medical Association, 1982.
8. Shott S: Statistics in veterinary research. J Am Vet Med Assoc *187*:138–141, 1985.

TEXT OBJECTIVES

After studying this text and working the problems, you should be able to:

1. Explain the process of statistical inference

2. Select appropriate statistical methods for most data sets

3. Interpret results from most of the commonly used statistical tests

4. Evaluate most statistical analyses reported in the medical and health care literature

5. Carry out basic calculations needed to obtain many statistical results

6. Interpret SPSS and SAS output for many commonly used statistical procedures

7. Recognize data analysis problems that require consultation with a statistician

CONTENTS

EXPERIMENTAL DESIGN

Bad experimental designs create problems that cannot be corrected by any statistical procedure, however sophisticated. As Dingle states[1]:

> No intelligent person would underestimate the importance of mathematics in science or question the necessity for its correctness, but it cannot bring truth out of error. If it is applied to truth it will produce truth, and if it is applied to error it will almost certainly produce error.

For this reason, we begin by discussing some elementary principles of experimental design. Health professionals who understand these principles can avoid errors when designing their own experiments, and they can detect design errors in medical and health care research by others.*

---

*Our discussion of experimental design is necessarily brief. For more detail, the reader may want to consult Gore and Altman,[2] which provides an excellent discussion of problems associated with medical experimental designs.

1.1 CONFOUNDED EFFECTS

Experimental design refers to the structure of an experiment; specifically, the experimental procedures, the selection of subjects, and the allocation of subjects to different experimental procedures. The goal of sound experimental design is the elimination of *confounded effects*, which occur when the effects of the treatments are so hopelessly mixed up with the effects of something else that treatment effects cannot be separated out and analyzed.

Suppose a nurse wants to determine whether a new urinary catheter is less likely to result in urinary tract infection (UTI) than a standard catheter. She selects 40 patients requiring long-term urinary catheterization and uses the new catheter on 17 of the patients who are predisposed to UTI. The standard catheter is used for the other 23 patients, who are not predisposed to UTI. After six weeks, the nurse compares the percentage of patients using the new catheter who develop UTI with the percentage of patients using the standard catheter who develop UTI.

The design of this experiment guarantees that the effect of the new catheter will be confounded with the effect of predisposition to UTI. Even if the new catheter reduces the risk of UTI, the percentage of patients with this catheter who develop UTI may be larger than the percentage of patients with the standard catheter who develop UTI. Patients with the new catheter are more predisposed to UTI than the other patients, and this may cancel out the infection-reducing properties of the new catheter. The experiment creates a bias against the new catheter.

When this sort of confounding is present, no statistical method can repair the damage and the experiment has no value. If the conclusions of confounded experiments are accepted, the medical and health care consequences may be quite harmful. Beneficial treatments may be ignored or useless treatments adopted.

Four precautions are essential for a sound experimental design:

1. Control groups
2. Placebos or sham procedures
3. Double-blind or single-blind procedures
4. Random assignment of subjects to treatment and control groups

We will discuss the rationale for each of these precautions, as well as the possible consequences of omitting them.

1.2 CONTROL GROUPS

A *control group* is a group of subjects who are left untreated or are treated with standard methods. A *treatment group* is a group of subjects who are given the treatment being studied. The reasoning behind the use of control groups is straightforward: if you have nothing with which to compare a treatment group, you cannot determine whether the treatment works. A report on insulin pump therapy, for example, found that the average glycosylated hemoglobin concentration improved in 83% of 127 diabetic patients who used insulin pumps.[3] What does this tell us about the effectiveness of insulin pumps? Without a control group, there is not much we can say. It is possible that 83% of these patients also would have improved on conventional treatment and with the close monitoring imposed on human research subjects.

Researchers sometimes attempt to reduce the cost of their studies by omitting control groups. The additional cost of using a control group, however, is small compared with the potential cost of a faulty design. The results of a bad experiment may have to be thrown out, making the entire experiment a waste of time and money.

1.3 PLACEBOS AND SHAM PROCEDURES

The control and treatment groups should be as similar as possible. Ideally, they should differ only with respect to the treatment of interest. Many experiments use placebos or sham procedures to increase the similarity of treatment and control groups. *Placebos* are inert substances administered in the same way as treatment medications. *Sham procedures* closely resemble treatment procedures but are not intended to provide effective treatment.

Placebo injections were used in a study of the effectiveness of ampicillin prophylaxis in clean surgical procedures.[4] Infection rates for two groups of animals that underwent clean surgical procedures were compared. The treatment group received two intramuscular injections of ampicillin and the control group received two intramuscular injections of normal saline solution (the placebo). If placebo injections had not been used, the effect of ampicillin would have been confounded with the effect of using an injection as a method of administration. Since any injection carries a slight risk of infection, failure to use placebo injections would have created a slight bias against ampicillin prophylaxis.

A sham procedure was used in a study of acute pancreatitis in the dog.[5] Acute hemorrhagic pancreatitis was induced in six dogs by infusing oleic acid into the pancreas. Four control dogs were sham-operated, using the same anesthetic protocol and surgical approach but omitting the acid infusion. If sham operations had not been done, the effect of pancreatitis would have been confounded with the effect of surgery. Lethargy, depression, and ascites were observed after surgery in the dogs with pancreatitis but not in the control dogs. Because sham surgeries were done, we can rule out the possibility that these differences were due to the surgery rather than to pancreatitis.

1.4 BLIND PROCEDURES

A study is *double blind* if neither the researchers nor the subjects know which subjects are in the control group and which are in the treatment groups until the study has ended. In a *single-blind* study, the researchers do not know which subjects are controls and which are being treated, but each subject knows which group she is in.* Double-blind procedures are always better than single-blind procedures, although double-blind procedures are not always possible. If one treatment is surgical and the

*Studies in which the researcher, but not the subject, knows the subject's treatment status are also called single blind.

other is medical, patients obviously will know which treatment group they are in.

The purpose of blind procedures is the reduction of bias. If patients know that they were given placebos, they may exaggerate symptoms that they would dismiss if they knew that they were given drugs. If a researcher knows a patient's treatment status, the patient's responses and the researcher's interpretation of patient responses can be affected, thereby biasing the results. Researcher bias is of particular concern in medicine and health care, since clinical signs and laboratory results are often amenable to different interpretations. This sort of bias is not necessarily intentional, but it can subconsciously influence the interpretations of even the most conscientious researcher. Consider the study of ampicillin prophylaxis described earlier. This experiment was a blind study: the surgeons who evaluated wounds for infection were not told which injection (ampicillin or placebo) was given. The possibility that evaluations were biased by knowledge of the injection was eliminated. Such bias could not have been ruled out if blind procedures had not been used, since the determination of wound infection is not always clear-cut.

Blind procedures cannot always be used. The pancreatitis study could not have been blind if the surgeons evaluated the animals after surgery. A surgeon obviously knows whether she induced pancreatitis or performed a sham operation. However, blind procedures could have been used if persons other than the surgeons evaluated the dogs after surgery. In some experiments, the nature of the treatment makes blind procedures impossible. A study comparing the effectiveness of video and lecture descriptions of colostomy care can be single blind but not double blind, as patients know which presentation they witnessed. Experiments without double-blind procedures must be interpreted with caution whenever knowledge of treatment status could bias the responses of subjects or researchers.

1.5 RANDOMIZATION

Randomization, or *random assignment*, is the assignment of subjects to treatment and control groups by using some chance-governed mechanism. For example, subjects might be randomly assigned by tossing a coin and letting "heads" dictate assignment to the control group and "tails" dictate assignment to the treatment group. We will describe the mechanics of randomization in Chapter 5. Here our concern is the rationale for randomization.

If confounded effects are to be avoided, the control and treatment groups must be similar with respect to any characteristic that could affect the results (age, sex, race, general health, etc.). It might seem that the best way to do this is to deliberately make the groups similar with respect to all charac-

teristics that seem important. The researcher could try to assign subjects so that all groups have similar racial compositions, similar medical problems, similar ages, and so forth. If there are many characteristics to distribute evenly between groups, however, it is quite difficult to do so. In addition, researchers rarely know all of the characteristics that could influence the results. Characteristics that were not taken into account when subjects were assigned to groups may later turn out to be important, producing confounded effects.

Yet another problem is *selection bias*—bias in the assignment of subjects to treatment and control groups. Selection bias is almost inevitable when the researcher decides which subjects are to be assigned to treatment and control groups, and it need not be conscious to have an effect. Suppose the treatment group will be subjected to extremely unpleasant chemotherapy. The researcher assigning patients to treatment and control groups may, out of sympathy, assign to the treatment group only patients in good physical condition. If this is done, the effect of chemotherapy will be confounded with the effect of good physical condition, creating a bias in favor of chemotherapy.

These problems can often be avoided by the random assignment of subjects. Human selection bias is eliminated by randomization, since the researcher does not decide which subjects go into treatment groups and which into control groups. Practical difficulties are reduced, since randomization is easy to carry out. If large enough groups are used (ideally, at least 100 subjects per group for a two-group experiment[2]), the treatment and control groups are likely to be similar. When small groups are used, randomization can produce dissimilar groups. The chance of getting dissimilar groups increases as the group size decreases. Experimenters should always check to make sure that their groups are similar with respect to characteristics that might be important. If random assignment produces obviously dissimilar treatment and control groups, rerandomization should be carried out if possible. Even when the groups used are small, however, randomization is essential to eliminate human bias when assigning subjects to groups.

1.6 OBSERVATIONAL STUDIES

Many medical and health care studies are observational rather than experimental. In an experimental study, the researcher assigns subjects to the groups studied, using randomization or some other method. In an observational study, the researcher cannot assign subjects to the groups studied. Studies comparing people who have a disease with healthy people are necessarily observational. A researcher cannot ethically assign certain people to a disease group and then induce the disease. Instead, he obtains a group of people who already have the disease and compares these people with a group of people who do not have the disease.

Many observational studies have produced invaluable information, and most human diseases cannot be studied in any other way—but a high risk of confounded effects is always involved. Suppose the estradiol levels of women with uterine cancer are compared with the estradiol levels of women without uterine cancer. If the estradiol levels of the two groups differ, the difference may be due to some factor other than uterine cancer. Because women cannot be randomly assigned to cancer and no-cancer groups, confounded effects are a major concern.

Confounding is evident in an observational study of the effect of aerobic exercise on maternal self-esteem and physical discomfort during pregnancy.[6] Thirty-one women attending prenatal exercise classes were compared with 22 women attending childbirth preparation classes. The exercise group had higher self-esteem scores and lower discomfort scores, on average, than the nonexercise group. But we cannot conclude that aerobic exercise during pregnancy results in higher self-esteem and lower discomfort. Table 1.1 shows that the exercise and nonexercise groups differ with respect to education, income, and occupation—all characteristics that affect both self-esteem and expression of discomfort. Because the effect of exercise is confounded with the effects of education, income, and occupation, we cannot attribute higher self-esteem or lower discomfort to exercise.

Observational studies must always be closely examined for confounding. Even if no obvious confounding is evident, the results of such studies must be interpreted with caution, since confounded effects may result from characteristics that were not measured. Whenever possible, the results of observational studies should be confirmed or disconfirmed by well-designed experimental studies. If this is not possible, the use of various nonexperimental or quasi-experimental designs can sometimes reduce the risk of confounding. Information about such designs can be found in other texts.[7]

TABLE 1.1 SOCIOECONOMIC CHARACTERISTICS OF EXERCISE AND NONEXERCISE GROUPS

Characteristic	Exercise Group No.	Exercise Group %	Nonexercise Group No.	Nonexercise Group %
Education Less than college degree	6	19.4	13	59.1
Income Less than $30,000	6	19.4	15	68.2
Occupation Unemployed or nonprofessional	18	58.1	17	77.3

1.7 CONSEQUENCES OF DESIGN FLAWS

If data are analyzed improperly, they can always be reanalyzed correctly (preferably before publication). If data are based on an experiment with fundamental design flaws, nothing can be done to correct the damage resulting from confounded effects. The only remedy is to repeat the experiment, using a sound design. This unpleasant fact causes considerable consternation among researchers who hope that their badly designed experiments can be patched up statistically. It simply cannot be done. Just as some patients are beyond medical repair, some data sets are beyond statistical repair. The best strategy is prevention: avoid confounded experiments whenever possible.

SUMMARY

The purpose of good experimental design is the elimination of confounded effects. When confounded effects are present, no amount of statistical manipulation can repair the damage. Ideally, four precautions should be taken to obtain sound experimental designs: control groups, placebos or sham procedures, double-blind or single-blind procedures, and random assignment. For practical and ethical reasons, not all of these precautions can be used in every study. Because observational studies lack some of these precautions, their results must be interpreted with caution. Nonetheless, many observational studies have produced invaluable information.

PROBLEMS

For the studies described in problems 1 through 9, indicate whether sound experimental designs were used and describe any design problems that are evident. Also discuss biases or confounding that might have arisen from design deficiencies. Essential information about the design is omitted in some of the studies, and this should be noted. Such omissions are all too common in the medical and health care literature.[8, 9]

1. "This prospective study was designed to evaluate the efficacy of cisplatin in treating cancer-associated hypercalcemia in humans. Thirteen patients with severe hypercalcemia refractory to rehydration were treated with a 24-hour infusion of cisplatin, 100 mg/m^2. Serial measurements of serum calcium and tumor size were made following cisplatin treatment and compared with pretreatment values. Nine patients (69%) achieved normocalcemia after treatment with cisplatin; and mean [average] duration of benefit was 38 days in these patients. ... We conclude that cisplatin can control malignant hypercalcemia for relatively long periods."[10]

2. "The purpose of this study was to compare the effect of three methods of chest tube management on mediastinal drainage volume in cardiac surgery patients: (1) a standard single-lumen thoracic catheter with suction of -20 cm H_2O and intermittent chest tube stripping (standard method), (2) the standard method with addition of venting poststripping pressures over -20 cm H_2O (venting method), and (3) use of a sump catheter with no stripping (sump method). ... Thirty men undergoing closed mediastinal drainage after first-time cardiac surgery were studied, 10 in each group. ... Data was collected first for the standard method because it created the least disruption in usual agency practice, second for the venting method, and last for the sump method, which represented the greatest change from usual routines."[11]

3. "Seventy-eight patients having at least one impacted mandibular third molar extracted were assigned randomly to one of the following four treatment groups:
   —Acetaminophen 1,000 mg before surgery and acetaminophen 650 mg at fixed intervals of 4 and 8 hours after surgery.
   —Placebo (lactose) before surgery and acetaminophen 650 mg at fixed intervals of 4 and 8 hours after surgery.
   —Acetaminophen 1,000 mg before surgery and acetaminophen 650 mg taken as needed for pain after surgery.
   —Placebo (lactose) before surgery and acetaminophen 650 mg taken as needed for pain after surgery.
The medications and schedules were coded so that neither the surgeon nor the research assistant who collected the data knew the assigned treatment group. The acetaminophen 1,000 mg and placebo were prepared as identically appearing capsules and administered 30 minutes before surgery."[12]

4. "Three hundred patients who underwent elective, interval or emergency appendectomy at four participating hospitals were entered into the study. ... All patients received 1 gram of metronidazole per rectum at least 40 minutes prior to operation and at intervals of 12 hours for five days postoperatively. Patients were randomized to receive 2 grams of cefotetan intravenously just before induction of anesthesia (group 1) or no further antibiotic (group 2). ... Details of the antibiotics given were recorded on a data sheet kept separate from the patient notes. Wounds were examined daily until the patient left the hospital and again at outpatient review four weeks later. Wound infection was defined as the presence of pus, wound disruption or serous discharge from which bacteria were cultured."[13]

5. "The first [method] (experimental group) was based on a new approach which claimed that postpartum breast discomfort in non-breastfeeding women would be reduced if milk was extracted from the breasts. The second approach (hospital policy group) involved adhering to the normal hospital routine which was a combination of traditional methods. ... Non-breastfeeding women admitted to Ward A were assigned to the experimental group ($N = 95$), and non-breastfeeding women admitted to Ward B acted as the control or hospital policy group ($N = 57$). ... Three times daily, participants entered details on the questionnaire relating to self-assessment of pain, use of analgesia and methods employed in supressing lactation."[14]

6. "The Medical Research Council trial of treatment of hypertension in the elderly is a randomized placebo-controlled study designed to show whether antihypertensive therapy is associated with a reduced incidence of stroke in men and women aged 65 to 74 years with mean [average] systolic pressures sustained at screening in the range of 160 to 209 mm Hg. The treatment groups used are hydrochlorothiazide together with amiloride or a placebo, or atenolol or a placebo. ... At all follow-up visits, patients were asked if they had noticed certain symptoms possibly as a result of adverse reactions to the drugs (joint pain, lethargy, nausea, dizziness, headache, etc.) and were given an opportunity to mention other problems. ... [The study] was of a single-blind design."[15]

7. "All newborns of consenting parents at Rochester Methodist Hospital were randomized to one of two ophthalmic prophylaxis treatment groups, either 1% silver nitrate or 1% tetracycline hydrochloride ophthalmic solution. ... Parents and physicians were kept blind to the actual agent employed in the delivery room for prophylaxis. ... Almost exactly the same proportion of two-week-old infants in both treatment groups had a history of ongoing eye discharge."[16]

8. "Tail amputation was used to treat dogs affected with perianal fistulas. The described surgical technique was applied to clinical cases over a five-and-one-half-year period. ... Data was collected on 25 dogs by means of examination and telephone survey. Complications included incomplete resolution of the fistulas (five dogs) emergence of new fistulas (five dogs), anal stricture (one dog), anal sac abscessation (one dog), and wound dehiscence (one dog). Of the 13 cases with complications, nine did not require additional surgery to alleviate the symptoms. The data indicates that tail amputation is a viable first choice of treatment for perianal fistulas."[17]

9. "This experimental design study was instituted with two sample groups of a population of traumatic head-injured patients utilizing two health care facilities ... The first sample consisted of 15 patients who were admitted to a setting that employed a controlled structured sensory-stimulation program for head injured patients. This was the experimental group. The control group consisted of 15 head-injured patients who received nursing care that did not include planned, structured sensory stimulation. ... The patients in the control group were matched on a one-to-one basis with the patients in the experimental group on the basis of sex, age range, approximate type of injury, Glasgow Coma Scale Score, and length of time post injury. ... Scores of cognitive function in the experimental group were compared to those of the control group."[18]

10. Find (1) an article in a medical or health care journal that describes a badly designed experiment and (2) one that describes a well-designed experiment. Discuss the problems evident in the badly designed study and describe confounding or biases that might result from these problems. Describe possible confounding or biases that were avoided in the well-designed study.

11. Design an experiment to investigate a question of interest to you. Describe in detail all of the safeguards against confounding that you could use. If some of the safeguards described in this chapter cannot be used, describe the types of confounding or bias that might result. Discuss steps you could take to reduce the chance of confounding or bias.

REFERENCES

1. Dingle H: Quoted in Bean WB: A critique of criticism in medicine and the biological sciences. Perspect Biol Med *1*:224–232, 1958 (reprinted Arch Intern Med *134*:858–861, 1974).
2. Gore SM, Altman DG: Statistics in Practice. London: British Medical Association, 1982.
3. Mecklenburg RS, Benson EA, Benson JW, et al: Long-term metabolic control with insulin pump therapy. Report of experience with 127 patients. N Engl J Med *313*:465–468, 1985.
4. Vasseur PB, Paul HA, Enos ER, et al: Infection rates in clean surgical procedures: A comparison of ampicillin prophylaxis vs a placebo. J Am Vet Med Assoc *187*:825–827, 1985.
5. Jacobs RM, Murtaugh RJ, DeHoff WD: Review of the clinicopathological findings of acute pancreatitis in the dog: Use of an experimental model. J Am Anim Hosp Assoc *21*:795–800, 1985.
6. Wallace AM, Boyer DB, Dan A, et al: Aerobic exercise, maternal self-esteem, and physical discomforts during pregnancy. J Nurs-Midwif *31*:255–262, 1986.
7. Oyster CK, Hanten WP, Llorens LA: Introduction to Research: A Guide for the Health Science Professional. Philadelphia: Lippincott, 1987.
8. DerSimonian R, Charette LJ, McPeek B, et al: Reporting on methods in clinical trials. N Engl J Med *306*:1332–1337, 1982.
9. Jacobsen BS, Meininger JC: Randomized experiments in nursing: The quality of reporting. Nurs Res *35*:379–382, 1986.
10. Lad TE, Mishoulam HM, Shevrin DH, et al: Treatment of cancer-associated hypercalcemia with cisplatin. Arch Intern Med *147*:329–332, 1987.
11. Duncan CR, Erickson RS, Weigel RM: Effect of chest tube management on drainage after cardiac surgery. Heart Lung *16*:1–9, 1987.
12. Moore PA, Werther JR, Seldin EB, et al: Analgesic regimens for third molar surgery: Pharmacologic and behavioral considerations. J Am Dent Assoc *113*:739–744, 1986.
13. Wilson RG, Taylor EW, Lindsay G, et al: A comparative study of cefotetan and metronidazole against metronidazole alone to prevent infection after appendectomy. Surg Gynecol Obstet *164*:447–451, 1987.
14. Webster J: Lactation supression: A pilot study. Austr J Adv Nurs *4*:36–40, 1986.
15. Medical Research Council Working Party: Comparison of the antihypertensive efficacy and adverse reactions to two doses of bendrofluazide and hydrochlorothiazide and the effect of potassium supplementation on the hypotensive action of bendrofluazide: Substudies of the Medical Research Council's trials of treatment of mild hypertension. J Clin Pharmacol *27*:271–277, 1987.
16. Hick JF, Block DJ, Ilstrup DM: A controlled study of silver nitrate prophylaxis and the incidence of nasolacrimal duct obstruction. J Ophthal Nurs Technol *5*:61–62, 1986.
17. van Ee RT, Palminteri A: Tail amputation for treatment of perianal fistulas in dogs. J Am Anim Hosp Assoc *23*:95–100, 1987.
18. Kater KM: Response of head-injured patients to sensory stimulation. West J Nurs Res *11*:20–33, 1989.

2

DESCRIPTIVE STATISTICS

CHAPTER OBJECTIVES

After studying this chapter and working the problems,
you should be able to:

1. Calculate and interpret simple descriptive statistics

2. Determine whether the mean, median, and mode are appropriate

3. Distinguish among nominal, ordinal, interval, and ratio data

4. Recognize skewed and symmetric histograms

Statistics is often defined as the science of collecting, analyzing, and interpreting data. This is accurate enough, but another definition better reflects the importance of statistics: statistics is "the study and informed application of methods of reaching conclusions about the world from fallible observations."[1] Unlike other methods, statistics can sometimes provide the probability of getting observations that are way off base. (We will have more to say about this in Chapter 6 when we discuss confidence intervals.) No method can offer certainty, but statistics at least can tell you what your odds are.

(the *sample*) to all possible observations of interest (the *population*).*

Before we consider statistical inference, we need to look at some common descriptive statistics. This requires a certain amount of notation. Statistical notation is often bewildering at first, but the effort required to learn it is far less than the effort required to struggle through lengthy verbal descriptions of formulas. Notation is nothing more than a convenience, a form of shorthand. Anyone who can learn the intricacies of medical terminology can also learn statistical notation.

The customary representation for data values is

$$x_1, x_2, x_3, x_4, \ldots, x_n$$

2.1 DESCRIPTIVE STATISTICS

Descriptive statistics are numerical or graphical summaries of data. An average is a descriptive statistic; so is a line chart. Most descriptive statistics are easily understood and often are not very interesting in themselves. What is usually of interest are the *inferences* that can be drawn from descriptive statistics. *Statistical inference* is the process of generalizing from the data collected by the researcher

---

*In some studies, only descriptive statistics are of interest, and inferences to a population are not made. Administrators studying cost-control measures at the Minicare Health Maintenance Organization (HMO) might be concerned only with the effectiveness of these measures at Minicare. In this case, they would not attempt to generalize their results to the population of all HMOs similar to Minicare.

where x_1 represents the first observation, x_2 the second observation, and so on, with x_n representing the last observation. The letter n denotes the total number of observations. Because many statistical procedures involve addition, we also need notation to represent addition. The Greek letter Σ (sigma) is used for this purpose. The expression

$$\sum_{i=1}^{n} x_i$$

means "the sum of all n observations" ($x_1 + x_2 + \cdots + x_n$). The "$i = 1$" under the Σ tells us to start adding with the first observation (x_1), and the n on top of the Σ tells us to stop adding with the last observation (x_n).

2.2 MEASURES OF CENTRAL TENDENCY

Loosely speaking, measures of central tendency are numbers that represent some "central value" that the data seem to be grouped around. Since there are different notions of what a central value is, there are different measures of central tendency. The most familiar measure is the sample *mean*, or arithmetic average. The sample mean is denoted by $\bar{x}$ (pronounced "x bar") and is the sum of all the observations, divided by the number of observations:

$$\bar{x} = \frac{\sum_{i=1}^{n} x_i}{n} \qquad (2.1)$$

Example 2.1 _____

A study of chronic asthma resulting from toluene diisocyanate (TDI) exposure reported the time interval from TDI exposure to onset of symptoms for seven workers with TDI asthma.[2] These time intervals are shown in Table 2.1.

Applying formula (2.1), we obtain a mean time interval of 23.07 months for these seven workers:

$$\bar{x} = \frac{(1.00 + 0.46 + 12.00 + 120.00 + 24.00 + 0.03 + 4.00)}{7}$$

$$= \frac{161.49}{7} = 23.07$$

_____

Means have an important limitation: they are excessively influenced by data values far outside the range of most of the data. This is evident for the mean time interval obtained in Example 2.1. Five of the time intervals are between 0.03 and 12.00 months, but there is one extremely large time interval of 120.00 months that greatly affects the mean. If the mean is calculated without including this

TABLE 2.1 TIME INTERVAL FROM TDI EXPOSURE TO ONSET OF SYMPTOMS

Worker	Time Interval (months)
1	1.00
2	0.46
3	12.00
4	120.00
5	24.00
6	0.03
7	4.00

unusually large time interval, we get 6.92 months:

$$\bar{x} = \frac{(1.00 + 0.46 + 12.00 + 24.00 + 0.03 + 4.00)}{6}$$

$$= \frac{41.49}{6} = 6.92$$

This mean is much smaller than the original mean of 23.07 months, indicating the strong influence of the large time interval.

When data consist of survival times, the mean usually cannot be calculated. Consider the survival times in Table 2.2 for patients with acute lymphoblastic leukemia.[3] Two of these survival times have a "+" sign after them, indicating that the patient survived for *at least* the number of months given. Exact survival times often cannot be obtained because patients are lost to follow-up or they are still alive at the end of the study. Survival times for such patients are called *censored data*. Because they are not exact survival times, they cannot be averaged.

The same problem often occurs when any *waiting time*, the time until the occurrence of some event, is studied. Survival times are waiting times, since they are the times until the occurrence of death. If the time until recurrence of disc disease after disc surgery is studied, patients may still be free of disc disease at the end of the study, they may be lost to follow-up, or they may die before disc disease re-

TABLE 2.2 SURVIVAL TIME FOR PATIENTS WITH ACUTE LYMPHOBLASTIC LEUKEMIA

Patient No.	Survival Time (months)
1	17
2	9
3	17
4	23
5	11
6	15+
7	6
8	13
9	13
10	28+
11	15

curs. Censored observations usually result when waiting times are studied, making the mean inappropriate.* The TDI time intervals of Example 2.1 are not censored because the sample consists of workers with symptoms. If a sample of workers with TDI exposure was followed for several years to determine whether symptoms developed, censored data would probably result.

Censored data can also arise when concentrations of a substance are measured. If some of the concentrations are below the detection limit of the measuring equipment, we know that these concentrations are less than the detection limit, but we do not know their exact values. Means cannot be obtained for any type of censored data.

Another measure of central tendency, the *median*, is much less affected by extreme data values than the mean. The median is a middle number that is calculated by arranging the data in increasing order and finding the value in the middle of the sorted data. When the number of observations is even, there are two middle values, and the median is the average of these two values. The median time interval in Example 2.1 is 4.00 months, since 4.00 is the middle number for the sorted time intervals:

$$0.03 \quad 0.46 \quad 1.00 \quad \underline{4.00} \quad 12.00 \quad 24.00 \quad 120.00$$

For the time interval data, the median seems to be a more reasonable measure of central tendency than the mean. If we compute the median after removing the extremely large time interval, the median changes only a little, from 4.00 months to 2.50 months $((1.00 + 4.00)/2 = 2.50)$:

$$0.03 \quad 0.46 \quad \underline{1.00} \quad \underline{4.00} \quad 12.00 \quad 24.00$$

The extremely large time interval of 120 months has much less influence on the median than on the mean. When the median and the mean are quite different, as they are for the time interval data, both should be reported.[†]

Example 2.2

The blood pressure measurements shown in Table 2.3 were recorded for a dog with glomerulonephritis. Readings were taken every 20 to 90 seconds for 10 minutes.

TABLE 2.3   BLOOD PRESSURE FOR DOG WITH GLOMERULONEPHRITIS

Time	Blood Pressure (mm Hg) (Systolic / Diastolic)
19:27	141/58
19:28	128/63
19:28	135/69
19:29	117/58
19:30	106/55
19:31	103/64
19:32	117/74
19:32	128/82
19:33	118/86
19:34	121/70
19:35	115/60
19:35	123/74
19:36	109/86

The median systolic blood pressure is 118, the middle number of the sorted systolic blood pressures:

103 106 109 115 117 117 <u>118</u> 121 123 128 128 135 141

The median diastolic blood pressure is 69, the middle number of the sorted diastolic blood pressures:

55 58 58 60 63 64 <u>69</u> 70 74 74 82 86 86

For these data, the means are quite close to the medians, with the mean systolic blood pressure equal to 120.1 and the mean diastolic blood pressure equal to 69.2.

Another commonly used measure of central tendency is the *mode*, the most frequently occurring data value. To find the mode, we determine how often each data value occurs. Data may have more than one mode. Such data are called *bimodal* if two modes are present. Data with only one mode are called *unimodal*.

Example 2.3

A study examined the effect of patient instruction booklets on the retention of treatment information by multiple sclerosis patients.[5] Table 2.4 shows the scores on a treatment information test for 10 patients who received instruction manuals. To find the modal test score, we determine the frequency with which each test score occurs. The score 16 occurs five times, and as no other score occurs as frequently, the mode is 16.

The test-score data are unimodal. An example of bimodal data is provided by the systolic blood pressures in Example 2.2. These data have two modes, 117 and 128, since each of these values occurs twice and all of the other values occur only once. The

---

*Survival times and other waiting times usually cannot be analyzed by statistical procedures based on means, such as *t* tests (Chapter 7) or analysis of variance (Chapters 8, 9, and 13). Instead, statistical methods called *survival analysis* are used to analyze waiting times. Information about these methods can be found in other texts.[4]

[†]Medians for survival times and other waiting times are obtained using special methods from survival analysis.

TABLE 2.4   TEST SCORE AFTER RECEIVING INSTRUCTION BOOKLET*

Patient No.	Score
1	16
2	12
3	9
4	14
5	16
6	17
7	16
8	13
9	16
10	16

*Perfect score = 17

diastolic blood pressures have three modes: 58, 74, and 86.

A mode with many values is not a useful measure of central tendency. The extreme case is a data set in which each value occurs only once. For such data, there are as many modes as there are observations, as each value occurs with equal frequency (once). We say that such data have no mode.

The mode is often appropriate for *nominal* data, data that consist of arbitrary numerical labels for categories. The race codes 1 = black, 2 = Hispanic, 3 = Asian, and 4 = white result in nominal data. Means and medians are not appropriate for nominal data, since the numbers used are arbitrary and have no real numerical meaning. We could just as well code race with 10 = black, 15 = Hispanic, 20 = Asian, and 25 = white. Unlike the mean or median, the mode does make sense as a measure of central tendency for nominal data. If the modal race code is 1, blacks are the largest racial group in the sample.

Other types of data for which measures of central tendency are obtained include ordinal, interval, and ratio data. *Ordinal* data consist of rankings according to some criterion. Apgar scores are ordinal, as are the following headache pain ratings:

1 = no headache pain
2 = slight headache pain
3 = moderate headache pain
4 = severe headache pain

These rankings indicate an ordering of pain (4 indicates worse pain than 3, and so on), but they are still arbitrary. Other ordered numbers could be used just as well. For this reason, we cannot say that the distance between severe headache pain and moderate headache pain is 1. We can only say that severe headache pain is worse than moderate headache pain. Modes and medians are appropriate measures of central tendency for ordinal data. Although some researchers prefer not to calculate means for ordinal data, mean ranks are the basis for many nonparametric statistical tests (see Chapter 11). There

is no statistical reason not to obtain means for ordinal data.

Like ordinal data, *interval* data are ordered, but they allow us to compute distances. The zero point for interval data is arbitrary, however. Temperatures provide the classic example of interval data. Although distances between temperatures can be calculated, the zero point depends on which scale is used (e.g., Celsius or Fahrenheit). *Ratio* data are also ordered, with distances that make sense, and have a nonarbitrary zero point. Blood pressures are ratio data, since a blood pressure of 0 is not arbitrary. Weights are ratio data, since the zero point on all weight scales must be the same. Means, medians, and modes are all appropriate measures of central tendency for interval and ratio data.

2.3   MEASURES OF VARIABILITY

Measures of central tendency are incomplete data summaries, even if all of them are calculated. Two sets of data can have exactly the same mean, median, and mode, yet differ greatly in the variability of the observations. It is usually important to determine how much the observations vary—whether they are close together or far apart.

Example 2.4

Suppose a nurse anesthetist has evaluated two new short-acting anesthetics. She reports the following durations of anesthesia (in minutes) for 10 patients:

| *Anesthetic 1:* | 20.0 | 20.5 | 20.5 | 22.5 | 23.0 |
| *Anesthetic 2:* | 0 | 20.5 | 20.5 | 21.0 | 44.5 |

The anesthetics produced the same mean duration of anesthesia (21.3 minutes), the same median duration (20.5 minutes), and the same modal duration (20.5 minutes). But a glance at the data should convince you that the anesthetics are quite different: anesthetic 2 seems to produce a much more variable response than anesthetic 1. This difference in variability makes anesthetic 1 preferable to anesthetic 2, if the drugs are otherwise comparable in terms of side effects, cost, and so on. If we had ignored variability, we would have overlooked an important difference between these anesthetics.

Measures of variability are numbers that represent the degree to which observations vary. The simplest measure of variability is the *range*, the difference between the largest data value and the smallest data value:

range = largest value − smallest value

For the anesthetic-1 durations of Example 2.4, the range is 3.0 minutes. For the anesthetic-2 durations, the range is 44.5 minutes, reflecting the greater variability of these data.

Though easy to calculate, the range is not a very useful measure of variability, since it is based on only two of the data values. A much better measure of variability is given by the sample *variance* s^2, which is defined by the formula

$$s^2 = \frac{\sum\limits_{i=1}^{n}(x_i - \bar{x})^2}{n - 1} \tag{2.2}$$

We will first translate this formula into steps for calculation, then consider why s^2 makes sense as a measure of variability. Formula (2.2) indicates that s^2 is calculated as follows:

STEP 1.   Find the mean of the data.

STEP 2.   Subtract the mean from each observation to get n differences.

STEP 3.   Square each of the differences obtained in step 2.

STEP 4.   Add all the squared differences obtained in step 3.

STEP 5.   Divide the sum of the squared differences by $n - 1$ (the total number of observations minus 1).

These steps can be done efficiently by setting them up in a table, as in Tables 2.5 and 2.6 for the anesthetic data. The sample variance can be calcu-

lated even more efficiently by using a computer with statistical software or a calculator with statistical function keys.

Note that the anesthetic-2 variance is much larger than the anesthetic-1 variance, as we would expect. In general, the more variable the data, the larger the variance.

Now let us examine the s^2 formula to see how s^2 measures variability. Suppose first that all of the observations are identical—all equal to some constant number c. Then the sample mean must also equal c, so each term $(x_i - \bar{x})^2$ in the sample variance formula is $(c - c)^2 = 0$, and $s^2 = 0$. If there is no variability, the sample variance is 0, as it should be. Now suppose that some of the observations are different, but all are close together. Then all of the observations must be close to the sample mean, so all of the terms $(x_i - \bar{x})^2$ must be small, making s^2 small. Finally, suppose that some of the observations are quite far apart. Then some of the observations must be far from the sample mean, so some of the terms $(x_i - \bar{x})^2$ must be large, making s^2 large. In this way, the sample variance reflects the degree of variability in the data.

One disadvantage of the sample variance is its units, which are the *square* of the units of the data, not the original units (e.g., milliliters squared rather than milliliters). This defect is remedied by working with the sample *standard deviation* s, the positive square root of the sample variance:

$$s = \sqrt{s^2} \tag{2.3}$$

For the anesthetic data in Example 2.4, the standard deviations are $\sqrt{1.82 \text{ min}^2} = 1.35$ min for anesthetic 1 and $\sqrt{248.32 \text{ min}^2} = 15.76$ min for anesthetic 2. Because the square root is taken, s is in the same units as the data. This is the reason standard deviations are usually reported rather than variances.

How do we interpret standard deviations? When deciding whether a standard deviation is large or small, we need to take the units of the data into account. A standard deviation of 729 is large if the data are measured in hundreds but is small if the data are measured in 10 thousands. In general, a standard deviation as big as the mean is considered large.

TABLE 2.5   ANESTHETIC-1 CALCULATIONS

$x_i - \bar{x}$	$(x_i - \bar{x})^2$
$20.0 - 21.3 = -1.3$	$(-1.3)^2 = 1.69$
$20.5 - 21.3 = -0.8$	$(-0.8)^2 = 0.64$
$20.5 - 21.3 = -0.8$	$(-0.8)^2 = 0.64$
$22.5 - 21.3 = 1.2$	$(1.2)^2 = 1.44$
$23.0 - 21.3 = 1.7$	$(1.7)^2 = 2.89$
	Sum = 7.30

$$\text{Anesthetic-1 variance} = \frac{7.30}{5 - 1} = 1.82$$

TABLE 2.6   ANESTHETIC-2 CALCULATIONS

$x_i - \bar{x}$	$(x_i - \bar{x})^2$
$0 - 21.3 = -21.3$	$(-21.3)^2 = 453.69$
$20.5 - 21.3 = -0.8$	$(-0.8)^2 = 0.64$
$20.5 - 21.3 = -0.8$	$(-0.8)^2 = 0.64$
$21.0 - 21.3 = -0.3$	$(-0.3)^2 = 0.09$
$44.5 - 21.3 = 23.2$	$(23.2)^2 = 538.24$
	Sum = 993.30

$$\text{Anesthetic-2 variance} = \frac{993.30}{5 - 1} = 248.32$$

2.4   FREQUENCY DISTRIBUTIONS

It is often necessary to obtain an idea of how the data are distributed—whether they clump toward large values, tend to be either very large or very small, spread out evenly over a wide range of values, and so forth. This information is given by a *frequency distribution*, a list of intervals followed by a list of frequencies. *Frequencies* give the number of observations that fall into each interval. To construct a frequency distribution, we divide the range

TABLE 2.7 LVEF (%) FOR 30 DIABETIC PATIENTS

68	76	78	71	67
76	94	53	58	60
76	82	64	61	62
67	82	65	74	40
68	57	68	64	71
76	78	52	78	60

TABLE 2.8 FREQUENCY DISTRIBUTION WITH INTERVAL LENGTH OF 5 FOR LVEF DATA

LVEF (%)	No. of Patients
40–44	1
45–49	0
50–54	2
55–59	2
60–64	6
65–69	6
70–74	3
75–79	7
80–84	2
85–89	0
90–94	1

TABLE 2.9 FREQUENCY DISTRIBUTION WITH INTERVAL LENGTH OF 10 FOR LVEF DATA

LVEF (%)	No. of Patients
40–49	1
50–59	4
60–69	12
70–79	10
80–89	2
90–99	1

of observed values into intervals and count the number of observations that fall into each interval.*

Example 2.5

In a study of abnormal cardiac function in diabetic patients, the resting left ventricular ejection fraction (LVEF) for 30 insulin-dependent diabetics was measured.[6] The data are shown in Table 2.7.

Two frequency distributions for these data are shown in Tables 2.8 and 2.9. The first frequency distribution (Table 2.8) has an interval length of 5 and the second frequency distribution (Table 2.9) has an interval length of 10.

Many frequency distributions can be constructed from the same data set, and there is usually no

---

*Some data sets have so few distinct values that intervals are not used in the frequency distribution. Instead, the frequency distribution consists of a list of *numbers* followed by a list of frequencies that give the number of observations equal to each number. Frequency distributions of this type are shown in Chapter 10.

TABLE 2.10 PLASMA GH (ng/ml) FOR PATIENTS WITH ACROMEGALY

51.2	40.5	5.2	10.9	9.7
3.6	27.2	3.1	12.4	3.0
108.0	11.4	41.9	99.3	20.9
49.2	292.3	78.7	14.4	38.5
19.8	27.5	19.4	47.3	144.1

"best" frequency distribution. The amount of detail needed in a frequency distribution depends on the purpose of the research and the nature of the data. Extremely detailed frequency distributions should usually be avoided. The goal is to summarize the data, not to describe every facet. In some cases, you may need to construct several frequency distributions before you find one that is satisfactory. All frequency distributions must have nonoverlapping intervals that cover all the data values.

Once you have decided on the number of intervals, the interval length is found by dividing the range by the number of intervals, then rounding off the result. If the range is 107.5 and the number of intervals is 16, the interval length is $107.5/16 = 6.72$, which is rounded off to 7. Intervals usually should be of the same length, although adjacent intervals with low frequencies are sometimes combined into one large interval. This is done in Example 2.6.

Example 2.6

The data in Table 2.10 are the plasma growth hormone (GH) levels for 25 patients with acromegaly.[7] Two frequency distributions for these data are shown in Tables 2.11 and 2.12. In the second frequency distribution (Table 2.12), the last eight intervals of the first frequency distribution (Table 2.11) are combined into one large interval. Information is always lost when intervals are combined in this way. If this matters, intervals should not be combined. It may be important to know that exactly one patient had a GH level greater than 274.9, and that information cannot be obtained from the second frequency distribution.

TABLE 2.11 FREQUENCY DISTRIBUTION WITHOUT COMBINED FINAL INTERVAL FOR PLASMA GH

Plasma GH (mean ng/ml)	No. of Patients
0.0–24.9	12
25.0–49.9	7
50.0–74.9	1
75.0–99.9	2
100.0–124.9	1
125.0–149.9	1
150.0–174.9	0
175.0–199.9	0
200.0–224.9	0
225.0–249.9	0
250.0–274.9	0
275.0–299.9	1

TABLE 2.12 FREQUENCY DISTRIBUTION WITH COMBINED FINAL INTERVAL FOR PLASMA GH

Plasma GH (mean ng/ml)	No. of Patients
0.0–24.9	12
25.0–49.9	7
50.0–74.9	1
75.0–99.9	2
100.0–299.9	3

TABLE 2.14 PERCENTAGE FREQUENCY DISTRIBUTION AND PERCENTAGE CUMULATIVE FREQUENCY DISTRIBUTION FOR LVEF

LVEF (%)	% of Patients	Cumulative % of Patients
40–49	3.3	3.3
50–59	13.3	16.7
60–69	40.0	56.7
70–79	33.3	90.0
80–89	6.7	96.7
90–99	3.3	100.0

A *cumulative frequency distribution* is a list of intervals followed by a list of cumulative frequencies. *Cumulative frequencies* give the number of observations in each interval or any of the preceding intervals. Table 2.13 shows a frequency distribution and cumulative frequency distribution for the LVEF data of Example 2.5. The cumulative frequencies in this table are obtained by adding the frequencies for each interval and its preceding intervals. Thus, the first cumulative frequency is 1, the second cumulative frequency is $1 + 4 = 5$, the third cumulative frequency is $1 + 4 + 12 = 17$, the fourth cumulative frequency is $1 + 4 + 12 + 10 = 27$, and so on.

Cumulative frequency distributions can be used to determine the number of observations less than certain values. From Table 2.13, we see that 17 of the 30 patients had LVEF values less than 70% and 27 patients had LVEF values less than 80%.

Frequency distributions and cumulative frequency distributions sometimes list percentages of observations instead of numbers of observations. A frequency distribution based on percentages lists the percentage of observations in each interval. A cumulative frequency distribution based on percentages lists the percentages of observations in each interval or any of the preceding intervals. Some frequency distributions and cumulative frequency distributions list both numbers and percentages.

Table 2.14 shows the percentage frequency distribution and the percentage cumulative frequency distribution for the LVEF data. The percentages can be calculated from the frequency distribution and the cumulative frequency distribution in Table 2.13. The first percentage in Table 2.14 is calculated as $(1/30) \times 100 = 3.3\%$, the second percentage is

calculated as $(4/30) \times 100 = 13.3\%$, and so on. The first cumulative percentage in Table 2.14 is calculated as $(1/30) \times 100 = 3.3\%$, the second cumulative percentage is calculated as $(5/30) \times 100 = 16.7\%$, and so on.

2.5 HISTOGRAMS

Histograms are frequency distributions that have been turned into graphs. They allow the viewer to quickly determine how the data are distributed. To construct a histogram, you draw the interval bound-

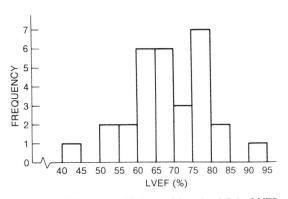

Figure 2.1 Histogram with interval length of 5 for LVEF data

TABLE 2.13 FREQUENCY DISTRIBUTION AND CUMULATIVE FREQUENCY DISTRIBUTION FOR LVEF

LVEF (%)	No. of Patients	Cumulative No. of Patients
40–49	1	1
50–59	4	5
60–69	12	17
70–79	10	27
80–89	2	29
90–99	1	30

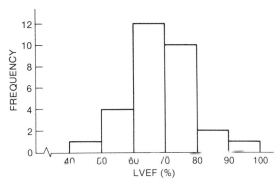

Figure 2.2 Histogram with interval length of 10 for LVEF data

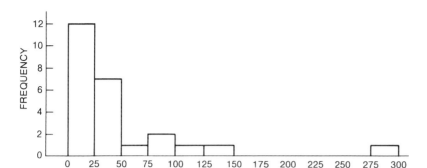

Figure 2.3 Histogram with equal intervals for plasma GH data

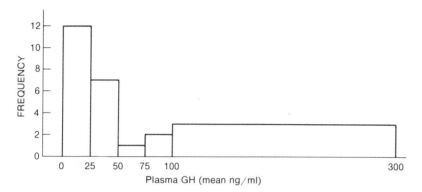

Figure 2.4 Incorrect histogram with unequal intervals for plasma GH data

aries on a horizontal line and the frequencies on a vertical line. Nonoverlapping intervals that cover all of the data values must be used. Bars are then drawn over the intervals in such a way that the *areas* of the bars are all proportional in the same way to their interval frequencies. If all of the intervals have the same length, this can be done by drawing each bar so that its height is equal to its interval frequency. The area of each bar is the interval length times the interval frequency, so all areas are proportional in the same way to their interval frequencies.

Histograms can be constructed in this way from the frequency distributions of LVEF (Tables 2.8 and 2.9) and from the first frequency distribution of plasma GH (Table 2.11). These histograms are shown in Figures 2.1 through 2.3. We cannot say that either of the histograms in Figures 2.1 and 2.2 is statistically better than the other. The amount of detail required usually determines which histogram is preferable, and this depends on the purpose of the research and the nature of the data. A histogram should not be so detailed that it fails to give a quick impression of the distribution of the data, nor should it go to the other extreme by lumping all of the observations under a single bar.

When the interval lengths are not all equal, constructing a histogram becomes a bit more complicated. Suppose we again draw each bar so that its height is equal to its interval frequency. Then the area of each bar is still the interval length times the

interval frequency. The bars are no longer proportional to the interval frequencies in the same way because the interval lengths are not the same. The longer intervals are given undue weight in the graph, as can be seen in the incorrectly drawn histogram in Figure 2.4. This histogram is based on the second frequency distribution of plasma GH (Table 2.12) and it has the height of each bar equal to its interval frequency. But the last interval is eight times longer than the other intervals, and the histogram incorrectly suggests that over half of the patients have plasma GH levels between 100 and 300. In fact, only 12% of the patients have plasma GH levels in this interval.

A correct histogram for the frequency distribution in Table 2.12 can be drawn by reducing the height of the last bar. Since the last interval is eight times longer than all the other intervals, its bar should be eight times shorter than its interval frequency. Shortening the bar in this way produces the correctly drawn histogram in Figure 2.5. This histogram accurately represents the distribution of the plasma GH levels.

The general procedure for drawing histograms with unequal intervals is as follows: First, determine which interval length is most common. Intervals with this length will be your base intervals. For each base interval, draw the bar so that its height is equal to its interval frequency. Once this has been done for all of the base intervals, go back to the remaining intervals. If an interval is *b* times *longer* than

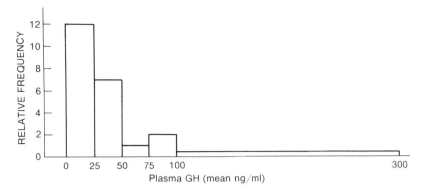

Figure 2.5 Correct histogram with unequal intervals for plasma GH data

```
Count   Midpoint

    1     42.50  |XXXXX
    0     47.50  |
    2     52.50  |XXXXXXXXXX
    2     57.50  |XXXXXXXXXX
    6     62.50  |XXXXXXXXXXXXXXXXXXXXXXXXXXXXXX
    6     67.50  |XXXXXXXXXXXXXXXXXXXXXXXXXXXXXX
    3     72.50  |XXXXXXXXXXXXXX
    7     77.50  |XXXXXXXXXXXXXXXXXXXXXXXXXXXXXXXXXXXX
    2     82.50  |XXXXXXXXXX
    0     87.50  |
    1     92.50  |XXXXX
               I....+....I....+....I....+....I....+....I....+....I
               0         2         4         6         8        10
                              Histogram Frequency
```

Figure 2.6 SPSS/PC histogram with interval length of 5 for LVEF data

the base intervals, the height of the bar is its *interval frequency divided by b*. If an interval is *shorter* than the base intervals, so that its length is the base-interval length divided by some number c, the height of its bar is its *interval frequency times c*. If these height adjustments are made, the areas of the bars will all be proportional in the same way to their interval frequencies.

2.6 COMPUTER HISTOGRAMS

A computer can be used to generate histograms much faster than they can be drawn by hand. A graphics package, together with a plotter, produces histograms that look like those in Figures 2.1 through 2.3. If a printer is used instead of a plotter to obtain histograms, the format is usually slightly different. The statistical software package SPSS/PC* has a FREQUENCIES program that produces histograms like those shown in Figures 2.6

through 2.8. These histograms are the SPSS/PC versions of those in Figures 2.1 through 2.3. The bars are drawn horizontally rather than vertically in SPSS/PC histograms, but the histograms are interpreted in the same way as before. The column labeled "Midpoint" gives the midpoints of the histogram intervals used. In Figure 2.6, the midpoints indicate that the intervals used are 40.00–44.99, 45.00–49.99, 50.00–54.99, and so on. The "Count" column lists the number of observations in each interval.

2.7 QUICK HISTOGRAMS

Histograms drawn for publication usually have the bar format shown in Figures 2.1 through 2.3 and Figure 2.5. Less elaborate, easily sketched histograms are useful for obtaining a rough idea of how the data are distributed. Such quick histograms can be drawn very easily for data sets with fewer than 40 observations. A computer should be used for larger data sets. In the quick-histogram format, a single observation is represented by an X, and the X's are stacked to form the bars. The construction

---

*The operation of SPSS/PC is described in several texts and manuals.[8-10]

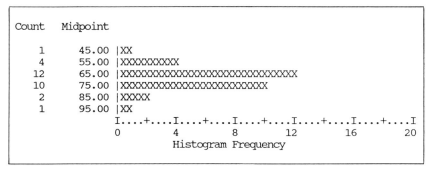

Figure 2.7 SPSS/PC histogram with interval length of 10 for LVEF data

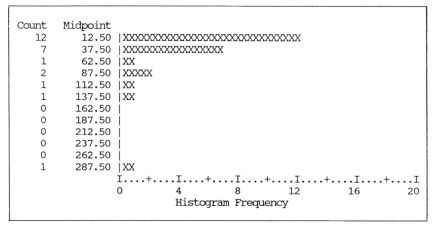

Figure 2.8 SPSS/PC histogram with equal intervals for GH data

TABLE 2.15   DIFFERENCE BETWEEN STANDING AND SUPINE HEART RATES (beats/min)

28	−1	13	26
35	29	17	2
29	13	−3	3
10	24	14	0
9	7	7	
9	0	22	
−17	19	14	

```
-20 - -11 |X
-10 - -1  |XX
   0 - 9  |XXXXXXX
  10 - 19 |XXXXXX
  20 - 29 |XXXXX
  30 - 39 |X
```

Figure 2.9 Quick histogram for heart rate data

of quick histograms is best understood by looking at examples.

Example 2.7

In a study of the effect of postural changes on heart rate and blood pressure, the heart rate changes shown in Table 2.15 were reported.[11] These values are the differences between standing and supine heart rates for 25 healthy women. A quick histogram with an interval length of 10 is shown in Figure 2.9. Since the interval −20 − −11 has one X, there is one observation in this interval. There are

two observations in the interval −10 − −1, eight observations in the interval 0−9, and so on.

Example 2.8

A study examined the results of autologous bone marrow transplantation for patients with acute non-lymphocytic leukemia.[12] Table 2.16 shows the number of days after transplantation before an absolute neutrophil count (ANC) greater than 0.5×10^9/liter was attained for 20 patients. A quick histogram with an interval length of 5 is shown in Figure 2.10.

TABLE 2.16 TIME (days) TO ATTAIN ANC GREATER THAN 0.5 × 10⁹/liter

21	31	27	42
16	44	37	20
20	24	27	29
24	35	29	27
63	28	42	46

```
15 – 19 |X
20 – 24 |XXXXX
25 – 29 |XXXXXX
30 – 34 |X
35 – 39 |XX
40 – 44 |XXX
45 – 49 |X
50 – 54 |
55 – 59 |
60 – 64 |X
```

Figure 2.10 Quick histogram for time data

2.8 SYMMETRY AND SKEWNESS

Some histograms and frequency distributions can be classified as symmetric or skewed. A histogram and its frequency distribution are *symmetric* if a vertical line through the center of the histogram divides it into halves that are mirror images of each other. (A horizontal line is used to divide quick histograms and computer histograms.) The histograms in Figures 2.11 and 2.12 are exactly symmetric and the histogram in Figure 2.13 is about as nearly symmetric as real data usually get.

If most of the observations in a histogram are clumped toward one end, with the observations at the other end forming a stretched-out tail, the histogram and its frequency distribution are *skewed*. A *negatively skewed* histogram, also called a histogram *skewed to the left*, is skewed with the tail on the left. Figures 2.14 and 2.15 show negatively skewed histograms. A *positively skewed* histogram, also called a histogram *skewed to the right*, is skewed with the tail on the right. Figures 2.8 and 2.10 show positively skewed histograms. Some distributions are neither symmetric nor skewed. A histogram for such a distribution is shown in Figure 2.16.

We have described only the most commonly used descriptive statistics. Other numerical and graphical data summaries are sometimes used. Information

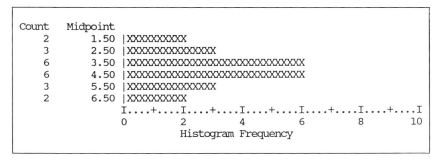

```
Count   Midpoint
   2       1.50   |XXXXXXXXXX
   3       2.50   |XXXXXXXXXXXXXX
   6       3.50   |XXXXXXXXXXXXXXXXXXXXXXXXXXXX
   6       4.50   |XXXXXXXXXXXXXXXXXXXXXXXXXXXX
   3       5.50   |XXXXXXXXXXXXXX
   2       6.50   |XXXXXXXXXX
                  I....+....I....+....I....+....I....+....I....+....I
                  0        2        4        6        8       10
                           Histogram Frequency
```

Figure 2.11 Symmetric SPSS/PC histogram

```
Count   Midpoint
   3      50.00   |XXXXXXXXXXXXXX
   6      70.00   |XXXXXXXXXXXXXXXXXXXXXXXXXXXX
   5      90.00   |XXXXXXXXXXXXXXXXXXXXXXX
   2     110.00   |XXXXXXXXXX
   1     130.00   |XXXXX
   2     150.00   |XXXXXXXXXX
   5     170.00   |XXXXXXXXXXXXXXXXXXXXXXX
   6     190.00   |XXXXXXXXXXXXXXXXXXXXXXXXXXXX
   3     210.00   |XXXXXXXXXXXXXX
                  I....+....I....+....I....+....I....+....I....+....I
                  0        2        4        6        8       10
                           Histogram Frequency
```

Figure 2.12 Symmetric SPSS/PC histogram

```
Count   Midpoint
  1        8.00  |XXXXX
  2       10.00  |XXXXXXXXXX
  7       12.00  |XXXXXXXXXXXXXXXXXXXXXXXXXXXXXXXXXXXXX
  8       14.00  |XXXXXXXXXXXXXXXXXXXXXXXXXXXXXXXXXXXXXXXXXX
  2       16.00  |XXXXXXXXXX
  1       18.00  |XXXXX
                 I....+....I....+....I....+....I....+....I....+....I
                 0         2         4         6         8        10
                              Histogram Frequency
```

Figure 2.13   SPSS/PC histogram of intraocular pressure (mm Hg) for 21 contact lens wearers[13]

```
Count   Midpoint
  1        5.00  |XXXXX
  3       15.00  |XXXXXXXXXXXXXXX
  4       25.00  |XXXXXXXXXXXXXXXXXXXX
  7       35.00  |XXXXXXXXXXXXXXXXXXXXXXXXXXXXXXXXXXXXX
                 I....+....I....+....I....+....I....+....I....+....I
                 0         2         4         6         8        10
                              Histogram Frequency
```

Figure 2.14   SPSS/PC histogram of weight (kg) of 15 dogs with pathological fracture of a long bone[14]

```
Count   Midpoint
  1        1.75  |XXXXXXXXXX
  1        2.25  |XXXXXXXXXX
  2        2.75  |XXXXXXXXXXXXXXXXXXXX
  5        3.25  |XXXXXXXXXXXXXXXXXXXXXXXXXXXXXXXXXXXXXXXXXXXXXXXXXXXX
  4        3.75  |XXXXXXXXXXXXXXXXXXXXXXXXXXXXXXXXXXXXXXXXXX
  2        4.25  |XXXXXXXXXXXXXXXXXXXX
                 I....+....I....+....I....+....I....+....I....+....I
                 0         1         2         3         4         5
                              Histogram Frequency
```

Figure 2.15   SPSS/PC histogram of albumin (mg/100 ml) for 15 patients with cirrhosis[15]

```
Count   Midpoint
  4       25.00  |XXXXXXXXXXXXXXXXXXXX
  4       35.00  |XXXXXXXXXXXXXXXXXXXX
  2       45.00  |XXXXXXXXXX
  1       55.00  |XXXXX
  1       65.00  |XXXXX
  1       75.00  |XXXXX
  2       85.00  |XXXXXXXXXX
  2       95.00  |XXXXXXXXXX
  3      105.00  |XXXXXXXXXXXXXXX
  5      115.00  |XXXXXXXXXXXXXXXXXXXXXXXXX
  6      125.00  |XXXXXXXXXXXXXXXXXXXXXXXXXXXXXX
  7      135.00  |XXXXXXXXXXXXXXXXXXXXXXXXXXXXXXXXXXXXX
                 I....+....I....+....I....+....I....+....I....+....I
                 0         2         4         6         8        10
                              Histogram Frequency
```

Figure 2.16   SPSS/PC histogram that is neither symmetric nor skewed

about these descriptive statistics can be found in other texts.[16]

SUMMARY

Descriptive statistics are numbers or graphs that summarize data. The most commonly used descriptive statistics concern central tendency or variability. Measures of central tendency include the mean, median, and mode. Unlike the median, the mean is heavily influenced by extreme values. The appropriateness of a measure of central tendency depends in part on whether the data are nominal, ordinal, interval, or ratio. Measures of variability include the range, variance, and standard deviation. Because the standard deviation has the same units as the data, it is preferred to the variance.

Frequency distributions and cumulative frequency distributions are tables that summarize the distribution of the data. Frequency distributions are often converted into graphs called histograms, which allow the viewer to quickly evaluate the distribution of the data. A histogram is symmetric if its two halves are mirror images of each other. A histogram is skewed if most of the data are clumped at one end and the remaining data form a stretched-out tail at the other end. Some histograms are neither symmetric nor skewed.

FORMULAS FOR FREQUENTLY USED DESCRIPTIVE STATISTICS

Sample mean: $\bar{x} = \dfrac{\sum\limits_{i=1}^{n} x_i}{n}$

Sample variance: $s^2 = \dfrac{\sum\limits_{i=1}^{n} (x_i - \bar{x})^2}{n-1}$

Sample standard deviation: $s = \sqrt{s^2}$

PROBLEMS

1. The white blood cell counts ($\times 10^3/mm^3$) for 10 dogs with pyometra are as follows[17]:

14.1 37.4 26.7 33.8 43.1 42.1 25.2 34.8 18.4 13.2

a. Construct a combined frequency and cumulative frequency distribution (based on frequencies, not percentages) and a quick histogram for these data. Use an interval length of 10 and start the first interval with 10. Comment briefly on the shape of the histogram.

b. Calculate the mean, median, variance, and standard deviation for these data. How discrepant are the mean and median? Are the data extremely variable? Would the mode be a useful measure of central tendency for these data?

2. In a study of decubitis ulcer care, the following information was recorded.[18]

Decubitis ulcer stage:
  1 = skin red but unbroken
  2 = skin red and broken
  3 = loss of full thickness of skin
  4 = loss of full thickness of skin and invasion of deeper tissues
Age
Sex: 1 = female, 2 = male
Source of admission: 1 = home
  2 = skilled nursing facility
  3 = family or friend's home
Number of medications
Size of ulcer: open area length × width (longest axis)

Classify the data for each of these quantities as nominal, ordinal, interval, or ratio.

3. The following data are the preoperative prolactin levels (ng/ml) for 18 women with prolactinomas.[19]

77 43 34 61 212 74 49 37 295 130 67 152 500 232 350 833 147 168

Draw a histogram for these data, using the intervals 0–99, 100–199, 200–299, and 300–849. Comment briefly on the shape of the histogram.

4. The following data are the survival times in months since the start of radiotherapy for six cats with intranasal tumors.[20] Can the mean be calculated for these data?

6 14* 41 2 41 12*   (* = still alive)

5. The average preprandial serum glucose values (mg/dl) for 39 stroke patients are shown in the following.[21] Thirteen of these patients died or failed to improve and 26 improved.

Died/not improved:
  85 92 115 137 177 198 215 257 273 280 295 307 377 ($s^2 = 8357.8$)

Improved:
  68 72 76 85 87 90 93 94 94 95 97 98 103 105 105 107 114 117 118 119 123 124 127 151 159 217 ($s^2 = 949.7$)

a. Construct combined frequency and cumulative frequency distributions (based on frequencies, not percentages) and quick histograms for these groups. For the died/not improved group, use an interval length of 60 and begin with 80. For the improved group, use an interval length of 20 and begin with 60. Compare the histograms for the two groups.

b. Calculate the means, medians, modes (if they exist), and standard deviations for the two groups. (Note that the variances are given with the data.) Are the two groups similar with respect to variability? Compare the means for the two groups. What does the difference between these means suggest?

6. Suppose the nursing staff of a small surgery department consists of one highly paid supervisor and four poorly paid nurses. If the nurses asked for a raise, what statistic would they use to support their claim that they are underpaid? What statistic would the hospital administration use to support its claim that the nurses are well paid?

7. The following data are the alkaline phosphatase values (mU/ml) for eight patients with fatty livers and 10 patients with cirrhosis.[22]

Fatty liver:
 49 62 70 99 108 116 117 183 ($s = 42.2$)

Cirrhosis:
 50 88 92 98 130 139 150 152 187 202
 ($s = 47.2$)

a. Construct combined frequency and cumulative frequency distributions (based on frequencies, not percentages) and quick histograms for these groups. Try various interval lengths, if necessary, to obtain good histograms. Compare the histograms for the two groups.

b. Calculate the means and medians for these groups. Are the two groups similar with respect to variability? (Note that the standard deviations are given with the data.) Compare the means for the two groups.

8. In a study of cobalamin deficiency, neurologic abnormalities were coded according to the following scale.[23]

 0 = no neurologic abnormalities
 1 = paresthesia with negative neurological exam
 2 = no neurological symptoms but impairment of position or vibration sense on exam
 3 = combined systems disease or severe cerebral dysfunction responsive to cobalamin treatment
 4 = severe advanced combined systems disease

The diagnosis was also recorded and can be coded as follows:

 1 = pernicious anemia
 2 = tropical sprue

The abnormality and diagnosis data for 25 Hispanic patients in the study are as follows:

Neurologic abnormality:
 2 3 0 0 1 2 0 1 0 0 3 0 1 0 0 0 1 0 4
 0 0 0 2 0 0

Diagnosis:
 1 1 2 1 2 1 2 1 1 1 1 1 1 1 2 2 2 1 1
 1 1 2 2 2 2

Calculate and interpret all *appropriate* measures of central tendency for these data.

9. A study evaluated the use of the dexamethasone suppression test (DST) to differentiate chronic schizophrenia from major depression with psychosis.[24] The cortisol levels ($\mu g/dl$) shown here were obtained 17 hours after 26 patients with chronic schizophrenia or major depression with psychosis ingested 2 mg of dexamethasone. All patients were in a drug-free acute-exacerbation phase of illness.

Major depression with psychosis:
 5.7 6.7 10.2 11.4 14.1 14.4 ($s^2 = 13.3$)
Chronic schizophrenia:
 0.6 0.7 0.7 0.8 0.8 0.9 0.9 0.9 0.9 1.0 1.1 1.2
 1.2 1.5 1.6 1.8 1.8 2.1 3.0 3.9 ($s^2 = 0.7$)

a. Construct combined frequency and cumulative frequency distributions (based on frequencies, not percentages) and quick histograms for these groups. Try various interval lengths, if necessary, to obtain good histograms. Compare the histograms for the two groups. What percentage of patients with chronic schizophrenia have cortisol levels below 5 $\mu g/dl$? What percentage of patients with major depression with psychosis have cortisol levels below 5 $\mu g/dl$? Do the data support the author's statement that "the 2-mg DST in the drug-free acute-exacerbation phase can differentiate between major depression with psychosis and chronic schizophrenia?"

b. Calculate the means, medians, modes (if they exist), and standard deviations for the two groups. (Note that the variances are given with the data.) What does the difference between the group means suggest?

10. In a study of equine colic, hemostatic profiles were obtained for 30 horses with clinical colic.[25] The following data are the antithrombin values for these horses, measured as percentages of a normal antithrombin value. An antithrombin percentage below 100 indicates an antithrombin value less than the normal value and a percentage above 100 indicates an antithrombin value greater than the normal value.

Horses with colitis or severe diarrhea (group 1):
51 53 54 56 60 90 100 127 $(s^2 = 804.4)$

Horses with torsion or obstruction of the intestine (group 2):
76 83 87 89 100 100 113 116 120 122 130 143 $(s^2 = 426.6)$

Horses with impaction of the intestine (group 3):
84 89 93 103 105 105 105 106 107 111 $(s^2 = 78.8)$

    a. Construct combined frequency and cumulative frequency distributions (based on frequencies, not percentages) and quick histograms for these groups. Try various interval lengths, if necessary, to obtain good histograms. Compare the histograms for these groups.

    b. Calculate the means, medians, modes (if they exist), and standard deviations for all three groups. (Note that the variances are given with the data.) Are the groups similar with respect to variability? What do the differences between the group means suggest?

11. The following data are the times before relapse for 28 cancer patients who underwent bone marrow transplantation.[26] Can the mean be calculated for these data?

1 33* 1† 12 1.5 20 14 25* 24* 21* 22* 21 21*

5 18* 18* 17* 9 16* 15* 3† 7 13* 1† 7 5 5* 5*

(*alive with no relapse before end of follow-up; †dead before relapse occurred)

REFERENCES

1. Kruskal W: Statistics, Moliere, and Henry Adams. Amer Scient 55:416–428, 1967.
2. Moller DR, Brooks SM, McKay RT, et al: Chronic asthma due to toluene diisocyanate. Chest 90:494–499, 1986.
3. Hirata J, Katsuno M, Kaneko S, et al: Clinical significance of human bone marrow stromal cell colonies in acute leukemias. Leuk Res 10:1441–1445, 1986.
4. Lee E: Statistical Methods for Survival Data Analysis. Belmont: Wadsworth, 1980.
5. Young FK, Brooks BR: Patient teaching manuals improve retention of treatment information—A controlled clinical trial in multiple sclerosis. J Neurosci Nurs 18:26–28, 1986.
6. Zola B, Kahn JK, Juni JE, et al: Abnormal cardiac function in diabetic patients with autonomic neuropathy in the absence of ischemic heart disease. J Clin Endocrinol Metab 63:208–214, 1986.
7. Shibasaki T, Hotta M, Masuda A, et al: Studies on the response of growth hormone (GH) secretion to GH-releasing hormone, thyrotropin-releasing hormone, gonadotropin-releasing hormone, and somatostatin in acromegaly. J Clin Endocrinol Metab 63:167–173, 1986.
8. Norusis MJ: The SPSS Guide to Data Analysis for SPSS/PC+. Chicago: SPSS, 1988.
9. Norusis MJ, SPSS Inc.: SPSS/PC+ V3.0 Base Manual for the IBM PC/XT/AT and PS/2. Chicago: SPSS, 1989.
10. Norusis MJ, SPSS Inc.: SPSS/PC+ Advanced Statistics V3.0 for the IBM PC/XT/AT and PS/2. Chicago: SPSS, 1989.
11. Moore KI, Newton K: Orthostatic heart rates and blood pressures in healthy young women and men. Heart Lung 15:611–617, 1986.
12. Yeager AM, Kaizer H, Santos GW, et al: Autologous bone marrow transplantation in patients with acute nonlymphocytic leukemia, using ex vivo marrow treatment with 4-hydroperoxycyclophosphamide. N Engl J Med 315:141–147, 1986.
13. Insler MS, Robbins RG: Intraocular pressure by noncontact tonometry with and without soft contact lenses. Arch Ophthalmol 105:1358–1359, 1987.
14. Boulay JP, Wallace LJ, Lipowitz AJ: Pathological fracture of long bones in the dog. J Am Anim Hosp Assoc 23:297–303, 1987.
15. Stanek B, Renner F, Sedlmayer A, et al: Effect of captopril on renin and blood pressure in cirrhosis. Eur J Clin Pharmacol 33:249–254, 1987.
16. Remington RD, Schork MA: Statistics with Applications to the Biological and Health Sciences. 2nd ed. Englewood Cliffs: Prentice-Hall, 1985.
17. Meyers-Wallen VN, Goldschmidt MH, Flickinger GL: Prostaglandin $F_{2\alpha}$ treatment of canine pyometra. J Am Vet Med Assoc 189:1557–1561, 1986.
18. Kurzuk-Howard G, Simpson L, Palmieri A: Decubitis ulcer care: A comparative study. West J Nurs Res 7:58–79, 1985.
19. Blake RE, Maroulis GB, Sherman BM, et al: Prolactinoma and adrenal androgens. J Reprod Med 31:675–679, 1986.
20. Straw RC, Withrow SJ, Gellette EL, et al: Use of radiotherapy for the treatment of intranasal tumors in cats: Six cases (1980–1985). J Am Vet Med Assoc 189:927–929, 1986.
21. Berger L, Hakim AM: The association of hyperglycemia with cerebral edema in stroke. Stroke 17:865–871, 1986.
22. Schuller A, Solis-Herruzo JA, Moscat J, et al: The fluidity of liver plasma membranes from patients with different types of liver injury. Hepatology 6:714–717, 1986.
23. Stabler SP, Marcell PD, Podell ER, et al: Assay of methylmalonic acid in the serum of patients with cobalamin deficiency using capillary gas chromatography-mass spectrometry. J Clin Invest 77:1606–1612, 1986.
24. Clower CG: The 2-mg dexamethasone suppression test in differentiating major depression with psychosis from schizophrenia. J Clin Psychopharmacol 6:363–365, 1986.
25. Johnstone IB, Crane S: Hemostatic abnormalities in equine colic. Am J Vet Res 47:356–358, 1986.
26. Or R, Matzner Y, Konijn AM: Serum ferritin in patients undergoing bone marrow transplantation. Cancer 60:1127–1131, 1987.

3

PROBABILITY

CHAPTER OBJECTIVES

After studying this chapter and working the problems, you should be able to:

1. Calculate and interpret sample probabilities
2. Explain the concepts of conditional probability, disjoint events, and independent events
3. Check for independence of events in a sample
4. Compare conditional probabilities

We will focus on interpreting probabilities as well as calculating them. The ideas in this chapter and the next two chapters are fundamental. If you understand them, you will have the tools you need to understand statistical inference. Many people find ideas about probability difficult to grasp at first, but probability docs become clear after some study —and it makes a great deal of sense once you understand it.

3.1 PROBABILITY

Most people have some notion of what probability means, having watched lottery drawings or played cards. Health professionals must often appeal to probabilities in discussions with patients, although they may not realize that they are talking about probabilities. If a patient wants to know whether he will survive a risky thoracic surgery, you cannot ethically guarantee him that he will. Instead, you might tell him that the death rate for this surgery is about one in 100. In doing so, you would have given him a probability—1/100. What exactly does this probability mean? Both you and the patient would know enough about probability to feel somewhat

reassured by this number, although a number like 1/10,000 would be vastly more reassuring. You would interpret the number 1/100 as follows: "I expect this patient to survive surgery, but I won't be entirely surprised if he doesn't, and I won't feel relaxed about this case until the surgery is over." This is a reasonable interpretation, but why? To understand this, we need to define probability more precisely than it is defined in everyday use.

A *probability* can be thought of as a proportion that enables people to make intelligent guesses about future events. Suppose you want to predict the response of an apprehensive patient to a nurse's explanation of medical procedures. Suppose also that you somehow know that 73% of all apprehensive patients are less anxious after the nurse's explanation. If a nurse explains medical procedures to a randomly selected apprehensive patient,* you can

---

*We will describe the mechanics of random selection in Chapter 5. For now, we will suppose that all apprehensive patients in the United States were assigned numbers that were mixed up in a huge bin. A patient then was selected by drawing her number from the bin.

say that the probability that the patient will be less anxious after the explanation is 0.73.

A probability can also be viewed as *the long-run proportion of times some event of interest will occur.* Suppose you are asked a three-choice question concerning a subject you know nothing about. Since you have to guess, you have only a one in three (1/3) chance of choosing the right answer. If you are asked 10 such questions, it would not be very surprising for you to get half of them right just by "luck." If you are asked 50 such questions, it would be quite surprising if you got half of them right, but 40% correct would not be extremely unusual. If you are asked 1000 such questions, it is almost certain that the proportion of correct answers will be very close to 1/3. The more questions asked, the closer the proportion of correct answers will usually be to 1/3. The proportion of correct answers eventually stabilizes at 1/3, the probability of a correct answer for any particular question.

Similarly, a 1/100 probability of a thoracic-surgery death can be interpreted as the long-run proportion of patients undergoing this surgery who die. When you tell a patient that the death rate for this type of surgery is one in 100, you are telling him that the proportion of patients who die from this surgery is about 1/100, when a large number of surgeries is considered.

3.2 CALCULATION OF SAMPLE PROBABILITIES

The probabilities of interest are usually population probabilities rather than sample probabilities. (Recall that the sample consists of the data collected by the researcher and the population consists of all observations of interest.) A nurse does not really want to know that seven of 30 patients with a new type of central venous catheter developed inflammation at the placement site. What she wants to know is the *population* probability that patients with this catheter will develop inflammation at the placement site. This population probability can never be determined, since the catheter cannot be placed in every patient who needs one. But sample probabilities are often good estimates of population probabilities.

For this reason, sample probabilities are frequently computed. Most sample probabilities can be calculated easily. The formula is quite simple. The probability of an event, denoted by P(Event), is given by

$$P(\text{Event})$$

$$= \frac{\text{no. of observations for which event occurs}}{\text{total no. of observations}} \quad (3.1)$$

In our sample of 30 patients with the new central venous catheter, the sample probability that a patient will develop inflammation at the placement site is

$$P(\text{Inflammation})$$

$$= \frac{\text{no. of patients who develop inflammation at placement site}}{\text{total no. of patients}}$$

$$= \frac{7}{30} = 0.23$$

Example 3.1

A study of confusional states in hospitalized elderly patients evaluated 170 elderly patients admitted for treatment of traumatic hip fractures.[1] Although none of these patients had a history of mental impairment prior to injury, 60 of them showed mild confusion during the five-day postoperative period, 27 showed moderate or severe confusion during this time, and 83 showed no confusion. For this sample of 170 patients, the probability of mild confusion is

$$P(\text{Mild confusion})$$

$$= \frac{\text{no. of patients showing mild confusion}}{\text{total no. of patients}}$$

$$= \frac{60}{170} = 0.35$$

The sample probability of moderate or severe confusion is

$$P(\text{Moderate or severe confusion})$$

$$= \frac{\text{no. of patients showing moderate or severe confusion}}{\text{total no. of patients}}$$

$$= \frac{27}{170} = 0.16$$

The sample probability of no confusion is

$$P(\text{No confusion})$$

$$= \frac{\text{no. of patients showing no confusion}}{\text{total no. of patients}}$$

$$= \frac{83}{170} = 0.49$$

What do these probabilities mean? First, they are estimates of population probabilities. They estimate the population probability that elderly hip-fracture patients show mild confusion during the five-day postoperative period, the population probability that elderly hip-fracture patients show moderate or severe confusion, and the population probability that elderly hip-fracture patients show no confusion. Here the population is the theoretical population that would result if all elderly hip-fracture patients similar to those in the study were admitted for treatment.

In the second interpretation of these probabilities, we assume that a patient's record is selected at random from the records of these 170 patients. If this is done, the probability of selecting a patient with mild confusion is 0.35, the probability of selecting a patient with moderate or severe confusion is 0.16, and the probability of selecting a patient with no confusion is 0.49.

Example 3.2

A study investigated the effect of prolonged exposure to bright light on retinal damage in premature infants.[2] Eighteen of 21 premature infants exposed to bright light developed retinopathy, while 21 of 39 premature infants exposed to reduced light levels developed retinopathy. For this sample, the probability of developing retinopathy is

$$P(\text{Retinopathy}) = \frac{\text{no. of infants with retinopathy}}{\text{total no. of infants}}$$

$$= \frac{18 + 21}{21 + 39} = \frac{39}{60} = 0.65$$

3.3 CONDITIONAL PROBABILITIES

In the retinopathy study described in Example 3.2, the primary concern is comparison of the bright-light infants with the reduced-light infants. We want to know whether the probability of retinopathy for the bright-light infants differs from the probability of retinopathy for the reduced-light infants. These probabilities are *conditional probabilities*, probabilities based on the knowledge that some event has occurred. We want to compare the probability of retinopathy, given that the infant was exposed to bright light, with the probability of retinopathy, given that the infant was exposed to reduced light. Exposure to bright light and exposure to reduced light are *conditioning events*, events we want to take into account when calculating conditional probabilities.

Conditional probabilities are denoted by $P(\text{Event}|\text{Conditioning event})$ (read as "the probability of the event, given the conditioning event"). The formula for calculating a sample conditional probability is easy to use:

$P(\text{Event}|\text{Conditioning event})$

$$= \frac{\substack{\text{no. of observations for which event} \\ \text{and conditioning event both occur}}}{\substack{\text{no. of observations for which} \\ \text{conditioning event occurs}}} \quad (3.2)$$

For the retinopathy data, the conditional probability of retinopathy, given exposure to bright light, is

$P(\text{Retinopathy}|\text{Exposure to bright light})$

$$= \frac{\substack{\text{no. of infants with retinopathy exposed} \\ \text{to bright light}}}{\text{no. of infants exposed to bright light}}$$

$$= \frac{18}{21} = 0.86$$

and

$P(\text{Retinopathy}|\text{Exposure to reduced light})$

$$= \frac{\substack{\text{no. of infants with retinopathy exposed} \\ \text{to reduced light}}}{\text{no. of infants exposed to reduced light}}$$

$$= \frac{21}{39} = 0.54$$

These conditional probabilities suggest that premature infants exposed to bright light have a higher risk of retinopathy than premature infants exposed to reduced light. For this sample of 60 infants, the risk of retinopathy is obviously higher for infants exposed to bright light, but the question of interest concerns the population. In the population consisting of all premature infants similar to those in the study, do infants exposed to bright light have a higher risk of retinopathy than infants exposed to reduced light? In later chapters, we will discuss methods for using sample data to answer questions like this.

Example 3.3

A study of pet ownership among heart-attack survivors found that three of the 53 survivors who owned pets died within a year after their heart attacks.[3] Eleven of the 39 survivors without pets died within a year after their heart attacks. Using formula (3.2), we can calculate the conditional probabilities of obvious interest:

$P(\text{Die within a year}|\text{Own a pet})$

$$= \frac{\text{no. of pet owners who die within a year}}{\text{no. of pet owners}}$$

$$= \frac{3}{53} = 0.06$$

$P(\text{Die within a year}|\text{Don't own a pet})$

$$= \frac{\text{no. of non-pet owners who die within a year}}{\text{no. of non-pet owners}}$$

$$= \frac{11}{39} = 0.28$$

These conditional probabilities indicate that heart-attack survivors who own pets are much less likely to die within a year than are heart-attack survivors who do not own pets. Although pet owners clearly have a lower risk of death than do non-pet owners in this sample, what we really want to know is whether pet owners have a lower risk of death than non-pet owners in the population of all heart-attack survivors.

Another formula for calculating conditional probabilities is sometimes used instead of formula (3.2):

P(Event|Conditioning event)

$$= \frac{P(\text{Both event and conditioning event})}{P(\text{Conditioning event})} \quad (3.3)$$

P(Both event and conditioning event) is the probability that the event and the conditioning event both occur. Formulas (3.3) and (3.2) always give the same answer, subject to rounding error.* If all the data are available, formula (3.2) is easier to use than formula (3.3) because it requires less calculation. Formula (3.3) is used to calculate conditional probabilities from other probabilities when the information needed for formula (3.2) is not available. Suppose that 12% of the children at a hospital are receiving steroid therapy, and that 7% of the children at this hospital are receiving steroid therapy and have nosocomial infections. Formula (3.3) can be used to calculate the conditional probability of nosocomial infection, given treatment with steroids, for children at this hospital:

P(Nosocomial infection|Treatment with steroids)

$$= \frac{P(\text{Both nosocomial infection and treatment with steroids})}{P(\text{Treatment with steroids})}$$

$$= \frac{0.07}{0.12} = 0.58$$

Example 3.4

A study of inflatable penile prostheses (IPPs) reported that 12% of the patients studied had Scott IPPs and experienced mechanical failures, while 4% of the patients had Mentor IPPs and experienced mechanical failures.[4] Of the patients studied, 42% had the Scott IPP implanted and 58% had the Mentor IPP implanted. What is the conditional probability of mechanical failure, given that the Scott IPP was implanted? What is the conditional probability of mechanical failure, given that the

Mentor IPP was implanted? Applying formula (3.3), we get

P(Mechanical failure|Scott IPP)

$$= \frac{P(\text{Mechanical failure and Scott IPP})}{P(\text{Scott IPP})}$$

$$= \frac{0.12}{0.42} = 0.29$$

and

P(Mechanical failure |Mentor IPP)

$$= \frac{P(\text{Mechanical failure and Mentor IPP})}{P(\text{Mentor IPP})}$$

$$= \frac{0.04}{0.58} = 0.07$$

For these patients, the Mentor IPP has a much lower probability of mechanical failure than the Scott IPP.

3.4 PROPERTIES OF PROBABILITIES

There are certain properties of probabilities that are often useful when carrying out probability calculations. We will concentrate on the use of these properties and omit their proofs.

PROPERTY 1. Probabilities are always between 0 and 1. For any event

$$0 \leq P(\text{Event}) \leq 1^*$$

This property provides a check on probability calculations. If a negative probability or a probability greater than 1 is calculated, there is an error somewhere. This should make sense to you, as most people would find "probabilities" like -0.33 or 2.78 rather strange.

PROPERTY 2. For any two events

P(Event 1 or event 2)

$$= P(\text{Event 1}) + P(\text{Event 2}) \quad (3.4)$$

$$- P(\text{Both event 1 and event 2})$$

P(Event 1 or event 2) is the probability that event 1 occurs or event 2 occurs or both events occur. P(Both event 1 and event 2) is the probability that both events occur. Sample probabilities of the form

---

*Formula (3.3) does not work if the probability of the conditioning event is 0, since we cannot divide by 0. The conditional probability makes no sense then anyway. Such "conditional probabilities" would be "probabilities" like P(Caesarean|68 fetuses) or P(Slipped disc|Body length of 961 meters).

*The symbol " $\leq$ " means "is less than or equal to." The symbol " $\geq$," which we will use in the next chapter, means "is greater than or equal to."

P(Both event 1 and event 2) are calculated as follows:

P(Both event 1 and event 2)

$$= \frac{\text{no. of observations for which event 1 and event 2 both occur}}{\text{total no. of observations}} \quad (3.5)$$

Example 3.5

The data in Table 3.1 are the results of electrocardiograms (ECGs) and radionuclide angiocardiograms (RAs) for 19 patients with post-traumatic myocardial contusion.[5] A "+" indicates abnormal results and a "−" indicates normal results. Suppose we want to find the sample probability that either the ECG or the RA is abnormal. To calculate this probability, we can apply formulas (3.4), (3.1), and (3.5):

P(ECG abnormal or RA abnormal)

$$= P(\text{ECG abnormal}) + P(\text{RA abnormal})$$
$$- P(\text{Both ECG and RA abnormal})$$
$$= \frac{17}{19} + \frac{9}{19} - \frac{7}{19} = \frac{19}{19} = 1$$

We cannot calculate the sample probability that either the ECG or the RA is abnormal by adding the number of patients with abnormal ECGs to the number with abnormal RAs and then dividing the sum by 19. If we try this, we get $(17 + 9)/19 = 26/19 = 1.4$, which must be wrong by Property 1. The problem here is the seven patients whose ECGs and RAs are both abnormal. We count these patients twice when we add the 17 patients with abnormal ECGs to the nine patients with abnormal RAs. Formula (3.4) corrects for this sort of double counting by subtracting P(Both event 1 and event 2).

Example 3.6

In a study of bronchoalveolar lavage for diagnosing pneumonia, specimens were obtained by open-lung biopsy (OLB), bronchoscopy, and needle aspiration (NA), and then cultured for cytomegalovirus (CMV).[6] Some of the results are shown in Table 3.2. A "+" indicates that the culture was positive for CMV and a "−" indicates that it was negative for CMV. Suppose we want to find the sample probability that the OLB culture is positive or the bronchoscopy culture is positive, the sample probability that the OLB culture is positive or the NA culture is positive, and the sample probability that the bronchoscopy culture is positive or the NA culture is positive.

To calculate the sample probability that the OLB culture is positive or the bronchoscopy culture is positive, we can use formulas (3.4), (3.1), and (3.5):

P(Positive OLB culture or positive bronchoscopy culture)

$$= P(\text{Positive OLB culture})$$
$$+ P(\text{Positive bronchoscopy culture})$$
$$- P(\text{Both positive OLB culture and positive bronchoscopy culture})$$
$$= \frac{8}{13} + \frac{5}{13} - \frac{5}{13} = \frac{8}{13} = 0.62$$

TABLE 3.1   ECG AND RA ABNORMALITIES*

Patient No.	ECG	RA
1	−	+
2	+	−
3	+	−
4	+	−
5	+	−
6	+	−
7	+	+
8	+	+
9	+	+
10	+	+
11	+	−
12	+	−
13	−	+
14	+	−
15	+	+
16	+	+
17	+	−
18	+	−
19	+	+

* + = abnormal, − = normal

TABLE 3.2   CMV CULTURE RESULT*

Patient No.	Open-Lung Biopsy	Bronchoscopy	Needle Aspiration
1	+	+	+
2	+	+	+
3	−	−	−
4	+	+	+
5	−	−	−
6	+	−	+
7	+	−	+
8	+	+	−
9	−	−	−
10	−	−	−
11	+	−	−
12	−	−	−
13	−	+	+

* + = positive, − = negative

Similarly,

$$P(\text{Positive OLB culture or positive NA culture})$$

$$= P(\text{Positive OLB culture})$$

$$+ P(\text{Positive NA culture})$$

$$- P(\text{Both positive OLB culture and}$$

$$\text{positive NA culture})$$

$$= \frac{8}{13} + \frac{6}{13} - \frac{6}{13} = \frac{8}{13} = 0.62$$

and

$$P(\text{Positive bronchoscopy culture or positive}$$

$$\text{NA culture})$$

$$= P(\text{Positive bronchoscopy culture})$$

$$+ P(\text{Positive NA culture})$$

$$- P(\text{Both positive bronchoscopy culture}$$

$$\text{and positive NA culture})$$

$$= \frac{5}{13} + \frac{6}{13} - \frac{4}{13} = \frac{7}{13} = 0.54$$

PROPERTY 3. If two events cannot both happen at the same time, then

$$P(\text{Event 1 or event 2})$$
$$= P(\text{Event 1}) + P(\text{Event 2}) \qquad (3.6)$$

Events that cannot occur simultaneously are called *disjoint*. Formula (3.6) works *only* when the two events are disjoint, but formula (3.4) works whether the events are disjoint or not. If you are not certain that two events are disjoint, use formula (3.4) to compute probabilities of the form P(Event 1 or event 2).

How can we tell whether two events are disjoint? This is not a statistical issue at all. Determining whether events are disjoint requires nonstatistical information and common sense. Since two events are disjoint if they cannot both happen at the same time, we need to decide whether it is possible for the two events of interest to occur at the same time. If the events cannot occur simultaneously, they are disjoint. If they can occur simultaneously, they are not disjoint. The events "patient is male" and "patient has a gunshot wound" are not disjoint. A male patient can have a gunshot wound, so these events can happen at the same time. The events "patient is male" and "patient has ovarian cysts" are disjoint. No male patient can have ovarian cysts, so these events cannot both happen at the same time.

Example 3.7

In a study of home care for cancer patients, the primary tumor sites shown in Table 3.3 were reported for 123 patients.[7] Suppose we want to find the sample probability that a patient has the pri-

TABLE 3.3   PRIMARY TUMOR SITES

Primary Tumor Site	No. of Patients
Lung	34
Colon	21
Breast	19
Head and neck	7
Pancreas	6
Gynecological	5
Lymphoma	4
Other	27

mary tumor site in the lung or colon and the sample probability that a patient has the primary tumor site in the breast or pancreas.

A patient cannot have the primary tumor site simultaneously in the lung and colon, so the events "primary tumor site in lung" and "primary tumor site in colon" are disjoint. We can use formula (3.6) to find the probability that a patient in this study has the primary tumor site in the lung or colon:

$$P(\text{Primary tumor site in lung or colon})$$

$$= P(\text{Primary tumor site in lung})$$

$$+ P(\text{Primary tumor site in colon})$$

$$= \frac{34}{123} + \frac{21}{123} = \frac{55}{123} = 0.45$$

A patient also cannot have the primary tumor site in both the breast and pancreas, so the events "primary tumor site in breast" and "primary tumor site in pancreas" are disjoint. By formula (3.6),

$$P(\text{Primary tumor site in breast or pancreas})$$

$$= P(\text{Primary tumor site in breast})$$

$$+ P(\text{Primary tumor site in pancreas})$$

$$= \frac{19}{123} + \frac{6}{123} = \frac{25}{123} = 0.20$$

There is a more general version of formula (3.6). Suppose that *n* events are *pairwise disjoint*; that is, no two of them can happen at the same time. Then

$$P(\text{Event 1 or event 2 or event 3 or } \ldots \text{ or event } n)$$
$$= P(\text{Event 1}) + P(\text{Event 2}) \qquad (3.7)$$
$$+ P(\text{Event 3}) + \cdots + P(\text{Event } n)$$

If events are not pairwise disjoint, formula (3.7) *cannot* be used.

We can use formula (3.7) and Table 3.3 to find the sample probability that the primary tumor site is in the lung, colon, or breast. Since the primary tumor site cannot simultaneously be in the lung and colon, or in the lung and breast, or in the colon and breast, the events "primary tumor site in lung," "primary tumor site in colon," and "primary tumor site in breast" are pairwise disjoint. Applying formula (3.7), we get

P(Primary tumor site in lung or colon or breast)

$= P$(Primary tumor site in lung)

$+ P$(Primary tumor site in colon)

$+ P$(Primary tumor site in breast)

$= \dfrac{34}{123} + \dfrac{21}{123} + \dfrac{19}{123} = \dfrac{74}{123} = 0.60$

PROPERTY 4. The probability of the *opposite event*, which happens when a given event does *not* occur, is

$$P(\text{Opposite event}) = 1 - P(\text{Event})^* \quad (3.8)$$

Example 3.8

In a study of onion-induced hemolytic anemia, six dogs were fed a large quantity of dehydrated onions.[8] Two days later, 33% of these dogs showed intravascular hemolysis. What is the sample probability that a dog does *not* show intravascular hemolysis? Since the events "intravascular hemolysis" and "no intravascular hemolysis" are opposite events, we can use formula (3.8):

P(No intravascular hemolysis)

$= 1 - P$(Intravascular hemolysis)

$= 1 - 0.33 = 0.67$

3.5 INDEPENDENCE

One of the most important concepts in probability theory is the idea of independence. Informally speaking, two events are *independent* if knowing whether one of the events has occurred tells you nothing about whether the other event will occur. If you know that a patient has appendicitis, this tells you nothing about whether he has a broken toe. The events "patient has appendicitis" and "patient has a broken toe" are independent. The fact that a patient has appendicitis has nothing to do with the presence or absence of a broken toe. But if you know that a patient has appendicitis, you are fairly sure that the patient has abdominal pain. The events "patient has appendicitis" and "patient has abdominal pain" are *not* independent.

Formally, two events are independent if

$$P(\text{Event 1}|\text{Event 2}) = P(\text{Event 1}) \quad (3.9)$$

In other words, conditioning on one event does not

change the probability of the other event. For patients with appendicitis, we have

P(Patient has a broken toe|Patient has appendicitis)

$= P$(Patient has a broken toe)

The probability P(Patient has a broken toe) is the nonconditional probability that a patient has a broken toe (the proportion of all patients in the world who have broken toes). If you were asked for the probability that a patient has a broken toe, given that he has appendicitis, you would say that this probability is just the proportion of all patients who have broken toes.

For the events "patient has abdominal pain" and "patient has appendicitis," we have

P(Patient has abdominal pain|Patient has appendicitis)

$\neq P$(Patient has abdominal pain)*

The conditional probability of abdominal pain, given appendicitis, is much higher than the nonconditional probability of abdominal pain (the proportion of all patients in the world with abdominal pain). The equality (3.9) does not hold, and this confirms what we already know—the events "patient has abdominal pain" and "patient has appendicitis" are not independent.

Often common sense and nonstatistical knowledge will tell you whether two events are independent. You can also determine whether two events are independent by calculating the two probabilities in (3.9) and checking whether these probabilities are equal. *If P(Event 1|Event 2) is equal to P(Event 1), the events are independent. If P(Event 1|Event 2) does not equal P(Event 1), the events are not independent.* Let us illustrate this rule by considering the retinopathy data of Example 3.2 again. The sample conditional probability of retinopathy, given exposure to bright light, is 0.86, and the overall sample probability of retinopathy is 0.65. Since 0.86 does not equal 0.65,

P(Retinopathy|Exposure to bright light)

$\neq P$(Retinopathy)

The equality (3.9) does not hold, and the events "retinopathy" and "exposure to bright light" are *not* independent for this sample of 60 infants.

Example 3.9

In a study of optic-nerve degeneration in Alzheimer's disease, postmortem examinations were conducted on 10 Alzheimer's patients.[9] Table 3.4 shows the distribution of these patients according to sex and evidence of optic-nerve degeneration. From this table, we see that four patients were females

---

*Opposite events are also called *complementary events*.

*The symbol " $\neq$ " means "is not equal to."

TABLE 3.4 DISTRIBUTION OF ALZHEIMER'S PATIENTS ACCORDING TO SEX AND OPTIC-NERVE DEGENERATION

Sex	Optic-Nerve Degeneration	
	Present	Not Present
Female	4	1
Male	4	1

TABLE 3.5 DISTRIBUTION OF PATIENTS ACCORDING TO DEVICE USED AND PRESENCE OF INFILTRATION

Device	Infiltration	
	Present	Not Present
IMED	12	29
AVI Guardian	2	37

with optic-nerve degeneration, four patients were males with optic-nerve degeneration, and so on.

Are the events "patient has optic-nerve degeneration" and "patient is female" independent for this sample of 10 patients? To determine this, we need to calculate P(Optic-nerve degeneration|Female) and P(Optic-nerve degeneration). If these sample probabilities are equal, the events are independent for this sample of 10 patients. If these sample probabilities are not equal, the events are not independent for this sample of 10 patients. Applying formula (3.2), we get

P(Optic-nerve degeneration|Female)

$$= \frac{\text{no. of females with optic-nerve degeneration}}{\text{no. of females}}$$

$$= \frac{4}{4 + 1} = \frac{4}{5} = 0.80$$

Applying formula (3.1), we get

P(Optic-nerve degeneration)

$$= \frac{\text{no. of patients with optic-nerve degeneration}}{\text{total no. of patients}}$$

$$= \frac{4 + 4}{4 + 1 + 4 + 1} = \frac{8}{10} = 0.80$$

Since P(Optic-nerve degeneration|Female) is equal to P(Optic-nerve degeneration), the equality (3.9) holds. The events are independent for this sample of 10 patients.

Example 3.10

A study compared two volumetric infusion devices, the IMED 928 and the AVI Guardian 100.[10] Table 3.5 shows the distribution of 80 patients according to device type and infiltration at the intravenous site.

The obvious question of interest concerns which device (if either) presents a greater risk of infiltration. If the events "infiltration" and "IMED use" are independent, it does not matter which device is used as far as infiltration is concerned. To determine whether these events are independent for this sample of 80 patients, we need to calculate P(Infiltration|IMED use) and P(Infiltration). If these probabilities are equal, the events are inde-

pendent. If these probabilities are not equal, the events are not independent. Applying formula (3.2), we get

P(Infiltration|IMED use)

$$= \frac{\begin{array}{c}\text{no. of patients with infiltration who}\\\text{used IMED device}\end{array}}{\text{no. of patients who used IMED device}}$$

$$= \frac{12}{12 + 29} = \frac{12}{41} = 0.29$$

Applying formula (3.1), we get

$$P(\text{Infiltration}) = \frac{\text{no. of patients with infiltration}}{\text{total no. of patients}}$$

$$= \frac{2 + 12}{12 + 29 + 2 + 37} = \frac{14}{80} = 0.18$$

Since 0.29 does not equal 0.18, we conclude that infiltration and IMED use are not independent for this sample. If we know nothing about a patient who will be randomly selected from this sample, our probability of infiltration is 0.18. If we are told that a patient will be randomly selected from those using the IMED device, our probability of infiltration is higher—0.29. The type of device matters when predicting infiltration.

We would have reached the same conclusion if we had calculated and compared P(Infiltration|Guardian use) and P(Infiltration). Using formula (3.2), we obtain

P(Infiltration|Guardian use)

$$= \frac{\begin{array}{c}\text{no. of patients with infiltration who}\\\text{used Guardian device}\end{array}}{\text{no. of patients who used Guardian device}}$$

$$= \frac{2}{2 + 37} = \frac{2}{39} = 0.05$$

Since 0.05 does not equal 0.18, infiltration and Guardian use are not independent for this sample. Again, we conclude that the type of device matters. Comparing the sample conditional probabilities P(Infiltration|IMED use) and P(Infiltration| Guardian use), we conclude that the risk of infiltration is much higher for patients using the IMED than for patients using the Guardian in this sample.

Without using an appropriate method for statistical inference, we cannot say that the risk of infiltration is higher for patients using the IMED than for patients using the Guardian in the population of all patients similar to those in the study. Statistical inferences of this sort will be discussed in later chapters.

Example 3.11

The data in Table 3.6 concern the severity of microscopic lesions in the renal pelvis of 12 female dogs with urinary tract infections.[11] A "+" indicates inflammation and a "−" indicates no inflammation. In this sample, does the presence of inflammation in the left renal pelvis tell us anything about the presence of inflammation in the right renal pelvis? This question is an informal way of asking whether the events "inflammation in right renal pelvis" and "inflammation in left renal pelvis" are independent. If these events are independent, knowing that inflammation is present in the left renal pelvis tells us nothing about whether inflammation is present in the right renal pelvis.

Applying formulas (3.2) and (3.1), we can calculate the probabilities needed to determine whether independence holds:

$P($Inflammation in right renal pelvis|Inflammation in left renal pelvis$)$

$$= \frac{\text{no. of dogs with inflammation in right and left renal pelvis}}{\text{no. of dogs with inflammation in left renal pelvis}}$$

$$= \frac{7}{8} = 0.88$$

$P($Inflammation in right renal pelvis$)$

$$= \frac{\text{no. of dogs with inflammation in right renal pelvis}}{\text{total no. of dogs}}$$

$$= \frac{7}{12} = 0.58$$

Since 0.88 does not equal 0.58, we conclude that inflammation in the right renal pelvis is not independent of inflammation in the left renal pelvis for this sample of 12 dogs. If we know nothing about a dog that will be randomly selected from these 12 dogs, our probability of inflammation in the right renal pelvis is 0.58. If we are told that a dog will be randomly selected from those with inflammation in the left renal pelvis, our probability of inflammation in the right renal pelvis is much higher—0.88.

TABLE 3.6 SEVERITY OF MICROSCOPIC LESIONS IN THE RENAL PELVIS OF DOGS WITH URINARY TRACT INFECTIONS

	Renal Pelvis	
Dog No.	Left	Right
1	−	−
2	+	−
3	+	+
4	+	+
5	+	+
6	+	+
7	+	+
8	−	−
9	−	−
10	−	−
11	+	+
12	+	+

An important consequence of independence is the following. If two events are independent,

$$P(\text{Both event 1 and event 2}) \tag{3.10}$$
$$= P(\text{Event 1})P(\text{Event 2})$$

This formula works *only* when the two events are independent. It should *never* be used when there is the slightest doubt about independence.

Example 3.12

Suppose you are asked to identify an organelle in a muscle cell and another organelle in a nerve cell. You have forgotten exactly what these organelles are, but you have narrowed the muscle-cell organelle down to three possibilities (one of which is correct) and the nerve-cell organelle down to four possibilities (one of which is correct). If your answer to one question has no effect on your answer to the other question, the events "correct identification of muscle-cell organelle" and "correct identification of nerve-cell organelle" are independent. We can then apply formula (3.10) to find the probability that you correctly identify both organelles.

$P($Correctly identify both organelles$)$

$$= P(\text{Correctly identify muscle-cell organelle})$$
$$\times P(\text{Correctly identify nerve-cell organelle})$$
$$= \frac{1}{3} \times \frac{1}{4} = \frac{1}{12} = 0.08$$

Your chance of correctly identifying both organelles is rather small.

Formula (3.10) can be generalized. If n events are independent,

$$P(\text{Event 1 and event 2 and event 3 and}$$
$$\ldots \text{and event } n)$$
$$= P(\text{Event 1})P(\text{Event 2})P(\text{Event 3}) \qquad (3.11)$$
$$\ldots P(\text{Event } n)$$

Like formula (3.10), formula (3.11) can be used *only* for independent events.

Example 3.13

A veterinarian stopped buying vaccines from a drug company after having problems with its intranasal *Bordetella* (kennel cough) vaccine. Although the company claimed that the reaction rate for this vaccine was one in 10, he observed severe reactions in all of the 10 dogs he vaccinated. Is his mistrust of the vaccine justified, given the responses of these 10 dogs? To answer this, we need to consider how reasonable the claimed reaction rate of $1/10$ is in light of the veterinarian's experience. Suppose for the moment that the reaction rate is, in fact, $1/10$, so the veterinarian and the dogs he vaccinated were just unlucky. How likely is it that 10 out of 10 dogs will have bad reactions, assuming a reaction rate of $1/10$? We can use formula (3.11) to calculate the probability we need if we realize that (1) the probability of a bad reaction in a single dog is $1/10$, and (2) the response of one dog to the vaccine is independent of the responses of other dogs to the vaccine.

By formula (3.11),

$$P(\text{All 10 dogs react badly})$$
$$= P(\text{Dog 1 reacts badly and dog 2 reacts badly}$$
$$\text{and } \ldots \text{ and dog 10 reacts badly})$$
$$= P(\text{Dog 1 reacts badly})P(\text{Dog 2 reacts badly})$$
$$\ldots P(\text{Dog 10 reacts badly})$$
$$= \left(\frac{1}{10}\right)^{10} = 0.0000000001$$

Because this probability is so small, the number of reactions seen by the veterinarian is extremely unlikely if the reaction rate is really $1/10$. The company's claim seems unreasonable, and the veterinarian's mistrust appears well founded.

3.6 BAYES' RULE*

Sometimes the conditional probability we have is the reverse of the conditional probability we want. Suppose that we know the probability of persistent

diarrhea, given Crohn's disease. When presented with a patient with persistent diarrhea, we would rather know the probability of Crohn's disease, given persistent diarrhea. Bayes' rule can sometimes be used to get the conditional probability we want from the conditional probability we do not want.

Let us abbreviate "event 1" as E1, "event 2" as E2, and "opposite of event 1" as opp. E1. The simple form of Bayes' rule consists of the following formula*:

$$P(E1 \mid E2) \qquad (3.12)$$
$$= \frac{P(E2 \mid E1)P(E1)}{[P(E2 \mid E1)P(E1) + P(E2 \mid \text{Opp. E1})P(\text{Opp. E1})]}$$

This formula is not self-evident, and we will not prove it. Instead, we will concentrate on using Bayes' rule. Although Bayes' rule strikes many people as horrendously complicated, it is not nearly as bad as it looks. Using it is just a tedious bookkeeping procedure in which you have to pay careful attention to what goes where. The use of Bayes' rule is best understood by working through examples.

Example 3.14

In a study of risk factors for patient falls, the following probabilities were obtained for a sample of 631 hospitalized patients aged 60 or older.[13]

$$P(\text{Sleeplessness} \mid \text{Fall}) = 0.60$$
$$P(\text{Sleeplessness} \mid \text{No fall}) = 0.36$$
$$P(\text{No sleeplessness} \mid \text{Fall}) = 0.40$$
$$P(\text{No sleeplessness} \mid \text{No fall}) = 0.64$$
$$P(\text{Fall}) = 0.52$$
$$P(\text{No fall}) = 0.48$$

What is the probability of falling, given sleeplessness, for this sample of patients? We can use Bayes' rule to obtain this probability. We will calculate $P(\text{Fall} \mid \text{Sleeplessness})$ first. If we think of "fall" as E1 and "sleeplessness" as E2, we can apply formula (3.12) to get

$$P(\text{Fall} \mid \text{Sleeplessness})$$
$$= \frac{P(\text{Sleeplessness} \mid \text{Fall})P(\text{Fall})}{[P(\text{Sleeplessness} \mid \text{Fall})P(\text{Fall}) + P(\text{Sleeplessness} \mid \text{No fall})P(\text{No fall})]}$$
$$= \frac{(0.60)(0.52)}{[(0.60)(0.52) + (0.36)(0.48)]}$$
$$= \frac{0.31}{0.48} = 0.65$$

---

*This section is not needed for later material and can be omitted.

*There is a more general form of Bayes' rule, which we will not consider. Further information can be found in other texts.[12]

For this sample of patients, the probability of falling, given that sleeplessness is present, is fairly high. What about the probability of falling, given that sleeplessness is *not* present? We can use Bayes' rule again to find the probability of falling, given no sleeplessness, for this sample of patients. Here we will let "fall" be E1 and "no sleeplessness" be E2. Applying formula (3.12), we get

$P(\text{Fall} | \text{No sleeplessness})$

$$= \frac{P(\text{No sleeplessness} | \text{Fall}) P(\text{Fall})}{\left[\begin{array}{l} P(\text{No sleeplessness} | \text{Fall}) P(\text{Fall}) + \\ P(\text{No sleeplessness} | \text{No fall}) P(\text{No fall}) \end{array}\right]}$$

$$= \frac{(0.40)(0.52)}{[(0.40)(0.52) + (0.64)(0.48)]}$$

$$= \frac{0.21}{0.52} = 0.40$$

For this sample of patients, the probability of falling, given that sleeplessness is present, is larger than the probability of falling, given that sleeplessness is not present.

Example 3.15

In a study of ischemic heart disease (IHD), the following sample probabilities were obtained.[14]

$P(\text{Current cigarette smoker} | \text{IHD}) = 0.53$

$P(\text{Current cigarette smoker} | \text{No IHD}) = 0.38$

$P(\text{Not current cigarette smoker} | \text{IHD}) = 0.47$

$P(\text{Not current cigarette smoker} | \text{No IHD}) = 0.62$

$P(\text{IHD}) = 0.08$

$P(\text{No IHD}) = 0.92$

What is the sample probability of IHD, given that the patient is a current cigarette smoker? What is the sample probability of IHD, given that the patient is *not* a current cigarette smoker? We have all the information we need to use Bayes' rule. Let us abbreviate "current cigarette smoker" as CCS. We will find $P(\text{IHD} | \text{CCS})$ first. Treating IHD as E1 and CCS as E2, we apply formula (3.12) to get

$P(\text{IHD} | \text{CCS})$

$$= \frac{P(\text{CCS} | \text{IHD}) P(\text{IHD})}{\left[\begin{array}{l} P(\text{CCS} | \text{IHD}) P(\text{IHD}) + \\ P(\text{CCS} | \text{No IHD}) P(\text{No IHD}) \end{array}\right]}$$

$$= \frac{(0.53)(0.08)}{[(0.53)(0.08) + (0.38)(0.92)]}$$

$$= \frac{0.042}{0.392} = 0.11$$

There is an 11% chance of IHD for current cigarette smokers in this sample.

The probability of IHD for nonsmokers in this sample can be obtained by treating IHD as E1 and "not CCS" as E2. Applying formula (3.12), we get

$P(\text{IHD} | \text{Not CCS})$

$$= \frac{P(\text{Not CCS} | \text{IHD}) P(\text{IHD})}{\left[\begin{array}{l} P(\text{Not CCS} | \text{IHD}) P(\text{IHD}) + \\ P(\text{Not CCS} | \text{No IHD}) P(\text{No IHD}) \end{array}\right]}$$

$$= \frac{(0.47)(0.08)}{[(0.47)(0.08) + (0.62)(0.92)]}$$

$$= \frac{0.038}{0.608} = 0.06$$

In this sample, subjects who are current cigarette smokers have a larger probability of IHD than subjects who are not current cigarette smokers.

Example 3.16

A study examined side effects after metrizamide myelography and lumbar laminectomy.[15] Some of the patients underwent laminectomy and myelography on the same day (same-day laminectomy group) and others underwent laminectomy at least two days after myelography (delayed laminectomy group). The following sample probabilities concerning nausea were obtained:

$P(\text{Same-day laminectomy} | \text{Nausea}) = 0.67$

$P(\text{Same-day laminectomy} | \text{No nausea}) = 0.35$

$P(\text{Delayed laminectomy} | \text{Nausea}) = 0.33$

$P(\text{Delayed laminectomy} | \text{No nausea}) = 0.65$

$P(\text{Nausea}) = 0.48$

$P(\text{No nausea}) = 0.52$

We would like to compare $P(\text{Nausea} | \text{Same-day laminectomy})$ and $P(\text{Nausea} | \text{Delayed laminectomy})$. Both of these probabilities can be calculated by using Bayes' rule. Let us find $P(\text{Nausea} | \text{Same-day laminectomy})$ first. We will abbreviate "same-day laminectomy" as SDL. Treating "nausea" as E1 and SDL as E2 in formula (3.12), we get

$P(\text{Nausea} | \text{SDL})$

$$= \frac{P(\text{SDL} | \text{Nausea}) P(\text{Nausea})}{\left[\begin{array}{l} P(\text{SDL} | \text{Nausea}) P(\text{Nausea}) + \\ P(\text{SDL} | \text{No nausea}) P(\text{No nausea}) \end{array}\right]}$$

$$= \frac{(0.67)(0.48)}{[(0.67)(0.48) + (0.35)(0.52)]}$$

$$= \frac{0.32}{0.50} = 0.64$$

In this sample, patients who underwent same-day laminectomy had a fairly high probability of nausea.

Now let us calculate $P(\text{Nausea} | \text{Delayed laminectomy})$. We will abbreviate "delayed laminectomy" as DL. Letting "nausea" correspond to E1 and DL to E2 in formula (3.12), we get

$$P(\text{Nausea} | \text{DL})$$

$$= \frac{P(\text{DL} | \text{Nausea}) P(\text{Nausea})}{[P(\text{DL} | \text{Nausea}) P(\text{Nausea}) + P(\text{DL} | \text{No nausea}) P(\text{No nausea})]}$$

$$= \frac{(0.33)(0.48)}{[(0.33)(0.48) + (0.65)(0.52)]}$$

$$= \frac{0.16}{0.50} = 0.32$$

Patients in this sample who underwent delayed laminectomy had a much smaller probability of nausea than patients who underwent same-day laminectomy.

An obvious drawback to Bayes' rule is the fact that the information needed to use it is often unavailable. Suppose that we want to find the probability of a certain disease, given certain neurological signs. If we do not know the overall proportion of people with the disease, we cannot use Bayes' rule, since $P(\text{Disease})$ must be known. When the necessary information is available or can be estimated, however, Bayes' rule is extremely useful.

3.7 PROBABILITY PITFALLS

Certain probability mistakes crop up so often that they warrant special attention here.

1. The Independence-Disjointness Confusion. People unaccustomed to probability calculations frequently confuse independence and disjointness. They apply the independence formula (3.10) when the disjointness formula (3.6) is required, and vice versa. The "and" in probabilities of the form

$$P(\text{Both event 1 and event 2})$$

seems to bring to mind addition, and students incorrectly try to compute such probabilities by adding $P(\text{Event 1})$ and $P(\text{Event 2})$. If independence has been demonstrated, the correct formula for calculating probabilities of this form is (3.10), which involves multiplication. If independence has not been demonstrated, the correct formula is (3.5).

Addition of probabilities is done when *disjoint* events are connected by "*or*," as in probabilities of the form

$$P(\text{Event 1 or event 2})$$

If you have difficulty with a probability calculation, check to make sure that you have not confused independence and disjointness.

Once you fully understand independence and disjointness, it is hard to make this error, since *disjoint events cannot be independent* (unless one event has probability 0). Suppose that event 1 and event 2 are disjoint and that $P(\text{Event 1})$ and $P(\text{Event 2})$ are both greater than 0. If event 2 has occurred, we know that event 1 has *not* occurred, since disjoint events cannot both happen at the same time. Hence,

$$P(\text{Event 1} | \text{Event 2}) = 0$$

Since $P(\text{Event 1})$ does not equal 0, the equality (3.9) does not hold. Event 1 and event 2 are not independent.

2. The Gambler's Fallacy. This fallacy is the superstitious belief that the repeated occurrence of an event increases the chance that the opposite event will occur. If a fair coin comes up heads eight times in a row, many people believe that the probability of tails on the ninth toss is greater than $1/2$. The eight preceding heads are somehow supposed to influence the outcome on the ninth toss, making tails more likely in order to balance out the large number of heads. In fact, coin tosses are independent, so the outcome on one toss has no effect on the outcome on another toss. The probability of tails on the ninth toss is always $1/2$, no mater what the eight previous outcomes were.

The gambler's fallacy is widespread, and health professionals sometimes succumb to it. Suppose that four consecutive esophageal surgeries performed by a surgeon have gone well. Suppose also that the complication rate for this surgery is $1/5$. The surgeon may believe that her next surgery is almost certain to cause trouble: the four successful surgeries mean she is due for problems. The reasoning is fallacious, but here things are more complicated than they are for coin tosses. Because the surgeries are performed by the same surgeon, their outcomes may not be independent. The previous four surgeries could have increased the surgeon's skill, so the chance of complications for the fifth esophageal surgery might be *reduced*. On the other hand, the surgeon's expectation that trouble is likely might become a self-fulfilling prophecy, subconsciously steering her toward complications during the fifth surgery. But there is no law of probability that dictates that four successful surgeries are likely to be followed by a surgery with complications. A history of successful surgeries cannot, by itself, reduce the chance that the next surgery will be successful.

3. The Fifty-Fifty Fallacy. This fallacy is the belief that events are equally likely when only two events are possible. The fifty-fifty fallacy is encountered in such statements as the following.

> "Either my home will be burglarized while I'm on vacation or it won't, so the chance of a burglary is 50%."
>
> "Either Mr. Kravitz shows up at 4:00 today or he doesn't, so there's a 50% chance that he will keep his 4:00 appointment."
>
> "Either this patient recovers or she doesn't, so she has a 50% chance of recovering."

A moment's thought should convince you that the fact that there are only two possible events tells you nothing about the probabilities of the events.

SUMMARY

The probability of an event is the long-run proportion of times the event will occur. Sample probabilities are often calculated in order to estimate population probabilities. Conditional probabilities are of particular interest in medicine and health care, since they give the probability of an event given that some other event has occurred. When events are disjoint or independent, probability calculations involving the events can often be simplified. Sometimes a desired conditional probability can be obtained from the reverse conditional probability by using Bayes' rule. Common probability pitfalls are the independence-disjointness confusion, the gambler's fallacy, and the fifty-fifty fallacy.

COMMONLY USED PROBABILITY FORMULAS

Sample probability:

$$P(\text{Event}) = \frac{\text{no. of observations for which event occurs}}{\text{total no. of observations}}$$

Sample conditional probability:

$P(\text{Event} | \text{Conditioning event})$

$$= \frac{\text{no. of observations for which event and conditioning event both occur}}{\text{no. of observations for which conditioning event occurs}}$$

Sample conditional probability:

$P(\text{Event} | \text{Conditioning event})$

$$= \frac{P(\text{Both event and conditioning event})}{P(\text{Conditioning event})}$$

For ANY two events:

$P(\text{Both event 1 and event 2})$

$$= \frac{\text{no. of observations for which event 1 and event 2 both occur}}{\text{total no. of observations}}$$

For ANY two events:

$P(\text{Event 1 or event 2})$

$$= P(\text{Event 1}) + P(\text{Event 2}) - P(\text{Both event 1 and event 2})$$

For DISJOINT events only:

$$P(\text{Event 1 or event 2}) = P(\text{Event 1}) + P(\text{Event 2})$$

For PAIRWISE DISJOINT events only:

$P(\text{Event 1 or event 2 or event 3 or } \ldots \text{ or event } n)$

$$= P(\text{Event 1}) + P(\text{Event 2}) + P(\text{Event 3}) + \cdots + P(\text{Event } n)$$

For INDEPENDENT events only:

$$P(\text{Both event 1 and event 2}) = P(\text{Event 1})P(\text{Event 2})$$

For INDEPENDENT events only:

$P(\text{Event 1 and event 2 and event 3 and } \ldots \text{ and event } n)$

$$= P(\text{Event 1})P(\text{Event 2})P(\text{Event 3}) \ldots P(\text{Event } n)$$

PROBLEMS

1. In a study of nursing care of skeletal pins, data were collected on the following characteristics.[16]

General physical condition: good, fair, poor
Movement of limb: yes, no
Medications: antibiotics, anticoagulants, oral hypoglycemic agents, insulin, steroids, vitamins
Existing physical disorders: endocrine disease, circulatory disease, respiratory disease, digestive disease, blood disease, genitourinary disease, nervous system disease, musculoskeletal disease, skin disease, mental disease
Drainage at pin: none, clear, purulent

Which of these characteristics concern disjoint events?

2. A study evaluated the use of vincristine to treat idiopathic thrombocytic purpura.[17] The responses of 10 patients are shown in Table 3.7. Are the events "sustained response," "transient response," and "no response" disjoint? Calculate the following sample probabilities, if possible. If a probability cannot be calculated, indicate what further information is needed to calculate the probability.
  - a. P(Sustained response)
  - b. P(Transient response)
  - c. P(Transient or sustained response)
  - d. P(No response)

TABLE 3.7 RESPONSE OF PATIENTS TO VINCRISTINE

Patient No.	Response
1	Sustained
2	Transient
3	Sustained
4	None
5	Transient
6	Sustained
7	Transient
8	Sustained
9	Sustained
10	Transient

3. A study examined the association between chemical conjunctivitis and the use of wet-look hair-styling products.[18] Twenty-one patients who used these products complained of various ocular symptoms, some of which are shown in Table 3.8. Are the events in Table 3.8 disjoint? Calculate the following sample probabilities, if possible. If a probability cannot be calculated, indicate what further information is needed to calculate the probability.
  - a. P(Tearing)
  - b. P(Itching)
  - c. P(Tearing or itching)

TABLE 3.8 OCULAR COMPLAINTS OF PATIENTS

Symptom	No. of Patients
Tearing	8
Redness	6
Itching	2

4. Twenty-one patients with aggressive non-Hodgkin's lymphoma were treated with a high-dose combination chemotherapy regimen.[19] After treatment, 16 patients showed a complete response, three patients showed a partial response, and two patients died. Are the events "complete response," "partial response," and "death" disjoint? Calculate the following sample probabilities, if possible. If a probability cannot be calculated, indicate what further information is needed to calculate the probability.
  - a. P(Complete response)
  - b. P(Partial response)
  - c. P(Complete or partial response)

5. The data in Table 3.9 were reported in a study of locoweed poisoning and congestive heart failure in cattle.[20] A " + " indicates that edema and swelling were present. A " − " indicates that edema and swelling were not present. Are the events "edema and swelling in jaw," "edema and swelling in neck," and "edema and swelling in brisket" disjoint? Calculate the following sample probabilities, if possible. If a probability cannot be calculated, indicate what further information is needed to calculate the probability.
  - a. P(Edema and swelling in jaw or neck)
  - b. P(Edema and swelling in jaw or brisket)
  - c. P(Edema and swelling in neck or brisket)

TABLE 3.9 EDEMA AND SWELLING IN CALVES FED LOCOWEED

| Calf No. | Location of Edema and Swelling | | |
	Jaw	Neck	Brisket
1	+	+	+
2	+	+	+
3	−	−	−
4	+	+	+
5	+	+	+
6	+	+	+
7	+	+	−
8	+	+	+
9	+	+	+
10	+	+	+

6. The effect of early discharge of low-birthweight infants was examined in a randomized clinical trial.[21] The 40 control group infants were discharged according to routine nursery criteria, and the 39 early-discharge infants were discharged before they weighed 2200 grams. Table 3.10 shows the distribution of infants according to group and outcome with respect to need for acute-care visits or rehospitalization.

    a. Calculate and compare P(Acute-care visits|Early discharge) and P(Acute-care visits|Routine discharge) for this sample.

    b. Calculate and compare P(Rehospitalization|Early discharge) and P(Rehospitalization|Routine discharge) for this sample.

    c. Do these data suggest that early discharge of infants like those in the study will result in increased illness?

TABLE 3.10 DISTRIBUTION OF INFANTS ACCORDING TO OUTCOME AND GROUP

Outcome	Early-Discharge Group	Control Group
Acute-care visits	29	36
Rehospitalization	10	10

7. A study investigated the effect of dental treatment on the ST segment of the electrocardiogram (ECG).[22] During the anesthesia and surgery phases of routine dental extractions, ECGs were obtained for 19 patients with cardiac disease and 18 patients without cardiac disease. The ECGs were then evaluated for ST-segment depression by a cardiologist who did not know the patients' medical condition. The distribution of patients according to ST-segment depression and cardiac disease is shown in Table 3.11.

    a. Calculate and compare P(ST depression|Cardiac disease) and P(ST depression|No cardiac disease) for this sample.

    b. Do these data suggest that a cardiac patient undergoing routine dental extraction should be concerned about ST-segment depression?

TABLE 3.11 DISTRIBUTION OF PATIENTS ACCORDING TO PRESENCE OF ST-SEGMENT DEPRESSION AND CARDIAC DISEASE STATUS

ST-Segment Depression	Cardiac Disease	
	Present	Absent
Present	12	2
Absent	7	16

8. In a randomized clinical study, the use of acupuncture for relieving the pain of primary dys-

menorrhea was evaluated.[23] Patients with primary dysmenorrhea were randomly assigned to one of four groups:

    (1) The acupuncture group, which was treated by placing needles at appropriate acupuncture points

    (2) The placebo acupuncture group, which was treated by placing needles at nonacupuncture points

    (3) The control group, which received no treatments other than those used before entering the study

    (4) The visitation group, which received no treatments other than those used before entering the study but had extra visits with the physician during the study

Table 3.12 shows the distribution of 43 patients according to response and treatment group.

    a. Calculate and compare the following sample probabilities:
P(Improvement|Acupuncture)
P(Improvement|Placebo acupuncture)
P(Improvement|No additional treatment)
P(Improvement|Extra visits but no additional treatment)

    b. Do these data suggest that acupuncture is effective for relieving menstrual pain?

TABLE 3.12 DISTRIBUTION OF PATIENTS ACCORDING TO RESPONSE AND TREATMENT GROUP

Response	Treatment Group			
	Acupuncture	Placebo Acupuncture	Control	Visitation
Improvement	10	4	2	1
No improvement	1	7	9	9

9. The association between video display terminal (VDT) use and adverse health conditions was examined in an epidemiologic study.[24] Table 3.13 shows the distribution of 812 clerical workers according to industry type, VDT use, and headaches.

    a. Calculate and compare P(Headaches|No VDT use) and P(Headaches|7 or more hours of VDT use) for the sample of workers from computer and data processing industries, public utilities, and state departments.

    b. Calculate and compare P(Headaches|No VDT use) and P(Headaches|7 or more hours of VDT use) for the sample of workers from banks, communications industries, and hospitals.

c. Do these data suggest that the risk of headache for heavy VDT users differs from the risk of headache for non-VDT users? If so, does the type of industry matter?

TABLE 3.13 DISTRIBUTION OF CLERICAL WORKERS ACCORDING TO INDUSTRY TYPE, VDT USE, AND HEADACHES

Industry Type	Daily VDT Use (hours)	No. of Workers	No. of Workers with Headaches
Computer and data processing, public utilities, state departments	0	199	16
	7 or more	332	50
Banking, communications, hospitals	0	185	24
	7 or more	96	9

10. A randomized, double-blind study evaluated the effectiveness of topical antibiotic treatment of impetigo.[25] Children with impetigo were randomly assigned to receive either 2% mupirocin in polyethylene glycol or the vehicle polyethylene glycol alone. The distribution of 36 children according to treatment and outcome is shown in Table 3.14.

a. Are the events "cure" and "treatment with mupirocin" independent for this sample?

b. If the events "cure" and "treatment with mupirocin" are not independent for this sample, calculate and compare $P(\text{Cure}|\text{Treatment with mupirocin})$ and $P(\text{Cure}|\text{Treatment with vehicle})$.

c. Do these data suggest that mupirocin is effective for the treatment of impetigo?

TABLE 3.14 DISTRIBUTION OF CHILDREN ACCORDING TO TREATMENT AND OUTCOME

Treatment	Outcome		
	Cured	Improved	Failure
Mupirocin in vehicle	14	3	0
Vehicle alone	8	8	3

11. In a trial of streptokinase in myocardial infarction, 1741 patients with symptoms of acute myocardial infarction were randomly assigned to receive a one-hour infusion of either streptokinase or placebo.[26] Table 3.15 shows the distribution of patients according to survival outcome and group.

a. Are the events "death" and "treatment with streptokinase" independent for this sample?

b. If the events "death" and "treatment with streptokinase" are not independent for this sample, calculate and compare

$P(\text{Death}|\text{Treatment with streptokinase})$ and $P(\text{Death}|\text{Treatment with placebo})$.

c. Do these data suggest that the use of streptokinase for treating myocardial infarctions greatly reduces the risk of death within 21 days?

TABLE 3.15 DISTRIBUTION OF PATIENTS ACCORDING TO SURVIVAL OUTCOME AND GROUP

Outcome	Group	
	Streptokinase	Placebo
Died within 21 days	54	63
Survived at least 21 days	805	819

12. The effect of perineal massage on perineal laceration and the need for episiotomy was examined.[27] Twenty women were randomly assigned to a massage group or a control group, and those in the massage group were instructed to practice perineal massage for the last six weeks of pregnancy. The distribution of women according to group and perineal outcome is shown in Table 3.16.

a. Are the events "intact perineum" and "massage" independent for this sample?

b. If the events "intact perineum" and "massage" are not independent for this sample, calculate and compare $P(\text{Intact perineum}|\text{Massage})$ and $P(\text{Intact perineum}|\text{No massage})$.

c. Do these data suggest that women who use perineal massage have a lower risk of episiotomy or perineal laceration than women who do not use perineal massage?

TABLE 3.16 DISTRIBUTION OF WOMEN ACCORDING TO GROUP AND PERINEAL OUTCOME

Group	Perineal Outcome	
	Intact	Episiotomy or Laceration
Massage	9	1
No massage	2	8

13. A study evaluated the effectiveness of child restraint devices in preventing death and injury by analyzing traffic accident data for New Mexico.[28] Table 3.17 shows the distribution of 20,972 children under five years of age involved in motor vehicle accidents according to accident outcome and restraint category.

a. Are the events "death" and "restraint" independent for this sample?

b. If the events "death" and "restraint" are not independent for this sample, calculate and compare $P(\text{Death}|\text{Restraint})$ and $P(\text{Death}|\text{No restraint})$.

c. Are the events "nonfatal injury" and "restraint" independent for the 20,934 children who were not killed?

d. If the events "nonfatal injury" and "restraint" are not independent for the 20,934 children who were not killed, calculate and compare P(Nonfatal injury|Restraint) and P(Nonfatal injury|No restraint).

e. Do these data suggest that restrained children are less likely to suffer death or nonfatal injury than nonrestrained children?

TABLE 3.17 DISTRIBUTION OF CHILDREN ACCORDING TO ACCIDENT OUTCOME AND RESTRAINT CATEGORY

Accident Outcome	Restraint Category	
	Restrained	Not Restrained
Fatal	2	36
Not fatal	4,552	16,382
Nonfatal injury	321	2,242
No injury or death	4,231	14,140

14. A clinical and experimental study examined the results of cardiopulmonary resuscitation (CPR) in cats.[29] Table 3.18 shows the distribution of 10 cats according to length of CPR efforts and outcome.

a. Are the events "alive" and "less than 5 min CPR" independent for this sample?

b. If the events "alive" and "less than 5 min CPR" are not independent for this sample, calculate and compare P(Alive|Less than 5 min CPR) and P(Alive|5 to 15 min CPR).

c. Do the data suggest that the probability of surviving when less than five minutes of CPR is done differs from the probability of surviving when 5 to 15 minutes of CPR is done?

d. Calculate P(Both alive and less than 5 min CPR). Can formula (3.10) be used?

TABLE 3.18 DISTRIBUTION OF CATS ACCORDING TO LENGTH OF CPR EFFORTS AND OUTCOME

Length of CPR Efforts (min)	Outcome	
	Alive After Four Hours	Dead Within Four Hours
Less than 5	1	1
5 to 15	4	4

15. In a study of sorbitol intolerance, healthy volunteers ingested 10 grams of sorbitol.[30] The distribution of 40 sorbitol-intolerant volunteers according to race and symptoms of intolerance is given in Table 3.19. Calculate the following probabilities for the sorbitol-intolerant subjects, if possible. If a probability cannot be calculated, indicate what further information is needed to calculate the probability.

a. P(Both Asian Indian and affected by bloating)

b. P(Both black and affected by cramping)

c. P(Both white and affected by diarrhea)

d. P(Both affected by bloating and affected by cramping)

TABLE 3.19 DISTRIBUTION OF SUBJECTS ACCORDING TO RACE AND SYMPTOMS OF INTOLERANCE

Race	Bloating		Abdominal Cramping		Diarrhea	
	Present	Absent	Present	Absent	Present	Absent
Asian Indian	22	3	14	11	8	17
Black	4	0	1	3	2	2
White	10	1	6	5	3	8

16. A study compared Abbott and Wellcome ELISA tests for detection of serum antibodies to the human immunodeficiency virus.[31] Table 3.20 shows the distribution of 932 ELISA tests according to the Abbott results and the Wellcome results. Calculate the following sample probabilities, if possible. If a probability cannot be calculated, indicate what further information is needed to calculate the probability.

a. P(Both Abbott test negative and Wellcome test positive)

b. P(Both Abbott test positive and Wellcome test negative)

c. P(Both Abbott test equivocal and Wellcome test positive)

d. P(Both Abbott test equivocal and Wellcome test negative)

e. Do the data suggest that the Abbott and Wellcome tests are frequently inconsistent?

TABLE 3.20 DISTRIBUTION OF ELISA TESTS ACCORDING TO ABBOTT RESULTS AND WELLCOME RESULTS

Abbott Results	Wellcome Results	
	Positive	Negative
Positive	223	0
Negative	2	684
Equivocal	10	13

17. A study evaluated the use of computed tomography (CT) for the diagnosis of blunt intestinal and mesenteric injuries.[32] The CT findings for 15 patients with blunt abdominal trauma requiring surgery are shown in Table 3.21. A "+" indicates that the finding was present. A "−" indicates that the finding was absent. Calculate the following sample probabilities, if possible. If a probability cannot be calculated, indicate what further information is needed to calculate the probability.

    a. P(Both thickened bowel wall and thickened mesentery)

    b. P(Both thickened bowel wall and peritoneal fluid)

    c. P(Both thickened mesentery and free air)

    d. P(Both peritoneal fluid and free air)

TABLE 3.21 CT FINDINGS FOR PATIENTS WITH BLUNT ABDOMINAL TRAUMA*

| | Findings | | | |
Patient	Thickened Bowel Wall	Thickened Mesentery	Peritoneal Fluid	Free Air
EM	+	+	+	−
DS	+	−	+	−
DK	−	+	−	−
HG	+	+	+	−
AR	+	+	+	+
RM	+	+	+	−
ML	+	−	+	+
JP	+	+	−	−
VM	−	−	+	−
KL	+	+	+	−
JS	−	+	+	−
TK	−	+	+	−
JA	+	+	+	−
RR	+	+	+	−
RR	+	+	+	+

* + = present, − = absent

18. In a study of idiopathic anaphylaxis, 73 patients with episodes of life-threatening anaphylactoid reactions were evaluated.[33] Table 3.22 shows the number of patients with various symptoms of anaphylaxis at the time of presentation. Calculate the following sample probabilities, if possible. If a probability cannot be calculated, indicate what further information is needed to calculate the probability.

    a. P(Both angioedema and upper airway obstruction)

    b. P(Both urticaria and pruritis)

    c. P(Both upper airway obstruction and bronchospasm)

TABLE 3.22 SYMPTOMS OF ANAPHYLAXIS AT TIME OF PRESENTATION

Symptom	No. of Patients
Angioedema	69
Upper airway obstruction	52
Urticaria	44
Pruritis	36
Bronchospasm	27

19. The following sample probabilities were obtained in a randomized, double-blind study of the effect of in-line filtration on infusion phlebitis.[34]

P(Filter|Phlebitis) = 0.52
P(Filter|No phlebitis) = 0.47
P(No filter|Phlebitis) = 0.48
P(No filter|No phlebitis) = 0.53
P(Phlebitis) = 0.28
P(No phlebitis) = 0.72

    a. Use Bayes' rule to find P(Phlebitis|Filter) for this sample.

    b. Use Bayes' rule to find P(Phlebitis|No filter) for this sample.

    c. Do these data suggest that the risk of phlebitis when filtration is done is lower than the risk of phlebitis when filtration is not done?

20. A study examined the relationship between gold sodium thiomalate (GSTM) use and hematuria in patients with rheumatoid arthritis.[35] The following sample probabilities were obtained.

P(GSTM|Hematuria) = 0.56
P(GSTM|No hematuria) = 0.56
P(Placebo|Hematuria) = 0.44
P(Placebo|No hematuria) = 0.44
P(Hematuria) = 0.35
P(No hematuria) = 0.65

    a. Use Bayes' rule to find P(Hematuria|GSTM) for this sample.

    b. Use Bayes' rule to find P(Hematuria|Placebo) for this sample.

    c. Do these data suggest that arthritis patients who use GSTM have a higher risk of hematuria than patients who do not use GSTM?

21. The use of scintigraphy to detect total obstruction of the common bile duct was evaluated.[36] If the gallbladder, the bile duct, and intestinal activity could not be visualized during scintigraphy, total obstruction was suspected. The following sample probabilities were obtained.

P(Nonvisualization|Total obstruction) = 1
P(Nonvisualization|Partial or no obstruction) = 0.005
P(Visualization|Total obstruction) = 0
P(Visualization|Partial or no obstruction) = 0.995
P(Total obstruction) = 0.06
P(Partial or no obstruction) = 0.94

    a. Use Bayes' rule to find P(Total obstruction|Nonvisualization) for this sample.

    b. Use Bayes' rule to find P(Partial or no obstruction|Visualization) for this sample.

c. Do these data suggest that scintigraphy is an accurate method for detecting total obstruction of the bile duct?

REFERENCES

1. Williams MA, Campbell EB, Raynor WJ, et al: Predictors of acute confusional states in hospitalized elderly patients. Res Nurs Health 8:31–40, 1985.
2. Glass P, Avery GB, Subramanian KNS, et al: Effect of bright light in the hospital nursery on the incidence of retinopathy of prematurity. N Engl J Med 313:401–404, 1985.
3. Beck A, Katcher A: Between Pets and People. New York: Putnam, 1983.
4. Merrill DC: Clinical experience with Mentor inflatable penile prosthesis in 206 patients. Urology 28:185–189, 1986.
5. Flancbaum L, Wright J, Siegel JH: Emergency surgery in patients with post-traumatic myocardial contusion. J Trauma 26:795–803, 1986.
6. Springmeyer SC, Hackman RC, Holle R, et al: Use of bronchoalveolar lavage to diagnose acute diffuse pneumonia in the immunocompromised host. J Infect Dis 154:604–610, 1986.
7. Coyle N, Monzillo E, Loscalzo M, et al: A model of continuity of care for cancer patients with pain and neuro-oncologic complications. Canc Nurs 8:111–119, 1985.
8. Harvey JW, Rackear D: Experimental onion-induced hemolytic anemia in dogs. Vet Pathol 22:387–392, 1985.
9. Hinton DR, Sadun AA, Blanks JC, et al: Optic-nerve degeneration in Alzheimer's disease. N Engl J Med 315:485–487, 1986.
10. Engler MM, Engler MB: Comparative evaluation of intravenous therapy regulating devices. Heart Lung 15:262–267, 1986.
11. Ling GV, Cullen JM, Kennedy PC, et al: Relationship of upper and lower urinary tract infection and bacterial invasion of uroepithelium to antibody-coated bacteria test results in female dogs. Am J Vet Res 46:499–504, 1985.
12. Remington RD, Schork MA: Statistics with Applications to the Biological and Health Sciences. 2nd ed. Englewood Cliffs: Prentice-Hall, 1985.
13. Janken JK, Reynolds BA, Swiech K: Patient falls in the acute care setting: Identifying risk factors. Nurs Res 35:215–219, 1986.
14. Meade TW, Mellows, S, Brozovic M, et al: Haemostatic function and ischaemic heart disease: Principal results of the Northwick Park Heart Study. Lancet 2:533–537, 1986.
15. Jones AG, Meinecke E, Becker J, et al: Side effects following metrizamide myelography and lumbar laminectomy. J Neurosci Nurs 19:90–94, 1987.
16. Sproles KJ: Nursing care of skeletal pins: A closer look. Orthopaed Nurs 4:11–20, 1985.
17. Manoharan A: Slow infusion of vincristine in the treatment of idiopathic thrombocytopenic purpura. Am J Hematol 21:135–138, 1986.
18. Kupchock S, Thom H, Minowski J: "Wet-look" hairstyle linked to ocular complaints. J Ophthal Nurs Technol 4:27–29, 1985.
19. Hainsworth JD, Wolff SN, Stein RS, et al: Effects of mega-COMLA (cyclophosphamide, cytarabine, vincristine, and methotrexate followed by leucovorin and prednisone) plus CHOP (cyclophosphamide, doxorubicin, vincristine, and prednisone) in the treatment of lymphoid neoplasms with very poor prognosis. Canc Treat Rep 70:953–958, 1986.
20. James LF, Hartley WJ, Nielsen D, et al: Locoweed (Oxytropis sericea) poisoning and congestive heart failure in cattle. J Am Vet Med Assoc 189:1549–1556, 1986.
21. Brooten D, Kumar S, Brown LP, et al: A randomized clinical trial of early hospital discharge and home follow-up of very-low-birth-weight infants. N Engl J Med 315:934–939, 1986.
22. Hasse AL, Heng MK, Garrett NR: Blood pressure and electrocardiographic response to dental treatment with use of local anesthesia. J Am Dent Assoc 113:639–642, 1986.
23. Helms JM: Acupuncture for the management of primary dysmenorrhea. Obstet Gynecol 69:51–56, 1987.
24. Rossignol AM, Morse EP, Summers VM, et al: Video display terminal use and reported health symptoms among Massachusetts clerical workers. J Occup Med 29:112–118, 1987.
25. Eells LD, Mertz PM, Piovanetti Y, et al: Topical antibiotic treatment of impetigo with mupirocin. Arch Dermatol 122:1273–1276, 1986.
26. I.S.A.M. Study Group: A prospective trial of intravenous streptokinase in acute myocardial infarction (I.S.A.M.): Mortality, morbidity, and infarct size at 21 days. N Engl J Med 314:1465–1471, 1986.
27. Avery MD, Burket BA: Effect of perineal massage on the incidence of episiotomy and perineal laceration in a nurse-midwifery service. J Nurs-Midwif 31:128–134, 1986.
28. Sewell CM, Hull HF, Fenner J, et al: Child restraint law effects on motor vehicle accident fatalities and injuries: The New Mexico experience. Pediatrics 78:1079-1084, 1986.
29. Gilroy BA, Dunlop DJ, Shapiro HM: Outcome from cardiopulmonary resuscitation in cats: Laboratory and clinical experience. J Am Anim Hosp Assoc 23:133–139, 1987.
30. Jain NK, Patel VP, Pitchumoni CS: Sorbitol intolerance in adults. Prevalence and pathogenesis on two continents. J Clin Gastroenterol 9:317–319, 1987.
31. Evans RP, Shanson DC, Mortimer PP: Clinical evaluation of Abbott and Wellcome enzyme linked immunosorbent assays for detection of serum antibodies to human immunodeficiency virus (HIV). J Clin Pathol 40:552–555, 1987.
32. Donohue JH, Federle MP, Griffiths BG, et al: Computed tomography in the diagnosis of blunt intestinal and mesenteric injuries. J Trauma 27:11–17, 1987.
33. Boxer M, Greenberger PA, Patterson R: Clinical summary and course of idiopathic anaphylaxis in 73 patients. Arch Intern Med 147:269–272, 1987.
34. Adams SD, Killien M, Larson, E: In-line filtration and infusion phlebitis. Heart Lung 15:134–140, 1986.
35. Leonard PA, Bienz SR, Clegg DO, et al: Hematuria in patients with rheumatoid arthritis receiving gold and D-penicillamine. J Rheumatol 14:55–59, 1987.
36. Lecklitner ML, Austin AR, Benedetto AR, et al: Positive predictive value of cholescintigraphy in common bile duct obstruction. J Nucl Med 27:1403–1406, 1986.

4

RANDOM VARIABLES
AND DISTRIBUTIONS

CHAPTER OBJECTIVES

*After studying this chapter and working the problems,
you should be able to:*

1. Explain the concepts of random variables, distributions, and independence

2. Recognize nonindependent data

3. Recognize extremely nonnormal data

4. Obtain standard normal tail probabilities from a table

5. Determine whether a random variable has a binomial distribution

6. Obtain binomial probabilities from a table

Most statistical procedures involve the use of random variables, and a failure to understand statistical methods often stems from a failure to understand random variables. Many students find the notation required for a discussion of random variables intimidating at first. For this reason, symbols are used in this chapter only when necessary. If you view statistical notation as nothing more than a foreign language, you should quickly become accustomed to it.

4.1 RANDOM VARIABLES

A random variable is a *potential* quantity whose values are determined by a chance-governed mechanism. We have already looked at several random

variables, although we did not use this term. Let us consider Example 3.12 again. In this example, there were three possible identifications of a muscle-cell organelle. Suppose we label these identifications 1, 2, and 3. Then your potential identification of the muscle-cell organelle is a random variable with the possible values 1, 2, and 3. Since you are guessing from these values, your answer is determined by the chance-governed mechanism of guessing.

Another random variable is obtained if we randomly select one of the patients in the acromegaly study of Example 2.6 and record her plasma GH level. Plasma GH is a random variable. We cannot know before selection what the plasma GH will be, and the plasma GH we get is determined by the chance-governed mechanism of random selection. In a sense, a random variable is a name for a potential number that is converted into a specific number when the chance-governed mechanism (e.g., guessing or random selection) takes place.

For convenience, random variables are often denoted by X, Y, or Z, or by

$$X_1, X_2, X_3, \ldots$$

For example, X could be used to represent the antinuclear antibody titer for a randomly selected patient.

A random variable is *discrete* if there are always gaps between possible values of the random variable. The random variable representing identification of the muscle-cell organelle is discrete, taking the values 1, 2, and 3 but no values between these numbers. A random variable is *continuous* if it can take any value between any two of its possible values (there are no gaps). The random variable representing plasma GH is continuous, since there are no impossible GH values between any two possible GH values.

4.2 DISTRIBUTIONS

The *distribution* of a random variable is a table, graph, or formula that gives the probabilities with which the random variable takes different values or ranges of values. The distribution of the organelle-identification random variable is given in Table 4.1. If a random variable is continuous, its distribution is described by its *frequency curve*, a curve used to find probabilities by calculating areas under the curve. Figure 4.1 shows the frequency curve for a random variable we will call X. Various probabilities obtained from this curve are also shown. From this

TABLE 4.1 DISTRIBUTION OF ORGANELLE-IDENTIFICATION RANDOM VARIABLE

Value	Probability of Value
1	1/3
2	1/3
3	1/3

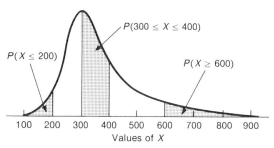

Figure 4.1 Frequency curve and various probabilities for X

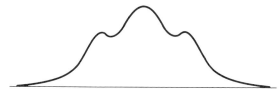

Figure 4.2 A symmetric distribution

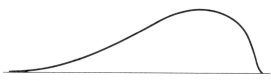

Figure 4.3 A negatively skewed distribution

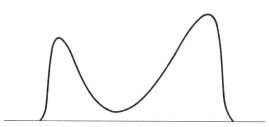

Figure 4.4 A distribution that is neither symmetric nor skewed

figure, we see that $P(300 \leq X \leq 400)$ is the area under the frequency curve between 300 and 400, $P(X \geq 600)$ is the area under the frequency curve above 600, and $P(X \leq 200)$ is the area under the frequency curve below 200.* Only the *area* under a frequency curve can be used to obtain probabilities. The height of the frequency curve cannot be used. The total area under a frequency curve is always 1, since the total area is the probability that the random variable takes any of its possible values.

The distributions of random variables, like frequency distributions, can be skewed, symmetric, or neither. Figure 4.2 shows the frequency curve for a symmetric distribution and Figure 4.3 shows the frequency curve for a distribution that is skewed to the left. Figure 4.4 shows a distribution that is neither symmetric nor skewed. A distribution with only one peak (like the distribution in Figure 4.3) is *unimodal*.

Most random variables have means, variances, and standard deviations. The mean of a random variable is a measure of central tendency for the random variable's possible values. The standard deviation and variance are measures of variability for the random variable's possible values. As you would

---

*The symbol " $\leq$ " means "is less than or equal to" and the symbol " $\geq$ " means "is greater than or equal to."

expect, the standard deviation of a random variable is simply the positive square root of its variance. The mean of a random variable is usually denoted by the Greek letter μ (mu, pronounced "mew"), the standard deviation by the Greek letter σ (sigma), and the variance by σ^2 (sigma squared).

Greek letters are also used to denote population means, standard deviations, and variances in order to distinguish them from the corresponding sample statistics. A *population mean* is denoted by μ, a *population standard deviation* by σ, and a *population variance* by σ^2. A *sample mean* is denoted by $\bar{x}$, a *sample standard deviation* by s, and a *sample variance* by s^2. Characteristics of a population or distribution, such as the mean and standard deviation of a population or random variable, are called *parameters*. Characteristics of a sample, such as the sample mean and sample standard deviation, are called *statistics*. The sample and population notation can be summarized as follows:

Characteristic	Population Parameter	Sample Statistic
Mean	μ	$\bar{x}$
Standard deviation	σ	s
Variance	σ^2	s^2

4.3 INDEPENDENCE

The concept of independence applies to random variables as well as events. Informally, two random variables X_1 and X_2 are *independent* if knowing the value of X_1 gives no information about the value of X_2, and vice versa. Suppose that we randomly select a patient from the Arthur A. Gletsky Memorial Hospital and measure his creatinine clearance. We then randomly select another patient from the Southern Northside Hospital and measure her creatinine clearance. When we do this, we obtain values for two independent random variables, Memorial creatinine clearance and Northside creatinine clearance. Knowing the Memorial creatinine clearance tells us nothing about the Northside creatinine clearance, and knowing the Northside creatinine clearance tells us nothing about the Memorial creatinine clearance.

Now suppose that we randomly select one patient and measure his creatinine clearance, and then measure his creatinine clearance again the next day. We obtain values for two random variables (day-1 creatinine clearance and day-2 creatinine clearance) that are *not* independent. Knowing a patient's creatinine clearance from the previous day usually gives us some idea of what his current creatinine clearance is. The day-1 creatinine clearance value provides information about the day-2 creatinine clearance value.

Formally, two random variables X_1 and X_2 are independent if

$$P(a \leq X_1 \leq b \quad \text{and} \quad c \leq X_2 \leq d)$$
$$= P(a \leq X_1 \leq b)P(c \leq X_2 \leq d)$$

for any numbers a, b, c, and d. This formal definition cannot be used in data analysis to determine whether independence holds. Instead, you must acquire a good grasp of the informal definition of independence and be able to use it to decide whether specific random variables are independent. This requires common sense and nonstatistical information as well as statistical understanding. If you are not sure whether particular random variables are independent, consult a statistician. You should never assume independence without very good reasons for doing so.

Why is it so important to be able to determine whether random variables are independent? As we will see in later chapters, many statistical procedures require *independent observations*. What does this mean? Suppose X_1 is the random variable representing the first observation collected (e.g., the plasma cortisol concentration for the first patient), X_2 is the random variable representing the second observation collected (e.g., the plasma cortisol concentration for the second patient), and so on, with X_n as the random variable representing the last observation collected (e.g., the plasma cortisol concentration for the last patient). Many statistical procedures require that $X_1, X_2, X_3, \ldots, X_n$ be independent: X_1 must be independent of $X_2, X_3, \ldots, X_n$; X_2 must be independent of $X_1, X_3, X_4, \ldots, X_n$; and so on.

This *assumption of independent observations* is one of the most frequently violated assumptions in medical and health care research. The consequences of ignoring violations of independence are not trivial. If statistical procedures requiring independent observations are applied to observations that are not independent, the results can be dangerously misleading.

Example 4.1

A study evaluated the use of a trace element supplement for low-birthweight preterm infants.[1] Table 4.2 shows the urine excretion of zinc at two time periods for five premature infants receiving the trace

TABLE 4.2   URINE ZINC EXCRETION (μg/day) FOR PREMATURE INFANTS

Infant No.	Time 1	Time 2
1	21	38
2	857	696
3	109	94
4	208	321
5	80	62

element supplement. Are these observations independent? The two zinc excretion measurements for any particular infant are not independent, since they were both obtained for the same infant. A glance at the data should convince you that knowing an infant's zinc excretion at one time gives you some idea of what her zinc excretion will be at the other time. An infant's zinc excretion at one time cannot be predicted perfectly from her zinc excretion at the other time, but approximate predictions can be made.

The observations for different infants are independent. The zinc excretion measurements for one infant tell us nothing about the zinc excretion measurements for any other infant. Since some of the observations are not independent, statistical procedures that require independence of all the observations cannot be used to analyze these data.

Example 4.2

Suppose one of your patients has six young children, whom he has refused to vaccinate against measles. If X_i is the random variable that equals 1 if the ith child develops measles within the next six months and equals 0 otherwise, are the random variables $X_1, X_2, X_3, \ldots, X_6$ independent? The answer is no. If one of the children has measles ($X_i = 1$ for some i), you can be fairly sure that at least some of the other children will also develop measles.

Example 4.3

The bronchodilating effect of nifedipine was evaluated in a double-blind, randomized study.[2] Table 4.3 shows the forced expiratory volume in one second (FEV_1) for 10 asthmatic subjects after administration of nifedipine, albuterol, or a placebo. Are these observations independent? The three FEV_1 values for any given subject are not independent, since they were all obtained for the same subject. Knowing a subject's FEV_1 after one drug gives us some idea of what her FEV_1 will be after another drug. *In general, repeated measurements of some quantity taken on the same subject are not independent.* The FEV_1 values for different subjects, how-

TABLE 4.4 AGE OF TRANSPLANT RECIPIENTS

Subject No.	Age (years)
1	47
2	56
3	52
4	57
5	51
6	39
7	58
8	32

ever, are independent. Statistical procedures that require independence of all the observations cannot be used to analyze these data.

Example 4.4

A study investigated a noninvasive method for early detection of graft rejection in heart transplant recipients.[3] Table 4.4 shows the ages of eight heart transplant recipients in which rejection occurred. Are these observations independent? Since the age of one transplant recipient tells us nothing about the age of another transplant recipient, the data are independent.

Example 4.5

Suppose a veterinarian evaluated the effect of a new anesthetic on feline heart rates by anesthetizing each of two cats 10 times and recording the heart rates when the cats were completely anesthetized. Are the resulting 20 observations independent? Since repeated measurements were obtained for the cats, not all of the observations are independent. Although heart rates from different cats are independent, heart rates from the same cat are not independent. Furthermore, 20 observations based on two cats are not equivalent to 20 observations obtained by anesthetizing each of 20 cats once. There is a much higher chance of getting two cats that respond abnormally to the anesthetic than there is of getting 20 cats that respond abnormally.

Suppose that 30% of cats consistently exhibit bradycardia when anesthetized with this drug. If two cats are randomly selected to be anesthetized, their responses to the anesthetic will be independent. By formula (3.10), the probability that both of them show bradycardia is

$P($Both cats show bradycardia$)$

$\quad = P($Cat 1 shows bradycardia and cat 2

$\qquad$ shows bradycardia$)$

$\quad = P($Cat 1 shows bradycardia$)$

$\qquad \times P($Cat 2 shows bradycardia$)$

$\quad = (0.30)(0.30) = 0.09$

TABLE 4.3 FEV₁ (l) AFTER ADMINISTRATION OF NIFEDIPINE, ALBUTEROL, OR PLACEBO

Patient No.	Nifedipine	Albuterol	Placebo
1	2.90	2.33	2.18
2	2.13	1.70	2.29
3	3.15	3.32	3.18
4	2.76	3.08	2.61
5	1.15	0.86	0.91
6	2.93	2.12	2.59
7	3.83	3.67	3.79
8	3.33	3.06	3.17
9	2.18	2.47	2.21
10	1.77	1.69	2.44

The chance that both cats will exhibit bradycardia is nearly one in 10.

If 20 cats are randomly selected, the probability that all 20 exhibit bradycardia is much smaller. Since the response of any cat is independent of the responses of the other cats, we can use formula (3.11) to obtain the probability

P(All 20 cats show bradycardia)

$\qquad = P$(Cat 1 shows bradycardia)

$\qquad\qquad \times P$(Cat 2 shows bradycardia) $\times$

$\qquad\qquad \cdots \times P$(Cat 20 shows bradycardia)

$\qquad = 0.30^{20} = 0.00000000003$

It is much easier to get misleading results with two subjects than with 20 subjects. Calculations like this should make clear the importance of obtaining a large enough sample of subjects. When used intelligently, designs with repeated measurements can be quite informative (see Chapter 9), but they cannot compensate for an inadequate sample size.

4.4 NORMAL DISTRIBUTIONS

Many random variables of interest in medicine and health care have distributions similar to *normal distributions*. Normal distributions are continuous distributions with bell-shaped frequency curves given by specific mathematical formulas. The formulas for normal frequency curves will not be described here. Instead, we will use some of the probabilities that can be obtained from normal frequency curves.

Let us first consider the *standard normal distribution*, which is the normal distribution that has a mean equal to 0 and a standard deviation equal to 1. The frequency curve for this distribution, shown in Figure 4.5, may look familiar to you as a "bell-shaped curve."

If a random variable Z has a standard normal distribution, almost any probability of interest can be calculated from areas under the standard normal frequency curve. We will limit ourselves to *tail probabilities*, which are probabilities calculated from areas in the tails of a distribution. *Upper-tail probabilities* are calculated from areas in the upper (right) tail of a distribution. *Lower-tail probabilities* are calculated from areas in the lower (left) tail of a

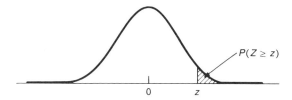

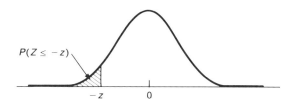

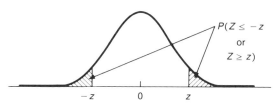

Figure 4.6 Standard normal tail probability areas

distribution. *Two-tailed probabilities* are calculated from areas in both tails of a distribution. Tail probabilities for standard normal distributions have the following forms.

Upper-tail probabilities: $P(Z \geq z)$
Lower-tail probabilities: $P(Z \leq -z)$
Two-tailed probabilities: $P(Z \leq -z \text{ or } Z \geq z)$

The letter z represents any positive number. In Figure 4.6, the areas under the standard normal frequency curve corresponding to tail probabilities are shown. Tail probabilities from several distributions will be needed to carry out statistical tests discussed in later chapters.

We do not have to calculate areas under the standard normal frequency curve to find standard normal tail probabilities. Instead, we can use Table E.2 in Appendix E. The column labeled "z" in this table lists some of the numbers used in standard normal probability statements. The column labeled

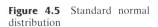

Figure 4.5 Standard normal distribution

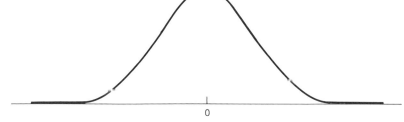

"Upper-tail prob." lists upper-tail probabilities, and the column labeled "Two-tailed prob." lists two-tailed probabilities. For example, if you want to find $P(Z \geq 1.20)$, where Z has a standard normal distribution, you first look up 1.20 in the z column. Since $P(Z \geq 1.20)$ is an upper-tail probability, you then go to the column for upper-tail probabilities. The number given in this column and in the row for the z value of 1.20 is the probability that $Z \geq 1.20$: $P(Z \geq 1.20) = 0.1151$.

Although there is no column for lower-tail probabilities, we can use the column for upper-tail probabilities to find lower-tail probabilities. Because the normal distribution is symmetric, $P(Z \leq -z) = P(Z \geq z)$. (Examine Figure 4.6 to convince yourself that this is true.) To find $P(Z \leq -0.83)$, for example, you first remember that $P(Z \leq -0.83) = P(Z \geq 0.83)$, and look up 0.83 in the z column. You then look up the probability in the upper-tail probability column to get $P(Z \leq -0.83) = 0.2033$.

Example 4.6

If Z has a standard normal distribution, what are the following probabilities?

1. $P(Z \geq 3.55)$. Using the column for upper-tail probabilities, we get 0.0002.

2. $P(Z \leq -1.11)$. Remembering that $P(Z \leq -1.11) = P(Z \geq 1.11)$ and using the column for upper-tail probabilities, we get 0.1335.

3. $P(Z \leq -1.63$ or $Z \geq 1.63)$. Using the column for two-tailed probabilities, we get 0.1031.

4. $P(Z \geq 4.71)$. The number 4.71 is not listed in the z column, since the highest z value given is 3.80. From the column for upper-tail probabilities, we get $P(Z \geq 3.80) = 0.0001$. Because 4.71 is farther out in the tail than 3.80, the area under the frequency curve above 4.71 must be less than the area above 3.80 (see Figure 4.7). Thus, we know that $P(Z \geq 4.71) < 0.0001$,* but we cannot get a more exact probability from this table. An exact probability could be obtained from a computer or a more extensive table.

5. $P(Z \geq 3.33)$. Since 3.33 is not listed in the z column, we use the closest z value, 3.35, to get an approximate probability from the column for upper-tail probabilities: $P(Z \geq 3.33) \cong P(Z \geq 3.35) = 0.0004$.†

Most normal distributions encountered in practice are *nonstandard normal distributions*, normal distributions with means other than 0 or standard deviations other than 1. Although nonstandard normal distributions, like the standard normal distribu-

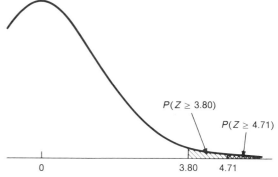

Figure 4.7 Comparison of $P(Z \geq 4.71)$ and $P(Z \geq 3.80)$

tion, are symmetric with one peak, their shapes differ when their standard deviations differ. The larger the standard deviation, the more spread out and less peaked the normal distribution. This is illustrated in Figure 4.8. Normal distributions with the same standard deviation but different means have the same shape but different locations. This is illustrated in Figure 4.9.

Because many statistical procedures require data from normal or approximately normal populations, it is important to be able to determine whether normality is a reasonable assumption for a data set. In Chapter 5, we will discuss the use of sample histograms for this purpose. It is often possible to see that data are nonnormal without examining a histogram. If your population values are discrete, you should immediately realize that the population is not exactly normal, since normal distributions are continuous. White blood cell counts cannot be exactly normally distributed, since they take only integer values. Because white blood cell counts have a wide range of values, their distribution might be *approximately* normal if it is symmetric and unimodal. Discrete data with only a few possible values cannot be even approximately normally distributed. In many cases, common sense will tell you that data do not come from a normal population.

The *medical* normality or abnormality of data *cannot* be used to distinguish between normal and nonnormal distributions. We cannot conclude that a random variable has a nonnormal distribution because it involves medically abnormal patients. *Statistical* normality refers only to a specific type of distribution and has nothing to do with medical normality. Thyroxine values for hyperthyroid patients are medically abnormal, but they might have a nearly normal distribution in the statistical sense. Thyroxine values for euthyroid patients are medically normal, but might have a statistically nonnormal distribution. *When we say that a random variable is normally distributed, we mean only that probabilities involving this random variable can be calculated from a normal frequency curve.* Statistical normality does *not* imply that the values of the random variable are medically normal.

---

*The symbol " < " means "is less than." The symbol " > ," which we will use in the next chapter, means "is greater than."

†The symbol " $\cong$ " means "is approximately equal to."

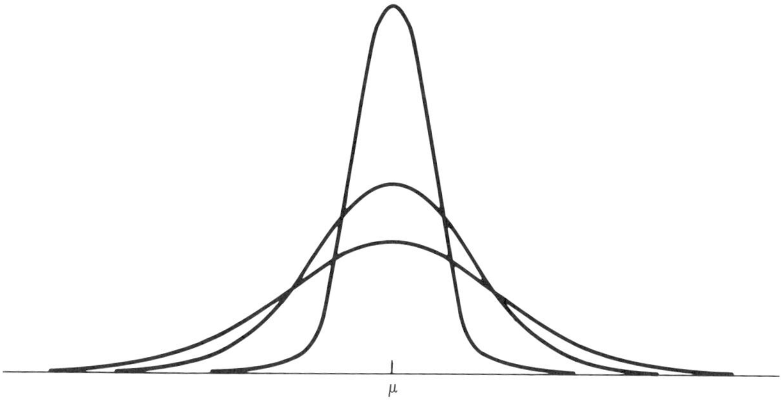

Figure 4.8 Normal distributions with the same mean but different standard deviations

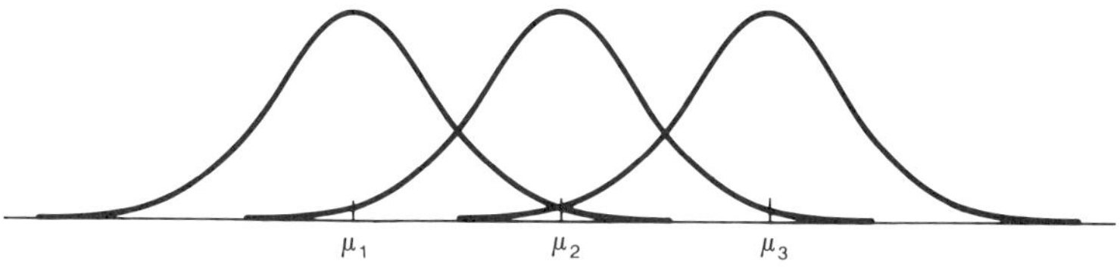

Figure 4.9 Normal distributions with the same standard deviation but different means

Example 4.7

In a study of pain management during hospice home care, the following scale was used to rate pain intensity.[4]

1 = none
2 = mild
3 = discomforting
4 = distressing
5 = horrible
6 = excruciating

Let X be the random variable representing the pain-intensity rating. Could X have a normal distribution? Since X takes only the values 1, 2, 3, 4, 5, and 6, it is discrete and has only a few possible values. X is not even approximately normally distributed.

Example 4.8

A study evaluated the effectiveness of respiratory teaching programs for patients with chronic obstructive pulmonary disease.[5] In this study, values were obtained for the following random variables:

X_1 = health status on discharge (1 = self-care, 2 = partially dependent, 3 = totally dependent)

X_2 = mental health on discharge (1 = alert, 2 = occasionally alert, 3 = confused, 4 = disoriented)

X_3 = reason for readmission (0 = no readmission, 1 = chronic obstructive pulmonary disease, 2 = alcoholism, 3 = other)

Could any of these random variables have a normal distribution? Since all three random variables are discrete and have only a few possible values, none of them has a normal distribution.

Example 4.9

An experienced surgeon is to perform a hypophysectomy on a patient with Cushing's disease. Let X equal 1 if the patient survives the surgery and 0 otherwise. Could X have a normal distribution? Since X has only two possible values, 0 and 1, it is not even approximately normally distributed.

4.5 BINOMIAL DISTRIBUTIONS

Example 4.9 concerns a random variable that takes only two possible values. Such random variables are common in medicine and health care: a patient either survives brain surgery or does not; a woman is either pregnant or not pregnant; an accident victim either has a fractured skull or does not.

Medical and health care research often involves a sequence of such random variables. Suppose we randomly select five patients with hepatic failure. Then each patient either recovers or dies. If we let X_i have the value 1 if the ith patient recovers and 0 if the ith patient dies, we have five random variables: X_1, X_2, X_3, X_4, and X_5. These random variables are independent. Since the patients were selected randomly, the death or recovery of one patient tells us nothing about the death or recovery of another patient. Random selection also ensures that the probability of getting a patient who will recover is the same for the first, second, third, fourth, and fifth selections. This probability is equal to the population proportion of patients with hepatic failure who recover. Let us assume this proportion is 0.3.

We would like to calculate such probabilities as P(All five patients recover) and P(One patient recovers or no patients recover). Since the number of patients who recover is the sum of all the X_i's, we need to know the distribution of this sum in order to obtain these probabilities. If we let Y equal the sum of the X_i's, then we want to find the probabilities

$$P(\text{All five patients recover}) = P(Y = 5)$$

$$P(\text{One patient recovers or no patients recover})$$
$$= P(Y \leq 1)$$

It can be shown (although we will not do so) that Y has a distribution called the binomial distribution with parameters $n = 5$ and $p = 0.3$. The parameters of a binomial distribution are simply characteristics of the distribution that distinguish it from other binomial distributions.

In general, a random variable Y has a *binomial distribution with parameters n and p* if Y is the sum of n random variables $X_1, X_2, X_3, \ldots, X_n$ such that all of the following conditions hold.

Each X_i takes only the values 0 and 1 (4.1)

All of the X_i's are independent (4.2)

The probability that X_i equals 1 is the same for all of the X_i's, and this (4.3)
probability is equal to p

The parameter n is the number of X_i's, and p is the probability that X_i is equal to 1. Just as there are infinitely many normal distributions, with different means and standard deviations, there are infinitely many binomial distributions, with different parameters n and p.

If a random variable Y has a binomial distribution, Table E.3 in Appendix E can be used to find probabilities concerning Y when the parameters n and p are in the table. If Y is the number of patients out of five who recover from hepatic failure, we can use Table E.3 to find $P(Y = 5)$ as follows. Since n is 5, we first find the block of numbers corresponding to $n = 5$ in the table. (The n values are listed in the first column.) We then find our p of 0.3 in the first row of the table, which lists values of p. The probabilities for our random variable Y are those in the block of numbers for $n = 5$ and in the column for $p = 0.3$. The second column, headed by k, tells us what probabilities are listed. All of the probabilities in Table E.3 have the form $P(Y = k)$. To find $P(Y = 5)$ for our patients with hepatic failure, we look in the row for $k = 5$ (in the block for $n = 5$) and in the column for $p = 0.3$ to

get 0.0024. The probability that all five patients recover is very small.

How do we find $P(Y \leq 1)$ using Table E.3? Although this probability is not given directly in the table, we can calculate it by adding appropriate probabilities in the table. The random variable Y takes only integer values, so the event "$Y \leq 1$" is the same as the event "$Y = 0$ or $Y = 1$." The events "$Y = 0$" and "$Y = 1$" are disjoint, since we cannot simultaneously have no patients recover and exactly one patient recover. By formula (3.6),

$$P(Y \leq 1) = P(Y = 0 \text{ or } Y = 1)$$
$$= P(Y = 0) + P(Y = 1)$$

Looking in the rows for $k = 0$ and $k = 1$ (in the block for $n = 5$) and in the column for $p = 0.3$, we get $P(Y = 0) = 0.1681$ and $P(Y = 1) = 0.3601$. Thus,

$$P(Y \leq 1) = 0.1681 + 0.3601 = 0.5282$$

The chance that one patient recovers or no patient recovers is slightly greater than 50%.

Since binomial distributions concern counts (the number of times something happens), the number k in Table E.3 is always an integer.* For the same reason, k is always nonnegative and less than or equal to n. You cannot remove kidney stones from 5.7 patients, nor can you detect signs of drug toxicity in -31 patients. You also cannot diagnose congestive heart failure in 15 patients if you have examined only 12 patients, so k cannot be greater than n. If k is not an integer, or k is negative, or k is larger than n, no table is needed to find $P(Y = k)$ when Y has a binomial distribution. In all of these cases, $P(Y = k) = 0$.

Example 4.10

Suppose the proportion of patients with spinal cord injury (SCI) who develop severe pressure sores after discharge is 0.15, and six randomly selected patients with SCI are discharged. If the number of SCI patients who develop severe pressure sores has a binomial distribution, what is the probability that at least one of the six patients will develop severe pressure sores? The parameters of this binomial distribution are $n = 6$ (since there are six patients) and $p = 0.15$ (since the probability of severe pressure sores is 0.15).

Let Y be the number of patients who develop severe pressure sores. We can use Table E.3 to find $P(Y \geq 1)$. There are two ways to calculate this probability, a long way and a short way. If we do it the long way, we proceed as follows. Since Y takes only integer values up to 6, the event "$Y \geq 1$" is the

_____

Integers are the numbers $0, 1, 2, \ldots$ and $-1, -2, -3, \ldots$.

same as the event "$Y = 1$ or $Y = 2$ or $Y = 3$ or $Y = 4$ or $Y = 5$ or $Y = 6$." The events "$Y = 1$," "$Y = 2$," "$Y = 3$," "$Y = 4$," "$Y = 5$," and "$Y = 6$" are pairwise disjoint. The number of patients who develop pressure sores cannot be both 1 and 2 at the same time, or both 1 and 3 at the same time, and so on. We can apply formula (3.7) to get

$$P(Y \geq 1) = P(Y = 1 \text{ or } Y = 2 \text{ or } Y = 3 \text{ or } Y = 4$$
$$\text{or } Y = 5 \text{ or } Y = 6)$$
$$= P(Y = 1) + P(Y = 2) + P(Y = 3)$$
$$+ P(Y = 4) + P(Y = 5) + P(Y = 6)$$

Thus, we can find $P(Y = 1)$, $P(Y = 2)$, $P(Y = 3)$, $P(Y = 4)$, $P(Y = 5)$, and $P(Y = 6)$ in Table E.3 and add them to obtain $P(Y \geq 1)$. Looking in the $n = 6$ block and in the $p = 0.15$ column, we get

$$P(Y \geq 1) = 0.3994 + 0.1762 + 0.0414 + 0.0055$$
$$+ 0.0004 + 0.0000$$
$$= 0.6229$$

The short way of finding $P(Y \geq 1)$ can be used if we realize that the events "$Y = 0$" and "$Y \geq 1$" are opposite events. Applying formula (3.8), we get

$$P(Y \geq 1) = 1 - P(Y = 0)$$

If we calculate $P(Y \geq 1)$ in this way, we need to look up only one probability, $P(Y = 0)$. Using Table E.3, we get

$$P(Y \geq 1) = 1 - 0.3771 = 0.6229$$

The probability that at least one SCI patient will develop severe pressure sores is fairly high.

Example 4.11

Suppose the probability of sexual dysfunction after recovery from severe head trauma is 0.80, and nine randomly selected patients with severe head trauma are discharged. If the number of patients who experience sexual dysfunction has a binomial distribution, what is the probability that eight or nine patients will experience sexual dysfunction?

Let Y be the number of patients with sexual dysfunction. Then Y has a binomial distribution with parameters $n = 9$ and $p = 0.8$. Although $n = 9$ is listed in Table E.3, $p = 0.8$ is not listed. No p greater than 0.5 is listed in this table. We can still use Table E.3 if we restate the problem in terms of the number of patients who do *not* experience sexual dysfunction. By formula (3.8), the probability that a patient does *not* experience sexual dysfunction is

$$P(\text{No sexual dysfunction})$$
$$= 1 - P(\text{Sexual dysfunction})$$
$$= 1 - 0.8 = 0.2$$

Table E.3 does list $p = 0.2$. We now need to realize that the event "eight or nine patients with sexual dysfunction" is the same as the event "one patient without sexual dysfunction or no patients without sexual dysfunction." Thus,

$$P(\text{Eight or nine patients with sexual dysfunction})$$
$$= P(\text{One patient without sexual dysfunction or}$$
$$\text{no patients without sexual dysfunction})$$

If X is the number of patients *without* sexual dysfunction, X has a binomial distribution with parameters $n = 9$ and $p = 0.2$. We want to find $P(X = 1$ or $X = 0)$. The events "$X = 1$" and "$X = 0$" are disjoint, since the number of patients without sexual dysfunction cannot be both 1 and 0. By formula (3.6),

$$P(X = 1 \text{ or } X = 0) = P(X = 1) + P(X = 0)$$

From Table E.3, looking under $n = 9$ and $p = 0.2$, we get

$$P(X = 1 \text{ or } X = 0) = 0.3020 + 0.1342 = 0.4362$$

The probability that eight or nine patients will experience sexual dysfunction is 0.4362.

What if you want a binomial probability involving parameters that are not in Table E.3, and you cannot resolve the problem as we did in Example 4.11? You have several options. You can find a more complete table, use a computer, or consult a statistician. You can also calculate the probability yourself, using a probability formula for binomial distributions. This formula and information about its use can be found in other texts.[6]

Example 4.12

A physician plans to randomly select 11 male patients with blastomycosis and record the changes in the serum testosterone concentration after administering ketoconazole. If Y is the total testosterone change (the sum of the 11 testosterone changes), does Y have a binomial distribution?

It is clear that Y is the sum of 11 random variables. If X_i is the testosterone change for the ith patient, Y is the sum of $X_1, X_2, X_3, \ldots,$ and X_{11}. Since the patients were randomly selected, the X_i's are independent. Knowing the testosterone change for one patient tells us nothing about the testosterone change for another patient. But the zero-one condition (4.1) does not hold. Each X_i can take values other than 0 or 1, and Y does not have a binomial distribution.

It is not necessary to check conditions (4.1) through (4.3) if Y can have noninteger values. This fact alone implies that Y does not have a binomial distribution, since binomially distributed random variables can take only integer values.

Example 4.13

A randomly selected patient at Saint Oscar Hospital will be asked on five successive days whether she is satisfied with the nursing care provided. Let X_i equal 1 if she says she is satisfied on the ith day and 0 otherwise. If Y is the sum of the five X_i's, Y is the random variable representing the number of days the patient reports being satisfied. Does Y have a binomial distribution?

Even though Y is the sum of five random variables that can take only the values 0 and 1, the independence of these random variables is highly suspect. If you know, for example, that the patient was satisfied on the first three days, you expect her to be satisfied on the fourth and fifth days. The independence condition (4.2) does not appear to hold, and it is not reasonable to assume that Y has a binomial distribution.

Example 4.14

Four surgeons at a hospital have certain probabilities of performing various surgical procedures without any complications. These probabilities are shown in Table 4.5. On a busy afternoon, each surgical procedure is to be done by the surgeon indicated in Table 4.5. If Y is the number of surgical procedures performed without complications, does Y have a binomial distribution?

To answer this, we need to examine Y more closely. Certainly Y is the sum of four random variables that can take only the values 0 and 1. Let X_1 equal 1 if there are no TURP complications and 0 otherwise. Let X_2 equal 1 if there are no mastectomy complications and 0 otherwise. Let X_3 equal 1 if there are no cruciate-repair complications and 0 otherwise. Let X_4 equal 1 if there are no valve-replacement complications and 0 otherwise. Then Y is the sum of these X_i's.

Since each surgery is performed by a different surgeon on a different patient, we expect the X_i's to be independent. Knowing whether there will be complications for one surgery should not tell us anything about whether there will be complications for another surgery. We can reasonably assume that the zero-one condition (4.1) and the independence condition (4.2) hold. But the same-probability condition (4.3) does not hold, since the X_i's do not

have the same probability of being equal to 1. For X_1, this probability is 0.97; for X_2, it is 0.80; for X_3, it is 0.88; and for X_4, it is 0.71. Y does not have a binomial distribution.

Example 4.15

Suppose the proportion of patients with myocardial infarction (MI) who are anxious and depressed after recovery is 0.71. If 15 MI patients are randomly selected, and Y is the number of patients who are anxious and depressed after recovery, does Y have a binomial distribution?

Let X_i equal 1 if the ith patient is anxious and depressed and 0 otherwise. Then Y is the sum of the X_i's, so the zero-one condition (4.1) holds. Since the patients were randomly selected, the X_i's are independent and the independence condition (4.2) holds. Knowing whether one patient will be anxious and depressed tells us nothing about whether another patient will be anxious and depressed. Random selection also ensures that the probability of getting a patient who will be anxious and depressed is the same for the first, second, third, ..., and 15th selections, so the same-probability condition (4.3) holds. Y has a binomial distribution with parameters $n = 15$ and $p = 0.71$.

Binomial distributions and normal distributions are only two of infinitely many types of distributions. Random variables of interest in medicine and health care often have entirely different distributions. Probabilities for such distributions cannot be calculated from binomial or normal tables. We will describe some of these distributions in later chapters, but our coverage of distributions is limited primarily to those needed to carry out statistical tests. The reader with a strong interest in distributions should consult a textbook on probability theory.[*]

SUMMARY

Most statistical methods involve the use of random variables, which are potential quantities whose values are determined by some chance-governed mechanism. The distribution of a random variable is a table, graph, or formula that gives the probabilities with which the random variable takes different values or ranges of values. Random variables are independent if knowing the value of one random variable gives no information about the other random variables. The concept of independent random variables is extremely important because many statistical procedures require independent observations.

TABLE 4.5 PROBABILITIES OF NO COMPLICATIONS FOR VARIOUS SURGICAL PROCEDURES

Surgical Procedure	P(No complications)
Transurethral resection of prostate (TURP) (surgeon 1)	0.97
Mastectomy (surgeon 2)	0.80
Cruciate-ligament repair (surgeon 3)	0.88
Mitral-valve replacement (surgeon 4)	0.71

---

[*]Hoel et al.[7] present a concise introduction to probability theory, although their text requires calculus.

Normal distributions and binomial distributions are frequently encountered in medicine and health care. Many statistical procedures require normal or approximately normal populations. If data are discrete, with only a few possible values, the corresponding population cannot be even approximately normal. A random variable has a binomial distribution if it is the sum of independent random variables that take only the values 0 and 1 and have the same probability of being equal to 1. Many other types of distributions are also used in statistics.

PROBLEMS

1. A study evaluated at-home intravenous immunoglobulin replacement therapy by self-administration.[8] Table 4.6 shows the minimum and maximum IgG levels after at least six months of intravenous γ-globulin for five patients. Are these observations independent?

2. In a study of factors related to the development of postcardiotomy psychosis, patients undergoing open heart surgery were evaluated for psychosis by using a behavioral checklist.[9] The raters' scores for the item evaluating sleep are shown in Table 4.7 for 10 patients. Are these scores independent?

3. A study of aluminum-related bone disease in hemodialysis patients reported the total dialysate aluminum exposure values shown in Table 4.8.[10] Are these observations independent?

4. A clinical study evaluated the use of intra-aortic balloon pumping (IABP) for managing low

TABLE 4.6   MINIMUM AND MAXIMUM IgG LEVELS

Patient No.	Minimum IgG (mg/dl)	Maximum IgG (mg/dl)
1	783	1398
2	607	1518
3	733	1846
4	358	975
5	334	712

TABLE 4.7   RATERS' SCORES FOR SLEEP ITEM

Patient No.	Rater A	Rater B
1	4	3
2	2	3
3	3	2
4	3	3
5	3	3
6	2	3
7	4	3
8	4	3
9	2	2
10	3	3

TABLE 4.8   TOTAL DIALYSATE ALUMINUM EXPOSURE (g)

Patient No.	Exposure	Patient No.	Exposure
1	8.8	13	1.5
2	9.9	14	1.1
3	10.3	15	2.3
4	9.5	16	2.2
5	6.0	17	5.1
6	5.8	18	1.2
7	5.9	19	1.3
8	4.9	20	2.1
9	9.6	21	1.3
10	10.6	22	0
11	28.7	23	0.5
12	4.1	24	0.7

TABLE 4.9   DECREASE IN PEAK SYSTOLIC PRESSURE AND END-DIASTOLIC PRESSURE

Patient No.	Decrease in Peak Systolic Pressure (mm Hg)	Decrease in End-Diastolic Pressure (mm Hg)
1	6	14
2	1	4
3	3	5
4	3	5
5	5	13
6	3	11
7	2	4
8	3	11
9	2	4
10	3	6
11	4	7
12	5	5
13	2	4

cardiac output in pediatric patients.[11] Table 4.9 shows the decrease in peak systolic pressure and the decrease in end-diastolic pressure for 13 children who underwent IABP. Are these observations independent?

5. Assume that the random variable Z has a standard normal distribution. Use Table E.2 to find the following upper-tail probabilities. If an exact probability cannot be obtained from the table, estimate the probability as closely as you can.
   a. $P(Z \geq 0.45)$
   b. $P(Z \geq 2.59)$
   c. $P(Z \geq 3.98)$
   d. $P(Z \geq 2.67)$

6. Assume that the random variable Z has a standard normal distribution. Use Table E.2 to find the following lower-tail probabilities. If an exact probability cannot be obtained from the table, estimate the probability as closely as you can.
   a. $P(Z \leq -0.07)$
   b. $P(Z \leq -1.84)$
   c. $P(Z \leq -8.73)$
   d. $P(Z \leq -3.04)$

7. Assume that the random variable Z has a standard normal distribution. Use Table E.2 to find the following two-tailed probabilities. If an exact probability cannot be obtained from the table, estimate the probability as closely as you can.
  a. $P(Z \leq -0.21 \text{ or } Z \geq 0.21)$
  b. $P(Z \leq -2.00 \text{ or } Z \geq 2.00)$
  c. $P(Z \leq -2.81 \text{ or } Z \geq 2.81)$
  d. $P(Z \leq -4.72 \text{ or } Z \geq 4.72)$

8. In a study of the quality of life for cancer patients, values were obtained for the following random variables.[12]

X_1 = assistance in daily living (1 = yes, 0 = no)
X_2 = pain (1 = pain-free, 2 = occasional pain, 3 = frequent pain, 4 = persistent pain)
X_3 = quality of life (1 = worst, 2, 3, 4 = midpoint, 5, 6, 7 = best)

Could any of these random variables have a normal or approximately normal distribution?

9. In a study of the effect of cimetidine on gastric hemorrhage in dogs, values were obtained for the following random variables.[13]

X_1 = weight (kg)
X_2 = fecal hemoglobin concentration (mg/g)
X_3 = severity of gastric mucosal lesions (0 = no lesions, 1 = petechial hemorrhages, 2 = petechial to linear hemorrhages, 3 = linear to ecchymotic hemorrhages, 4 = suffusive hemorrhage)

Could any of these random variables have a normal or approximately normal distribution?

10. Suppose the probability of renal insufficiency after open heart surgery is 0.05. Eight patients undergoing open heart surgery are randomly selected, and the number of patients who develop renal insufficiency is recorded. Let Y be the random variable representing the number of patients who develop renal insufficiency. Does Y have a binomial distribution? If Y does not have a binomial distribution, indicate which of the conditions (4.1) through (4.3) fail to hold. If Y has a binomial distribution, specify the parameters n and p and use Table E.3 to find the following probabilities.
  a. $P(8 \text{ patients develop renal insufficiency})$
  b. $P(\text{No patients develop renal insufficiency})$
  c. $P(2 \text{ or fewer patients develop renal insufficiency})$

11. Suppose that the proportion of pregnant women who believe that breast self-examination (BSE) is an effective way to detect early breast cancer is 0.75. Twelve pregnant women are randomly selected for an interview about BSE. All of the women are brought together for the interview, and a nurse asks whether they believe that BSE is effective for the early detection of breast cancer. The women are encouraged to discuss this question with each other before answering it. Let Y be the random variable representing the number of women who believe that BSE is effective. Does Y have a binomial distribution? If Y does not have a binomial distribution, indicate which of the conditions (4.1) through (4.3) fail to hold. If Y has a binomial distribution, specify the parameters n and p and use Table E.3 to find the following probabilities.
  a. $P(12 \text{ women believe that BSE is effective})$
  b. $P(2 \text{ or more women believe that BSE is effective})$
  c. $P(7 \text{ or 8 women believe that BSE is effective})$

12. Suppose the probability of elevated aspartate aminotransferase (AST) levels is 0.95 for patients with infectious mononucleosis. The AST levels for seven randomly selected patients with infectious mononucleosis are to be obtained. Let Y be the random variable representing the sum of the AST values for all seven patients. Does Y have a binomial distribution? If Y does not have a binomial distribution, indicate which of the conditions (4.1) through (4.3) fail to hold. If Y has a binomial distribution, specify the parameters n and p and use Table E.3 to find the following probabilities.
  a. $P(Y \text{ is greater than 7000})$
  b. $P(Y \text{ is less than 500})$
  c. $P(Y \text{ is greater than 2000})$

13. Suppose the probability of a second stroke within two weeks is 0.10 for patients with cardioembolic stroke. Three patients with cardioembolic stroke are randomly selected and carefully monitored for evidence of a second stroke. Let Y be the random variable representing the number of patients who have a second stroke. Does Y have a binomial distribution? If Y does not have a binomial distribution, indicate which of the conditions (4.1) through (4.3) fail to hold. If Y has a binomial distribution, specify the parameters n and p and use Table E.3 to find the following probabilities.
  a. $P(3 \text{ patients have a second stroke})$
  b. $P(1 \text{ or 2 patients have a second stroke})$
  c. $P(\text{No patients have a second stroke})$

14. Suppose the probability of displacement is 0.15 for a silicone nasogastric tube and 0.05 for a polyvinyl nasogastric tube. Twenty patients with nasogastric tubes are randomly selected and watched for tube displacement. Nine of these patients have the silicone tube and 11 have the polyvinyl tube. Let Y be the random variable representing the number of patients with tube displacement. Does Y have a binomial distribution? If Y does not have a binomial distribution, indicate which of the conditions (4.1) through (4.3) fail to hold. If Y has a binomial distribution, specify the parameters n and p and use Table E.3 to find the following probabilities.

    a. P(1 or more patients have tube displacement)

    b. P(10 patients have tube displacement)

    c. P(1 or 2 patients have tube displacement)

15. Suppose the probability that a cat will object violently to vaccination is 0.05. Fifteen cats scheduled for routine vaccination are randomly selected and placed in wire cages in an examination room. Each cat is vaccinated in the presence of the other cats, and the cat's reaction to vaccination is observed. Let Y be the random variable representing the number of cats who react violently to vaccination. Does Y have a binomial distribution? If Y does not have a binomial distribution, indicate which of the conditions (4.1) through (4.3) fail to hold. If Y has a binomial distribution, specify the parameters n and p and use Table E.3 to find the following probabilities.

    a. P(1, 2, or 3 cats react violently)

    b. P(1 cat reacts violently)

    c. P(More than 3 cats react violently)

16. Suppose the probability of anticipatory nausea before chemotherapy is 0.30 for cancer patients undergoing chemotherapy. Nine cancer patients are randomly selected and asked about nausea before chemotherapy. Let Y be the random variable representing the number of patients who report anticipatory nausea. Does Y have a binomial distribution? If Y does not have a binomial distribution, indicate which of the conditions (4.1) through (4.3) fail to hold. If Y has a binomial distribution, specify the parameters n and p and use Table E.3 to find the following probabilities.

    a. P(No patients report anticipatory nausea)

    b. P(2, 3, or 4 patients report anticipatory nausea)

    c. P(3 or more patients report anticipatory nausea)

REFERENCES

1. Friel JK, Penney S, Reid DW, et al: Zinc, copper, manganese, and iron balance of parenterally fed very low birth weight preterm infants receiving a trace element supplement. J Paren Enter Nutr 12:382–386, 1988.
2. Schwartzstein RS, Fanta CH: Orally administered nifedipine in chronic stable asthma. Comparison with an orally administered sympathomimetic. Am Rev Respir Dis 134:262–265, 1986.
3. Zbilut JP, Murdock DK, Lawson L, et al: Use of power spectral analysis of respiratory sinus arrhythmia to detect graft rejection. J Heart Transplant 7:280–288, 1988.
4. Austin C, Cody CP, Eyres PJ, et al: Hospice home care pain management. Four critical variables. Canc Nurs 9:58–65, 1986.
5. Howard JE, Davies JL, Roghmann KJ: Respiratory teaching of patients: How effective is it? J Adv Nurs 12:207–214, 1987.
6. Huntsberger DV, Billingsley P: Elements of Statistical Inference. 6th ed. Boston: Allyn & Bacon, 1987.
7. Hoel PG, Port SC, Stone CJ: Introduction to Probability Theory. Boston: Houghton Mifflin, 1971.
8. Ashida ER, Saxon A: Home intravenous immunoglobulin therapy by self-administration. J Clin Immunol 6:306–309, 1986.
9. Quinless FW, Cassese M, Atherton N: The effect of selected preoperative, intraoperative, and postoperative variables on the development of postcardiotomy psychosis in patients undergoing open heart surgery. Heart Lung 14:334–341, 1985.
10. O Connor M, Garrett P, Dockery M, et al: Aluminum-related bone disease. Correlation between symptoms, osteoid volume, and aluminum staining. Am J Clin Pathol 86:168–174, 1986.
11. Webster H, Veasy LG: Intra-aortic balloon pumping in children. Heart Lung 14:548–555, 1985.
12. Morris JN, Sherwood S: Quality of life of cancer patients at different stages in the disease trajectory. J Chron Dis 40:545–553, 1987.
13. Boulay JP, Lipowitz AJ, Klausner JS: Effect of cimetidine on aspirin-induced gastric hemorrhage in dogs. Am J Vet Res 47:1744–1746, 1986.

5

SAMPLES AND SAMPLING DISTRIBUTIONS

CHAPTER OBJECTIVES

After studying this chapter and working the problems, you should be able to:

1. Obtain random samples by using a random number table

2. Randomize subjects by using a random number table

3. Explain the concepts of sampling distributions and statistical inference

4. Explain why the central limit theorem is important

5. Determine whether sample histograms are consistent with normal or approximately normal populations

We have referred repeatedly to random sampling, using only an informal definition. We now need to define random sampling more precisely and describe a practical method for selecting random samples. We will also describe a method for randomly assigning subjects to different treatment groups. In addition, we will discuss sampling distributions and the central limit theorem. Because sampling distributions are the basis for statistical inference, they are the most important topic in this chapter.

5.1 RANDOM SAMPLES

Recall that the purpose of statistical inference is to use a sample to reach conclusions about a population. If you want to know the population mean μ, you estimate μ with the sample mean $\bar{x}$. This sort of inference works best if you have a *probability sam-*

ple, a sample obtained in a way that ensures that every member of the population has a known, nonzero probability of being included in the sample. The most important type of probability sample for our purposes is the *simple random sample*, hereinafter referred to as the random sample. A random sample is obtained in a way that ensures the following.

1. Every member of the population has the same probability of being included in the sample.
2. Different members of the population are selected independently (that is, selection of one member has no effect on selection of another member).

Taking every fifth name from a list of patients will *not* produce a random sample. If we know that the fifth patient was selected, we know that the fourth patient was not selected, so members of the population were not selected independently. Samples obtained by taking every kth name in a list are called *systematic samples*.

Sometimes a population is divided into groups called *strata* and random samples are taken from these strata and combined to get a *stratified random sample*. This is often done when the researcher wants to be sure that she will have specified numbers of subjects from each stratum. A population of patients with squamous cell carcinoma could be divided into four strata: females with metastases, females without metastases, males with metastases, and males without metastases. If we want 50 patients from each stratum, we randomly select 50 patients from each stratum to get a stratified random sample of 200 patients.*

Selecting a random sample requires a listing of the population of interest. When such a list is available, we can use a *random number table* to obtain a random sample. A random number table is a table of numbers constructed by a process that ensures that both of the following hold.

1. In any position in the table, each of the numbers 0 through 9 has probability 1/10 of occurring.
2. The occurrence of any number in one part of the table is independent of the occurrence of any number in any other part of the table (knowing the numbers in one part of the table tells us nothing about the numbers in another part of the table).

Table E.1 in Appendix E is a random number table. The use of such a table to select a random sample can best be understood by studying an example.

Example 5.1

Suppose our population consists of the 21 patients in Table 5.1, and we want to obtain a random sample of 10 of them. We will first assign four consecutive, two-digit numbers to each patient, as shown in Table 5.1. We then go to Table E.1 and haphazardly select a page of the table and a starting point on the page (e.g., by tossing a paper clip onto the page). The starting point should be chosen in this way in order to avoid bias. If you want the patient E. Beasley in your sample and you deliberately look for a starting point, you may subconsciously choose a starting point that includes one of her numbers, 00–03.

Let us start with the second page of Table E.1, in the sixth column and the ninth row of digits. Beginning here, we can go up, down, or across. Let us arbitrarily decide to go across to the right. Reading the first two digits, we get 47. Since 47 was assigned to C. Pflugel, he is the first member of our sample. The next two digits, going across to the right, give us 45, which also belongs to C. Pflugel, so this number is thrown out. Moving across to the next pair of

*Information about this type of sampling and other sampling methods can be found in other texts.[1]

TABLE 5.1   POPULATION OF PATIENTS AND THEIR ASSIGNED NUMBERS

Patient	Assigned Numbers	Patient	Assigned Numbers
E. Beasley	00–03	C. Pflugel	44–47
P. McGirt	04–07	F. Junkroski	48–51
T. Dreeze	08–11	J. Mudge	52–55
S. Tootooian	12–15	S. Ribstein	56–59
B. Osnoss	16–19	A. Volgi	60–63
C. Crater	20–23	J. Unfried	64–67
E. Scheib	24–27	L. Nazey	68–71
W. Wenckus	28–31	H. Kwartowski	72–75
G. Hoogenboom	32–35	L. Glunz	76–79
M. Eidlhuber	36–39	T. Leeth	80–83
T. Zych	40–43		

TABLE 5.2   SELECTED RANDOM NUMBERS AND RESULTING RANDOM SAMPLE

Random Number	Sampled Patient
47	C. Pflugel
45	None (45 selects C. Pflugel again)
49	F. Junkroski
86	None (no patient has number 86)
38	M. Eidlhuber
15	S. Tootooian
18	B. Osnoss
98	None (no patient has number 98)
73	H. Kwartowski
45	None (45 selects C. Pflugel again)
80	T. Leeth
50	None (50 selects F. Junkroski again)
93	None (no patient has number 93)
33	G. Hoogenboom
92	None (no patient has number 92)
50	None (50 selects F. Junkroski again)
86	None (no patient has number 86)
61	A. Volgi
76	L. Glunz

digits, we get 49, which belongs to F. Junkroski, who becomes the second member of our sample. We continue in this fashion until we obtain 10 patients. The digits obtained, and the resulting sample, are shown in Table 5.2.

The random selection procedure in Example 5.1 can be modified in various ways as long as each member of the population is assigned different numbers and all members are assigned the same number of numbers. We cannot assign 10 numbers to E. Beasley and then assign only five numbers to each of the other members of the population. If we did this, E. Beasley would be more likely to be selected than other patients. We could have assigned each patient a single two-digit number (e.g., E. Beasley—01, P. McGirt—02, etc.), and this would have produced a random sample through use of the random number table. If we had done this, we would have thrown out most of the selected random numbers, since most would not have been assigned to any patient. It would have taken much longer to get our random sample.

Once a random sample is obtained, we can compute *sample statistics*, which are any measures calculated from the sample (such as the sample mean $\bar{x}$, the sample standard deviation s, or the sample survival rate). These statistics can be used to estimate the corresponding *population parameters*, which are any population characteristics of interest (such as the population mean μ, the population standard deviation σ, or the population survival rate). There is no method of sampling, short of selecting the entire population, that guarantees that sample statistics will equal their corresponding population parameters. In fact, sample statistics almost never equal their corresponding population parameters. If a random sample is used, however, we can make statements (with certain levels of confidence) about how close a sample statistic is to its corresponding population parameter. We can also use sample statistics to test hypotheses about population parameters. We will have more to say about this in Chapters 6 and 7.

Random samples cannot be obtained from most populations of interest in medical and health care research because these populations usually cannot be enumerated in a list. We cannot obtain a random sample of all men in the United States with gynecomastia, since there is no list of U.S. men with gynecomastia. The best we can usually do is try to make sure that our sample is not biased. A sample must accurately reflect the population about which we want to draw conclusions. If our population consists of all patients in the United States with hyperkalemia, we cannot reasonably make inferences about this population if our sample contains only white males. We might be able to generalize to the population of white males with hyperkalemia. If a nonrandom sample accurately reflects the population of interest, statistical procedures can still be used as guidelines for statistical inference.

5.2 RANDOMIZATION

Whether a sample is random or not, randomization should be used when subjects must be assigned to different treatment groups. A table of random numbers provides an efficient way to do this. Suppose our sample consists of the 21 patients in Table 5.1 and we want to randomly assign these patients as follows to three groups.

Group 1 (asthma information booklet 1): eight patients
Group 2 (asthma information booklet 2): eight patients
Group 3 (no information booklet): five patients

To make this random assignment, we will select a two-digit random number from Table E.1 for each patient. Any duplicate numbers will be thrown out, so each patient will have a unique random number. We will then assign the patients with the eight largest numbers to Group 1, the patients with the eight next largest numbers to Group 2, and the patients with the five smallest numbers to Group 3.

Let us choose an arbitrary starting point in Table E.1, say the fourth column and 12th row on the first page of this table. Starting at this point, we obtain 44, which we assign to E. Beasley. Going down in the table this time, we get 76 as our next number, which we assign to P. McGirt. Continuing in this

TABLE 5.3 SAMPLE OF PATIENTS AND THEIR SELECTED RANDOM NUMBERS

Patient	Random Number	Patient	Random Number
E. Beasley	44	C. Pflugel	47
P. McGirt	76	F. Junkroski	68
T. Dreeze	57	J. Mudge	63
S. Tootooian	97	S. Ribstein	28
B. Osnoss	61	A. Volgi	X̶, X̶, 41
C. Crater	55	J. Unfried	06
E. Scheib	86	L. Nazey	37
W. Wenckus	08	H. Kwartowski	96
G. Hoogenboom	01	L. Glunz	92
M. Eidlhuber	46	T. Leeth	X̶, 51
T. Zych	94	.	

TABLE 5.4 SAMPLE OF PATIENTS, SORTED RANDOM NUMBERS, AND GROUP ASSIGNMENTS

Group 1		Group 2		Group 3	
PATIENT	RANDOM NUMBER	PATIENT	RANDOM NUMBER	PATIENT	RANDOM NUMBER
S. Tootooian	97	B. Osnoss	61	L. Nazey	37
H. Kwartowski	96	T. Dreeze	57	S. Ribstein	28
T. Zych	94	C. Crater	55	W. Wenckus	08
L. Glunz	92	T. Leeth	51	J. Unfried	06
E. Scheib	86	C. Pflugel	47	G. Hoogenboom	01
P. McGirt	76	M. Eidlhuber	46		
F. Junkroski	68	E. Beasley	44		
J. Mudge	63	A. Volgi	41		

fashion, we obtain the random number assignments shown in Table 5.3. Crossed-out numbers in this table were thrown out because they duplicated previously selected numbers. Table 5.4 shows the sorted random numbers and the resulting group assignments.

The benefits of randomization were discussed in Chapter 1. When subjects are randomly assigned to groups, the chance of confounding is reduced. This allows us to reasonably attribute differences among groups to the treatments.

5.3 SAMPLING DISTRIBUTIONS

Having determined what a random sample is, we can now examine the distributions of statistics calculated from random samples. The *sampling distribution* of a statistic for samples of a given size is the distribution of this statistic when all samples of that size from a population are considered. This definition requires you to think of sample statistics as random variables, an important idea that many people find difficult at first.

Let us consider the sample mean, $\bar{x}$. You are accustomed to thinking of $\bar{x}$ as a specific number calculated from a specific sample. If we consider only one sample, this is correct. If we consider more than one sample, we need to think of $\bar{x}$ differently. The value of $\bar{x}$ usually changes as the sample changes. When we select different samples from a population, we generally get different values for $\bar{x}$. Thus, $\bar{x}$ has a set of possible values and is converted into a specific value by the chance-governed mechanism of selecting a random sample. By the definition of a random variable, $\bar{x}$ is a random variable.

The same reasoning shows that any sample statistic (such as s^2, s, or the sample success rate) is a random variable.* Because sample statistics are random variables, they have distributions. The distribution of a sample statistic is called its *sampling distribution*. If we take all possible samples of size 10 from a population and calculate $\bar{x}$ for each sample, we obtain the sampling distribution of $\bar{x}$ for samples of size 10 from this population. *The concept of sampling distributions underlies all of statistical inference* (the use of sample statistics to reach conclusions about population parameters). *It is essential that you become accustomed to the idea that sample statistics are random variables.* The following example may help you view sample statistics in this way.

Example 5.2

In a study of thyroid neoplasia following radiation treatment for Hodgkin's lymphoma, the latency pe-

riods for five patients were reported.[2] Table 5.5 shows these times in years from last radiation treatment to detection of thyroid neoplasia.

Suppose the records of these five patients constitute our population. The mean latency period for this population is $\mu = 11.6$, as you can verify by adding the five latency periods and dividing the sum by 5. Now suppose that we want to know the population mean, but we cannot obtain the records for all five patients. This is unrealistic, but we need a simplified example in order to show the rationale for statistical inference. Let us assume that severe budget cuts restrict us to a random sample of two of these records. All we can do is use our sample mean to estimate the population mean.

If we use the sample mean x as an estimate, how well will we do? This depends on the sample we get. It can be shown that there are 10 possible samples of size 2 from this population. Each of these 10 samples has a sample mean, and different samples produce different sample means. Examination of Table 5.6, which shows the values of $\bar{x}$ for all 10 possible samples, should make this clear. The values of $\bar{x}$ shown in this table differ for different samples. Thus, *the value of our estimate $\bar{x}$ depends on which sample we get.*

We can use Table 5.6 to find out anything we want to know about the sampling distribution of $\bar{x}$ for samples of size 2 from the neoplasia population. The population mean μ is 11.6, and we want to use $\bar{x}$ to estimate this mean. What is the chance of getting an $\bar{x}$ value that is a good estimate of μ? An

TABLE 5.5   LATENCY PERIOD FOR PATIENTS WITH THYROID NEOPLASIA

Patient	Latency Period (years)
MG	14
AR	9
SJ	11
PK	16
BL	8

TABLE 5.6   SAMPLING DISTRIBUTION OF $\bar{x}$ FOR SAMPLES OF SIZE 2

Sample No.	Patients in Sample	$\bar{x}$
1	MG, AR	11.5
2	MG, SJ	12.5
3	MG, PK	15.0
4	MG, BL	11.0
5	AR, SJ	10.0
6	AR, PK	12.5
7	AR, BL	8.5
8	SJ, PK	13.5
9	SJ, BL	9.5
10	PK, BL	12.0

---

*Of course, the specific value of a statistic for a particular sample is not a random variable. Such a number is one possible value of a random variable, obtained when the random variable is converted into a number by selecting a specific random sample.

$\bar{x}$ value is a good estimate of μ if it is close to μ. Let us arbitrarily consider $\bar{x}$ close to the population mean 11.6 if $\bar{x}$ differs from 11.6 by no more than two years.

What is the probability that $\bar{x}$ will be within two years of μ? Since $11.6 - 2 = 9.6$ and $11.6 + 2 = 13.6$, we want to find the probability that $\bar{x}$ will be between 9.6 and 13.6. There are seven sample means in Table 5.6 that are between 9.6 and 13.6, so there are seven sample means that are within two years of μ. We can apply formula (3.1) to calculate the probability that $\bar{x}$ is within two years of μ. Treating each sample as an "observation" in formula (3.1), we get

$P(\bar{x}$ differs from μ by at most 2$)$

$$= P(\bar{x} \text{ is between } 11.6 - 2 \text{ and } 11.6 + 2)$$

$$= P(\bar{x} \text{ is between } 9.6 \text{ and } 13.6)$$

$$= \frac{\text{no. of samples for which } \bar{x} \text{ is between } 9.6 \text{ and } 13.6}{\text{total no. of samples}}$$

$$= \frac{7}{10} = 0.70$$

We have a 70% chance of getting a value of $\bar{x}$ within two years of μ.

What is the chance of getting a value of $\bar{x}$ even closer to μ, say, within one year of μ? Here we want to find the probability that $\bar{x}$ differs from 11.6 by no more than one year. Five of the means in Table 5.6 are between $11.6 - 1 = 10.6$ and $11.6 + 1 = 12.6$. Applying (3.1) again, we get

$P(\bar{x}$ differs from μ by at most 1$)$

$$= P(\bar{x} \text{ is between } 11.6 - 1 \text{ and } 11.6 + 1)$$

$$= P(\bar{x} \text{ is between } 10.6 \text{ and } 12.6)$$

$$= \frac{\text{no. of samples for which } \bar{x} \text{ is between } 10.6 \text{ and } 12.6}{\text{total no. of samples}}$$

$$= \frac{5}{10} = 0.50$$

We have only a 50% chance of getting a sample mean value within one year of μ.

What is the chance of getting a value of $\bar{x}$ exactly equal to μ? None of the sample means in Table 5.6 is equal to 11.6, so the probability that $\bar{x}$ is exactly equal to μ is 0. We have no chance at all of getting a sample mean that is identical to the population mean. Seventy percent of the time, however, a random sample of two patients from this population will produce a value of $\bar{x}$ within two years of μ.

What happens the other 30% of the time? If we are very unlucky, we will get the third or seventh random sample. The third sample produces an $\bar{x}$ value equal to 15.0. We will then overestimate the population mean μ by more than three years. The seventh sample produces an $\bar{x}$ value equal to 8.5, and we will underestimate μ by more than three years. Selecting a random sample is like gambling,

with bad estimates instead of financial losses as the penalty for unlucky choices.

In this example, we have treated the sample statistic $\bar{x}$ as a random variable. We have calculated probabilities involving $\bar{x}$, and these calculations make sense only if we view $\bar{x}$ as a random quantity whose value is determined by the sample we select. All statistical inference rests on the concept of sample statistics as random variables.

The usefulness of a sample estimate increases as the sample size increases. In general, the larger the sample, the better our chance of getting an estimate that is close to the population parameter we want to estimate. Another factor that affects the accuracy of a sample estimate is the variability of the population values from which we are sampling. If the population values are extremely variable, the sample estimate will also be quite variable, unless very large sample sizes are used.

If we know the distribution of a sample statistic, we can assess how well it works as an estimate of a population parameter. We do not have much confidence in a highly variable sample estimate, since the chance of getting an estimate value close to the population parameter is small. We have much more confidence in a sample estimate with low variability. Such a statistic is likely to have values close to the population parameter it estimates.

Let us consider the sampling distribution of $\bar{x}$. This statistic has a sampling distribution with the following properties, which we will not prove.

PROPERTY 1. If random samples of size n are taken from any population with mean μ, the mean of $\bar{x}$ is also μ.* In Example 5.2, the mean of $\bar{x}$ for samples of size 2 is equal to the population mean of 11.6. This can be seen by adding all 10 possible values of $\bar{x}$ and dividing the sum by 10.

PROPERTY 2. If random samples of size n are taken from any infinitely large population with standard deviation σ, the standard deviation of $\bar{x}$ is $\sigma/\sqrt{n}$.† The *estimated* standard deviation of $\bar{x}$ is $s/\sqrt{n}$. The standard deviation or estimated standard deviation of any sample statistic is called its *standard error*. This term is used frequently in the medical and health care literature.

PROPERTY 3. If random samples are taken from any normal population, $\bar{x}$ has a normal distribution.

The second property implies that the variability of $\bar{x}$ depends on both the sample size and the

---

*A sample statistic whose mean is equal to the population parameter it estimates is *unbiased*. The sample mean $\bar{x}$ is an unbiased estimate of μ.

†When random samples of size n are taken from a *finite* population, the standard deviation of $\bar{x}$ is not equal to $\sigma/\sqrt{n}$. Formulas for the standard deviation of $\bar{x}$ in this case can be found in other texts.[1]

variability of the population. The larger the sample size, the smaller the standard deviation $\sigma/\sqrt{n}$ of $\bar{x}$ and the smaller the variability of $\bar{x}$. This makes sense intuitively. Sample means based on large samples should be more trustworthy (less variable) than sample means based on small samples. In addition, the smaller the population standard deviation σ, the smaller the standard deviation $\sigma/\sqrt{n}$ of $\bar{x}$ and the smaller the variability of $\bar{x}$. This also makes sense intuitively. Sample means based on samples from slightly variable populations should be more trustworthy than sample means based on samples from highly variable populations.

5.4 THE CENTRAL LIMIT THEOREM

Many statistical procedures assume that $\bar{x}$ has a normal distribution. From the previous section, we know that the sample mean has a normal distribution if it is based on samples from a normal population. What happens when samples are taken from nonnormal populations, as they frequently are in medical and health care research? In many cases, we can appeal to the *central limit theorem*, one of the most important results in statistics. This theorem often allows us to apply statistical methods that require normally distributed sample means to nonnormal data. The central limit theorem can be stated as follows.

> *The central limit theorem.* If sufficiently large random samples are taken from any infinitely large population with a finite variance, $\bar{x}$ has an approximately normal distribution.*

How large is "sufficiently large" in the central limit theorem? This depends on how nonnormal the population is. If the population is continuous, unimodal, and fairly symmetric, a sample size as small

---

*This theorem is by no means obvious, and its proof is well beyond the scope of this text.

as 5 may be large enough. If the population is extremely skewed, a sample size of 30 or more may be needed. The more nonnormal a population is, the larger the sample size needed to apply the central limit theorem. If you are not sure whether the central limit theorem applies to a particular sample, consult a statistician.

Since researchers usually do not know the distributions of the populations from which they sample, they use their samples to evaluate how closely population distributions resemble normal distributions. This is done by examining a histogram of the sample data to see whether the histogram is consistent with sampling from a normal population. When doing this, you must take the sample size into account. If the sample is large (say, $n \geq 25$), the histogram should resemble a bell-shaped curve. In other words, the sample histogram should be fairly symmetric and unimodal to be consistent with a normal population.

If the sample size is quite small (say, $n \leq 10$), a skewed histogram is not necessarily inconsistent with sampling from a normal population. Extreme skewness makes the assumption of normality questionable, but it is possible to get samples with grossly nonnormal histograms from normal populations. This possibility becomes less likely as the sample size increases. Histograms based on fewer than five observations are generally not useful for evaluating normality.

Example 5.3 _____

The histograms in Figures 5.1 through 5.4 were obtained for data from medical and health care journals. None of the data sets concern discrete random variables with only a few possible values, so we cannot rule out normality on these grounds. Instead, we need to evaluate the histograms. Which of these histograms (if any) are consistent with sampling from a normal population?

Let us consider Figure 5.1 first. Since the sample size is 30 and the histogram is quite skewed, it is not reasonable to assume that this sample came from a

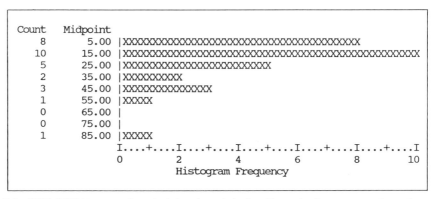

```
Count   Midpoint
   8       5.00  |XXXXXXXXXXXXXXXXXXXXXXXXXXXXXXXXXXXXXXXX
  10      15.00  |XXXXXXXXXXXXXXXXXXXXXXXXXXXXXXXXXXXXXXXXXXXXXXXXXXXX
   5      25.00  |XXXXXXXXXXXXXXXXXXXXXXXXXX
   2      35.00  |XXXXXXXXXX
   3      45.00  |XXXXXXXXXXXXXXX
   1      55.00  |XXXXX
   0      65.00  |
   0      75.00  |
   1      85.00  |XXXXX
                 I....+....I....+....I....+....I....+....I....+....I
                 0        2        4        6        8        10
                           Histogram Frequency
```

Figure 5.1   SPSS/PC histogram of survival time (months) after diagnosis of recurrence of rectal cancer for 30 patients[3]

```
Count  Midpoint
   4      4.00  |XXXXXXXXXXXXXXXXXXXX
   8      6.00  |XXXXXXXXXXXXXXXXXXXXXXXXXXXXXXXXXXXXXXXX
   4      8.00  |XXXXXXXXXXXXXXXXXXXX
   2     10.00  |XXXXXXXXXX
   5     12.00  |XXXXXXXXXXXXXXXXXXXXXXXXX
   2     14.00  |XXXXXXXXXX
                I....+....I....+....I....+....I....+....I....+....I
                0         2         4         6         8        10
                          Histogram Frequency
```

Figure 5.2 SPSS/PC histogram of HLTV-III ratio for 25 homosexual men with immune thrombocytopenia[4]

```
Count  Midpoint
   1     22.00  |XXXXX
   5     26.00  |XXXXXXXXXXXXXXXXXXXXXXXXX
   6     30.00  |XXXXXXXXXXXXXXXXXXXXXXXXXXXXXX
   3     34.00  |XXXXXXXXXXXXXXX
   2     38.00  |XXXXXXXXXX
   1     42.00  |XXXXX
   2     46.00  |XXXXXXXXXX
                I....+....I....+....I....+....I....+....I....+....I
                0         2         4         6         8        10
                          Histogram Frequency
```

Figure 5.3 SPSS/PC histogram of activated partial thromboplastin time for 20 patients[5]

```
Count  Midpoint
   3     87.00  |XXXXXXXXXXXXXXX
   3     89.00  |XXXXXXXXXXXXXXX
   5     91.00  |XXXXXXXXXXXXXXXXXXXXXXXXX
   7     93.00  |XXXXXXXXXXXXXXXXXXXXXXXXXXXXXXXXXXX
   6     95.00  |XXXXXXXXXXXXXXXXXXXXXXXXXXXXXX
   3     97.00  |XXXXXXXXXXXXXXX
   3     99.00  |XXXXXXXXXXXXXXX
                I....+....I....+....I....+....I....+....I....+....I
                0         2         4         6         8        10
                          Histogram Frequency
```

Figure 5.4 SPSS/PC histogram of percentage of ideal body weight for 30 cirrhotic patients[6]

```
Count  Midpoint
   2      6.50  |XXXXXXXXXXXXXXXXXXXX
   1      7.50  |XXXXXXXXXX
   0      8.50  |
   0      9.50  |
   0     10.50  |
   0     11.50  |
   0     12.50  |
   0     13.50  |
   0     14.50  |
   4     15.50  |XXXXXXXXXXXXXXXXXXXXXXXXXXXXXXXXXXXXXXXX
                I....+....I....+....I....+....I....+....I....+....I
                0         1         2         3         4         5
                          Histogram Frequency
```

Figure 5.5 SPSS/PC histogram of seven hypothetical values

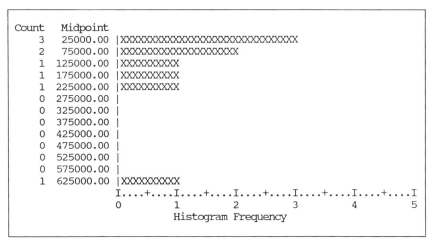

Figure 5.6 SPSS/PC histogram of serum endogenous polymerase (cpm) for nine HBsAg carriers[7]

normally distributed population. Figure 5.2 shows a histogram for a sample of 25 patients. Although the histogram is not skewed, it is not bell-shaped either, and it seems inconsistent with sampling from a normal population. The histogram in Figure 5.3, based on a sample of 20 patients, is skewed and appears inconsistent with sampling from a normal population. Figure 5.4 shows a fairly symmetric histogram based on a sample of 30 patients. This histogram seems consistent with sampling from a normal or approximately normal population.

Most statisticians would agree that the sample sizes in Figures 5.1 through 5.4 are large enough to justify applying the central limit theorem to these nonnormal samples. We can reasonably assume that the sample mean $\bar{x}$ is approximately normally distributed in each case. Suppose we obtained the histogram in Figure 5.5 or in Figure 5.6. These histograms suggest such extremely nonnormal populations that the sample sizes are not large enough to justify using the central limit theorem. With these data sets, we cannot assume that $\bar{x}$ is approximately normally distributed.

is random or not, a random number table should be used for randomization if subjects are to be assigned to different groups.

When a sample is obtained, sample statistics are frequently used to estimate population parameters. The distribution of a sample statistic is called the sampling distribution of the statistic. Sample statistics can be thought of as random variables that usually have different values for different samples. The concept of sample statistics as random variables is extremely important because it is the basis for statistical inference.

When random samples are taken from a population with a known mean and standard deviation, the mean and standard deviation of the sample mean can be obtained. The central limit theorem states that the sample mean has an approximately normal distribution if sufficiently large random samples are taken from an infinitely large population with a finite variance. This theorem often allows us to apply statistical methods that require normally distributed sample means to nonnormal data. Sample histograms can be used to evaluate the normality or nonnormality of a population.

SUMMARY

Statistical inference is the process of reaching conclusions about a population by examining a sample from the population. This type of inference works best if the sample is a probability sample. The most important type of probability sample is the random sample, which can be obtained by using a listing of the population and a random number table. Random samples cannot be used for most medical and health care research, since there is usually no listing of the population. As long as the sample is not biased, statistical inference can be based on nonrandom samples. Whether the sample

PROBLEMS

1. Use the random number table and the assigned patient numbers in Table 5.1 to obtain a random sample of size 15 from the population of patients in Table 5.1. To get an answer you can check, start with the last two digits (99) on the first page of Table E.1 and go up.

2. Use the random number table to randomly assign the 21 patients in Table 5.1 to two groups with the following group sizes.

Group 1: 10 patients
Group 2: 11 patients

To get an answer you can check, start with the first two digits (30) on the fourth page of Table E.1 and go across. Assign the patients with the 10 largest numbers to Group 1.

3. Use the random number table to randomly assign the 21 patients in Table 5.1 to three groups with the following group sizes:

Group 1: 6 patients
Group 2: 6 patients
Group 3: 9 patients

TABLE 5.7   SERUM CALCIUM LEVEL FOR HYPERCALCEMIC PATIENTS

Patient	Serum Calcium (mg /dl)
RR	24.0
PB	16.8
DS	20.0
FT	13.2
MK	14.4

TABLE 5.8   SAMPLING DISTRIBUTION OF $\bar{x}$ FOR SAMPLES OF SIZE 3

Sample No.	Patients in Sample	$\bar{x}$
1	RR, PB, DS	20.3
2	RR, PB, FT	18.0
3	RR, PB, MK	18.4
4	RR, DS, FT	19.1
5	RR, DS, MK	19.5
6	RR, FT, MK	17.2
7	PB, DS, FT	16.7
8	PB, DS, MK	17.1
9	PB, FT, MK	14.8
10	DS, FT, MK	15.9

To get an answer you can check, start with the two digits (33) in the first row and the 11th and 12th columns on the third page of Table E.1 and go down. Assign the patients with the six largest numbers to Group 1, the patients with the six next largest numbers to Group 2, and the patients with the nine smallest numbers to Group 3.

4. In a study of hypercalcemic patients with adult T-cell lymphoma, the serum calcium levels in Table 5.7 were reported.[8] Suppose that the records of these five patients constitute our population, but we can obtain only a random sample of three records. There are 10 possible samples of size 3 from this population. The means for these samples are shown in Table 5.8. The population mean μ is 17.7.

Calculate the following probabilities, assuming that a random sample of size 3 is to be selected from this population.

a. The probability that $\bar{x}$ is equal to μ, which is the probability that $\bar{x}$ is equal to 17.7.

b. The probability that $\bar{x}$ differs from μ by no more than 1 mg/dl, which is the probability that $\bar{x}$ is between 16.7 and 18.7.

c. The probability that $\bar{x}$ differs from μ by no more than 2 mg/dl, which is the probability that $\bar{x}$ is between 15.7 and 19.7.

d. For this example, is $\bar{x}$ close to μ for most samples? Consider $\bar{x}$ close to μ if $\bar{x}$ differs from μ by no more than 2 mg/dl.

5. The histogram in Figure 5.7 is based on a sample of 40 pediatric patients.[9] Is this histogram consistent with sampling from a normal or approximately normal distribution? Why or why not?

6. The histogram in Figure 5.8 is based on a sample of 18 physicians.[10] Is this histogram consistent with sampling from a normal or approximately normal distribution? Why or why not?

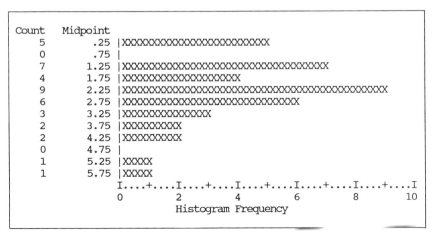

```
Count  Midpoint
    5      .25  |XXXXXXXXXXXXXXXXXXXXXXXXX
    0      .75  |
    7     1.25  |XXXXXXXXXXXXXXXXXXXXXXXXXXXXXXXXXXX
    4     1.75  |XXXXXXXXXXXXXXXXXXXX
    9     2.25  |XXXXXXXXXXXXXXXXXXXXXXXXXXXXXXXXXXXXXXXXXXXXX
    6     2.75  |XXXXXXXXXXXXXXXXXXXXXXXXXXXXX
    3     3.25  |XXXXXXXXXXXXXX
    2     3.75  |XXXXXXXXX
    2     4.25  |XXXXXXXXX
    0     4.75  |
    1     5.25  |XXXXX
    1     5.75  |XXXXX
              I....+....I....+....I....+....I....+....I....+....I
              0         2         4         6         8        10
                            Histogram Frequency
```

Figure 5.7 SPSS/PC histogram of number of narcotic doses per postoperative day given to pediatric patients

```
Count   Midpoint
    2       8.90  |XXXXXXXXXXXXXXXXXXXX
    2       9.70  |XXXXXXXXXXXXXXXXXXXX
    5      10.50  |XXXXXXXXXXXXXXXXXXXXXXXXXXXXXXXXXXXXXXXXXXXXXXXXXXX
    3      11.30  |XXXXXXXXXXXXXXXXXXXXXXXXXXXXXX
    4      12.10  |XXXXXXXXXXXXXXXXXXXXXXXXXXXXXXXXXXXXXXXX
    1      12.90  |XXXXXXXXXX
    1      13.70  |XXXXXXXXXX
                  I....+....I....+....I....+....I....+....I....+....I
                  0         1         2         3         4         5
                              Histogram Frequency
```

Figure 5.8 SPSS/PC histogram of average patient length of stay (days) for physicians

```
Count   Midpoint
    1       6.00  |XXXXXXXXXX
    4       8.00  |XXXXXXXXXXXXXXXXXXXXXXXXXXXXXXXXXXXXXXXXXX
    4      10.00  |XXXXXXXXXXXXXXXXXXXXXXXXXXXXXXXXXXXXXXXXXX
    1      12.00  |XXXXXXXXXX
                  I....+....I....+....I....+....I....+....I....+....I
                  0         1         2         3         4         5
                              Histogram Frequency
```

Figure 5.9 SPSS/PC histogram of percent bone porosity for hypothyroid patients after thyroid replacement

```
Count   Midpoint
    2       7.50  |XXXXXXXXXX
    1      12.50  |XXXXX
    3      17.50  |XXXXXXXXXXXXXXX
    4      22.50  |XXXXXXXXXXXXXXXXXXXX
    4      27.50  |XXXXXXXXXXXXXXXXXXXX
    4      32.50  |XXXXXXXXXXXXXXXXXXXX
    2      37.50  |XXXXXXXXXX
    2      42.50  |XXXXXXXXXX
    6      47.50  |XXXXXXXXXXXXXXXXXXXXXXXXXXXXXX
                  I....+....I....+....I....+....I....+....I....+....I
                  0         2         4         6         8        10
                              Histogram Frequency
```

Figure 5.10 SPSS/PC histogram of serum iron (μg/dl) for hospitalized horses with pseudo-iron deficiency

```
Count   Midpoint
   12      75.00  |XXXXXXXXXXXXXXXXXXXXXXXXXXXXXXXXXX
    8     105.00  |XXXXXXXXXXXXXXXXXXXXXX
    3     135.00  |XXXXXXXX
    1     165.00  |XX
    0     195.00  |
    1     225.00  |XX
                  I....+....I....+....I....+....I....+....I....+....I
                  0         4         8        12        16        20
                              Histogram Frequency
```

Figure 5.11 SPSS/PC histogram of time in recovery room for pediatric patients

7. The histogram in Figure 5.9 is based on a sample of 10 hypothyroid patients.[11] Is this histogram consistent with sampling from a normal or approximately normal distribution? Why or why not?

8. The histogram in Figure 5.10 is based on a sample of 28 horses.[12] Is this histogram consistent with sampling from a normal or approximately normal distribution? Why or why not?

9. The histogram in Figure 5.11 is based on a sample of 25 pediatric patients.[13] Is this histogram consistent with sampling from a normal or approximately normal distribution? Why or why not?

REFERENCES

1. Cochran WG: Sampling Techniques. 3rd ed. New York: Wiley, 1977.
2. McHenry C, Jarosz H, Calandra D, et al: Thyroid neoplasia following radiation therapy for Hodgkin's lymphoma. Arch Surg *122*:684–686, 1987.
3. Wanebo HJ, Gaker GL, Whitehill R, et al: Pelvic recurrence of rectal cancer. Options for curative resection. Ann Surg *205*:482–495, 1987.
4. Abrams DI, Kiprov DD, Goedert JJ, et al: Antibodies to human T-lymphotropic virus type III and development of the acquired immunodeficiency syndrome in homosexual men presenting with immune thrombocytopenia. Ann Intern Med *104*:47–50, 1986.
5. Molyneaux RD, Papciak B, Rorem DA: Coagulation studies and the indwelling heparinized catheter. Heart Lung *16*:20–23, 1987.
6. Cavallo-Perin P, Bruno A, Nuccio P, et al: Feedback inhibition of insulin secretion is altered in cirrhosis. J Clin Endocrinol Metal *63*:1023–1027, 1986.
7. Jenison SA, Lemon SM, Baker LN, et al: Quantitative analysis of hepatitis B virus DNA in saliva and semen of chronically infected homosexual men. J Infect Dis *156*:299–307, 1987.
8. Dodd RC, Winkler CF, Williams ME, et al: Calcitriol levels in hypercalcemic patients with adult T-cell lymphoma. Arch Intern Med *146*:1971–1972, 1986.
9. Burokas L: Factors affecting nurses' decisions to medicate pediatric patients after surgery. Heart Lung *14*:373–379, 1985.
10. Panniers TL: Severity of illness, quality of care, and physician practice as determinants of hospital resource consumption. QRB *13*:158–165, 1987.
11. Coindre J, David J, Riviere L, et al: Bone loss in hypothyroidism with hormone replacement. A histomorphometric study. Arch Intern Med *146*:48–53, 1986.
12. Smith JE, Cipriano JE, DeBowes R, et al: Iron deficiency and pseudo-iron deficiency in hospitalized horses. J Am Vet Med Assoc *188*:285–287, 1986.
13. Wehner RJ, Gilbert DH: Premedication of children with droperidol-glycopyrrolate versus meperidine-glycopyrrolate: Results of a blind study. AANA J *53*:504–507, 1985.

6

ESTIMATION

CHAPTER OBJECTIVES

After studying this chapter and working the problems, you should be able to:

1. Explain what a confidence interval means

2. Calculate and interpret confidence intervals for population proportions, differences between population proportions, population means, and differences between population means

3. Recognize data that violate assumptions required for confidence intervals

We have now covered the background needed to understand how inferences about population parameters can be made from sample statistics. In this chapter, we will discuss *estimation*, the use of sample statistics to estimate population parameters. The calculations required are fairly easy and rarely cause difficulty. The most common sources of trouble are the rationale for estimation and the interpretation of estimates. The rationale for estimation is based on sampling distributions, discussed in the previous chapter. If you understand sampling distributions, estimation will make sense to you.

6.1 CONFIDENCE INTERVALS

A study found that 94% of 54 women with premenstrual syndrome (PMS) had signs of thyroid hypofunction.[1] If all women similar to those in the study were tested for thyroid dysfunction, what proportion would show signs of thyroid hypofunction? For the sample of 54 patients, the proportion with thyroid hypofunction is 0.94. What does this tell us about the population proportion of women with

PMS who are hypothyroid? The number 0.94 is a *point estimate*, an estimate consisting of a single number. It is not reasonable to assume that the population proportion is exactly 0.94. The probability of getting a sample statistic value that is exactly equal to the corresponding population parameter is usually quite small. It may be reasonable to assume that 0.94 is *close to* the population proportion. The probability of getting a sample statistic value that is close to the corresponding population parameter is sometimes quite high.

We would like to use a point estimate to obtain an *interval estimate*. An interval estimate is a range of numbers that we hope includes the population parameter we want to estimate. One possible interval estimate for the population proportion of women with PMS who are hypothyroid consists of all the numbers from 0.92 to 0.96. We can write this estimate as the interval (0.92, 0.96). The *endpoints* of this interval estimate are 0.92 and 0.96. Another interval estimate is (0.89, 0.99)—all the numbers from 0.89 to 0.99. The endpoints of this interval estimate are 0.89 and 0.99. If the unknown population proportion p is 0.92, p is included in both of these interval estimates. If the unknown population proportion p is 0.86, p is not included in either of these interval estimates.

Ideally, we would like to be completely certain that the population parameter of interest is included in our interval estimate. This is too much to ask for. We have to settle for something less than certainty, namely, *confidence levels*. For example, we are 95% sure that an interval estimate includes the population parameter if the interval estimate is a 95% confidence interval.* A *95% confidence interval* is an interval estimate constructed in such a way that the interval will include the population parameter 95% of the time. In other words, 95% of all possible samples will produce 95% confidence intervals that include the population parameter. Five per cent of all possible samples will produce 95% confidence intervals that do *not* include the population parameter.

We can also obtain 99% confidence intervals, in which we have 99% confidence, 90% confidence intervals, in which we have 90% confidence, and so on. In fact, we can construct a confidence interval for any confidence level we want.† The customary confidence levels are 90%, 95%, 99%, and 99.9%. The methods used to construct confidence intervals depend on the population parameter estimated. We will consider confidence intervals for the following population parameters:

1. Population proportions
2. Differences between population proportions
3. Population means
4. Differences between population means

6.2 CONFIDENCE INTERVALS FOR POPULATION PROPORTIONS

Let us again consider the PMS data. We want an interval estimate of the population proportion p of women with PMS who are hypothyroid. To get this estimate, we can construct a confidence interval for p, using the sample proportion of women with PMS who are hypothyroid. We will denote sample proportions by $\hat{p}$ (pronounced "p hat") in order to distinguish them from population proportions. (The hat symbol " ˆ " is used to denote sample estimates of population parameters.)

To obtain a confidence interval for a population proportion, we also need a table of upper-tail probabilities from the standard normal distribution. If Z has a standard normal distribution, the α *upper percentage point* of the standard normal distribution is the number z_α such that

$$P(Z \geq z_\alpha) = \alpha$$

The symbol "α" is the Greek letter alpha.

For example, the 0.05 upper percentage point for the standard normal distribution is the number $z_{.05}$ such that

$$P(Z \geq z_{.05}) = 0.05$$

To find $z_{.05}$, we use Table E.2. Since an upper-tail probability is involved, we use the column for upper-tail probabilities, but we use the table in a different way than we used it in Chapter 4. In Chapter 4, we were given a z value and we looked up the corresponding upper-tail probability. Here we are given an upper-tail probability and we look up the corresponding z value. We first find 0.05 *in the column for upper-tail probabilities*, then read across to the z column. The number *in the z column* and in the row corresponding to 0.05 in the column for upper-tail probabilities is $z_{.05}$, so we get $z_{.05} = 1.645$. In other words, 1.645 is the 0.05 upper percentage point of the standard normal distribution:

$$P(Z \geq 1.645) = 0.05$$

If we want to find the 0.01 upper percentage point of the standard normal distribution, we first look up 0.01 *in the column for upper-tail probabilities*. We then read across to the z column and find the number *in the z column* and in the row corresponding to 0.01 in the column for upper-tail probabilities. When we do this, we get $z_{.01} = 2.326$. Thus, the 0.01 upper percentage point for the standard normal distribution is 2.326:

$$P(Z \geq 2.326) = 0.01$$

It can be shown (using the central limit theorem) that the sample proportion $\hat{p}$ has an approximately normal distribution with mean p and estimated standard deviation

$$s_{\text{prop}} = \sqrt{\frac{\hat{p}(1 - \hat{p})}{n}} \qquad (6.1)$$

when the sample is large enough. Although we will not prove it, this implies that a $100(1 - \alpha)\%$ confidence interval for p is given by the formula

$$\left(\hat{p} - (z_{\alpha/2})(s_{\text{prop}}), \quad \hat{p} + (z_{\alpha/2})(s_{\text{prop}}) \right) \quad (6.2)$$

The symbol $z_{\alpha/2}$ refers to the $\alpha/2$ upper percentage point of the standard normal distribution. If Z

---

*The phrase "95% sure" may sound odd at first, but similar phrases are commonly used. A physician may say she is "quite sure" that her diagnosis is correct, or "somewhat sure," or "not very sure." If you are 95% sure, you are very sure but not certain.

†The only 100% confidence interval is the interval containing all possible values of the population parameter. For example, a 100% confidence interval for a population proportion is all the numbers from 0 to 1, or (0, 1). This interval is certain to include the population proportion, but does not tell us anything.

has a standard normal distribution, $P(Z \geq z_{\alpha/2}) = \alpha/2$. For example, if $1 - \alpha = 0.95$, $\alpha = 0.05$, $\alpha/2 = 0.025$, and a 95% confidence interval for p is given by the formula

$$\left(\hat{p} - (z_{.025})(s_{prop}), \quad \hat{p} + (z_{.025})(s_{prop}) \right)$$

If formula (6.2) is used to obtain interval estimates of the population proportion p, interval estimates that include p will be produced about $100(1 - \alpha)\%$ of the time. Since $\hat{p}$ usually has different values for different samples, confidence intervals for the population proportion usually have different values for different samples. Suppose a 95% confidence interval for the population proportion p is to be obtained. Approximately 95% of all possible samples will produce 95% confidence intervals that include p. About 5% of all possible samples will produce 95% confidence intervals that do not include p. If we use formula (6.2) to obtain a 95% confidence interval for p, we get an interval estimate that includes p about 95% of the time. This is why we are 95% sure, or 95% confident, that an interval estimate calculated by using formula (6.2) includes p.

To use formula (6.2), we first decide what confidence level we want. Our α is then 1 minus our confidence level. If we want to be 90% sure that our interval estimate includes p, we want a confidence level of 0.90 and our α is 0.10. We then look up $z_{\alpha/2}$ in Table E.2, calculate $\hat{p}$ and s_{prop} from our data, and use these values and the sample size in formula (6.2).

Let us do this for the PMS data. The sample size is 54 and $\hat{p}$ is 0.94. To get a 90% confidence interval for the population proportion of women with PMS who are hypothyroid, we use $\alpha = 0.10$. Since $\alpha/2$ is 0.05, we look up $z_{.05}$ in Table E.2 and find $z_{.05} = 1.645$. The estimated standard deviation of $\hat{p}$ is

$$s_{prop} = \sqrt{\frac{(0.94)(1 - 0.94)}{54}}$$

$$= \sqrt{\frac{(0.94)(0.06)}{54}} = 0.032$$

Using these values in formula (6.2), we get the interval estimate

$$(0.94 - (1.645)(0.032), 0.94 + (1.645)(0.032))$$

$$(0.94 - 0.05, 0.94 + 0.05)$$

$$(0.89, 0.99)$$

Our 90% confidence interval for p is (0.89, 0.99).

We are 90% sure that the population proportion of women with PMS who are hypothyroid is between 0.89 and 0.99. We will never know whether the interval estimate (0.89, 0.99) actually includes the population proportion p or not. If we were

unlucky, we got one of the samples that produces a 90% confidence interval that does not include p. Since this happens only about 10% of the time, we are 90% sure that the interval (0.89, 0.99) does include p. We could be wrong, however. This is always a risk when we make inferences from a sample to a population. Because we see only a sample, our inferences about the population can be wrong. By calculating a 90% confidence interval, we use a method that produces correct interval estimates 90% of the time. We know the odds in favor of a correct interval estimate, but we never know whether we actually obtained a correct interval estimate.

Let us calculate 95% and 99% confidence intervals for the population proportion of women with PMS who are hypothyroid. For a 95% confidence interval, α is 0.05, so $\alpha/2$ is 0.025 and $z_{.025}$ is 1.96. Applying formula (6.2), we get the interval estimate

$$(0.94 - (1.96)(0.032), 0.94 + (1.96)(0.032))$$

$$(0.94 - 0.06, 0.94 + 0.06)$$

$$(0.88, 1.00)$$

Our 95% confidence interval for p is (0.88, 1.00).

To calculate a 99% confidence interval, we use an α of 0.01, so $\alpha/2$ is 0.005 and $z_{.005}$ is 2.576. Using formula (6.2), we get the interval estimate

$$(0.94 - (2.576)(0.032), 0.94 + (2.576)(0.032))$$

$$(0.94 - 0.08, 0.94 + 0.08)$$

$$(0.86, 1.02)$$

Since proportions cannot be greater than 1, we can replace the endpoint 1.02 with the endpoint 1. Our 99% confidence interval for p is then (0.86, 1). We are 99% sure that the interval (0.86, 1) includes p, and we are 95% sure that the interval (0.88, 1) includes p. In other words, we are 99% sure that the population proportion of women with PMS who are hypothyroid is between 0.86 and 1. We are 95% sure that the population proportion of women with PMS who are hypothyroid is between 0.88 and 1.

When a confidence interval for a population proportion is calculated, it is possible to get a negative endpoint or an endpoint greater than 1. Since proportions must be between 0 and 1, a negative endpoint should be replaced by 0, and an endpoint greater than 1 should be replaced by 1. For example, the confidence interval $(-0.09, 0.34)$ for a population proportion should be replaced by the interval (0, 0.34).

Confidence intervals for population proportions are based on the following assumptions about the data.

1. Random Sampling. Although a random sample is preferable, confidence intervals for a population proportion may be obtained when the sample is not random. The sample must not be biased, however.

2. Independent Observations. This assumption must *not* be violated. If the observations are not independent, a confidence interval for the population proportion cannot be obtained.

3. Sufficiently Large Sample. Samples as small as 10 are usually adequate. If $\hat{p}$ is quite close to 0 or 1, a larger sample is required. The closer $\hat{p}$ is to 0 or 1, the larger the sample needed. A statistician should be consulted if you are not sure whether your sample is large enough.

The assumption of independent observations appears to hold for the PMS data. Knowing whether one woman is hypothyroid tells us nothing about whether another woman is hypothyroid. The sample size of 54 is sufficiently large, given a $\hat{p}$ of 0.94, so the third assumption is satisfied. The women studied were not a random sample of all women with PMS, but random sampling is not essential. Because the second and third assumptions are satisfied, confidence intervals for the population proportion are appropriate.

Example 6.1

In a study of nasoenteral tube displacement, 213 tubes placed in 105 hospitalized patients were monitored.[2] Nine per cent of these tubes were found to be out of position. Can we use the sample proportion of displaced nasoenteral tubes to obtain a confidence interval for the population proportion of displaced nasoenteral tubes?

There are more than twice as many tubes as patients, so some patients had more than one tube. We have repeated measurements for some patients, and repeated measurements on the same patient are not independent. If we know that a patient's last three tubes were displaced, this gives us some idea of whether his next tube will be displaced. A confidence interval for the population proportion cannot be obtained.

If more information were available, we could base a confidence interval on the sample proportion of patients with displaced tubes. This would allow us to estimate the population proportion of hospitalized patients with displaced tubes. By using patients rather than tubes as the unit of analysis, we would eliminate the repeated measurements that produce nonindependent observations.

6.3 CONFIDENCE INTERVALS FOR DIFFERENCES BETWEEN POPULATION PROPORTIONS

In medical and health care research, we often want to compare two proportions. If one sample of patients is treated with one drug and a second sample is treated with another drug, we want to compare the proportions of successfully treated patients in the two groups. Or we might want to compare the proportion of patients with one disease who recover with the proportion of patients with another disease who recover.

Comparison of proportions is required to assess the results of a study concerning the effect of neuroleptic drugs on behavior.[3] In this study, 24 demented elderly nursing home patients who took neuroleptic medications were compared with 24 similar nursing home patients who did not take neuroleptic medications. Fifty per cent of the drug patients were verbally abusive, as were 21% of the no-drug patients. These sample proportions are quite different, suggesting that demented elderly patients who are given neuroleptic drugs may be more likely to be verbally abusive. We want to use these sample proportions to make inferences about two theoretical populations, the populations that would result if all patients similar to those in the study either received neuroleptic drugs or did not receive neuroleptic drugs.

In general, we want to make inferences that allow us to compare two population proportions. Let p_1 be the proportion for the first population and p_2 the proportion for the second population. If we obtain a confidence interval for the difference $p_1 - p_2$ between the two population proportions, we can make inferences about the difference between these proportions. In this way, we can make inferences comparing the two population proportions. If the difference $p_1 - p_2$ is zero, the population proportions p_1 and p_2 are the same. If the difference $p_1 - p_2$ is not zero, the population proportions p_1 and p_2 are different.

To obtain a confidence interval for the difference between two population proportions, we need a sample of size n_1 from the first population and a sample of size n_2 from the second population. The sample sizes n_1 and n_2 need not be equal. From these samples, we obtain the sample proportions $\hat{p}_1$ and $\hat{p}_2$ and the sample estimate $\hat{p}_1 - \hat{p}_2$.

It can be shown (using the central limit theorem) that the sample difference $\hat{p}_1 - \hat{p}_2$ has an approximately normal distribution with mean $p_1 - p_2$ and estimated standard deviation

$$s_{\text{diff}} = \sqrt{\frac{\hat{p}_1(1 - \hat{p}_1)}{n_1} + \frac{\hat{p}_2(1 - \hat{p}_2)}{n_2}} \quad (6.3)$$

if the samples are independent and sufficiently large. Although we will not prove it, this implies that a $100(1 - \alpha)\%$ confidence interval for $p_1 - p_2$ is given by the formula

$$\begin{aligned} &((\hat{p}_1 - \hat{p}_2) - (z_{\alpha/2})(s_{\text{diff}}), \\ &(\hat{p}_1 - \hat{p}_2) + (z_{\alpha/2})(s_{\text{diff}})) \end{aligned} \quad (6.4)$$

As before, $z_{\alpha/2}$ is the $\alpha/2$ upper percentage point of the standard normal distribution.

The values of $\hat{p}_1$ and $\hat{p}_2$ depend on which samples are selected. Thus, the values of a $100(1 - \alpha)\%$

confidence interval for $p_1 - p_2$ also depend on which samples are selected. About $100(1 - \alpha)\%$ of all samples will produce $100(1 - \alpha)\%$ confidence intervals that include the population difference $p_1 - p_2$. If α is 0.01, approximately 99% of all possible samples will produce 99% confidence intervals that include $p_1 - p_2$. About 1% of all possible samples will produce 99% confidence intervals that do not include $p_1 - p_2$. We have no way of knowing whether or not a particular confidence interval includes $p_1 - p_2$. We can only be fairly certain that it does.

Let us obtain a 95% confidence interval from the drug data. If $\hat{p}_1$ is the sample proportion of drug patients who are verbally abusive and $\hat{p}_2$ is the sample proportion of no-drug patients who are verbally abusive,

$$\hat{p}_1 - \hat{p}_2 = 0.50 - 0.21 = 0.29$$

Since $\alpha = 0.05$, $\alpha/2 = 0.025$ and $z_{.025} = 1.96$. The estimated standard deviation (6.3) is

$$
\begin{aligned}
s_{\text{diff}} &= \sqrt{\frac{(0.50)(1 - 0.50)}{24} + \frac{(0.21)(1 - 0.21)}{24}} \\
&= \sqrt{0.0104 + 0.0069} \\
&= \sqrt{0.0173} = 0.13
\end{aligned}
$$

Using the required values in formula (6.4), we get our 95% confidence interval:

$$(0.29 - (1.96)(0.13), 0.29 + (1.96)(0.13))$$
$$(0.29 - 0.25, 0.29 + 0.25)$$
$$(0.04, 0.54)$$

We are 95% sure that the population difference $p_1 - p_2$ is between 0.04 and 0.54. Thus, we are 95% sure that this difference is positive. This means we are 95% sure that p_1 is larger than p_2. If p_1 were less than p_2, the difference $p_1 - p_2$ would be negative. We interpret the confidence interval as follows:

> We are 95% sure that p_1 is greater than p_2 and the difference between these population proportions is between 0.04 and 0.54. Thus, we are 95% sure that demented elderly nursing home patients given neuroleptic drugs are more likely to be verbally abusive than similar patients not given neuroleptic drugs. The drug patients might be slightly more likely to be verbally abusive ($p_1 - p_2$ might be as low as 0.04); or they might be much more likely to be verbally abusive ($p_1 - p_2$ might be as high as 0.54); or they might be moderately more likely to be verbally abusive ($p_1 - p_2$ might be one of the moderate values included in the interval between 0.04 and 0.54).

What constitutes a small, moderate, or large difference between proportions? Since proportions are quite small, a difference of 0.4 or more between two proportions is a large difference. A difference of $0.2 - 0.3$ is usually a moderate difference, and a difference of 0.1 or less is usually a small difference.

To obtain a 99% confidence interval for $p_1 - p_2$, we use $z_{.005} = 2.576$, since $\alpha/2 = 0.01/2 = 0.005$. All of the other quantities in formula (6.4) remain the same, so we get the 99% confidence interval

$$(0.29 - (2.576)(0.13), 0.29 + (2.576)(0.13))$$
$$(0.29 - 0.33, 0.29 + 0.33)$$
$$(-0.04, 0.62)$$

We are 99% sure that $p_1 - p_2$ is between -0.04 and 0.62. Because the lower endpoint is negative and the upper endpoint is positive, the confidence interval includes 0. We cannot say with 99% confidence that there is a difference between p_1 and p_2. Since 0 is included in the confidence interval, we cannot rule out the possibility that $p_1 - p_2 = 0$. At a lower confidence level (95%), we can say that there is a difference between p_1 and p_2. For these data, the conclusion we reach depends on the confidence level we use.

If both endpoints of a confidence interval for $p_1 - p_2$ are *positive*, we can be fairly sure that p_1 is *greater* than p_2. If both endpoints are *negative*, we can be fairly sure that p_1 is *less* than p_2. If the lower endpoint is negative and the upper endpoint is positive, 0 is included in the confidence interval and we cannot be sure that p_1 does not equal p_2. Whenever a confidence interval for $p_1 - p_2$ includes 0, we cannot say, at that confidence level, that the population proportions are different.

Because proportions are always between 0 and 1, the largest possible difference between any two proportions is $1 - 0 = 1$. The smallest possible difference between any two proportions is $0 - 1 = -1$. Confidence intervals for differences between proportions sometimes have endpoints less than -1 or greater than 1. When this happens, the value less than -1 should be replaced by -1, and the value greater than 1 should be replaced by 1. The confidence interval $(-1.23, -0.41)$ for a difference between population proportions should be changed to $(-1, -0.41)$. The confidence interval $(0.30, 1.07)$ for a difference between population proportions should be changed to $(0.30, 1)$.

Confidence intervals for differences between population proportions are based on the following assumptions.

1. Random Sampling. As before, random sampling is not essential as long as the samples are not biased.

2. Independent Samples. The observations in one sample must be independent of the observations in the other sample. If this assumption is violated, formula (6.4) cannot be used to obtain a confidence interval for $p_1 - p_2$.[*]

---

[*] A method for comparing proportions from nonindependent samples is discussed in Chapter 10. Other methods are described by Schlesselman.[4]

3. Independent Observations Within Each Sample. The observations within each sample must be independent. A confidence interval cannot be obtained for $p_1 - p_2$ if this assumption is violated.

4. Sufficiently Large Samples. Samples as small as 10 are usually adequate, unless $\hat{p}_1$ or $\hat{p}_2$ is quite close to 0 or 1. The closer $\hat{p}_1$ or $\hat{p}_2$ is to 0 or 1, the larger the sample size needed. If you are not sure whether your samples are large enough, consult a statistician.

All of these assumptions except the first appear to hold for the drug data. The observations in different samples are independent, since knowing whether patients in one group were verbally abusive tells us nothing about whether patients in the other group were verbally abusive. Observations within each sample are also independent. Knowing whether one patient in a sample was verbally abusive tells us nothing about whether another patient in that sample was verbally abusive. Finally, the samples are large enough, given sample proportions of 0.50 and 0.21.

Example 6.2

Suppose a patient given epidural analgesia after surgery complained of pain on one of seven postoperative days. Another patient was given injectable analgesics after the same surgery and complained of pain on six of seven postoperative days. The proportion of days on which the patient given epidural analgesia complained of pain is $1/7 = 0.14$. The proportion of days on which the patient given injectable analgesics complained of pain is $6/7 = 0.86$. Is a confidence interval appropriate to compare population proportions?

The two samples are independent, assuming the patients had no contact with each other. Knowing whether the patient given epidural analgesia reported pain tells us nothing about whether the patient given injectable analgesics reported pain. The observations within each sample are *not* independent because they are based on the same patient. We cannot use these data to obtain a confidence interval to compare population proportions.

If we want to evaluate the efficacy of epidural analgesia, we need to have more than one patient each in the epidural and no-epidural groups. We could then use a confidence interval to compare the proportion of epidural patients who complained frequently of pain with the proportion of no-epidural patients who complained frequently of pain.

Example 6.3

Suppose the response of 28 immunosuppressed patients to a series of tetanus vaccinations is studied. Ten of the patients were seropositive before vaccination and 23 were seropositive after vaccination. The prevaccination proportion of seropositive patients is $10/28 = 0.36$, and the postvaccination proportion of seropositive patients is $23/28 = 0.82$. Can we obtain a confidence interval for the difference between the prevaccination population proportion of seropositive patients and the postvaccination population proportion of seropositive patients?

The observations within each sample are independent, since the response of one patient to the vaccine tells us nothing about the response of another patient to the vaccine. The two samples are not independent. The same patients make up the prevaccination and postvaccination samples, so repeated measurements are obtained. We cannot use formula (6.4) to obtain a confidence interval for the difference between population proportions. Methods described in other texts can be used to compare proportions based on the same subjects by obtaining a confidence interval for the ratio of the population proportions.[4]

6.4 CONFIDENCE INTERVALS FOR POPULATION MEANS

A study of hypoxemia during the immediate postoperative period reported the fractions of ideal weight for 11 patients who became severely hypoxemic during transfer to the recovery room.[5] These data are shown in Table 6.1. Suppose we want to estimate the population mean fraction of ideal weight, where the population consists of all hypoxemic patients similar to those in the study. The sample mean fraction of 1.51 provides a point estimate of the population mean fraction μ, but an interval estimate of μ would be better.

If the data satisfy certain assumptions, we can obtain an interval estimate by constructing a confidence interval for the population mean μ. To do this, we need to use tables for a set of distributions called *t distributions*. These distributions are all symmetric and unimodal, with means of 0. Their frequency curves resemble the standard normal frequency curve, although *t* distributions have fatter tails (see Figure 6.1). The shape of a *t* distribution depends on a population parameter called the

TABLE 6.1 FRACTION OF IDEAL WEIGHT FOR 11 SEVERELY HYPOXEMIC PATIENTS

Patient No.	Fraction of Ideal Weight
1	1.64
2	0.98
3	1.57
4	1.41
5	1.40
6	1.75
7	2.26
8	1.30
9	1.63
10	1.29
11	1.33
Mean ± SD*	1.51 ± 0.33

*SD = standard deviation

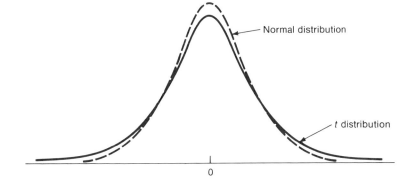

Figure 6.1 The t distribution with 5 degrees of freedom and the standard normal distribution

(number of) *degrees of freedom* (df), which can have the values 1, 2, 3, 4, ... The larger the degrees of freedom, the more closely a t distribution resembles the standard normal distribution.*

Table E.4 in Appendix E shows upper percentage points for selected t distributions. If t_d is a random variable having a t distribution with d degrees of freedom, the α *upper percentage point* for this t distribution is the number $t_{\alpha, d}$ such that

$$P(t_d \geq t_{\alpha, d}) = \alpha$$

For example, the 0.05 upper percentage point for the t distribution with 8 degrees of freedom is the number $t_{.05, 8}$ such that

$$P(t_8 \geq t_{.05, 8}) = 0.05$$

To get $t_{.05, 8}$ from Table E.4, we first find the row for 8 degrees of freedom. Degrees of freedom are listed in the first column of the table. We then find the column headed by 0.05. The number in the row for 8 degrees of freedom and in the column for 0.05 is $t_{.05, 8}$. We get $t_{.05, 8} = 1.860$, so

$$P(t_8 \geq 1.860) = 0.05$$

Table E.4 does not list all of the upper percentage points that might be needed. If we want to find $t_{.025, 73}$, we have to approximate, since Table E.4 does not list 73 degrees of freedom. The closest degrees of freedom in the table are 60, so we look up $t_{.025, 60}$. In the row for 60 degrees of freedom and in the column for 0.025, we find $t_{.025, 60} = 2.000$. Since $t_{.025, 73} \cong t_{.025, 60}$,[†]

$$P(t_{73} \geq 2.000) \cong 0.025$$

Now suppose we have a random sample of size n from a normal population, and we want to use the sample mean $\bar{x}$ to obtain an interval estimate of the population mean μ. Using methods outside the scope of this text, it can be shown that a $100(1 - \alpha)\%$ confidence interval for μ is given by the formula

$$\left(\bar{x} - (t_{\alpha/2, n-1}) \frac{s}{\sqrt{n}}, \bar{x} + (t_{\alpha/2, n-1}) \frac{s}{\sqrt{n}} \right) \quad (6.5)$$

Since the values of $\bar{x}$ and s are usually different for different samples, the confidence interval for μ is usually different for different samples. If 99% confidence intervals are used, 99% of all possible samples will produce 99% confidence intervals that include μ. One per cent of all possible samples will produce 99% confidence intervals that do *not* include μ. Since an interval estimate that includes μ will be produced 99% of the time, we are 99% sure that the 99% confidence interval we get includes μ.

Using the hypoxemia data, we can obtain a 99.9% confidence interval for the population mean fraction of ideal weight. Since the sample size n is 11, $n - 1 = 10$. Our α is 0.001, so $\alpha/2$ is 0.0005, and $t_{.0005, 10} = 4.587$. From Table 6.1, we get $\bar{x} = 1.51$ and $s = 0.33$. We apply formula (6.5) to obtain the 99.9% confidence interval

$$\left(1.51 - (4.587) \frac{0.33}{\sqrt{11}}, 1.51 + (4.587) \frac{0.33}{\sqrt{11}} \right)$$

$$(1.51 - 0.46, 1.51 + 0.46)$$

$$(1.05, 1.97)$$

We interpret this confidence interval by saying that we are 99.9% sure that the population mean fraction of ideal weight is between 1.05 and 1.97. We will never know whether μ is actually between 1.05 and 1.97, but we are 99.9% sure that it is. The confidence interval suggests that members of the population tend to be overweight, on average.

When confidence intervals are obtained, there is always a trade-off between precision and confidence. *The greater the confidence level, the wider the confidence interval*. The 99.9% confidence interval for the hypoxemia data is quite wide because of the high confidence level used. A confidence interval

---

*The t distributions are also called *Student's t distributions*, after the pseudonym "Student" of W. S. Gossett, who discovered them.

[†]Recall that the symbol " $\cong$ " means "is approximately equal to."

based on a lower confidence level would be narrower. This trade-off is also evident in the confidence intervals obtained from the PMS data. The 99% confidence interval for p is wider than the 95% confidence interval, which is wider than the 90% confidence interval. Whenever we increase the confidence level, we also increase the width of the confidence interval. This makes sense because a wide confidence interval pins down the population parameter less precisely than a narrow confidence interval does. Since a wide confidence interval contains more values, we have more confidence that it includes the population parameter.

Suppose we decide to settle for less confidence in order to get a more precise interval estimate of the hypoxemia population mean μ. If our confidence level is 95%, $\alpha = 0.05$, so $\alpha/2 = 0.025$ and $t_{.025, 10}$ = 2.228. Applying formula (6.5), we get the interval estimate

$$\left(1.51 - (2.228)\frac{0.33}{\sqrt{11}}, \ 1.51 + (2.228)\frac{0.33}{\sqrt{11}}\right)$$

$$(1.51 - 0.22, 1.51 + 0.22)$$

$$(1.29, 1.73)$$

The 95% confidence interval is much more precise than the 99.9% confidence interval. We interpret the 95% confidence interval by saying that we are 95% sure that the population mean fraction of ideal weight is between 1.29 and 1.73. Again, the confidence interval suggests that members of the population tend to be overweight, on average.

Other factors affecting the precision of confidence intervals are the variability of the data and the sample size. The more variable the data (i.e., the larger the standard deviation), the less precise the confidence interval. This makes sense. Estimates based on highly variable data are less trustworthy than estimates based on less variable data, and the confidence interval must be wider to compensate for this. In addition, large samples usually produce more precise confidence intervals than small samples. An estimate based on a large sample is more credible than an estimate based on a small sample.

Confidence intervals for population means are based on the following assumptions.

1. Random Sampling. If the sample is not biased, this assumption is not essential.

2. Independent Observations. If this assumption is violated, a confidence interval cannot be obtained for the population mean.

3. Sampling from a Normal Population. If the population does not appear to be exactly normal, a confidence interval can often be obtained for the population mean anyway. Thanks to the central limit theorem, a large enough sample size will compensate for a nonnormal population. The more nonnormal the population, the larger the sample size needed. If the population is extremely nonnormal (e.g., only a few values are possible), formula (6.5) should not be used to obtain a confidence interval for the population mean. A statistician should be consulted if you are not sure whether your sample is large enough to compensate for nonnormality.

Let us evaluate these assumptions for the hypoxemia data. The data cannot be a random sample (since there is no list of all patients with severe hypoxemia), but this is not crucial. Because the fraction of ideal weight for one patient tells us nothing about the fraction of ideal weight for another patient, the observations are independent. Do the data come from a normal population? A histogram of the data, shown in Figure 6.2, is consistent with a normal or approximately normal population. The data do not suggest any reason why a confidence interval cannot be obtained for the population mean.

Example 6.4

In a study of intra-articular fractures of the distal end of the radius, radiographs from 40 young adults with healed fractures were examined.[6] The severity of arthritis indicated by the radiographs can be rated as follows:

0 = not present
1 = minimal
2 = moderate

If the data are based on one fracture per patient, can a confidence interval be obtained for the population mean arthritis severity rating?

The ratings are independent, since the rating for one patient tells us nothing about the rating for

```
Count   Midpoint
    1       .75  |XXXXXXXXXX
    5      1.25  |XXXXXXXXXXXXXXXXXXXXXXXXXXXXXXXXXXXXXXXXXXXXXXXXXXXX
    4      1.75  |XXXXXXXXXXXXXXXXXXXXXXXXXXXXXXXXXXXXXXXXXX
    1      2.25  |XXXXXXXXXX
              I....+....I....+....I....+....I....+....I....+....I
              0         1         2         3         4         5
                        Histogram Frequency
```

Figure 6.2 SPSS/PC histogram of fraction of ideal weight

another patient. But the ratings are not even approximately normally distributed. With only three possible values, they are so extremely nonnormal that formula (6.5) cannot be used to obtain a confidence interval for the population mean rating. Instead, nonparametric methods described in other texts could be used to obtain a confidence interval for the population median rating.[7]

Example 6.5

Suppose a recent outbreak of antibiotic-resistant enteritis was linked to consumption of milk produced at the Swampfarm Dairy. Most of the cows at Swampfarm were treated with gentamicin shortly before the outbreak. As a result, several veterinarians investigated the concentration of gentamicin in milk two days after treatment with this antibiotic. Five cows were given gentamicin for one week. Two days after stopping gentamicin, the researchers collected milk from each cow and recorded the gentamicin concentration. After one month without antibiotic treatment, the same cows were used again to repeat the experiment. Can the resulting 10 concentrations be used to calculate a confidence interval for the population mean gentamicin concentration?

Concentrations from different cows are independent, but concentrations from the same cow are *not* independent. We cannot combine these 10 observations and calculate a confidence interval. If the population is normal or approximately normal, we can obtain a confidence interval for the population mean based on the five concentrations after the first treatment. These five observations are based on different cows and are independent. We can then obtain another confidence interval for the population mean based on the five concentrations after the second treatment, since these five observations are also independent. We can also calculate the average concentration for each cow by adding each cow's two concentrations and dividing the sum by two. A confidence interval for the population mean cow-average concentration can be obtained from this sample of five independent averages if the corresponding population of averages is normal.

6.5 CONFIDENCE INTERVALS FOR DIFFERENCES BETWEEN POPULATION MEANS

The comparison of means is one of the most common reasons for using statistical procedures in medical and health care research. When done properly, such comparisons are invaluable for determining the effects of treatments or diseases. In this chapter, we will describe three methods for comparing means. Each method is used under different circumstances, and use of the wrong method can produce extremely misleading results. Fortunately,

it is not difficult to determine which method should be used.

The first two methods we will discuss require two *independent* samples. The observations in one sample should tell us nothing about the observations in the other sample. We will call one of these methods the *pooled-variance confidence interval procedure* and the other the *separate-variance confidence-interval procedure*.

6.6 POOLED-VARIANCE CONFIDENCE INTERVALS FOR DIFFERENCES BETWEEN POPULATION MEANS

Suppose we have two independent samples from two normal populations with means μ_1 and μ_2 and *equal variances*. The variance of the first population is assumed to be equal to the variance of the second population. To compare the population means, we want to obtain a confidence interval for the difference $\mu_1 - \mu_2$ between the population means. From the first population, we have a sample of size n_1 with mean $\bar{x}_1$ and standard deviation s_1. From the second population, we have a sample of size n_2 with mean $\bar{x}_2$ and standard deviation s_2. The sample sizes n_1 and n_2 need not be equal.

To use the pooled-variance procedure, we need to compute an estimate of the common population standard deviation. Both of the sample standard deviations, s_1 and s_2, are estimates of the population standard deviation, and we will combine these two estimates into one *pooled estimate* of the population standard deviation. This pooled estimate, denoted by s_{pool}, is calculated as follows:

$$s_{pool} = \sqrt{\frac{(n_1 - 1)s_1^2 + (n_2 - 1)s_2^2}{n_1 + n_2 - 2}} \quad (6.6)$$

If we have independent random samples from two normal populations with equal variances, it can be shown that a $100(1 - \alpha)\%$ confidence interval for $\mu_1 - \mu_2$ is given by the formula

$$\left((\bar{x}_1 - \bar{x}_2) - (t_{\alpha/2, n_1+n_2-2})(s_{pool})\sqrt{\frac{1}{n_1} + \frac{1}{n_2}}, \right.$$
$$\left. (\bar{x}_1 - \bar{x}_2) + (t_{\alpha/2, n_1+n_2-2})(s_{pool})\sqrt{\frac{1}{n_1} + \frac{1}{n_2}} \right) \quad (6.7)$$

where $t_{\alpha/2, n_1+n_2-2}$ is the $\alpha/2$ upper percentage point of the t distribution with $n_1 + n_2 - 2$ degrees of freedom.

The interpretation of this confidence interval should sound familiar by now. If our confidence level is 98%, then 98% of all possible samples will produce 98% confidence intervals that include $\mu_1 - \mu_2$. Two per cent of all possible samples will produce 98% confidence intervals that do not include $\mu_1 - \mu_2$. We interpret a 98% confidence interval by saying that we are 98% sure that this interval estimate includes $\mu_1 - \mu_2$.

The pooled-variance confidence interval assumes that the population variances are equal. How can we check this assumption? If we do not know the population means, we usually do not know the population variances either. We do know the *sample* variances, and these are estimates of the population variances. As a rough guide, the following rule is helpful. If

$$0.5 \leq \frac{s_1^2}{s_2^2} \leq 2$$

assume that the population variances are equal. If s_1^2/s_2^2 is less than 0.5 or greater than 2, do *not* assume that the population variances are equal. If we cannot assume that the population variances are equal, a pooled-variance confidence interval should not be obtained. A separate-variance confidence interval (described in the next section) must be considered instead.

Pooled-variance confidence intervals are based on the following assumptions.

1. Random Sampling. As usual, random sampling is not essential if the samples are not biased.

2. Independent Samples. A pooled-variance confidence interval cannot be obtained for $\mu_1 - \mu_2$ if the samples are not independent.

3. Independent Observations Within Each Sample. If this assumption is violated, a confidence interval cannot be obtained for $\mu_1 - \mu_2$.

4. Sampling from Normal Populations. If the populations are not normal, a pooled-variance confidence interval can still be obtained for $\mu_1 - \mu_2$ if the samples are large enough to compensate for nonnormality. A pooled-variance confidence interval should not be obtained if the data are extremely nonnormal (e.g., if only a few values are possible). If you are not sure whether your samples are large enough to compensate for nonnormality, consult a statistician.

5. Equal Population Variances. A pooled-variance confidence interval cannot be obtained for $\mu_1 - \mu_2$ if the population variances are not equal or similar.

Example 6.6 _____

In a study of gonadal dysfunction in diabetic men, the serum total testosterone values shown in Table 6.2 were obtained for 11 diabetic men with primary organic impotence without vascular disease and for seven diabetic men with primary psychogenic impotence.[8] The men with organic impotence had a mean total testosterone of 524.0 ng/dl, while the men with psychogenic impotence had a mean total testosterone of 701.1 ng/dl. Can we obtain a pooled-variance confidence interval for the differ-

TABLE 6.2   SERUM TOTAL TESTOSTERONE FOR DIABETIC MEN

PATIENT No.	Primary Organic Impotence Without Vascular Disease SERUM TOTAL TESTOSTERONE (ng/dl)	PATIENT No.	Primary Psychogenic Impotence SERUM TOTAL TESTOSTERONE (ng/dl)
1	484	12	934
2	559	13	809
3	431	14	791
4	418	15	703
5	447	16	584
6	554	17	490
7	874	18	597
8	605		
9	399	Mean ± SD	701.1 ± 154.4
10	562		
11	431		
Mean ± SD*	524.0 ± 135.8		

*SD = standard deviation

ence between the population testosterone means? Here the first population consists of all diabetic men who are similar to those in the study and have primary organic impotence without vascular disease. The second population consists of all diabetic men who are similar to those in the study and have primary psychogenic impotence.

We need to determine whether the data satisfy the assumptions required. The samples are not random, but this is not essential. Since the testosterone values in one sample tell us nothing about the testosterone values in the other sample, the samples are independent. The observations within each sample are independent as well. Histograms of the sample testosterone levels, shown in Figures 6.3 and 6.4, suggest a slightly skewed population for the organic-impotence group and a normal or approximately normal population for the psychogenic-impotence group. The organic-impotence sample size of 11 is large enough to compensate for the degree of nonnormality indicated. To determine whether the equal-variance assumption is reasonable, we obtain the sample standard deviations from Table 6.2 and compute $s_1^2/s_2^2 = (135.8)^2/(154.4)^2 = 0.8$. Since $0.5 \leq 0.8 \leq 2$, it is reasonable to assume that the population variances are equal. We can obtain a pooled-variance confidence interval for $\mu_1 - \mu_2$.

We will calculate a 99% pooled-variance confidence interval for $\mu_1 - \mu_2$. We have $n_1 + n_2 - 2 = 11 + 7 - 2 = 16$ and $\alpha/2 = 0.01/2 = 0.005$. From Table E.4, we obtain $t_{.005, 16} = 2.921$. Applying formula (6.6) to calculate s_{pool}, we get

$$s_{\text{pool}} = \sqrt{\frac{(11-1)(135.8)^2 + (7-1)(154.4)^2}{11 + 7 - 2}}$$

$$= \sqrt{\frac{(10)(18441.6) + (6)(23839.4)}{16}} = 143.1$$

```
Count    Midpoint
   2      370.00  |XXXXXXXXXXXXXXXXXXXX
   4      490.00  |XXXXXXXXXXXXXXXXXXXXXXXXXXXXXXXXXXXXXXXXX
   4      610.00  |XXXXXXXXXXXXXXXXXXXXXXXXXXXXXXXXXXXXXXXXX
   0      730.00  |
   1      850.00  |XXXXXXXXXX
                  I....+....I....+....I....+....I....+....I....+....I
                  0         1         2         3         4         5
                           Histogram Frequency
```

Figure 6.3 SPSS/PC histogram of testosterone for diabetic men with primary organic impotence without vascular disease

```
Count    Midpoint
   1       400.00  |XXXXXXXXXX
   2       600.00  |XXXXXXXXXXXXXXXXXXXX
   3       800.00  |XXXXXXXXXXXXXXXXXXXXXXXXXXXXXX
   1      1000.00  |XXXXXXXXXX
                   I....+....I....+....I....+....I....+....I....+....I
                   0         1         2         3         4         5
                            Histogram Frequency
```

Figure 6.4 SPSS/PC histogram of testosterone for diabetic men with primary psychogenic impotence

Using these values in formula (6.7), we obtain a 99% confidence interval:

$$\left((524.0 - 701.1) - (2.921)(143.1)\sqrt{\frac{1}{11} + \frac{1}{7}} , \right.$$

$$\left. (524.0 - 701.1) + (2.921)(143.1)\sqrt{\frac{1}{11} + \frac{1}{7}} \right)$$

$$(-177.1 - 202.1, -177.1 + 202.1)$$

$$(-379.2, 25.0)$$

We are 99% sure that $\mu_1 - \mu_2$ is between -379.2 and 25.0. Since the lower endpoint is negative and the upper endpoint is positive, 0 is included in the confidence interval. At the 99% confidence level, we cannot rule out the possibility that $\mu_1 - \mu_2$ is equal to 0. Based on this confidence interval, we cannot say that the organic-impotence population and the psychogenic-impotence population have different testosterone means. If we use a lower confidence level, we might conclude that the population testosterone means are different.

Example 6.7

A study evaluated the use of whole-gut irrigation for the treatment of endotoxemia in active Crohn's disease.[9] Patients hospitalized for acute exacerba-

TABLE 6.3   ENDOTOXINS IN PLASMA (μg/l) FOR CONVENTIONAL AND IRRIGATION PATIENTS

Conventional Treatment			Irrigation		
	DAY OF HOSPITALIZATION			DAY OF HOSPITALIZATION	
PATIENT NO.	11	14	PATIENT NO.	11	14
1	11	0	10	11	3
2	0	0	11	0	0
3	2.5	0	12	0	0
4	12	0	13	0	1
5	20	10	14	0	0
6	4	6	15	3	7
7	7	0	16	0	8
8	11	8	17	3	3
9	11	8			
Mean ± SD*	6.1 ± 5.8			2.4 ± 3.4	

*SD = standard deviation

tion of Crohn's disease were randomly assigned to receive one of two treatments. Conventional treatment consisted of steroids and total parenteral nutrition. Irrigation treatment consisted of conventional treatment plus intestinal lavage with 5-aminosalicylic acid added to the lavage fluid. Table 6.3 shows the endotoxins in plasma for the conventional-treatment and irrigation-treatment patients. Can we obtain a pooled-variance confidence interval from these data for the difference between the conventional population endotoxin mean and the irrigation population endotoxin mean?

Since two endotoxin values were obtained for each patient, the data include repeated measurements. Observations for the same patient are not independent, and we cannot obtain a confidence interval for $\mu_1 - \mu_2$ based on all 34 observations.

We could split the data into two groups of data, day-11 observations and day-14 observations. This would produce two data sets, each consisting of independent observations. We could try to obtain two confidence intervals, one for the difference between the conventional population day-11 endotoxin mean and the irrigation population day-11 endotoxin mean, and one for the difference between the conventional population day-14 endotoxin mean and the irrigation population day-14 endotoxin mean. But the resulting data sets are so nonnormal that use of the pooled-variance confidence interval procedure is not justified. Instead, nonparametric methods described in other texts might be appropriate for obtaining a confidence interval for the difference between the day-11 population means and a confidence interval for the difference between the day-14 population means.[7]

If we averaged each patient's two endotoxin values, we would get 17 independent patient averages. The averaged values would have a more normal distribution than the original values. There is no statistical reason not to do this, but it does not make sense clinically. The day-14 observations were obtained later in hospitalization than the day-11 observations, and they do not measure the same thing as the day-11 observations. For this reason, the two sets of data should not be combined by averaging. We cannot obtain a pooled-variance confidence interval for $\mu_1 - \mu_2$.

6.7 SEPARATE-VARIANCE CONFIDENCE INTERVALS FOR DIFFERENCES BETWEEN POPULATION MEANS

Data often satisfy all of the assumptions for the pooled-variance procedure except the assumption of equal population variances. For such data, we can obtain a separate-variance confidence interval for $\mu_1 - \mu_2$. Because we cannot assume equal population variances, we need to use different degrees

of freedom for our t-distribution upper percentage points. The reason for this requires a proof that we will omit. Our degrees of freedom, which we will denote by f, are no longer $n_1 + n_2 - 2$. Instead, they are calculated according to the following formula.

$$f = \frac{\left(\dfrac{s_1^2}{n_1} + \dfrac{s_2^2}{n_2} \right)^2}{\dfrac{\left(\dfrac{s_1^2}{n_1} \right)^2}{n_1 - 1} + \dfrac{\left(\dfrac{s_2^2}{n_2} \right)^2}{n_2 - 1}} \qquad (6.8)$$

If you think this formula looks horrible, you are right. Using it is more painful than difficult, however. You simply have to keep track of where everything goes and what gets squared. Since f usually will not be an integer, and degrees of freedom must be an integer, you round f *down* to the closest integer smaller than f to obtain the degrees of freedom. If a computer with statistical software is available, it should be used to calculate f. There is no point in grinding f out by hand if you do not have to.

If we have two independent random samples from two normal populations, it can be shown that a $100(1 - \alpha)\%$ confidence interval for $\mu_1 - \mu_2$ is given by the formula

$$\left((\bar{x}_1 - \bar{x}_2) - \left(t_{\alpha/2, f} \right) \sqrt{\frac{s_1^2}{n_1} + \frac{s_2^2}{n_2}}, \right.$$

$$\left. (\bar{x}_1 - \bar{x}_2) + \left(t_{\alpha/2, f} \right) \sqrt{\frac{s_1^2}{n_1} + \frac{s_2^2}{n_2}} \right) \qquad (6.9)$$

where $t_{\alpha/2, f}$ is the $\alpha/2$ upper percentage point for the t distribution with f degrees of freedom.

We interpret this confidence interval in the usual way. If the confidence level is 90%, about 90% of all possible samples will produce 90% confidence intervals that include $\mu_1 - \mu_2$. Approximately 10% of all possible samples will produce 90% confidence intervals that do not include $\mu_1 - \mu_2$. We are 90% sure that the interval we calculate includes $\mu_1 - \mu_2$.

The separate-variance confidence interval does not use s_{pool}. It does not make sense to use this pooled estimate when the population variances are unequal, since we no longer have a common population standard deviation to estimate.

Separate-variance confidence intervals for $\mu_1 - \mu_2$ are based on the following assumptions.

1. Random Sampling. If the samples are not biased, random sampling is not essential.

2. Independent Samples. A separate-variance confidence interval cannot be obtained for $\mu_1 - \mu_2$ if the samples are not independent.

3. Independent Observations Within Each Sample. If the observations within each sample are not independent, a confidence interval cannot be obtained for $\mu_1 - \mu_2$.

4. Sampling from Normal Populations. If the samples are large enough to compensate for nonnormality, a separate-variance confidence interval can be obtained for $\mu_1 - \mu_2$ when the populations are not normal. A separate-variance confidence interval should not be obtained when the data are extremely nonnormal (e.g., if the data have only a few possible values). If you are not sure whether your samples are large enough to compensate for nonnormality, consult a statistician.

The separate-variance procedure does not assume that the population variances are *un*equal; it simply does not assume that they are equal. When the population variances are equal, it is *not* a mistake to obtain a separate-variance confidence interval. When the population variances are unequal, it *is* a mistake to obtain a pooled-variance confidence interval. If you have any reason to believe that the population variances are not equal, do not use the pooled-variance procedure.

Example 6.8

The serum progesterone levels for 29 women with ectopic pregnancies and 20 women with early intrauterine pregnancies are shown in Table 6.4.[10] For the women with normal pregnancies, the mean progesterone is 30.9 ng/ml. For the women with ectopic pregnancies, the mean progesterone is much lower—5.6 ng/ml. Can we obtain a confidence interval for the difference between the ectopic population progesterone mean and the normal population progesterone mean? Here the two populations consist of all women with ectopic pregnancies who are similar to those in the study and all women with early intrauterine pregnancies who are similar to those in the study.

As usual, the samples are not random, but this is not important. The samples are independent, since different women were used in the two samples and the progesterone levels for one sample tell us nothing about the progesterone levels for the other sample. The progesterone levels within each sample were obtained for different women and are independent. Histograms of the progesterone levels, shown in Figures 6.5 and 6.6, suggest nonnormal populations. The samples are large enough to compensate for this, however. Since the ratio of the sample variances is less than 0.5 $(s_1^2/s_2^2 = (3.6)^2/(6.9)^2 = 0.3)$, the pooled-variance procedure

TABLE 6.4   SERUM PROGESTERONE FOR WOMEN WITH ECTOPIC OR NORMAL PREGNANCY

Ectopic Pregnancy		Normal Pregnancy	
Patient No.	Progesterone (ng/ml)	Patient No.	Progesterone (ng/ml)
1	8.6	30	31.0
2	2.9	31	36.0
3	8.1	32	31.2
4	11.4	33	24.2
5	9.9	34	36.0
6	10.4	35	36.8
7	2.6	36	25.7
8	10.2	37	42.8
9	3.7	38	22.0
10	3.8	39	32.1
11	8.0	40	28.0
12	7.8	41	30.0
13	1.0	42	42.6
14	7.3	43	23.1
15	2.5	44	30.4
16	7.7	45	23.7
17	5.0	46	33.8
18	8.9	47	25.2
19	1.1	48	41.9
20	2.5	49	20.6
21	2.6		
22	3.7	Mean ± SD	30.9 ± 6.9
23	1.0		
24	8.3		
25	0.4		
26	2.8		
27	6.8		
28	12.9		
29	1.4		
Mean ± SD*	5.6 ± 3.6		

*SD = standard deviation

cannot be used. The separate-variance procedure is appropriate.

Let us obtain a 95% separate-variance confidence interval for $\mu_1 - \mu_2$. The degrees of freedom for our upper percentage point are, by formula (6.8),

$$
f = \frac{\left(\dfrac{(3.6)^2}{29} + \dfrac{(6.9)^2}{20} \right)^2}{\dfrac{\left(\dfrac{(3.6)^2}{29} \right)^2}{29 - 1} + \dfrac{\left(\dfrac{(6.9)^2}{20} \right)^2}{20 - 1}}
$$

$$
= \frac{(0.45 + 2.38)^2}{\dfrac{(0.45)^2}{28} + \dfrac{(2.38)^2}{19}}
$$

$$
= \frac{8.01}{0.007 + 0.298} = 26.3
$$

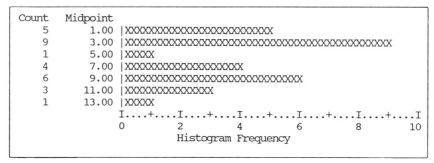

Figure 6.5 SPSS/PC histogram of progesterone for women with ectopic pregnancies

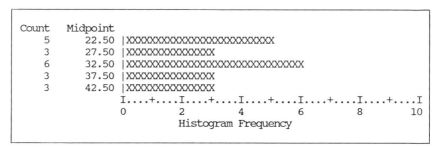

Figure 6.6 SPSS/PC histogram of progesterone for women with normal pregnancies

Rounding f down to the nearest integer, we get 26 degrees of freedom. Since $\alpha = 0.05$, $\alpha/2 = 0.025$ and $t_{.025, 26} = 2.056$. Applying formula (6.9), we get the 95% confidence interval

$$\left((5.6 - 30.9) - (2.056)\sqrt{\frac{(3.6)^2}{29} + \frac{(6.9)^2}{20}},\right.$$

$$\left.(5.6 - 30.9) + (2.056)\sqrt{\frac{(3.6)^2}{29} + \frac{(6.9)^2}{20}}\right)$$

$$(-25.3 - 3.5, -25.3 + 3.5)$$

$$(-28.8, -21.8)$$

Since both endpoints of the confidence interval are negative, we are 95% sure that $\mu_1 - \mu_2$ is negative. Hence, we are 95% sure that the ectopic-pregnancy population mean μ_1 is smaller than the normal-pregnancy population mean μ_2. We interpret the confidence interval as follows:

We are 95% sure that the progesterone mean for the ectopic-pregnancy population is smaller than the progesterone mean for the normal-pregnancy population and the difference between these population means is between -28.8 and -21.8. Thus, we are 95% sure that the ectopic-pregnancy popu-

lation progesterone mean is much smaller than the normal-pregnancy population progesterone mean.

When a confidence interval for $\mu_1 - \mu_2$ has two negative endpoints, we can be fairly sure that μ_1 is smaller than μ_2. If both endpoints are positive, we can be fairly sure that μ_1 is larger than μ_2. If the lower endpoint is negative and the upper endpoint is positive, 0 is included in the confidence interval and we cannot be sure that μ_1 does not equal μ_2.

Example 6.9

A study assessed the efficacy of metaprolol in the prevention and treatment of supraventricular tachycardia (SVT) after coronary artery bypass grafting.[11] Table 6.5 shows the day of onset of SVT for patients who developed SVT after surgery. For the 21 SVT episodes for the control patients, the average day of onset is 3.1. For the nine SVT episodes for the patients given metaprolol, the average day of onset is 4.1. Can we obtain a confidence interval for the difference between the control population mean day of onset and the metaprolol population mean day of onset?

As usual, we do not have random samples, but this is not crucial. The two samples appear to be independent, since the observations for one sample tell us nothing about the observations for the other

TABLE 6.5 DAY OF ONSET OF SVT AFTER OPERATION FOR METAPROLOL AND CONTROL PATIENTS

Control Group		Metaprolol Group	
PATIENT NO.	DAY OF ONSET	PATIENT NO.	DAY OF ONSET
1	2	19	1
2	4	20	4
3	2		6
4	2		8
	5	21	4
5	6	22	2
6	3		5
7	2	23	6
8	3	24	1
9	2		
10	6	Mean ± SD	4.1 ± 2.4
11	4		
12	1		
13	5		
14	2		
15	1		
16	1		
	2		
	3		
17	5		
18	4		
Mean ± SD*	3.1 ± 1.6		

*SD = standard deviation

TABLE 6.6 RESULTS OF ACTH STIMULATION TESTS IN HEALTHY DOGS

Dog No.	Baseline Cortisol (μg/dl)	Post-ACTH Cortisol (μg/dl)
1	2.9	9.1
2	1.8	11.0
3	1.3	9.5
4	7.2	15.3
5	5.3	8.4
6	3.3	11.7
7	3.3	14.1
8	1.9	7.9
9	1.7	10.7
10	2.6	6.6
11	2.4	12.1
12	3.7	9.7
13	3.5	11.5
14	2.2	7.8
15	11.7	18.4
16	1.4	9.2
17	1.3	8.2
18	1.1	8.2
19	1.5	9.6
20	1.5	7.3
Mean ± SD*	3.1 ± 2.5	10.3 ± 2.9

*SD = standard deviation

sample. Examination of Table 6.5, however, reveals repeated measurements on patients 4, 16, 20, and 22. These patients had more than one episode of SVT. Since repeated measurements on the same subject are not independent, the within-samples independence assumption is violated.

We could eliminate the repeated measurements by using only the day of onset for the first episode of SVT. This would produce 24 independent observations, but the normality assumption would not be reasonable. The resulting data would take only the values 1, 2, 3, 4, 5, and 6. We cannot obtain a pooled-variance or separate-variance confidence interval for the difference between the control population mean day of onset and the metaprolol population mean day of onset. If only the 24 independent observations are used, nonparametric methods described in other texts might be appropriate for obtaining a confidence interval for the difference between the control population mean and the metaprolol population mean.[7]

Example 6.10

In a study of adrenal-function testing in dogs, ACTH stimulation testing was done on 20 healthy dogs.[12] The resulting cortisol values are shown in Table 6.6. The mean baseline cortisol value for these dogs is

3.1 μg/dl, and the mean cortisol value one hour after ACTH injection is 10.3 μg/dl. Can we obtain a pooled-variance or separate-variance confidence interval for the difference between the population mean baseline cortisol and the population mean post-ACTH cortisol?

The within-samples independence assumption is satisfied, since the cortisol values for one dog tell us nothing about the cortisol values for another dog. The between-samples independence assumption does not hold. The two samples were obtained by taking two measurements on each dog, and these measurements cannot be considered independent. Knowing the baseline cortisol gives us some information about the post-ACTH cortisol. Neither the pooled-variance procedure nor the separate-variance procedure can be used to obtain a confidence interval for $\mu_1 - \mu_2$. In the next section, we will discuss a confidence-interval procedure that can be used for data such as these.

6.8 PAIRED-SAMPLES CONFIDENCE INTERVALS FOR DIFFERENCES BETWEEN POPULATION MEANS

Not all comparisons of population means are based on independent samples. Medical and health care research frequently involves before-versus-after studies, in which measurements taken before treatment are compared with measurements taken after treatment. Baseline measurements are obtained for each subject before treatment, and the measurements are repeated for each subject after treatment. The result is two *nonindependent* samples of observations, the before-treatment measurements and the after-treatment measurements. When such designs are used, the variability of the results is sometimes greatly reduced.

In general, *nonindependent samples result when two measurements of the same quantity are taken on the same subjects.* In Example 6.10, nonindependent samples were obtained by taking baseline cortisol measurements and post-ACTH cortisol measurements. Nonindependent samples can also be produced when each subject is deliberately paired with another subject on the basis of some important characteristic. A patient may be paired with his twin, or patients may be matched with respect to age, sex, length of illness, and so on.

If the pairing is successful, in the sense that paired subjects respond in a similar way, the measurements for paired subjects will not be independent. Knowing how one member of a pair responds will provide some information about how the other member of the pair responds. Using successfully paired subjects reduces variability, since each subject has a similar control for comparison. Samples obtained by pairing subjects or by measuring something twice are called *paired samples.*

Paired samples are quite useful for comparing means when analyzed correctly. A common mistake, seen all too often in print, is the use of independent-samples procedures to analyze paired samples. Because this error can produce extremely misleading results, it is important to be able to distinguish between paired and independent samples. How can we tell whether or not two samples are paired? This is entirely a matter of *experimental design.* If we are given two samples of numbers but no information about the design of the study, there is no way we can determine whether the observations were paired. If pairing was done or repeated measurements were obtained, any well-written report will say so. If no basis for pairing is described, it is usually safe to assume that subjects were not paired.

When paired samples are used, the appropriate procedure for obtaining confidence intervals for $\mu_1 - \mu_2$ is the *paired-samples procedure.* To use this method, we convert the two paired samples into a single sample of *differences.* For each pair of observations, we subtract one observation from the other to obtain the difference between the two observations. If the observations for the first sample are denoted by x_{1i} and the observations for the second sample by x_{2i}, we calculate the difference

$$d_i = x_{1i} - x_{2i}$$

for each pair. We end up with one sample of differences. Let us denote the mean of the differences by $\bar{d}$ and the standard deviation of the differences by s_d. It can be shown that the population mean of the differences is equal to $\mu_1 - \mu_2$ and that

$$\bar{d} = \bar{x}_1 - \bar{x}_2$$

Our point estimate of $\mu_1 - \mu_2$ is $\bar{d}$.

If the sample of *differences* is a random sample from a normal population, it can be shown that a $100(1 - \alpha)\%$ confidence interval for $\mu_1 - \mu_2$ is given by the formula

$$\left(\bar{d} - \left(t_{\alpha/2, n-1} \right) \frac{s_d}{\sqrt{n}}, \ \bar{d} + \left(t_{\alpha/2, n-1} \right) \frac{s_d}{\sqrt{n}} \right) \quad (6.10)$$

where n is the number of *differences.* We interpret this confidence interval in the usual way. If a 95% confidence level is used, 95% of all possible samples will produce confidence intervals that include $\mu_1 - \mu_2$. Five per cent of all possible samples will produce confidence intervals that do not include $\mu_1 - \mu_2$. For this reason, we are 95% sure that the 95% confidence interval we calculate includes $\mu_1 - \mu_2$.

Paired-samples confidence intervals are based on the following assumptions.

1. Random Sampling of Differences. As long as the sample is not biased, the differences need not be a random sample.

2. Paired Samples. A paired-samples confidence interval cannot be obtained for $\mu_1 - \mu_2$ if the samples are not paired.

3. Independent Differences. Knowing the value of one difference should not tell you anything about the value of another difference. If the differences are not independent, a confidence interval cannot be obtained for $\mu_1 - \mu_2$.

4. Sampling of Differences from a Normal Population. Ideally, the *differences* should come from a normal population. If the population of differences is not normal, a paired-samples confidence interval can still be obtained for $\mu_1 - \mu_2$ as long as the sample of differences is large enough to compensate for the nonnormality of the population. A paired-samples confidence interval should not be obtained if the data are extremely nonnormal (e.g., if the differences have only a few possible values). Consult a statistician if you are not sure whether the number of differences is large enough to compensate for a nonnormal population.

Example 6.11 _____

A study evaluated the effect of maternal care of hospitalized infants on maternal anxiety.[13] Fourteen

TABLE 6.7 SPIELBERGER TOTAL STATE ANXIETY BEFORE AND AFTER TIME IN A CBPU

Mother No.	Before CBPU	After CBPU	Difference (Before − After)
1	158	150	8
2	162	122	40
3	138	125	13
4	191	164	27
5	148	138	10
6	172	134	38
7	156	114	42
8	197	199	− 2
9	162	122	40
10	234	222	12
11	172	141	31
12	127	136	− 9
13	183	132	51
14	195	193	2
Mean ± SD*	171.1 ± 27.6	149.4 ± 33.0	21.6 ± 19.0

*SD = standard deviation

mothers spent 36 to 48 hours in a care-by-parent unit (CBPU) just before their infants were discharged from a neonatal intensive care unit. The Spielberger State Anxiety Inventory was used to measure maternal anxiety before spending time in a CBPU and after spending time in a CBPU. Table 6.7 shows total state anxiety scores before and after time in a CBPU.

The two samples are obviously paired, since two anxiety scores were obtained for each mother. Can we obtain a paired-samples confidence interval for the difference between the before-CBPU population mean anxiety score and the after-CBPU population mean anxiety score? Here the populations are the theoretical populations that would result if before-CBPU and after-CBPU anxiety scores were obtained for all mothers who are similar to those in the study and have infants in neonatal intensive care units.

The differences are not a random sample, but they appear to be independent, since the difference for one mother tells us nothing about the difference for another mother. A histogram of the *differences* is shown in Figure 6.7.* The histogram does not look exactly normal, but the sample is large enough to compensate for a slightly nonnormal population.

Since the data do not suggest any reason why a paired-samples confidence interval should not be obtained, we will obtain a 90% paired-samples confidence interval for $\mu_1 - \mu_2$. From Table 6.7, we get

---

*We do not obtain histograms for the original paired samples because no assumptions are made about the populations from which the paired samples were taken. Even if these populations are normal, this does *not* imply that the population of differences is normal.

$\bar{d} = 21.6$ and $s_d = 19.0$. Our α is 0.10, so $\alpha/2 = 0.05$ and $t_{.05,\,13} = 1.771$. Using formula (6.10), we obtain the 90% confidence interval

$$\left(21.6 - (1.771)\frac{19.0}{\sqrt{14}}, \, 21.6 + (1.771)\frac{19.0}{\sqrt{14}} \right)$$

$$(21.6 - 9.0, \, 21.6 + 9.0)$$

$$(12.6, 30.6)$$

Since both endpoints of the confidence interval are positive, we are 90% sure that the before-CBPU population anxiety score mean is larger than the after-CBPU population anxiety score mean. We interpret this confidence interval as follows:

> We are 90% sure that the before-CBPU population anxiety score mean is larger than the after-CBPU population anxiety score mean and that the difference between these population means is between 12.6 and 30.6. The difference might be small (as low as 12.6), moderate (no more than 30.6), or somewhere in between.

How do we determine whether a difference between population means is small, moderate, or large? This does not require any medical knowledge about the variable that is studied. Medical knowledge is needed only to assess the clinical importance of a difference. We evaluate the size of a difference in terms of the magnitude of the data. The anxiety scores from the maternal anxiety study have values between 122 and 234, with most values less than 170. For data such as these, a population mean difference of 12.6 is small and a difference of 30.6 is moderate. A difference of 60 would be large.

If the data had ranged between 0 and 10, a population mean difference of 12.6 would be quite large. If the data had ranged between 1000 and 3000, a population mean difference of 12.6 would be quite small. The units of the data must be considered when determining how large a population mean difference is. Judgments about the size of a difference may vary slightly. One person's small difference may be another person's moderate difference, and one person's moderate difference may be another person's large difference. Unless judgments about size are extremely discrepant, such disagreements are usually not important.

Example 6.12

In a study of gastric emptying, the retention of radiolabeled meals was measured at various times for eight healthy subjects.[14] Some of the results are shown in Table 6.8. Can we use the paired-samples procedure to obtain a confidence interval for the difference between the population mean retention

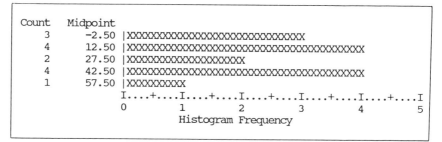

```
Count   Midpoint
  3     -2.50  |XXXXXXXXXXXXXXXXXXXXXXXXXXXXXX
  4     12.50  |XXXXXXXXXXXXXXXXXXXXXXXXXXXXXXXXXXXXXXXX
  2     27.50  |XXXXXXXXXXXXXXXXXXX
  4     42.50  |XXXXXXXXXXXXXXXXXXXXXXXXXXXXXXXXXXXXXXXX
  1     57.50  |XXXXXXXXXX
               I....+....I....+....I....+....I....+....I....+....I
               0         1         2         3         4         5
                              Histogram Frequency
```

Figure 6.7 SPSS/PC histogram of anxiety score difference

TABLE 6.8   RETENTION (%) OF RADIOLABELED MEALS AT 40 MINUTES AND 60 MINUTES

Subject No.	40 Min	60 Min	Subject No.	40 Min	60 Min
1	79	67	5	61	58
	55	47		71	55
	72	58		77	58
	82	72		54	32
2	76	48	6	90	58
	71	54		86	67
	79	68		59	41
	74	62		56	56
3	46	28	7	58	47
	55	43		66	29
	64	31		49	28
	61	45		73	57
4	40	27	8	62	44
	31	9		82	51
	56	28		66	50
	39	25		49	33

TABLE 6.9   PREOPERATIVE AND POSTOPERATIVE NEUROPSYCHOLOGICAL SCORES

Patient No.	Preop Score	Postop Score	Patient No.	Preop Score	Postop Score
1	3	2	21	1	2
2	2	1	22	3	3
3	0	0	23	0	0
4	3	2	24	3	3
5	2	1	25	1	1
6	4	1	26	0	0
7	2	1	27	0	0
8	2	1	28	3	3
9	3	0	29	0	0
10	4	1	30	1	1
11	3	2	31	2	2
12	1	0	32	3	3
13	4	0	33	1	1
14	3	1	34	3	3
15	3	2	35	3	3
16	2	1	36	3	3
17	3	4	37	3	3
18	1	2	38	2	2
19	1	1	39	1	1
20	3	4	40	3	3

at 40 minutes and the population mean retention at 60 minutes?

The samples are obviously paired, but four 40-minute and four 60-minute observations were obtained for each patient, based on four meals per patient. Each patient has four differences, and the differences for any given patient cannot be considered independent. Since the assumption of independent differences is not satisfied, we cannot obtain a paired-samples confidence interval for $\mu_1 - \mu_2$ using these 32 differences. We could split the data into four samples of eight differences: a meal-1 sample, a meal-2 sample, a meal-3 sample, and a meal-4 sample. Each of these four subsamples would satisfy the assumption of independent differences. If the normality assumption holds, a confidence interval could then be obtained from each subsample.

Example 6.13

Forty patients with normal-pressure hydrocephalus were evaluated before and after a ventriculoatrial shunt operation.[15] Table 6.9 shows the preoperative

and postoperative neuropsychological scores for these patients. The higher the score, the greater the degree of neurological and psychological impairment. Can a paired-samples confidence interval be obtained for the difference between the population preoperative mean neurological score and the population postoperative mean neurological score?

The study uses a before–after design, so the samples are paired. The differences are independent, since there is only one difference per patient and the difference for one patient tells us nothing about the difference for another patient. But the differences are extremely nonnormal, taking only the values 0, 1, 2, and 3. We cannot obtain a paired-samples confidence interval for the difference between the preoperative mean score and the postoperative mean score. Instead, nonparametric methods described in other texts might be appropriate for obtaining a confidence interval for the population median difference between the preoperative score and the postoperative score.[7]

The procedure used to compare two population means can greatly affect the results. For this reason, you should always clearly state which procedure was used. It is not enough to say that a 95% confidence interval was obtained for the difference between the population means. A person reading this statement has no way of knowing whether the correct procedure was used. Vague statements like this are common in medical and health care journals, making it impossible to evaluate many statistical analyses. A description of statistical methods should allow the reader to determine exactly what procedures were used. Further information about reporting statistical results is given in Appendix B.

6.9 ESTIMATION PITFALLS

Certain errors in estimation are common enough to warrant discussion here.

1. Misinterpretation of Confidence Intervals. The most common misinterpretation involves the mistaken notion that population parameters are random variables. Suppose that a 95% confidence interval for the population mean hematocrit for patients with a particular illness is (21, 34). Many people would interpret this confidence interval by saying that the probability that the population mean hematocrit is between 21 and 34 is 0.95. This is entirely wrong, since the population mean is a fixed number and not a random variable. *The fact that we do not know the value of μ does not make μ a random variable.*

If the unknown population mean hematocrit is actually 38, the probability that μ is between 21 and 34 is the probability that 38 is between 21 and 34. This probability is 0, since 38 is never between 21 and 34. If the unknown population mean hematocrit is actually 32, the probability that μ is between 21 and 34 is the probability that 32 is between 21 and 34. This probability is 1, since 32 is always between 21 and 34. The probability that a population parameter is between any two fixed numbers is either 0 or 1.

The correct way to interpret a 95% confidence interval is to say that you are 95% sure that the confidence interval includes the population parameter. Your confidence arises from the fact that 95% of all 95% confidence intervals do include the population parameter.

2. Violation of Independence Assumptions. Many people assume that there must be a way to statistically analyze a large number of repeated measurements on one or two subjects. As a result, they incorrectly apply statistical methods requiring independent observations to such data. If repeated measurements could be analyzed so simply, we would often need only one subject for research. Suppose that we want to estimate the population mean duration of arthritis-pain relief for a new anti-inflammatory drug, where the population consists of all patients with rheumatoid arthritis. We could select one patient with rheumatoid arthritis, give her the drug once a day for 50 consecutive days, and measure the duration of pain relief each day. In this way, we could obtain a sample of 50 observations.

Since the observations would not be independent, we could not use statistical procedures to generalize to the population of all patients with rheumatoid arthritis. It would not make sense if we could. Fifty observations from one patient are not equivalent to 50 observations from 50 patients. It is not difficult to select one patient whose response to a drug is consistently atypical, and such a patient would produce 50 misleading observations. But it is quite difficult to select 50 patients whose responses are atypical. Although several of the 50 patients might show unusual responses, their responses would usually be outweighed by the other, more typical responses and would have little effect on the sample mean. *We cannot make inferences about a population with more than one subject unless we have observations from more than one subject.*

3. Extreme Violations of Normality Assumptions. Because of the central limit theorem, data need not be exactly normally distributed in order for us to obtain confidence intervals for population means or differences between population means. But we cannot use these procedures to analyze data with only a few possible values. Extremely nonnormal data are often analyzed incorrectly in the medical and health care literature. Statistical procedures that are appropriate for such data are discussed in Chapters 10 and 11.

SUMMARY

Estimation is the use of sample statistics to estimate population parameters. A confidence interval is an interval estimate that is constructed in a way that ensures that the interval will contain the population parameter a specified percentage of the time. Confidence intervals for population proportions and for differences between population proportions are based on upper percentage points from the standard normal distribution. Confidence intervals for population means and for differences between population means are based on upper percentage points from t distributions. There are three types of confidence intervals for differences between population means: the pooled-variance confidence interval, the separate-variance confidence interval, and the paired-samples confidence interval. These confidence intervals require different assumptions.

Some confidence interval assumptions are more flexible than others. If the independence assumptions for a confidence interval are not met, the confidence interval cannot be obtained. If the normality assumptions for a confidence interval are not met, the confidence interval can still be obtained if approximate normality holds. Confidence intervals that require normality cannot be obtained if the data are extremely nonnormal.

We interpret a $100(1 - \alpha)\%$ confidence interval by saying that we are $100(1 - \alpha)\%$ sure that the confidence interval contains the population parameter. We do *not* say that the probability that the confidence interval contains the population parameter is $1 - \alpha$. If a confidence interval for the difference between population proportions or population means contains 0, we cannot say that the population proportions or population means are different. If a confidence interval for the difference between population proportions or population means does not contain 0, we are fairly sure that the population proportions or population means are different.

FORMULAS FOR QUANTITIES NEEDED TO OBTAIN CONFIDENCE INTERVALS

$$s_{\text{prop}} = \sqrt{\frac{\hat{p}(1 - \hat{p})}{n}}$$

$$s_{\text{diff}} = \sqrt{\frac{\hat{p}_1(1 - \hat{p}_1)}{n_1} + \frac{\hat{p}_2(1 - \hat{p}_2)}{n_2}}$$

$$s_{\text{pool}} = \sqrt{\frac{(n_1 - 1)s_1^2 + (n_2 - 1)s_2^2}{n_1 + n_2 - 2}}$$

$$s_d = \sqrt{\frac{\sum_{i=1}^{n} (d_i - \bar{d})^2}{n - 1}}$$

$$f = \frac{\left(\dfrac{s_1^2}{n_1} + \dfrac{s_2^2}{n_2}\right)^2}{\dfrac{\left(\dfrac{s_1^2}{n_1}\right)^2}{n_1 - 1} + \dfrac{\left(\dfrac{s_2^2}{n_2}\right)^2}{n_2 - 1}}$$

CONFIDENCE INTERVAL FORMULAS

Population parameter	$100(1 - \alpha)\%$ confidence interval
p	$(\hat{p} - (z_{\alpha/2})(s_{\text{prop}}), \hat{p} + (z_{\alpha/2})(s_{\text{prop}}))$
$p_1 - p_2$	$((\hat{p}_1 - \hat{p}_2) - (z_{\alpha/2})(s_{\text{diff}}), (\hat{p}_1 - \hat{p}_2) + (z_{\alpha/2})(s_{\text{diff}}))$
μ	$\left(\bar{x} - (t_{\alpha/2, n-1})\dfrac{s}{\sqrt{n}}, \bar{x} + (t_{\alpha/2, n-1})\dfrac{s}{\sqrt{n}}\right)$
$\mu_1 - \mu_2$	For INDEPENDENT samples, WITH equal-variance assumption $\left((\bar{x}_1 - \bar{x}_2) - (t_{\alpha/2, n_1+n_2-2})(s_{\text{pool}})\sqrt{\dfrac{1}{n_1} + \dfrac{1}{n_2}}, \right.$ $\left. (\bar{x}_1 - \bar{x}_2) + (t_{\alpha/2, n_1+n_2-2})(s_{\text{pool}})\sqrt{\dfrac{1}{n_1} + \dfrac{1}{n_2}}\right)$
$\mu_1 - \mu_2$	For INDEPENDENT samples, WITHOUT equal-variance assumption $\left((\bar{x}_1 - \bar{x}_2) - (t_{\alpha/2, f})\sqrt{\dfrac{s_1^2}{n_1} + \dfrac{s_2^2}{n_2}}, \right.$ $\left. (\bar{x}_1 - \bar{x}_2) + (t_{\alpha/2, f})\sqrt{\dfrac{s_1^2}{n_1} + \dfrac{s_2^2}{n_2}}\right)$
$\mu_1 - \mu_2$	For PAIRED samples $\left(\bar{d} - (t_{\alpha/2, n-1})\dfrac{s_d}{\sqrt{n}}, \bar{d} + (t_{\alpha/2, n-1})\dfrac{s_d}{\sqrt{n}}\right)$

PROBLEMS

Beginning with this chapter, most of the problems resemble real-life data analysis. Data do not come stamped with the names of appropriate statistical procedures, and these problems do not specify appropriate confidence interval procedures. Instead, data are presented and a question is asked. You must do the following.

1. Select an appropriate confidence-interval procedure. If no procedure discussed in this chapter is appropriate, indicate which assumptions are violated by the data.

2. If an appropriate procedure is described in this chapter, obtain a confidence interval. The confidence level is specified in the problem so you can check your answer.

3. If a confidence interval is obtained, *interpret* it. Your interpretation must answer the question asked in the problem.

In the real world, you would use a computer to obtain descriptive statistics and histograms. For this reason, descriptive statistics and histograms are provided when necessary. Unnecessary statistics and histograms are also given in some problems. Do not worry about slightly or moderately nonnormal histograms if the data have a large number of possible values. Unless the histogram is extremely nonnormal and the sample is very small, you can assume that the central limit theorem applies to the data.

1. Construct a flowchart that will help you determine which of the confidence interval procedures discussed in this chapter might be appropriate for particular data sets. The flowchart should begin as follows:

the morbidity was 59%. For 15 well-nourished patients, the morbidity was 20%. Do the data provide evidence that the malnourished population morbidity differs from the well-nourished population morbidity? Use a 95% confidence level.

3. A study evaluated the effect of diet on serum ammonia in epileptic patients receiving valproic acid (VPA) therapy.[17] Table 6.10 shows the serum ammonia levels after fasting and after an oral protein load for 10 epileptic patients on VPA therapy. Histograms are shown in Figures 6.8 through 6.10. Do the data provide evidence that the population serum ammonia mean after fasting differs from the population serum ammonia mean after an oral protein load? Use a 95% confidence level.

4. In a study of lorcainide use in patients taking digoxin, the antiarrhythmic effect of lorcainide was investigated.[18] Table 6.11 shows the number of premature ventricular depolarizations (PVDs) per hour for 12 patients while taking lorcainide or a placebo. Histograms are shown in Figures 6.11 through 6.13. Do the data provide evidence that the population mean number of PVDs when lorcainide is used differs from the population mean number of PVDs when the placebo is used? Use a 90% confidence level.

5. A study of verbal abuse of nurses found that 82% of 421 staff nurses reported experience with verbal abuse in their practice.[19] Can a 90% confidence interval be obtained from the data? If so, calculate and interpret this interval.

6. In a study of surgical treatment of Zollinger-Ellison syndrome (ZES), the ratio of basal acid output to maximal acid output (BAO/MAO) was reported for 32 patients with ZES.[20] These ratios are shown in Table 6.12. A histogram is shown in

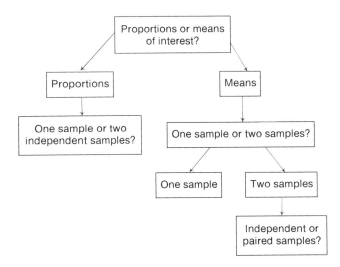

2. A study investigated the effect of malnutrition on morbidity after major gastrointestinal surgery for benign disease.[16] For 17 malnourished patients,

Figure 6.14. Can a 99% confidence interval be obtained from the data? If so, calculate and interpret this interval.

**TABLE 6.10 SERUM AMMONIA (µg/dl) AFTER FASTING
AND AFTER ORAL PROTEIN LOAD**

Patient No.	Fasting	Protein Load	Difference (Protein Load − Fasting)
1	58	58	0
2	107	185	78
3	54	145	91
4	62	214	152
5	33	93	60
6	126	58	− 68
7	90	375	285
8	66	205	139
9	85	180	95
10	143	426	283
Mean ± SD	82.4 ± 34.6	193.9 ± 123.4	111.5 ± 111.1

```
Count   Midpoint
  1       20.00  |XXXXXXXXXX
  4       60.00  |XXXXXXXXXXXXXXXXXXXXXXXXXXXXXXXXXXXXXXXXXX
  3      100.00  |XXXXXXXXXXXXXXXXXXXXXXXXXXXXXX
  2      140.00  |XXXXXXXXXXXXXXXXXXXX
               I....+....I....+....I....+....I....+....I....+....I
               0         1         2         3         4         5
                         Histogram Frequency
```

Figure 6.8 SPSS/PC histogram of serum ammonia after fasting

```
Count   Midpoint
  4      100.00  |XXXXXXXXXXXXXXXXXXXXXXXXXXXXXXXXXXXXXXXXXX
  4      200.00  |XXXXXXXXXXXXXXXXXXXXXXXXXXXXXXXXXXXXXXXXXX
  0      300.00  |
  2      400.00  |XXXXXXXXXXXXXXXXXXXX
               I....+....I....+....I....+....I....+....I....+....I
               0         1         2         3         4         5
                         Histogram Frequency
```

Figure 6.9 SPSS/PC histogram of serum ammonia after oral protein load

```
Count   Midpoint
  1      -50.00  |XXXXXXXXXX
  5       50.00  |XXXXXXXXXXXXXXXXXXXXXXXXXXXXXXXXXXXXXXXXXXXXXXXXXXXX
  2      150.00  |XXXXXXXXXXXXXXXXXXXX
  2      250.00  |XXXXXXXXXXXXXXXXXXXX
               I....+....I....+....I....+....I....+....I....+....I
               0         1         2         3         4         5
                         Histogram Frequency
```

Figure 6.10 SPSS/PC histogram of serum ammonia difference

TABLE 6.11 NUMBER OF PVDs PER HOUR FOR PATIENTS TAKING DIGOXIN WHEN GIVEN LORCAINIDE OR PLACEBO

Patient No.	Placebo	Lorcainide	Difference (Placebo − Lorcainide)
1	150	196	− 46
2	389	444	− 55
3	27	68	− 41
4	100	104	− 4
5	756	911	− 155
6	50	0	50
7	446	437	9
8	146	0	146
9	398	374	24
10	187	32	155
11	153	31	122
12	288	445	− 157
Mean ± SD	257.5 ± 209.5	253.5 ± 276.4	4.0 ± 103.9

```
Count   Midpoint
   7     100.00  |XXXXXXXXXXXXXXXXXXXXXXXXXXXXXXXXXXXX
   3     300.00  |XXXXXXXXXXXXXXX
   1    . 500.00  |XXXXX
   1     700.00  |XXXXX
                 I....+....I....+....I....+....I....+....I....+....I
                 0         2         4         6         8        10
                         Histogram Frequency
```

Figure 6.11 SPSS/PC histogram of number of PVDs per hour when given placebo

```
Count   Midpoint
   7     100.00  |XXXXXXXXXXXXXXXXXXXXXXXXXXXXXXXXXXXXX
   1     300.00  |XXXXX
   3     500.00  |XXXXXXXXXXXXXXX
   0     700.00  |
   1     900.00  |XXXXX
                 I....+....I....+....I....+....I....+....I....+....I
                 0         2         4         6         8        10
                         Histogram Frequency
```

Figure 6.12 SPSS/PC histogram of number of PVDs per hour when given lorcainide

```
Count   Midpoint
   2    -150.00  |XXXXXXXXXXXXXXXXXX
   4     -50.00  |XXXXXXXXXXXXXXXXXXXXXXXXXXXXXXXXXXXXX
   3      50.00  |XXXXXXXXXXXXXXXXXXXXXXXXXXX
   3     100.00  |XXXXXXXXXXXXXXXXXXXXXXXXXXX
                 I....+....I....+....I....+....I....+....I....+....I
                 0         1         2         3         4         5
                         Histogram Frequency
```

Figure 6.13 SPSS/PC histogram of PVD difference

TABLE 6.12 RATIO OF BASAL ACID OUTPUT TO MAXIMAL ACID OUTPUT FOR PATIENTS WITH ZES

0.92	1.00	0.61	1.00	0.96
0.88	0.57	0.63	0.92	0.68
0.82	0.53	0.83	0.76	0.73
0.94	0.98	0.61	1.00	0.80
0.67	1.00	0.94	0.52	
0.90	0.35	1.00	0.61	
0.64	0.57	0.62	0.80	

Mean ± SD 0.77 ± 0.18

7. In a study evaluating surgical repair of giant retinal tears, operations were performed on 27 eyes of 25 patients.[21] The surgery was successful for 89% of these eyes. Can a 95% confidence interval be obtained from the data? If so, calculate and interpret this interval.

8. A study examined the effect of zearalenone on the fertility of virgin dairy heifers.[22] For the 16 heifers randomly assigned to receive zearalenone, the conception rate was 62%. For the 15 heifers randomly assigned to receive a placebo, the conception rate was 87%. Do the data provide evidence that the zearalenone population conception rate differs from the placebo population conception rate? Use a 95% confidence level.

TABLE 6.13 NAUSEA SCORE FOR CANCER PATIENTS GIVEN CIS-PLATINUM DURING DAY OR NIGHT

	6:00 a.m.–6:00 p.m.	6:00 p.m.–6:00 a.m.
	41	47
	32	42
	48	37
	41	25
	53	33
	43	18
		42
Mean ± SD	43.0 ± 7.1	34.9 ± 10.3

```
Count    Midpoint
   1        .39   |XXXXX
   9        .56   |XXXXXXXXXXXXXXXXXXXXXXXXXXXXXXXXXXXXXXXXXXXXXXX
   7        .73   |XXXXXXXXXXXXXXXXXXXXXXXXXXXXXXXXXXX
   9        .90   |XXXXXXXXXXXXXXXXXXXXXXXXXXXXXXXXXXXXXXXXXXXXXXX
   6       1.07   |XXXXXXXXXXXXXXXXXXXXXXXXXXXXXX
                  I....+....I....+....I....+....I....+....I....+....I
                  0         2         4         6         8        10
                             Histogram Frequency
```

Figure 6.14 SPSS/PC histogram of BAO/MAO ratio

```
Count    Midpoint
   1       35.00  |XXXXXXXXXX
   4       45.00  |XXXXXXXXXXXXXXXXXXXXXXXXXXXXXXXXXXXXXXXXXX
   1       55.00  |XXXXXXXXXX
                  I....+....I....+....I....+....I....+....I....+....I
                  0         1         2         3         4         5
                             Histogram Frequency
```

Figure 6.15 SPSS/PC histogram of day nausea score

```
Count    Midpoint
   1       20.00  |XXXXXXXXXX
   2       30.00  |XXXXXXXXXXXXXXXXXXXX
   3       40.00  |XXXXXXXXXXXXXXXXXXXXXXXXXXXXXX
   1       50.00  |XXXXXXXXXX
                  I....+....I....+....I....+....I....+....I....+....I
                  0         1         2         3         4         5
                             Histogram Frequency
```

Figure 6.16 SPSS/PC histogram of night nausea score

9. In a study of cis-platinum–induced nausea and vomiting, the effect of time of cis-platinum administration on nausea and vomiting was investigated.[23] Table 6.13 shows the nausea scores for six cancer patients given cis-platinum between 6:00 a.m. and 6:00 p.m. (day group) and seven cancer patients given cis-platinum between 6:00 p.m. and 6:00 a.m. (night group). The higher the nausea score, the worse the nausea. Histograms are shown in Figures 6.15 and 6.16. Do the data provide evidence that the day population nausea score mean differs from the night population nausea score mean? Use a 90% confidence level.

10. A study evaluated the effectiveness of synthetic human calcitonin for treating Paget's disease of bone.[24] Fourteen patients with refractory Paget's disease were treated with synthetic human calcitonin and monitored for improvement. Table 6.14 shows the pain severity rating before and after treatment for these patients. Histograms are shown in Figures 6.17 through 6.19. Do the data provide evidence that the population pain score mean before calcitonin differs from the population pain score mean after calcitonin? Use a 90% confidence level.

TABLE 6.14 PAIN SEVERITY BEFORE AND AFTER TREATMENT*

Patient No.	Pain Severity		Difference (Initial − Final)
	INITIAL	FINAL	
1	3	3	0
2	2	1	1
3	2	1	1
4	3	0	3
5	2	1	1
6	2	2	0
7	2	0	2
8	2	1	1
9	3	2	1
10	1	0	1
11	1	1	0
12	3	1	2
13	3	1	2
14	1	0	1
Mean ± SD	2.1 ± 0.8	1.0 ± 0.9	1.1 ± 0.9

*0 = none, 1 = mild, 2 = moderate, 3 = severe

```
Count   Midpoint
  3        1.50  |XXXXXXXXXXXXXXX
  6        2.50  |XXXXXXXXXXXXXXXXXXXXXXXXXXXXXX
  5        3.50  |XXXXXXXXXXXXXXXXXXXXXXXXX
                 I....+....I....+....I....+....I....+....I....+....I
                 0        2        4        6        8        10
                          Histogram Frequency
```

Figure 6.17 SPSS/PC histogram of initial pain severity

```
Count   Midpoint
  4         .50  |XXXXXXXXXXXXXXXXXXX
  7        1.50  |XXXXXXXXXXXXXXXXXXXXXXXXXXXXXXXXXX
  2        2.50  |XXXXXXXXXX
  1        3.50  |XXXXX
                 I....+....I....+....I....+....I....+....I....+....I
                 0        2        4        6        8        10
                          Histogram Frequency
```

Figure 6.18 SPSS/PC histogram of final pain severity

```
Count   Midpoint
  3         .50  |XXXXXXXXXXXXXXX
  7        1.50  |XXXXXXXXXXXXXXXXXXXXXXXXXXXXXXXXXXXXXX
  3        2.50  |XXXXXXXXXXXXXXX
  1        3.50  |XXXXX
                 I....+....I....+....I....+....I....+....I....+....I
                 0        2        4        6        8        10
                          Histogram Frequency
```

Figure 6.19 SPSS/PC histogram of pain severity difference

TABLE 6.15 RESTING ENERGY EXPENDITURE (kcal / 24 hr) IN PATIENTS WITH ELD AND IN NORMAL SUBJECTS

	Patients with ELD	Normal Subjects
	2130	2180
	1590	2110
	1760	1970
	2090	1750
	1290	1620
	2080	1750
	1840	1500
	1430	1300
	1660	2310
	1490	1550
Mean ± SD	1736.0 ± 296.4	1804.0 ± 328.2

TABLE 6.16 CT ATROPHY RATING FOR SCHIZOPHRENIC PATIENTS*

Paranoid Schizophrenia		Undifferentiated Schizophrenia
3		2
3		3
1		2
3		3
4		1
2		
1	Mean ± SD	2.2 ± 0.8
Mean ± SD 2.4 ± 1.1		

*1 = normal, 2 = slight, 3 = mild, 4 = moderate

11. In a study of end-stage liver disease (ELD), the resting energy expenditure (REE) was measured for 10 patients with ELD and 10 unpaired normal subjects.[25] These data are shown in Table 6.15. Histograms are shown in Figures 6.20 and 6.21. Do the data provide evidence that the population REE mean for patients with ELD differs from the population REE mean for people without ELD? Use a 99% confidence level.

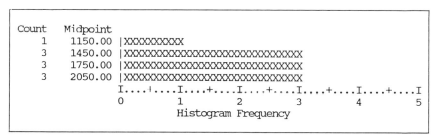

```
Count    Midpoint
   1     1150.00  |XXXXXXXXXX
   3     1450.00  |XXXXXXXXXXXXXXXXXXXXXXXXXXXXXX
   3     1750.00  |XXXXXXXXXXXXXXXXXXXXXXXXXXXXXX
   3     2050.00  |XXXXXXXXXXXXXXXXXXXXXXXXXXXXXX
                  I....+....I....+....I....+....I....+....I....+....I
                  0         1         2         3         4         5
                         Histogram Frequency
```

Figure 6.20 SPSS/PC histogram of REE in ELD patients

```
Count    Midpoint
   3     1450.00  |XXXXXXXXXXXXXXXXXXXXXXXXXXXXXX
   3     1750.00  |XXXXXXXXXXXXXXXXXXXXXXXXXXXXXX
   3     2050.00  |XXXXXXXXXXXXXXXXXXXXXXXXXXXXXX
   1     2350.00  |XXXXXXXXXX
                  I....+....I....+....I....+....I....+....I....+....I
                  0         1         2         3         4         5
                         Histogram Frequency
```

Figure 6.21 SPSS/PC histogram of REE in normal subjects

```
Count    Midpoint
   2       1.50  |XXXXXXXXXXXXXXXXXXXX
   1       2.50  |XXXXXXXXXX
   3       3.50  |XXXXXXXXXXXXXXXXXXXXXXXXXXXXXX
   1       4.50  |XXXXXXXXXX
                 I....+....I....+....I....+....I....+....I....+....I
                 0         1         2         3         4         5
                        Histogram Frequency
```

Figure 6.22 SPSS/PC histogram of CT atrophy rating for patients with paranoid schizophrenia

TABLE 6.17   FLEA COUNTS FOR DOGS DIPPED WITH SSS OR WATER

	SSS Dip	Water Dip
	88	109
	30	13
	26	121
	49	142
	106	147
Mean ± SD	59.8 ± 35.6	106.4 ± 54.4

TABLE 6.18   FEV₁ (% PREDICTED) FOR ASTHMATICS AND NORMAL SUBJECTS BEFORE HISTAMINE

	Asthmatics	Normal Subjects
	83.6	90.2
	68.4	100.7
	103.4	118.3
	83.0	101.6
	85.0	87.1
	80.4	
Mean ± SD	84.0 ± 11.3	99.6 ± 12.2

12. In a study of regional brain function in schizophrenia, computed tomography (CT) brain atrophy ratings were obtained for seven patients with paranoid schizophrenia and five patients with undifferentiated schizophrenia.[26] These ratings are shown in Table 6.16. Histograms are shown in Figures 6.22 and 6.23. Do the data provide evidence that the population mean CT atrophy rating for paranoid schizophrenics differs from the population mean CT atrophy rating for undifferentiated schizophrenics? Use a 99% confidence level.

13. A study evaluated the effectiveness of Avon's Skin-So-Soft (SSS) as a flea repellent for dogs.[27] Table 6.17 shows the flea counts for 10 dogs one day after a sponge dip with SSS or water. Histograms are shown in Figures 6.24 and 6.25. Do the data provide evidence that the population flea count mean for dogs treated with SSS differs from the population flea count mean for dogs treated with water? Use a 95% confidence level.

Figure 6.23   SPSS/PC histogram of CT atrophy rating for patients with undifferentiated schizophrenia

Figure 6.24   SPSS/PC histogram of flea count for dogs dipped with SSS

Figure 6.25   SPSS/PC histogram of flea count for dogs dipped with water

```
Count   Midpoint
    1     72.50  |XXXXXXXXXX
    4     87.50  |XXXXXXXXXXXXXXXXXXXXXXXXXXXXXXXXXXXXXXXXXX
    1    102.50  |XXXXXXXXXX
             I....+....I....+....I....+....I....+....I....+....I
             0         1         2         3         4         5
                            Histogram Frequency
```

Figure 6.26 SPSS/PC histogram of FEV_1 for asthmatics

```
Count   Midpoint
    1     82.50  |XXXXXXXXXX
    3     97.50  |XXXXXXXXXXXXXXXXXXXXXXXXXXXXXX
    1    112.50  |XXXXXXXXXX
             I....+....I....+....I....+....I....+....I....+....I
             0         1         2         3         4         5
                            Histogram Frequency
```

Figure 6.27 SPSS/PC histogram of FEV_1 for normal subjects

TABLE 6.19 NITROGEN BALANCE BEFORE AND AFTER TPN AND VITAMIN TREATMENT

Patient No.	Nitrogen Balance (g/day)		Difference (Initial − Final)
	INITIAL	FINAL	
1	−3.4	10.1	−13.5
2	−7.5	2.3	−9.8
3	−6.2	10.9	−17.1
4	3.1	9.2	−6.1
5	2.9	11.5	−8.6
6	−6.0	5.0	−11.0
7	3.8	−0.7	4.5
8	1.7	7.0	−5.3
9	−9.6	−0.7	−8.9
10	0.0	3.7	−3.7
Mean ± SD	−2.1 ± 5.0	5.8 ± 4.6	−8.0 ± 5.9

14. In a study comparing the bronchoconstrictor activity of leukotriene E_4 and histamine, one-second forced expiratory volume (FEV_1) measurements were reported for six asthmatic subjects and five normal subjects before inhalation of histamine.[28] These data are shown in Table 6.18. Histograms are shown in Figures 6.26 and 6.27. Do the data provide evidence that the population FEV_1 mean for asthmatics differs from the population FEV_1 mean for nonasthmatics? Use a 90% confidence level.

15. In a study of parenteral vitamins in total parenteral nutrition (TPN), patients were given high daily vitamin doses with TPN.[29] Table 6.19 shows the nitrogen balance for 10 male patients before treatment and after 10 days of treatment. Histograms are shown in Figures 6.28 through 6.30. Do the data provide evidence that the population nitrogen balance mean after treatment differs from the

```
Count   Midpoint
    1    -10.50  |XXXXXXXXXX
    2     -7.50  |XXXXXXXXXXXXXXXXXXXXX
    2     -4.50  |XXXXXXXXXXXXXXXXXXXXX
    0     -1.50  |
    3      1.50  |XXXXXXXXXXXXXXXXXXXXXXXXXXXXXX
    2      4.50  |XXXXXXXXXXXXXXXXXXXXX
             I....+....I....+....I....+....I....+....I....+....I
             0         1         2         3         4         5
                            Histogram Frequency
```

Figure 6.28 SPSS/PC histogram of initial nitrogen balance

```
Count    Midpoint
   2        .50   |XXXXXXXXXXXXXXXXXXXX
   2       3.50   |XXXXXXXXXXXXXXXXXXXX
   2       6.50   |XXXXXXXXXXXXXXXXXXXX
   3       9.50   |XXXXXXXXXXXXXXXXXXXXXXXXXXXXXX
   1      12.50   |XXXXXXXXXX
                  I....+....I....+....I....+....I....+....I....+....I
                  0         1         2         3         4         5
                            Histogram Frequency
```

Figure 6.29 SPSS/PC histogram of final nitrogen balance

```
Count    Midpoint
   1      -15.60  |XXXXXXXXXX
   3      -11.60  |XXXXXXXXXXXXXXXXXXXXXXXXXXXXXX
   3       -7.60  |XXXXXXXXXXXXXXXXXXXXXXXXXXXXXX
   2       -3.60  |XXXXXXXXXXXXXXXXXXXX
   0         .40  |
   1        4.40  |XXXXXXXXXX
                  I....+....I....+....I....+....I....+....I....+....I
                  0         1         2         3         4         5
                            Histogram Frequency
```

Figure 6.30 SPSS/PC histogram of nitrogen balance difference

TABLE 6.20 NEUTROPHIL COUNT ($\times 10^9/l$) FOR PATIENTS WITH ACUTE OR CHRONIC SEVERE APLASTIC ANEMIA

	Acute AA	Chronic AA
	5.2	2.6
	5.9	2.6
	4.9	1.7
	2.3	2.2
	3.8	1.9
	2.4	2.7
	3.7	2.7
	1.6	2.7
	2.2	
Mean ± SD	3.6 ± 1.5	2.4 ± 0.4

population nitrogen balance mean before treatment? Use a 95% confidence level.

16. In a study of androstane therapy for treatment of aplastic anemia (AA), neutrophil counts were reported for nine patients with acute severe AA and eight patients with chronic severe AA.[30] These counts are shown in Table 6.20. Histograms are shown in Figures 6.31 and 6.32. Do the data provide evidence that the population mean neutrophil count for patients with acute severe AA differs from the population mean neutrophil count for patients with chronic severe AA? Use a 99% confidence level.

17. A study of cardiac dysfunction in β-thalassemia major reported the average hemoglobin levels for 22 patients with β-thalassemia major.[31] These values are shown in Table 6.21. A histogram is shown in Figure 6.33. Can a 90% confidence inter-

```
Count    Midpoint
   1       1.50   |XXXXXXXXXX
   3       2.50   |XXXXXXXXXXXXXXXXXXXXXXXXXXXXXX
   2       3.50   |XXXXXXXXXXXXXXXXXXXX
   1       4.50   |XXXXXXXXXX
   2       5.50   |XXXXXXXXXXXXXXXXXXXX
                  I....+....I....+....I....+....I....+....I....+....I
                  0         1         2         3         4         5
                            Histogram Frequency
```

Figure 6.31 SPSS/PC histogram of neutrophil count for patients with acute severe aplastic anemia

```
Count   Midpoint
   2      1.65  |XXXXXXXXXXXXXXXXXXXX
   3      2.35  |XXXXXXXXXXXXXXXXXXXXXXXXXXXXXX
   3      3.05  |XXXXXXXXXXXXXXXXXXXXXXXXXXXXXX
              I....+....I....+....I....+....I....+....I....+....I
              0         1         2         3         4         5
                         Histogram Frequency
```

Figure 6.32 SPSS/PC histogram of neutrophil count for patients with chronic severe aplastic anemia

TABLE 6.21 AVERAGE HEMOGLOBIN LEVELS (g/dl) FOR PATIENTS WITH β-THALASSEMIA MAJOR

9.3	8.9	9.6	7.7	11.4	9.5
10.3	10.3	9.5	8.4	11.1	10.9
10.3	10.2	10.8	8.7	10.2	
10.4	8.7	9.8	9.6	8.5	

Mean ± SD 9.7 ± 1.0

TABLE 6.22 NUMBER OF *ANCYLOSTOMA* WORMS RECOVERED AT POSTMORTEM

	Untreated Cats	Cats Given Ivermectin
	2	0
	5	0
	6	0
	4	0
	20	0
	3	0
Mean ± SD	6.7 ± 6.7	0.0 ± 0.0

val be obtained from the data? If so, calculate and interpret this interval.

18. In a study of the anthelmintic efficacy of ivermectin in cats, ivermectin was administered to naturally parasitized cats.[32] Table 6.22 shows the numbers of *Ancylostoma* spp worms recovered at the postmortem examination for six untreated cats and six cats given ivermectin. Histograms are shown in Figures 6.34 and 6.35. Do the data provide evidence that the population mean number of worms for untreated cats differs from the population mean number of worms for treated cats? Use a 95% confidence level.

19. A study evaluated an education program concerning fall prevention for elderly patients.[33] Table 6.23 shows the fall prevention test scores for eight elderly patients before and after the education program. Histograms are shown in Figures 6.36

```
Count   Midpoint
   1      7.75  |XXXXX
   5      8.65  |XXXXXXXXXXXXXXXXXXXXXXXXX
   6      9.55  |XXXXXXXXXXXXXXXXXXXXXXXXXXXXXX
   7     10.45  |XXXXXXXXXXXXXXXXXXXXXXXXXXXXXXXXXXX
   3     11.35  |XXXXXXXXXXXXXX
              I....+....I....+....I....+....I....+....I....+....I
              0         2         4         6         8        10
                         Histogram Frequency
```

Figure 6.33 SPSS/PC histogram of average hemoglobin

```
Count   Midpoint
   4      3.00  |XXXXXXXXXXXXXXXXXXXXXXXXXXXXXXXXXXXXXXXXX
   1      9.00  |XXXXXXXXXX
   0     15.00  |
   1     21.00  |XXXXXXXXXX
              I....+....I....+....I....+....I....+....I....+....I
              0         1         2         3         4         5
                         Histogram Frequency
```

Figure 6.34 SPSS/PC histogram of number of *Ancylostoma* worms recovered from untreated cats

```
Count    Midpoint
   6        .50 |XXXXXXXXXXXXXXXXXXXXXXXXXXXXXXX
                I....+....I....+....I....+....I....+....I....+....I
                0         2         4         6         8        10
                          Histogram Frequency
```

Figure 6.35 SPSS/PC histogram of number of *Ancylostoma* worms recovered from treated cats

TABLE 6.23 FALL PREVENTION TEST SCORE (% CORRECT) BEFORE AND AFTER EDUCATIONAL PROGRAM

Patient No.	Before Program	After Program	Difference (Before − After)
1	36	91	−55
2	45	100	−55
3	54	100	−46
4	36	81	−45
5	81	100	−19
6	27	63	−36
7	36	45	−9
8	18	27	−9
Mean ± SD	75.9 ± 28.1	41.6 ± 19.2	−34.2 ± 19.4

through 6.38. Do the data provide evidence that the population test score mean before the program differs from the population test score mean after the program? Use a 99% confidence level.

20. In a study of urinary steroid conjugates after administration of gonadotropin-releasing hormone (GnRH), five infertile women with secondary amenorrhea were given GnRH therapy.[34] The peak urinary estrogen conjugates for these women are shown in Table 6.24. A histogram is shown in Figure 6.39. Can a 99% confidence interval be obtained from the data? If so, calculate and interpret this interval.

21. In a study of liver transplantation for hepatic failure, the number of days in coma was reported for 29 patients with acute or subacute hepatic failure.[35] These data are shown in Table 6.25. Histograms are shown in Figures 6.40 and 6.41. Do the data provide evidence that the population mean number of days in coma for patients with acute hepatic failure differs from the population mean number of days in coma for patients with subacute hepatic failure? Use a 95% confidence level.

22. A study investigated the sleep patterns of elderly people in long-term-care facilities.[36] Patients were asked about their sleep patterns before and after admission to long-term care. Of the 102 patients studied, 36.2% reported that they always woke up at intervals before admission and 59.9% reported that they always woke up at intervals after

```
Count    Midpoint
   2       20.00 |XXXXXXXXXXXXXXXXXXXX
   4       40.00 |XXXXXXXXXXXXXXXXXXXXXXXXXXXXXXXXXXXXXXXXXX
   1       60.00 |XXXXXXXXXX
   1       80.00 |XXXXXXXXXX
                 I....+....I....+....I....+....I....+....I....+....I
                 0         1         2         3         4         5
                           Histogram Frequency
```

Figure 6.36 SPSS/PC histogram of test score before educational program

```
Count    Midpoint
   1       20.00 |XXXXXXXXXX
   1       40.00 |XXXXXXXXXX
   1       60.00 |XXXXXXXXXX
   1       80.00 |XXXXXXXXXX
   4      100.00 |XXXXXXXXXXXXXXXXXXXXXXXXXXXXXXXXXXXXXXXXXX
                 I....+....I....+....I....+....I....+....I....+....I
                 0         1         2         3         4         5
                           Histogram Frequency
```

Figure 6.37 SPSS/PC histogram of test score after educational program

```
Count    Midpoint
  2       -57.50   |XXXXXXXXXXXXXXXXXXX
  3       -42.50   |XXXXXXXXXXXXXXXXXXXXXXXXXXXXX
  0       -27.50   |
  3       -12.50   |XXXXXXXXXXXXXXXXXXXXXXXXXXXXX
                   I....+....I....+....I....+....I....+....I....+....I
                   0         1         2         3         4         5
                             Histogram Frequency
```

Figure 6.38   SPSS/PC histogram of test score difference

TABLE 6.24   PEAK URINARY ESTROGEN CONJUGATES

Patient	Cycle No.	Peak Estrogen Conjugates
SD	1	144
	2	102
ML	1	180
	2	310
KT	1	128
	2	120
	3	180
	4	690
	5	138
	6	124
	7	220
TB	1	184
	2	96
KA	1	158
	Mcan ⊥ SD	198.1 ± 151.9

TABLE 6.25   NUMBER OF DAYS IN COMA FOR PATIENTS WITH ACUTE OR SUBACUTE HEPATIC FAILURE

Acute	Subacute
3	0
0	0
0	4
0	0
2	0
4	0
2	1
0	0
0	0
0	4
7	0
4	0
0	0
5	
2	Mean ± SD 0.7 ± 1.5
0	
Mean ± SD 1.8 ± 2.2	

```
Count    Midpoint
  7       100.00   |XXXXXXXXXXXXXXXXXXXXXXXXXXXXXXXXXXXXXX
  5       200.00   |XXXXXXXXXXXXXXXXXXXXXXXXXXX
  1       300.00   |XXXXX
  0       400.00   |
  0       500.00   |
  0       600.00   |
  1       700.00   |XXXXX
                   I....+....I....+....I....+....I....+....I....+....I
                   0         2         4         6         8         10
                             Histogram Frequency
```

Figure 6.39   SPSS/PC histogram of peak estrogen conjugates

```
Count    Midpoint
  8        1.00   |XXXXXXXXXXXXXXXXXXXXXXXXXXXXXXXXXXXXXXXXXX
  4        3.00   |XXXXXXXXXXXXXXXXXXXX
  3        5.00   |XXXXXXXXXXXXXXX
  1        7.00   |XXXXX
                  I....+....I....+....I....+....I....+....I....+....I
                  0         2         4         6         8         10
                            Histogram Frequency
```

Figure 6.40   SPSS/PC histogram of days in coma for acute patients

```
Count   Midpoint
  11      1.00  |XXXXXXXXXXXXXXXXXXXXXXXXXXXX
   0      3.00  |
   2      5.00  |XXXXX
              I....+....I....+....I....+....I....+....I....+....I
              0        4        8       12       16       20
                        Histogram Frequency
```

Figure 6.41 SPSS/PC histogram of days in coma for subacute patients

**TABLE 6.26 INTRAOCULAR PRESSURE BEFORE
AND AFTER ALT**

Eye No.	Intraocular Pressure (mm Hg)		Difference
	PRE-ALT	POST-ALT	
1	20	15	5
2	22	18	4
3	21	21	0
4	23	13	10
5	20	17	3
6	14	14	0
7	15	13	2
8	21	20	1
9	20	14	6
10	23	14	9
11	22	17	5
12	15	8	7
13	28	23	5
14	17	18	−1
15	23	20	3
16	21	16	5
17	14	15	−1
18	20	13	7
19	27	28	−1
20	13	14	−1
21	17	15	2
22	22	16	6
23	18	18	0
24	20	20	0
25	17	13	4
26	22	22	0
27	19	22	−3
28	25	25	0
29	19	14	5
30	21	20	1
Mean ± SD	20.0 ± 3.7	17.2 ± 4.3	2.8 ± 3.3

```
Count   Midpoint
   3     14.00  |XXXXXXXXXXXXXX
   2     16.00  |XXXXXXXXX
   4     18.00  |XXXXXXXXXXXXXXXXXXX
   7     20.00  |XXXXXXXXXXXXXXXXXXXXXXXXXXXXXXXXX
   8     22.00  |XXXXXXXXXXXXXXXXXXXXXXXXXXXXXXXXXXXXXX
   3     24.00  |XXXXXXXXXXXXXX
   1     26.00  |XXXXX
   2     28.00  |XXXXXXXXX
              I....+....I....+....I....+....I....+....I....+....I
              0        2        4        6        8       10
                        Histogram Frequency
```

Figure 6.42 SPSS/PC histogram of pre-ALT intraocular pressure

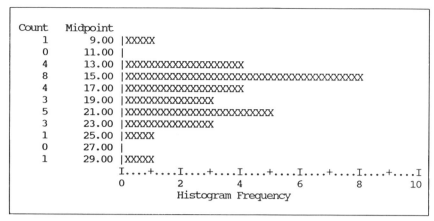

```
Count    Midpoint
  1         9.00  |XXXXX
  0        11.00  |
  4        13.00  |XXXXXXXXXXXXXXXXXXXX
  8        15.00  |XXXXXXXXXXXXXXXXXXXXXXXXXXXXXXXXXXXXXXXX
  4        17.00  |XXXXXXXXXXXXXXXXXXXX
  3        19.00  |XXXXXXXXXXXXXXX
  5        21.00  |XXXXXXXXXXXXXXXXXXXXXXXXX
  3        23.00  |XXXXXXXXXXXXXXX
  1        25.00  |XXXXX
  0        27.00  |
  1        29.00  |XXXXX
                  I....+....I....+....I....+....I....+....I....+....I
                  0         2         4         6         8        10
                          Histogram Frequency
```

Figure 6.43 SPSS/PC histogram of post-ALT intraocular pressure

```
Count    Midpoint
  1         3.00  |XXXXX
  4        -1.00  |XXXXXXXXXXXXXXXXXXXX
  8         1.00  |XXXXXXXXXXXXXXXXXXXXXXXXXXXXXXXXXXXXXXXX
  4         3.00  |XXXXXXXXXXXXXXXXXXXX
  7         5.00  |XXXXXXXXXXXXXXXXXXXXXXXXXXXXXXXXXXXXX
  4         7.00  |XXXXXXXXXXXXXXXXXXXX
  1         9.00  |XXXXX
  1        11.00  |XXXXX
                  I....+....I....+....I....+....I....+....I....+....I
                  0         2         4         6         8        10
                          Histogram Frequency
```

Figure 6.44 SPSS/PC histogram of intraocular pressure difference

admission. Do the data provide evidence that the population proportion of patients with sleep disturbances before admission differs from the population proportion of patients with sleep disturbances after admission? Use a 90% confidence level.

23. A study of blunt bovine and equine trauma reported that 69% of 134 patients admitted as a result of bovine or equine trauma had orthopedic injuries.[37] Can a 95% confidence interval be obtained from the data? If so, calculate and interpret this interval.

24. A study of anticipatory nausea in chemotherapy reported that 65% of 34 patients receiving cisplatin-based chemotherapy experienced anticipatory nausea.[38] Can a 99% confidence interval be obtained from the data? If so, calculate and interpret this interval.

25. A study evaluated argon laser trabeculoplasty (ALT) following failed trabeculectomy in patients with glaucoma.[39] Table 6.26 shows the intraocular pressure (IOP) before and after ALT for 30 eyes from 25 patients. Histograms are shown in Figures 6.42 through 6.44. Do the data provide evidence that the population IOP mean before ALT differs from the population IOP mean after ALT? Use a 95% confidence level.

REFERENCES

1. Brayshaw ND, Brayshaw DD: Thyroid hypofunction in premenstrual syndrome (correspondence). N Engl J Med *315*:1486–1487, 1986.

2. Metheny NA, Spies M, Eisenberg P: Frequency of nasoenteral tube displacement and associated risk factors. Res Nurs Health *9*:241–247, 1986.

3. Butler FR, Burgio LD, Engel BT: Neuroleptics and behavior: A comparative study. J Gerontol Nurs *13*:15–19, 1987.

4. Schlesselman JJ: Case-Control Studies. New York: Oxford, 1982.

5. Tyler IL, Tantisira B, Winter PM, et al: Continuous monitoring of arterial oxygen saturation with pulse oximetry during transfer to the recovery room. Anesth Analg *64*:1108–1112, 1985.

6. Knirk JL, Jupiter JB: Intra-articular fractures of the distal end of the radius in young adults. J Bone Joint Surg *68A*:647–659, 1986.

7. Conover WJ: Practical Nonparametric Statistics. 2nd ed. New York: Wiley, 1980.

8. Murray FT, Wyss HU, Thomas RG, et al: Gonadal dysfunction in diabetic men with organic impotence. J Clin Endocrinol Metab *65*:127–135, 1987.

9. Wellmann W, Fink PC, Benner F, et al: Endotoxaemia in active Crohn's disease. Treatment with whole gut irrigation and 5-aminosalicylic acid. Gut *27*:814–820, 1986.

10. Matthews CP, Coulson PB, Wild RA: Serum proges-

terone levels as an aid in the diagnosis of ectopic pregnancy. Obstet Gynecol *68*:390–394, 1986.

11. Janssen J, Loomans L, Harink J, et al: Prevention and treatment of supraventricular tachycardia shortly after coronary artery bypass grafting: A randomized open trial. Angiology *37*:601–609, 1986.

12. Moriello KA, Halliwell REW, Oakes M: Determination of thyroxine, triiodothyronine, and cortisol changes during simultaneous adrenal and thyroid function tests in healthy dogs. Am J Vet Res *48*:458–462, 1987.

13. Consolvo CA. Relieving parental anxiety in the care-by-parent unit. JOGN Nurs *15*:154–159, 1986.

14. Brophy CM, Moore JG, Christian PE, et al: Variability of gastric emptying measurements in man employing standardized radiolabeled meals. Dig Dis Sci *31*:799–806, 1986.

15. Thomsen AM, Borgesen SE, Bruhn P, et al: Prognosis of dementia in normal-pressure hydrocephalus after a shunt operation. Ann Neurol *20*:304–310, 1986.

16. Mughal MM, Meguid MM: The effect of nutritional status on morbidity after elective surgery for benign gastrointestinal disease. J Paren Enter Nutr *11*:140–143, 1987.

17. Laub MC: Nutritional influence on serum ammonia in young patients receiving sodium valproate. Epilepsia *27*:55–59, 1986.

18. Giardina EV, Raby K, Saroff AL, et al: Antiarrhythmic effect of lorcainide in patients taking digoxin. J Clin Pharmacol *27*:378–383, 1987.

19. Cox HC: Verbal abuse in nursing: Report of a study. Nurs Manag *18*:47–50, 1987.

20. Norton JA, Collen MJ, Gardner JD, et al: Prospective study of gastrinoma localization and resection in patients with Zollinger-Ellison syndrome. Ann Surg *204*:468–479, 1986.

21. Kao GW, Peyman GA: Penetrating diathermy for retinal microincarceration in the management of giant retinal tears with inverted flaps. Retina *6*:135–145, 1986.

22. Weaver GA, Kurtz HJ, Behrens JC, et al: Effect of zearalenone on the fertility of virgin dairy heifers. Am J Vet Res *47*:1395–1397, 1986.

23. Martin JM: The influence of the time of administration on Cis-platinum induced nausea and vomiting. Oncol Nurs Forum *9*:26–32, 1982.

24. Altman RD, Collins-Yudiskas B: Synthetic human calcitonin in refractory Paget's disease of bone. Arch Intern Med *147*:1305–1308, 1987.

25. Shanbhogue RLK, Bistrian BR, Jenkins RL, et al: Resting energy expenditure in patients with end-stage liver disease and in normal population. J Paren Enter Nutr *11*:305–308, 1987.

26. Gur RE, Resnick SM, Alavi A, et al: Regional brain function in schizophrenia. I. A positron emission tomography study. Arch Gen Psychiatry *44*:119–125, 1987.

27. Fehrer SL, Halliwell RE: Effectiveness of Avon's Skin-So-Soft® as a flea repellent on dogs. J Am Anim Hosp Assoc *23*:217–220, 1987.

28. Davidson AB, Lee TH, Scanlon PD, et al: Bronchoconstrictor effects of leukotriene E_4 in normal and asthmatic subjects. Am Rev Respir Dis *135*:333–337, 1987.

29. Dempsey DT, Mullen JL, Rombeau JL, et al: Treatment effects of parenteral vitamins in total parenteral nutrition patients. J Paren Enter Nutr *11*:229–237, 1987.

30. Gardner FH, Juneja HS: Androstane therapy to treat aplastic anaemia in adults: An uncontrolled pilot study. Br J Haematol *65*:295–300, 1987.

31. Koren A, Garty I, Antonelli D, et al: Right ventricular cardiac dysfunction in β-thalassemia major. Am J Dis Child *141*:93–96, 1987.

32. Blagburn BL, Hendrix CM, Lindsay DS, et al: Anthelmintic efficacy of ivermectin in naturally parasitized cats. Am J Vet Res *48*:670–672, 1987.

33. Gray-Vickrey M: Education to prevent falls. Geriatr Nurs *5*:179–183, 1984.

34. De Vane GW, Czekala NM, Shideler SE, et al: Monitoring gonadotropin-releasing hormone administration by measurement of urinary steroid conjugates. Obstet Gynecol *67*:710–717, 1986.

35. Peleman RR, Gavaler JS, Van Thiel DH, et al: Orthotopic liver transplantation for acute and subacute hepatic failure in adults. Hepatology *7*:484–489, 1987.

36. Clapin-French E: Sleep patterns of aged persons in long-term care facilities. J Adv Nurs *11*:57–66, 1986.

37. Busch HM, Cogbill TH, Landercasper J, et al: Blunt bovine and equine trauma. J Trauma *26*:559–560, 1986.

38. Coons HL, Leventhal H, Nerenz DR, et al: Anticipatory nausea and emotional distress in patients receiving cisplatin-based chemotherapy. Oncol Nurs Forum *14*:31–35, 1987.

39. Fellman RL, Starita RJ, Spaeth GL, et al: ALT. Argon laser trabeculoplasty following failed trabeculectomy. J Ophthal Nurs Technol *5*:65–68, 1986.

7

HYPOTHESIS TESTING

CHAPTER OBJECTIVES

After studying this chapter and working the problems, you should be able to:

1. Explain what hypothesis tests and *p*-values mean

2. Carry out and interpret hypothesis tests concerning population proportions, differences between population proportions, population means, and differences between population means

3. Recognize data that violate assumptions required for *Z* tests and *t* tests

4. Interpret SPSS and SAS *t* test output

5. Determine whether *Z* tests and *t* tests reported in the medical and health care literature are appropriate

Most statistical inference involves testing hypotheses about population parameters. A *hypothesis* is simply a statement about the world that can be tested. For example, we might want to test the hypothesis that the population mean serum uric acid level for men with gout is 11.6 mg/dl, using the serum uric acid levels for a sample of men with gout. In this chapter, we will describe procedures that allow us to evaluate whether data provide evidence against a hypothesis about a population parameter. No method short of examining the entire population enables us to determine with absolute certainty whether a hypothesis about a population parameter is true. We can only assess whether data provide evidence against a hypothesis. If the data provide evidence against a hypothesis, we reject the hypothesis. If the data do not provide evidence against a hypothesis, we cannot reject the hypothesis.

How do we decide whether data provide evidence against a hypothesis? We start by temporarily assuming that the hypothesis is true. We then determine how likely a data set like ours is, assuming the hypothesis is true. If data like ours are extremely unlikely, assuming the hypothesis is true, the data provide evidence against the hypothesis. If data like ours are not unlikely, assuming the hypothesis is true, the data do not provide evidence against the hypothesis.

A hypothesis test was done in Example 3.13 (p. 32), which concerned a series of bad reactions to a *Bordetella* vaccine. We temporarily assumed that the drug company's claimed reaction rate of 1/10 was correct. We then calculated the probability of getting 10 bad reactions in 10 dogs, assuming a reaction rate of 1/10. Since this probability is extremely small (0.0000000001), sample results like these are extremely unlikely if the reaction rate is really 1/10. For this reason, we rejected the hypothesis that the reaction rate is 1/10.

The *Bordetella*-vaccine example involves a hypothesis about a population proportion p, the population proportion of dogs that react badly to the vaccine. Hypotheses about other population parameters can also be tested, using appropriate methods. In this chapter, we will describe procedures for testing hypotheses about the following population parameters.

1. Population proportions
2. Differences between population proportions
3. Population means
4. Differences between population means

7.1 HYPOTHESES ABOUT POPULATION PROPORTIONS

A study of surgical treatment of aspergilloma found that the operative mortality for 32 patients with complex aspergillomas was 34%.[1] Suppose an internist believes that the population proportion of operative deaths is much higher and is equal to 0.60. Here the population is the theoretical population that would result if all complex-aspergilloma patients similar to those in the study were treated surgically. Do the data provide evidence that the population proportion of operative deaths is not equal to 0.60?

It may seem that no statistical procedure is necessary to decide whether the data provide evidence against a population proportion of 0.60. You might argue that a sample proportion of 0.34 is so far from 0.60 that we can dismiss the internist's claim without further discussion. But suppose a sample proportion of 0.33 had been obtained for a sample of only three patients. Could we still dismiss the internist's claim so easily? Or suppose a sample of size 32 had produced a sample proportion of 0.47. Is 0.47 far enough from 0.60 to warrant rejecting the internist's claim? Without a statistical test to settle matters, researchers could spend all of their time arguing about questions like these.

To carry out a statistical test, we begin by specifying the hypothesis we want to test. The hypothesis to be tested is called the *null hypothesis* and is denoted by H_0 (pronounced "H nought"). For the aspergilloma example, the null hypothesis states that the population proportion of operative deaths is 0.60. We can write this null hypothesis as

$$H_0: p = 0.60 \qquad (7.1)$$

We also need to specify an *alternative hypothesis*, which is the hypothesis we accept when we reject the null hypothesis. The alternative hypothesis is abbreviated as H_A (pronounced "H sub A;" the "sub" is short for "subscript"). For the aspergilloma

data, the alternative hypothesis is

$$H_A: p \neq 0.60^* \qquad (7.2)$$

If we reject the null hypothesis, we accept the alternative hypothesis that the population proportion of operative deaths does not equal 0.60.

Null hypotheses about a population proportion state that the population proportion is equal to some specific number p_0 (pronounced "p nought"). The number p_0 is specified by the researcher and is determined by the question he wants to answer. It is not derived by any statistical method. For the aspergilloma data, p_0 is 0.60. In general, the null hypothesis has the form

$$H_0: p = p_0 \qquad (7.3)$$

The usual alternative hypothesis H_A is

$$H_A: p \neq p_0 \qquad (7.4)$$

The alternative hypothesis (7.4) is *two-sided* in the sense that both of the possibilities "$p < p_0$" and "$p > p_0$" are included.[†] *One-sided* alternative hypotheses are sometimes used. These are hypotheses of the form

$$H_A: p > p_0 \qquad (7.5)$$

or

$$H_A: p < p_0 \qquad (7.6)$$

A test with a two-sided alternative hypothesis is called a *two-sided test* and a test with a one-sided alternative hypothesis is called a *one-sided test*.

One-sided alternative hypotheses should be used *only* when the excluded possibility ("$p < p_0$" for the alternative hypothesis (7.5) and "$p > p_0$" for the alternative hypothesis (7.6)) *cannot occur*, or the excluded possibility is of *absolutely no interest*. This means that one-sided tests should be done quite infrequently. We rarely know enough to rule out one of the possibilities, and we are usually interested in both possibilities. Because one-sided tests are usually inappropriate, they should be critically evaluated when encountered in the medical and health care literature.

Suppose that a physician is investigating an experimental drug for the control of epileptic seizures. She believes that 40% of epileptic patients are treated successfully with other drugs, and she wants to determine whether the population proportion of epileptic patients treated successfully with this drug is also equal to 0.40. If she works for the company that makes the new drug, she may argue that a

---

*The symbol "$\neq$" means "is not equal to."

[†]The symbol "$<$" means "is less than" and the symbol "$>$" means "is greater than."

one-sided test is justified because she is interested only in the possibility that the new drug is better than other drugs ($p > 0.40$). If the new drug is worse than other drugs ($p < 0.40$), she does not care about detecting this. A one-sided test might be appropriate for publication in an in-house company report, but it would not be appropriate for a medical or health care journal. Most medical and health care professionals would be quite interested in the possibility that the experimental drug is worse than other drugs.

In the Bordetella-vaccine example (Example 3.13 on p. 32), a one-sided test of the hypothesis H_0: $p = 1/10$ was done. The possibility that the reaction rate p is less than $1/10$ is of no interest to a veterinarian who is trying to decide whether he should stop using the vaccine. He is concerned only with the possibility that the reaction rate is greater than $1/10$. The manufacturer of the vaccine no doubt would prefer a two-sided test, since the company is interested in both a reaction rate greater than $1/10$ and a reaction rate less than $1/10$. The choice of a one-sided or two-sided test should be based not only on the interests of the researcher, but also on the interests of those who will read his results. When in doubt, use a two-sided test.

To test the null hypothesis (7.3), we use the *one-sample Z test*. This test is based on the one-sample Z statistic given by the formula

$$Z = \frac{\hat{p} - p_0}{s_{\text{prop}}} \qquad (7.7)$$

where $\hat{p}$ is the sample proportion and s_{prop} is defined as in Chapter 6:

$$s_{\text{prop}} = \sqrt{\frac{\hat{p}(1 - \hat{p})}{n}}$$

As before, n is the sample size.

Let us examine the one-sample Z statistic more closely to see why it makes sense as a test of H_0. The top part of Z is the difference $\hat{p} - p_0$, which is the difference between the sample proportion $\hat{p}$ and the hypothesized population proportion p_0. If the null hypothesis (7.3) is true, the population proportion is p_0, so $\hat{p}$ should usually be close to p_0. Thus, if the null hypothesis (7.3) is true, the difference $\hat{p} - p_0$ should usually be small in absolute value.* The bottom part of Z is the estimated standard deviation of $\hat{p}$, a fact we will not prove. A large standard deviation tends to make Z small in

absolute value and a small standard deviation tends to make Z large in absolute value.

A large Z statistic means that the difference between $\hat{p}$ and p_0 is large relative to the standard deviation of $\hat{p}$. In other words, a large Z means that the difference between $\hat{p}$ and p_0 is large relative to the variability of $\hat{p}$. This means that a large Z provides evidence against the null hypothesis (7.3). A large enough Z is grounds for rejecting this hypothesis. When Z is small, the difference between $\hat{p}$ and p_0 is small relative to the variability of $\hat{p}$. For this reason, a small Z does not provide evidence against the null hypothesis (7.3) and is not grounds for rejecting it.

How large does Z have to be for us to reject the null hypothesis? Suppose the Z statistic we calculate is so large that the probability of getting a Z statistic (7.7) at least as extreme as our calculated Z statistic is very small, if the null hypothesis (7.3) is true. Then our sample has produced results that are very unlikely if the null hypothesis (7.3) is true, and we reject this hypothesis. To test the null hypothesis (7.3), we need to find the probability of getting a one-sample Z statistic at least as extreme as the calculated one-sample Z statistic, assuming that the null hypothesis (7.3) is true.

For a two-sided test, this probability is the two-tailed probability.

$$P\left(\begin{array}{l} Z \text{ statistic} \leq -|z_{\text{calc}}| \quad \text{or} \\ Z \text{ statistic} \geq |z_{\text{calc}}| \end{array} \right) \qquad (7.8)$$

where z_{calc} is the calculated Z statistic and $|z_{\text{calc}}|$ is the absolute value of z_{calc}. It can be shown, using the central limit theorem, that the one-sample Z statistic has approximately a standard normal distribution if the null hypothesis (7.3) is true and the sample is large enough. We can use a standard normal table to find approximate probabilities of the form (7.8).

When a two-sided test is done, the probability (7.8) is the *p-value* for the calculated Z statistic. This p-value is the probability of getting a one-sample Z statistic at least as extreme as the calculated Z statistic if the null hypothesis (7.3) is true. Since we reject the null hypothesis (7.3) when the p-value is too small, the size of the p-value determines whether we reject or fail to reject this hypothesis. How small is too small? This is determined by the researcher. She decides, before testing, that p-values less than a particular value warrant rejection of the null hypothesis and p-values greater than or equal to that value do not warrant rejection of the null hypothesis.

This cutoff value is called the *significance level* and is denoted by α. The most common significance levels are 0.10, 0.05, 0.01, and 0.001. Significance levels greater than 0.10 are not used. Suppose we set our significance level at 0.05. If our p-value is 0.038, we reject the null hypothesis, since 0.038 is less than 0.05. If our p-value is 0.057, we cannot

---

*If a number is not negative, its *absolute value* is just its value. For example, the absolute value of 5.1 is 5.1 and the absolute value of 0 is 0. If a number is negative, its absolute value is its value without the negative sign. For example, the absolute value of -2.7 is 2.7.

reject the null hypothesis, since 0.057 is greater than 0.05.

If a one-sided test is done with the alternative hypothesis H_A: $p > p_0$, the p-value is the probability $P(Z \text{ statistic} \geq z_{calc})$. If the alternative hypothesis is H_A: $p < p_0$, the p-value is the probability $P(Z \text{ statistic} \leq z_{calc})$.* The p-values for two-sided tests are called *two-tailed p-values* and the p-values for one-sided tests are called *one-tailed p-values*. Because the standard normal distribution is symmetric, the two-tailed p-value for a calculated Z statistic (7.7) is equal to twice the one-tailed p-value *if the one-tailed p-value is less than or equal to 1/2*:

$$\text{two-tailed } p\text{-value} = 2(\text{one-tailed } p\text{-value}) \quad (7.9)$$

$$\text{one-tailed } p\text{-value} = \frac{\text{two-tailed } p\text{-value}}{2} \quad (7.10)$$

The relationships (7.9) and (7.10) hold whenever p-values are calculated from a symmetric distribution and the one-tailed p-value is less than or equal to 1/2. They do *not* hold if a nonsymmetric distribution is used to obtain p-values or if the one-tailed p-value is greater than 1/2.

Let us test the null hypothesis (7.1) for the aspergilloma data, using a 0.01 significance level. The sample proportion $\hat{p}$ is 0.34 and the sample size is 32, so

$$s_{prop} = \sqrt{\frac{(0.34)(1 - 0.34)}{32}}$$

$$= \sqrt{\frac{(0.34)(0.66)}{32}} = 0.084$$

Applying formula (7.7), we get the following calculated Z statistic.

$$Z = \frac{0.34 - 0.60}{0.084} = \frac{-0.26}{0.084} = -3.10$$

Our p-value is the two-tailed probability

$$P(Z \text{ statistic} \leq -3.10 \quad \text{or} \quad Z \text{ statistic} \geq 3.10)$$

which we obtain from Table E.2. We first find 3.10 in the z column, and then the number in the row for $z = 3.10$ and in the column for two-tailed probabilities. This number, which is 0.0019, is our p-value. How do we interpret this p-value? First, 0.0019 is less than 0.01, so we reject the null hypothesis (7.1) at the 0.01 significance level. Using a 0.01 significance level, we decide that the data provide evidence against the internist's claim that the population proportion of operative deaths is 0.60. Second, the probability of getting a one-sample Z statistic at

least as extreme as -3.10 is 0.0019, if the null hypothesis (7.1) is true. Only 0.19% of all possible samples produce calculated one-sample Z statistics at least as extreme as -3.10, if the null hypothesis (7.1) is true.

When we make a decision based on a hypothesis test, we never know whether our decision is correct. There are two kinds of mistakes we can make: (1) we can reject the null hypothesis when it is true, or (2) we can fail to reject the null hypothesis when it is false. The first mistake is called a *Type I error* and the second a *Type II error*. The best we can do is reduce the chance of making either of these errors. If the null hypothesis is true, the significance level is the probability of rejecting the null hypothesis. Since we decide what the significance level is, we control the probability of making a Type I error. Methods for controlling the probability of making a Type II error involve selecting an appropriate sample size. Some of these methods are described in Appendix A.

If the sample size is fixed, reducing the probability of making a Type I error increases the probability of making a Type II error, and reducing the probability of making a Type II error increases the probability of making a Type I error. When the sample size is fixed, the only way to reduce the chance of making a Type I error is to reject the null hypothesis less often, increasing the chance of making a Type II error. Similarly, the only way to reduce the chance of making a Type II error when the sample size is fixed is to reject the null hypothesis more often, increasing the chance of making a Type I error. We can reduce the chance of one type of error without increasing the chance of the other type of error only by increasing the sample size. But no sample size (short of sampling the entire population) reduces both of these probabilities to 0.

The one-sample Z test of the null hypothesis (7.3) requires the same assumptions as the confidence interval for population proportions described in Chapter 6.

1. Random Sampling. Although a random sample is preferable, the one-sample Z test may be done when the sample is not random. The sample must not be biased, however.

2. Independent Observations. This assumption must *not* be violated. If the observations are not independent, the one-sample Z test cannot be done.

3. Sufficiently Large Sample. The closer p_0 or $1 - p_0$ is to 0, the larger the sample required. As a rough guide, np_0 and $n(1 - p_0)$ should not be less than 5.

All of these assumptions, except random sampling, seem to hold for the aspergilloma data. The observations are independent, since knowing whether one patient died from surgery tells us nothing about whether another patient died from surgery. Both np_0 and $n(1 - p_0)$ are larger than 5, so the sample is large enough ($np_0 = 32(0.60) = 19.2$ and $n(1 - p_0) = 32(0.40) = 12.8$).

---

*If z_{calc} is negative, $P(Z \geq z_{calc})$ must be obtained indirectly from Table E.2 by using the relationship $P(Z \geq z_{calc}) = 1 - P(Z \leq z_{calc})$. If z_{calc} is positive, $P(Z \leq z_{calc})$ is obtained indirectly from Table E.2 by using the relationship $P(Z \leq z_{calc}) = 1 - P(Z \geq z_{calc})$.

The one-sample Z test and the confidence interval for the population proportion p are related. If we fail to reject the null hypothesis (7.3) at the significance level α, the number p_0 will be included in the $100(1 - \alpha)\%$ confidence interval for p. If we reject the null hypothesis (7.3) at the significance level α, the number p_0 will *not* be included in the $100(1 - \alpha)\%$ confidence interval for p. The 99% confidence interval for p based on the aspergilloma data will not include 0.60, since we rejected H_0: $p = 0.60$ at the 0.01 significance level.

If we reject the null hypothesis that the population proportion p is equal to p_0, we usually want to obtain a confidence interval for p. Because we have decided that p is not equal to p_0, we want to estimate p. For the aspergilloma data, the 99% confidence interval for p is (0.12, 0.56), which does not include 0.60. We are 99% sure that the population proportion of operative deaths is between 0.12 and 0.56.

Example 7.1

A study reported the results of 39 ear-canal ablation surgeries performed on 31 dogs and cats.[2] Thirty-six per cent of the 39 ablations were complicated by facial nerve damage. Can we use the one-sample Z test to test the hypothesis that the population proportion of ear ablations complicated by facial nerve damage is 0.30 (H_0: $p = 0.30$)?

Since 39 ablations were performed on 31 animals, bilateral ablations must have been done on eight animals. We have repeated observations for eight animals, and the independence of observations from the same animal is questionable at best. For this reason, the one-sample Z test cannot be used to test H_0: $p = 0.30$.

We can still use the one-sample Z test if we analyze the data differently. Let us split the data into right-ear ablations and left-ear ablations. Of the 16 right-ear ablations, 25% were complicated by facial nerve damage. Of the 23 left-ear ablations, 43% were complicated by facial nerve damage. All of the right-ear ablations are independent, since they were performed on different animals. For the same reason, all of the left-ear ablations are independent. We can calculate the one-sample Z statistic for the right-ear ablations to test the null hypothesis that the population proportion p_R of right-ear ablations complicated by facial nerve damage is 0.30 (H_0: $p_R = 0.30$). We can then calculate the one-sample Z statistic for the left-ear ablations to test the null hypothesis that the population proportion p_L of left-ear ablations complicated by facial nerve damage is 0.30 (H_0: $p_L = 0.30$).

7.2 HYPOTHESES ABOUT DIFFERENCES BETWEEN POPULATION PROPORTIONS

As we saw in Chapter 6, the comparison of proportions is often important in medical and health care research. One of the most commonly tested hypotheses about population proportions is the null hypothesis

$$H_0: p_1 = p_2 \qquad (7.11)$$

Suppose that patients with duodenal ulcers are randomly assigned to receive one of two H_2 antagonists. An obvious hypothesis of interest is the hypothesis that the population proportions of patients whose ulcers heal completely are the same. Here the populations are the theoretical populations that would result if all patients with duodenal ulcers were randomly assigned to receive one of the H_2 antagonists.

The usual alternative hypothesis when testing the null hypothesis (7.11) is two-sided:

$$H_A: p_1 \neq p_2 \qquad (7.12)$$

The one-sided alternative hypotheses (H_A: $p_1 > p_2$ and H_A: $p_1 < p_2$) are appropriate only when we can rule out the possibility "$p_1 < p_2$" or "$p_1 > p_2$" or when one of these possibilities is of no interest.

To test the null hypothesis (7.11), we use another Z test called the *two-sample Z test*. This test is based on the two-sample Z statistic given by the formula

$$Z = \frac{\hat{p}_1 - \hat{p}_2}{s_{\text{diff}}} \qquad (7.13)$$

As in Chapter 6, $\hat{p}_1$ and $\hat{p}_2$ are the sample proportions and s_{diff} is given by

$$s_{\text{diff}} = \sqrt{\frac{\hat{p}_1(1 - \hat{p}_1)}{n_1} + \frac{\hat{p}_2(1 - \hat{p}_2)}{n_2}}$$

where n_1 and n_2 are the sample sizes.

Why does it make sense to look at the two-sample Z statistic to test the null hypothesis (7.11)? The top part of the two-sample Z statistic is the difference between the sample proportions $\hat{p}_1$ and $\hat{p}_2$. If the population proportions p_1 and p_2 are the same, $p_1 - p_2 = 0$ and we expect the sample difference $\hat{p}_1 - \hat{p}_2$ to be small in absolute value most of the time. The bottom part of (7.13) is the estimated standard deviation of $\hat{p}_1 - \hat{p}_2$, a fact we will not prove. A large standard deviation tends to make Z small in absolute value and a small standard deviation tends to make Z large in absolute value.

Thus, Z is large when $\hat{p}_1 - \hat{p}_2$ is large relative to the variability of $\hat{p}_1 - \hat{p}_2$. A large Z, therefore, provides evidence against the null hypothesis (7.11). A small Z does not provide evidence against this hypothesis, since Z is small when $\hat{p}_1 - \hat{p}_2$ is small relative to the variability of $\hat{p}_1 - \hat{p}_2$.

When a two-sided test is done, the p-value for the calculated Z statistic is the two-tailed probability

$$P\left(\begin{array}{c} Z \text{ statistic} \leq -|z_{\text{calc}}| \quad \text{or} \\ Z \text{ statistic} \geq |z_{\text{calc}}| \end{array} \right) \qquad (7.14)$$

where z_{calc} is the value of the two-sample Z statistic calculated for the sample. If a one-sided test is done with the alternative hypothesis H_A: $p_1 > p_2$, the p-value is the probability $P(Z$ statistic $\geq z_{calc})$. If the alternative hypothesis is H_A: $p_1 < p_2$, the p-value is the probability $P(Z$ statistic $\leq z_{calc})$. As before, the two-tailed p-value is twice the one-tailed p-value, if the one-tailed p-value is less than or equal to $1/2$.

We reject the null hypothesis (7.11) when the p-value is less than the significance level α selected before carrying out the test. We fail to reject the null hypothesis (7.11) when the p-value is greater than or equal to the significance level α. It can be shown, using the central limit theorem, that the two-sample Z statistic has approximately a standard normal distribution if the null hypothesis (7.11) is true and the samples are independent and sufficiently large. Table E.2 can be used to obtain approximate p-values for two-sample Z statistics.

What do these p-values mean? The p-value (7.14) is the probability of getting a two-sample Z statistic at least as extreme as the calculated Z statistic if the null hypothesis (7.11) is true. If the p-value is small, the chance of getting a Z statistic at least as extreme as the calculated Z statistic is small, assuming that the null hypothesis (7.11) is true. A small p-value provides evidence against the null hypothesis. If the p-value is large, the chance of getting a Z statistic at least as extreme as the calculated Z statistic is large, assuming that the null hypothesis (7.11) is true. A large p-value does not provide evidence against the null hypothesis.

The two-sample Z test is based on the same assumptions as the confidence interval for differences between population proportions described in Chapter 6.

1. Random Sampling. As long as the samples are not biased, random sampling is not essential.

2. Independent Samples. If the observations in one sample are not independent of the observations in the other sample, the two-sample Z test cannot be done.*

3. Independent Observations Within Each Sample. The two-sample Z test cannot be done if the observations within each sample are not independent.

4. Sufficiently Large Samples. Unless $\hat{p}_1$ or $\hat{p}_2$ is very close to 0 or 1, samples as small as 10 are usually sufficient. The closer $\hat{p}_1$ or $\hat{p}_2$ is to 0 or 1, the larger the samples needed. If you are not sure whether your samples are large enough, consult a statistician.

---

*A method for comparing proportions from nonindependent samples is discussed in Chapter 10. Other methods are described by Schlesselman.[3]

There is a relationship between the two-sample Z test and the confidence interval for $p_1 - p_2$. If we reject the null hypothesis (7.11) at the significance level α, the $100(1 - \alpha)\%$ confidence interval for $p_1 - p_2$ will not include 0. If we fail to reject the null hypothesis (7.11) at the significance level α, the $100(1 - \alpha)\%$ confidence interval for $p_1 - p_2$ will include 0. The confidence interval always agrees with the results of the corresponding two-sample Z test. When we reject the null hypothesis (7.11), we often obtain a confidence interval to estimate $p_1 - p_2$, since we have concluded that $p_1 - p_2$ does not equal 0.

Example 7.2

A study investigated parental stress after a child's admission to the intensive care unit.[4] The subjects were 233 parents whose children's admissions were planned and 262 parents whose children's admissions were unexpected. Fifty-six per cent of the planned-admission parents and 75% of the unexpected-admission parents rated their children's condition as "extremely severe on admission." Can we use the two-sample Z test to test the hypothesis that the planned-admission population proportion of parents who rate their children's condition as extremely severe is the same as the unexpected-admission population proportion of parents who rate their children's condition as extremely severe? The planned-admission population consists of all parents similar to those in the study with children whose admission to the intensive care unit was planned. The unexpected-admission population consists of all parents similar to those in the study with children whose admission to the intensive care unit was unexpected.

If the parents did not have contact with each other, one parent's rating of her child's condition is unrelated to another parent's rating. Both of the independence assumptions appear to be satisfied. The samples are large enough and the lack of random samples is not a major problem. The two-sample Z test is appropriate.

We will obtain a two-sided test, since neither of the possibilities "$p_1 < p_2$" and "$p_1 > p_2$" can be ruled out and both are of interest. Let us use a 0.10 significance level. Using the sample proportions and sample sizes, we calculate s_{diff}:

$$s_{diff} = \sqrt{\frac{(0.56)(1 - 0.56)}{233} + \frac{(0.75)(1 - 0.75)}{262}}$$

$$= \sqrt{\frac{(0.56)(0.44)}{233} + \frac{(0.75)(0.25)}{262}}$$

$$= \sqrt{0.0018} = 0.042.$$

Applying formula (7.13), we obtain the calculated

two-sample Z statistic

$$Z = \frac{0.56 - 0.75}{0.042} = \frac{-0.19}{0.042} = -4.52$$

From Table E.2, our p-value is

$$P(Z \text{ statistic} \leq -4.52 \quad \text{or} \quad Z \text{ statistic} \geq 4.52)$$
$$< 0.0001$$

Since 0.0001 is less than 0.10, we reject the null hypothesis of equal population proportions. In fact, the p-value is so small that we would reject this hypothesis at any reasonable significance level. If the population proportions are equal, the probability of getting a two-sample Z statistic at least as extreme as -4.52 is less than 0.0001. In other words, sample results like ours are very unlikely if the two population proportions are equal. Less than 0.01% of all possible samples produce two-sample Z statistics at least as extreme as -4.52 if the population proportions are equal. The data provide evidence against the null hypothesis (7.11) and allow us to reject it.

Since we can reject the null hypothesis (7.11) at the 0.10 significance level, the 90% confidence interval for $p_1 - p_2$ based on these data cannot include 0. If we calculate a 90% confidence interval for $p_1 - p_2$, we get $(-0.26, -0.12)$.

Example 7.3

A randomized, controlled, double-blind study was conducted to determine whether intranasal alpha$_2$-interferon could prevent the spread of colds in families.[5] Sixty families were randomly assigned to receive either interferon or placebo nasal spray, resulting in interferon use by 79 family members and placebo use by 76 family members. When one or more members of a family showed signs of a cold, all of the healthy family members began using the spray and continued using it for seven days. In 23% of 222 seven-day uses of the placebo spray, the user caught a cold, as compared with 14% of 226 seven-day uses of the interferon spray. Can we use the two-sample Z test to test the null hypothesis that the interferon population proportion of uses in which the user catches a cold is equal to the placebo population proportion of uses in which the user catches a cold? Here the populations consist of the seven-day interferon and placebo spray uses that would result if all families similar to those in the study were randomly assigned to receive either interferon or a placebo.

Because the families presumably had no contact with each other, the placebo and interferon samples are independent. The observations within each sample are not independent. Since there are far more observations than subjects, many of the observations are repeated measurements on the same subjects. In addition, observations from members of the same family cannot be considered independent. When one family member has a cold, the probability that another family member will catch a cold increases. We cannot use sample proportions based on spray uses to test the null hypothesis that the corresponding population proportions are equal.

The data presented can be analyzed if we consider families, rather than individuals, to be the study subjects, and if we restrict the analysis to the first spraying episode for each family. Of the 28 evaluable families taking the placebo, 75% had at least one sprayer who caught a cold during the first spraying episode. Of the 26 evaluable families taking interferon, 27% had at least one sprayer who caught a cold during the first spraying episode. These sample proportions are based on observations from different families for a single spraying episode. Because the family observations are independent and the samples are large enough, the two-sample Z test can be used to compare population proportions. Here the populations consist of the family observations for the first spraying episode that would result if all families similar to those in the study were randomly assigned to receive either interferon or a placebo.

Example 7.4

In a study of psychological treatment of migraine, the effectiveness of stress-coping training (SCT) was evaluated.[6] Eight weeks after training, 81% of the 16 SCT patients reported that the training had reduced the frequency of their migraine headaches. Six months after training, 12 of the SCT patients were contacted again, and 43% of them reported that the training had reduced the frequency of their migraine headaches. Can we use the two-sample Z test to test the null hypothesis that the eight-week posttraining population proportion who report reduced headache frequency is equal to the six-month posttraining population proportion who report reduced headache frequency?

Within each sample, the observations are independent. Knowing one patient's evaluation of the training's effectiveness tells us nothing about another patient's evaluation. The observations in the second sample are not independent of the observations in the first sample. Because the 12 patients in the six-month sample were also in the eight-week sample, repeated measurements were obtained for these 12 patients. We cannot use the two-sample Z test. If we use only the data for the 12 patients who were in both samples, the McNemar test described in Chapter 10 can be used to test the hypothesis that the population proportions are equal.

7.3 HYPOTHESES ABOUT POPULATION MEANS

In a study of end-stage renal disease, the creatinine values shown in Table 7.1 were obtained for

TABLE 7.1 CREATININE FOR END-STAGE RENAL DISEASE PATIENTS UNDERGOING HEMODIALYSIS

Patient No.	Creatinine (mg/dl)
1	6.7
2	8.0
3	13.4
4	12.4
5	14.9
6	6.3
7	16.5
8	13.5
9	12.4
10	16.9
11	9.1
12	13.0
Mean ± SD	11.9 ± 3.6

12 end-stage renal disease patients undergoing hemodialysis.[7] These creatinine values have a mean of 11.9 mg/dl and a standard deviation of 3.6 mg/dl. A nephrology nurse believes that the population mean creatinine is 8.4 mg/dl. Do the data provide evidence against the hypothesis that the population mean creatinine is 8.4 mg/dl? Here the population consists of all end-stage renal disease patients (similar to those in the study) who are undergoing hemodialysis.

We want to test the null hypothesis that the population mean μ is equal to 8.4:

$$H_0: \mu = 8.4 \qquad (7.15)$$

Our alternative hypothesis is the two-sided hypothesis

$$H_A: \mu \neq 8.4 \qquad (7.16)$$

We have no reason to rule out either of the possibilities "$\mu < 8.4$" or "$\mu > 8.4$" and both are of interest.

Null hypotheses like (7.15) are fairly common in medical and health care research. In general, they have the form

$$H_0: \mu = \mu_0 \qquad (7.17)$$

where μ_0 (pronounced "mew nought") is a number specified by the researcher. The number μ_0 is not derived statistically but is determined by the question the researcher wants to answer. For the creatinine data, μ_0 is 8.4. The usual alternative hypothesis is two-sided:

$$H_A: \mu \neq \mu_0 \qquad (7.18)$$

The one-sided alternative hypotheses ($H_A: \mu > \mu_0$ and $H_A: \mu < \mu_0$) are rarely appropriate. We usually cannot rule out the possibility "$\mu < \mu_0$" or "$\mu >$

μ_0" and we are usually interested in both possibilities.

We test the null hypothesis (7.17) by using a *one-sample t-test*, which is based on the one-sample t statistic

$$t = \frac{\bar{x} - \mu_0}{s/\sqrt{n}} \qquad (7.19)$$

Let us examine this t statistic to see why it makes sense to use it for testing (7.17). The top part of the one-sample t statistic is the difference between the sample mean and the hypothesized population mean μ_0. If the null hypothesis (7.17) is true, the population mean μ is equal to μ_0, and $\bar{x}$ should usually be close to μ_0. Thus, the difference $\bar{x} - \mu_0$ should usually be small in absolute value if (7.17) is true. The bottom part of the one-sample t statistic is the estimated standard deviation of $\bar{x}$, as you may recall from Chapter 5. A large standard deviation tends to make the one-sample t statistic small in absolute value, and a small standard deviation tends to make it large in absolute value.

The one-sample t statistic is large when the difference between $\bar{x}$ and μ_0 is large relative to the variability of $\bar{x}$. A large one-sample t statistic provides evidence against the null hypothesis (7.17). A small one-sample t statistic means that the difference between $\bar{x}$ and μ_0 is small relative to the variability of $\bar{x}$, so a small one-sample t statistic does not provide evidence against the null hypothesis (7.17).

When a two-sided test is done, the p-value for the one-sample t test of the null hypothesis (7.17) is the two-tailed probability

$$P\left(\begin{array}{c} t \text{ statistic} \leq -|t_{\text{calc}}| \quad \text{or} \\ t \text{ statistic} \geq |t_{\text{calc}}| \end{array}\right) \qquad (7.20)$$

where t_{calc} is the value of the one-sample t statistic calculated for the sample. This p-value is the probability of getting a one-sample t statistic at least as extreme as the calculated t statistic if the null hypothesis (7.17) is true. If a one-sided test is done, with the alternative hypothesis $H_A: \mu > \mu_0$, the p-value is the probability $P(t \text{ statistic} \geq t_{\text{calc}})$. If the alternative hypothesis is $H_A: \mu < \mu_0$, the p-value is the probability $P(t \text{ statistic} \leq t_{\text{calc}})$. Because the t distribution is symmetric, the two-tailed p-value is equal to twice the one-tailed p-value when the one-tailed p-value is less than or equal to 1/2.

It can be shown that the one-sample t statistic has a t distribution with $n - 1$ degrees of freedom (df) if the null hypothesis (7.17) is true and the data are a random sample from a normal population. We can use Table E.4 to obtain approximate p-values for the one-sample t statistic, but we cannot get exact p-values from this table. Suppose we calculate a one-sample t statistic value of 3.24, based on a sample of size 7. Our two-tailed p-value is the two-tailed probability

$$P(t \text{ statistic} \leq -3.24 \quad \text{or} \quad t \text{ statistic} \geq 3.24)$$

Table E.4 involves upper-tail probabilities rather than two-tailed probabilities. But the t distribution is symmetric, so

$$P(t \text{ statistic} \leq -3.24 \quad \text{or} \quad t \text{ statistic} \geq 3.24)$$
$$= 2P(t \text{ statistic} \geq 3.24)$$

We can look up the approximate value of $P(t$ statistic $\geq 3.24)$ in Table E.4 and multiply this value by 2 to get our approximate p-value.

We first find the row corresponding to 6 $(7 - 1)$ degrees of freedom in Table E.4. We then find two *adjacent* numbers in this row such that 3.24 is between these numbers. The numbers we get are 3.143 and 3.372, which are the 0.01 and 0.0075 upper percentage points of the t distribution. Since 0.01 and 0.0075 are upper-tail probabilities and we want two-tailed probabilities, we multiply 0.01 and 0.0075 by 2 to get $2(0.01) = 0.02$ and $2(0.0075) = 0.015$. Our p-value is between 0.015 and 0.02:

$$0.015 < \text{two-tailed } p\text{-value} < 0.02 \quad (7.21)$$

Figure 7.1 shows the rationale behind the inequality (7.21). The area under the frequency curve above 3.24 is greater than the area above 3.372 (which is 0.0075) and is less than the area above 3.143 (which is 0.01). Hence,

$$P(t \text{ statistic} \geq 3.372) < P(t \text{ statistic} \geq 3.24)$$
$$< P(t \text{ statistic} \geq 3.143)$$

and

$$2P(t \text{ statistic} \geq 3.372) < 2P(t \text{ statistic} \geq 3.24)$$
$$< 2P(t \text{ statistic} \geq 3.143)$$

Exact p-values are much better than approximate p-values like (7.21), but a computer is usually needed to obtain them.

In general, Table E.4 is used as follows to find approximate two-tailed p-values for one-sample t statistics. We first locate the row for $n - 1$ degrees of freedom. If possible, we then find two *adjacent* numbers in this row such that $|t_{\text{calc}}|$ lies between them. The two-tailed p-value will lie between *twice* the upper-tail probabilities corresponding to these numbers. If t_{calc} is very large in absolute value, we will not find a number larger than $|t_{\text{calc}}|$ in the appropriate row ($n - 1$ degrees of freedom). When this happens, we find the largest number in the appropriate row. The two-tailed p-value will be *less* than *twice* the upper-tail probability corresponding to this number. If $|t_{\text{calc}}|$ is very small, we will not find a number smaller than $|t_{\text{calc}}|$ in the appropriate row. When this happens, we find the smallest number in the appropriate row. The two-tailed p-value will be *greater* than *twice* the upper-tail probability corresponding to this number. These possibilities are illustrated in the following example.

Example 7.5

What are the approximate two-tailed and one-tailed p-values for the following calculated t statistics?

1. $t_{\text{calc}} = 1.55$, $n = 12$. In the row for $12 - 1 = 11$ df, the two adjacent numbers that 1.55 lies between are 1.363 and 1.796. These correspond to the upper-tail probabilities 0.10 and 0.05. Multiplying these probabilities by 2, we get $2(0.10) = 0.20$ and $2(0.05) = 0.10$, so that

$$0.10 < \text{two-tailed } p\text{-value} < 0.20$$

If the one-sided alternative hypothesis is H_A: $\mu > \mu_0$, the one-tailed p-value is $P(t \geq 1.55)$, so

$$0.05 < \text{one-tailed } p\text{-value} < 0.10$$

If the one-sided alternative hypothesis is H_A: $\mu < \mu_0$, the one-tailed p-value is $P(t \leq 1.55)$. Because 1.55 is greater than 0, this probability involves both sides of the t distribution's frequency curve (see Figure 7.2) and is *not* a tail probability. Approximate nontail probabilities like this can be obtained indirectly from Table E.4, although we will

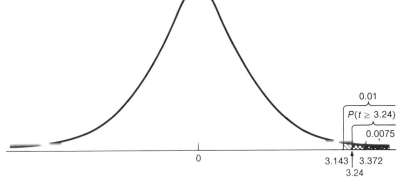

Figure 7.1 Some upper-tail probabilities for the t distribution with 6 degrees of freedom

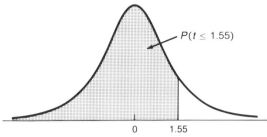

Figure 7.2 Area corresponding to $P(t \leq 1.55)$

not do so. It can be shown that probabilities of the form $P(t \leq t_{calc})$ are always greater than 0.5 when t_{calc} is greater than 0. This implies that $P(t \leq 1.55) > 0.5$. In the unlikely event that you need a more exact nontail probability, you can use a computer or consult a statistician.

2. $t_{calc} = -5.14$, $n = 20$. In the row for $20 - 1 = 19$ df, there is no number larger than $|t_{calc}| = 5.14$. The largest number in this row is 3.883, which corresponds to the upper-tail probability 0.0005. Multiplying this probability by 2, we get $2(0.0005) = 0.001$, so that

two-tailed p-value < 0.001

If the one-sided alternative hypothesis is H_A: $\mu < \mu_0$, the one-tailed p-value is $P(t \leq -5.14)$, so

one-tailed p-value < 0.0005

If the one-sided alternative hypothesis is H_A: $\mu > \mu_0$, the one-tailed p-value is $P(t \geq -5.14)$. This probability involves both sides of the t distribution (see Figure 7.3), since -5.14 is less than 0. Because $P(t \geq -5.14)$ is not a tail probability, we cannot obtain its approximate value directly from Table E.4. Probabilities of the form $P(t \geq t_{calc})$ are always greater than 0.5 when t_{calc} is less than 0, so $P(t \geq -5.24) > 0.5$. Although a more exact approximate one-tailed p-value can be obtained indirectly from Table E.4, we will not do so.

3. $t_{calc} = 0.16$, $n = 98$. There is no row for $98 - 1 = 97$ df, so we use the row for the closest degrees of freedom, 120. In this row, there is no number less than 0.16. The smallest number in this row is 0.254, which corresponds to the upper-tail probability 0.40.

Multiplying this probability by 2, we get $2(0.40) = 0.80$, so that

two-tailed p-value > 0.80

If the one-sided alternative hypothesis is H_A: $\mu > \mu_0$, the one-tailed p-value is $P(t \geq 0.16)$, so

one-tailed p-value > 0.40

If the one-sided alternative hypothesis is H_A: $\mu < \mu_0$, the one-tailed p-value is $P(t \leq 0.16)$. This probability is not a tail probability. Since 0.16 is greater than 0, $P(t \leq 0.16) > 0.5$. A more exact approximate one-tailed p-value can be obtained indirectly from Table E.4, but we will not do so.

4. $t_{calc} = 1.29$, $n = 125$. There is no row for $125 - 1 = 124$ df, so we use the row for the closest degrees of freedom, 120. The number 1.289 in this row is almost the same as t_{calc} and corresponds to the 0.10 upper-tail probability. Multiplying this probability by 2, we get $2(0.10) = 0.20$. Since t_{calc} is so close to 1.289,

two-tailed p-value $\cong 0.20$

If the one-sided alternative hypothesis is H_A: $\mu > \mu_0$, the one-tailed p-value is $P(t \geq 1.29)$, so

one-tailed p-value $\cong 0.10$

If the one-sided alternative hypothesis is H_A: $\mu < \mu_0$, the one-tailed p-value is $P(t \leq 1.29)$, which is not a tail probability. Because 1.29 is greater than 0, $P(t \leq 1.29) > 0.5$. A more exact one-tailed probability can be obtained indirectly from Table E.4.

As usual, p-values determine whether the data provide evidence against the null hypothesis. Before carrying out a one-sample t test, the researcher decides on a significance level α. If the p-value is less than α, the null hypothesis (7.17) is rejected at this significance level. If the p-value is greater than or equal to α, the null hypothesis (7.17) cannot be rejected at this significance level. As before, a small p-value means that test statistic values at least as extreme as the calculated test statistic are unlikely, if the null hypothesis is true.

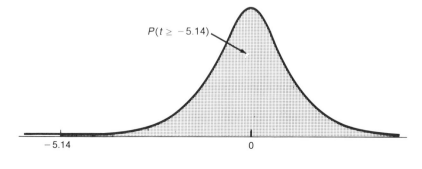

Figure 7.3 Area corresponding to $P(t \geq -5.14)$

The one-sample t test requires the same assumptions as the confidence interval for population means described in Chapter 6.

1. Random Sampling. If the sample is not biased, random sampling is not essential.

2. Independent Observations. One-sample t tests cannot be done if the observations are not independent.

3. Sampling from a Normal Population. Even if the population is not normal, one-sample t tests can often be done anyway. The sample must be large enough to compensate for a nonnormal population, however. If the population is extremely nonnormal (e.g., only a few values are possible), one-sample t tests cannot be done. Consult a statistician if you are not sure whether your sample is large enough to compensate for nonnormality.

As you might expect, the one-sample t test and the confidence interval for a population mean are related. If we reject the null hypothesis (7.17) at the significance level α, the $100(1 - \alpha)\%$ confidence interval for the population mean will not include the number μ_0. If we fail to reject the null hypothesis (7.17) at the significance level α, the $100(1 - \alpha)\%$ confidence interval for the population mean will include the number μ_0. Again, the hypothesis test and the corresponding confidence interval are consistent. When we reject the null hypothesis (7.17), we usually want to estimate the population mean with a confidence interval.

Let us return to the creatinine data. Is a one-sample t test appropriate for testing the null hypothesis that the population mean creatinine is 8.4? Although the data are not a random sample, this is not essential. The independence assumption appears to hold, since the creatinine for one patient tells us nothing about the creatinine for another patient. A histogram of the data, shown in Figure 7.4, suggests a slightly skewed population, but the sample is large enough to compensate for slight skewness. A one-sample t test seems appropriate for these data.

We will use a 0.05 significance level to test the null hypothesis (7.15). For these data, the sample mean is 11.9, the sample standard deviation is 3.6, and the sample size is 12. Using these values in

formula (7.19), we get the calculated one-sample t statistic

$$t = \frac{11.9 - 8.4}{3.6/\sqrt{12}} = \frac{3.5}{1.04} = 3.37$$

The degrees of freedom are $12 - 1 = 11$. In the row for 11 df in Table E.4, the two adjacent numbers that 3.37 lies between are 3.106 and 3.497. These correspond to the upper-tail probabilities 0.005 and 0.0025. Multiplying these probabilities by 2, we get $2(0.005) = 0.01$ and $2(0.0025) = 0.005$, so

$$0.005 < \text{two-tailed } p\text{-value} < 0.01$$

Since the p-value is less than 0.05, we reject the null hypothesis (7.15) at the 0.05 significance level. We would also reject this hypothesis at the 0.01 significance level because the p-value is less than 0.01. Less than 1% of all possible samples will produce a one-sample t statistic at least as extreme as 3.37 if the null hypothesis (7.15) is true. If a 0.005 significance level were used, we would not reject the null hypothesis (7.15), since the p-value is greater than 0.005.

Because we rejected the null hypothesis (7.15) at the 0.05 significance level, we are especially interested in estimating the population mean with a 95% confidence interval. The 95% confidence interval is (9.6, 14.2), which does not include the hypothesized population mean of 8.4. We are 95% sure that the population creatinine mean for end-stage renal disease patients undergoing hemodialysis is between 9.6 and 14.2.

Example 7.6

A study examined the effects of oxygen and hyperinflation on arterial oxygen tension after endotracheal suctioning.[8] Table 7.2 shows the baseline fraction of inspired oxygen (FI_{O_2}) for 28 patients in intensive care units after cardiac surgery. The mean of these FI_{O_2} values is 0.44 and the standard deviation is 0.07. Can we obtain a one-sample t test of the hypothesis that the population mean baseline FI_{O_2} is 0.50? Here the population consists of all patients similar to those in the study who are in intensive care units after cardiac surgery.

The observations are independent. Knowing one patient's FI_{O_2} value tells us nothing about another patient's FI_{O_2} value. But the data are extremely

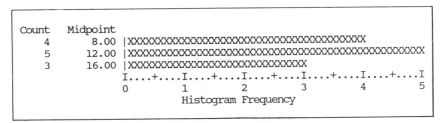

Figure 7.4 SPSS/PC histogram of creatinine

TABLE 7.2   BASELINE FI_{O_2} FOR PATIENTS AFTER CARDIAC SURGERY

Patient No.	Baseline FI_{O_2}
1	0.4
2	0.4
3	0.4
4	0.5
5	0.6
6	0.4
7	0.4
8	0.4
9	0.4
10	0.4
11	0.5
12	0.4
13	0.6
14	0.6
15	0.4
16	0.5
17	0.5
18	0.4
19	0.4
20	0.4
21	0.4
22	0.4
23	0.4
24	0.5
25	0.4
26	0.4
27	0.5
28	0.3
Mean ± SD	0.44 ± 0.07

TABLE 7.3   SERUM TOTAL CALCIUM (ADJUSTED FOR ALBUMIN) FOR FAMILY MEMBERS WITH BENIGN HYPERCALCEMIA

Patient No.	Serum Total Calcium (mmol/l)
1	2.63
2	2.51
3	2.60
4	2.65
5	2.56
6	2.77
Mean ± SD	2.62 ± 0.09

to use these data to test hypotheses about the population of patients with benign hypercalcemia.

7.4   HYPOTHESES ABOUT DIFFERENCES BETWEEN POPULATION MEANS

Population means are often compared by testing a null hypothesis of the form

$$H_0: \mu_1 - \mu_2 = \Delta_0 \qquad (7.22)$$

where Δ_0 (pronounced "delta nought") is a number specified by the researcher. Like p_0 and μ_0, Δ_0 is not derived statistically but is determined by the question the researcher wants to answer. Usually Δ_0 is 0, so the null hypothesis is

$$H_0: \mu_1 - \mu_2 = 0$$

This is the same as the null hypothesis

$$H_0: \mu_1 = \mu_2 \qquad (7.23)$$

The usual alternative hypothesis is the two-sided alternative

$$H_A: \mu_1 - \mu_2 \neq \Delta_0 \qquad (7.24)$$

When Δ_0 is 0, this is the alternative hypothesis

$$H_A: \mu_1 \neq \mu_2 \qquad (7.25)$$

One-sided alternative hypotheses ($H_A: \mu_1 - \mu_2 > \Delta_0$ and $H_A: \mu_1 - \mu_2 < \Delta_0$) are rarely appropriate. We usually cannot rule out one of the possibilities "$\mu_1 - \mu_2 > \Delta_0$" and "$\mu_1 - \mu_2 < \Delta_0$," and both possibilities are usually of interest.

We will describe three methods for testing the null hypothesis (7.22). Although all three methods use t tests, the t statistics are calculated differently and require different assumptions. The *pooled-variance t test* and the *separate-variance t test* require independent samples, whereas the *paired t test* requires paired samples. All too often, the wrong t

nonnormal, since the 28 observations have only four values. We cannot use the one-sample t statistic (7.19) to test the null hypothesis that the population mean FI_{O_2} is 0.50. We could test the hypothesis that the median FI_{O_2} is 0.50 by using the sign test described in Chapter 11.

Example 7.7

In a study of benign hypercalcemia and "benign hypocalcemia" in the same family, the serum total calcium was reported for 10 members of a single family.[9] Six of these family members had high serum total calcium values, as shown in Table 7.3. For these six total calcium values, the mean is 2.62 and the standard deviation is 0.09. Can we test the hypothesis that the population total calcium mean is 2.70 for the population of patients with benign hypercalcemia?

Because the data were obtained from members of the same family, the independence assumption does not hold. Knowing the total calcium value for one family member with benign hypercalcemia gives us some idea of the total calcium values for other family members with benign hypercalcemia. We cannot use these data to test hypotheses about the population mean. No statistical procedure allows us

test is selected, an error that can produce extremely misleading results. Such mistakes should be far less common than they are, as it is easy to determine which t test is appropriate.

7.5 THE POOLED-VARIANCE t TEST

The pooled-variance t test is based on the same assumptions as the pooled-variance confidence interval for $\mu_1 - \mu_2$ described in Chapter 6.

1. Random Sampling. As usual, random sampling is not crucial if the samples are not biased.

2. Independent Samples. If the samples are not independent, the pooled-variance t test cannot be done.

3. Independent Observations Within Each Sample. The pooled-variance t test cannot be done when the observations within each sample are not independent.

4. Sampling from Normal Populations. If the sample is large enough to compensate for nonnormality, the pooled-variance t test can be used when the population is not normal. This test should not be done if the data are extremely nonnormal (e.g., if only a few values are possible). If you are not sure whether your samples are large enough to compensate for nonnormality, consult a statistician.

5. Equal Population Variances. If there is any reason to believe that the population variances are not equal or similar, the pooled-variance t test should not be done.

As before, we determine whether the assumption of equal population variances is reasonable by examining the ratio of the sample variances. If this ratio is between 0.5 and 2, we can assume that the population variances are equal. If this ratio is less than 0.5 or greater than 2, the equal-variance assumption is questionable and the pooled-variance t test should not be done. The separate-variance t test must be considered instead.

The pooled-variance t statistic is given by

$$t = \frac{\bar{x}_1 - \bar{x}_2 - \Delta_0}{s_{\text{pool}}\sqrt{\dfrac{1}{n_1} + \dfrac{1}{n_2}}} \qquad (7.26)$$

where s_{pool} is the pooled estimate of the common population standard deviation introduced in Chapter 6.

$$s_{\text{pool}} = \sqrt{\frac{(n_1 - 1)s_1^2 + (n_2 - 1)s_2^2}{n_1 + n_2 - 2}}$$

It can be shown that the pooled-variance t statistic has a t distribution with $n_1 + n_2 - 2$ degrees of

freedom if the null hypothesis (7.22) is true and the data are independent random samples from normal populations. When a two-sided t test is used, the p-value for the pooled-variance t statistic is the two-tailed probability

$$P\left(\begin{array}{c} t \text{ statistic} \leq -|t_{\text{calc}}| \quad \text{or} \\ t \text{ statistic} \geq |t_{\text{calc}}| \end{array}\right) \qquad (7.27)$$

where t_{calc} is the calculated value of the pooled-variance t statistic (7.26). This p-value is the probability of getting a pooled-variance t statistic at least as extreme as the calculated t statistic if the null hypothesis (7.22) is true. If the one-sided alternative hypothesis H_A: $\mu_1 - \mu_2 > \Delta_0$ is used, the p-value is $P(t \text{ statistic} \geq t_{\text{calc}})$. If the alternative hypothesis H_A: $\mu_1 - \mu_2 < \Delta_0$ is used, the p-value is $P(t \text{ statistic} \leq t_{\text{calc}})$. As before, the two-tailed p-value is twice the one-tailed p-value when the one-tailed p-value is less than or equal to $1/2$. Approximate p-values for pooled-variance t statistics are obtained from Table E.4, using essentially the same procedure described for the one-sample t test. Only the degrees of freedom are different.

Like all of the test statistics described in this chapter, the pooled-variance t statistic (7.26) makes sense as a method for testing a hypothesis. The top part of this statistic measures the discrepancy between the sample value $\bar{x}_1 - \bar{x}_2$ and the hypothesized population value Δ_0. The bottom part is the estimated standard deviation of $\bar{x}_1 - \bar{x}_2$, a fact we will not prove. The absolute value of the pooled-variance t statistic is large when the difference between $\bar{x}_1 - \bar{x}_2$ and the hypothesized population value Δ_0 is large relative to the variability of $\bar{x}_1 - \bar{x}_2$. Thus, a large pooled-variance t statistic provides evidence against the null hypothesis (7.22). A small pooled-variance t statistic does not provide evidence against this hypothesis, since the pooled-variance t statistic is small when the difference between $\bar{x}_1 - \bar{x}_2$ and the hypothesized population value Δ_0 is small relative to the variability of $\bar{x}_1 - \bar{x}_2$.

We reject the null hypothesis (7.22) when the p-value (7.27) is less than the significance level α selected before carrying out the t test. If the p-value is greater than or equal to α, we cannot reject the null hypothesis (7.22) at this significance level.

The pooled-variance t test is closely related to the pooled-variance confidence interval for $\mu_1 - \mu_2$. If the null hypothesis (7.22) is rejected at the significance level α, the number Δ_0 will not be included in the $100(1 - \alpha)\%$ pooled-variance confidence interval for $\mu_1 - \mu_2$. If the null hypothesis (7.22) is not rejected at the significance level α, the $100(1 - \alpha)\%$ pooled-variance confidence interval for $\mu_1 - \mu_2$ will include the number Δ_0. Once again, the hypothesis test and the corresponding confidence interval are consistent. When the null hypothesis (7.22) is rejected, a confidence interval is often obtained to estimate $\mu_1 - \mu_2$.

TABLE 7.4 MORTALITY RATIO FOR HOSPITALS

Nurse Staffing Problems		No Nurse Staffing Problems	
HOSPITAL NO.	MORTALITY RATIO	HOSPITAL NO.	MORTALITY RATIO
1	0.84	9	0.59
2	0.88	10	0.90
3	0.93	11	0.92
4	1.00	12	0.96
5	1.04	13	1.10
6	1.13	Mean ± SD	0.89 ± 0.19
7	1.27		
8	1.58		
Mean ± SD	1.08 ± 0.24		

Example 7.8

A study investigated factors affecting patient outcome in intensive care units (ICUs).[10] For 13 tertiary care hospitals, the ratio of actual ICU deaths to predicted ICU deaths (the mortality ratio) was calculated. A mortality ratio less than 1 indicates fewer deaths than predicted. A mortality ratio greater than 1 indicates more deaths than predicted. Table 7.4 shows the mortality ratios for eight hospitals with nurse staffing problems and five hospitals without nurse staffing problems. Can a pooled-variance t test be used to test the hypothesis that the population mortality ratio means are the same for the staff-problem and no-staff-problem populations?

Since the mortality ratio for one hospital gives no information about the mortality ratio for another hospital, the observations appear to be independent. A histogram of mortality ratios for hospitals with nurse staffing problems (Figure 7.5) suggests a skewed population, but the sample is large enough to compensate for this. A histogram of mortality ratios for hospitals without nurse staffing problems (Figure 7.6) is consistent with sampling from a normal population. From Table 7.4, the ratio of the sample variances is $(0.24)^2/(0.19)^2 = 1.6$, so we can assume that the population variances are equal. Analysis of the data with a pooled-variance t test is justified.

Let us use a 0.10 significance level and a two-sided test of the null hypothesis (7.23). The pooled estimate s_{pool} is

$$s_{\text{pool}} = \sqrt{\frac{(8 - 1)(0.24)^2 + (5 - 1)(0.19)^2}{8 + 5 - 2}}$$
$$= 0.22$$

Using this value and the sample means in Table 7.4, we get the calculated pooled-variance t statistic

$$t = \frac{1.08 - 0.89}{0.22\sqrt{\dfrac{1}{8} + \dfrac{1}{5}}} = \frac{0.19}{0.13} = 1.46$$

The p-value is the two-tailed probability

$$P(t \text{ statistic} \le -1.46 \quad \text{or} \quad t \text{ statistic} \ge 1.46)$$

Using the row for $8 + 5 - 2 = 11$ df in Table E.4, we find that 1.46 lies between the adjacent numbers 1.363 and 1.796. These numbers correspond to the upper-tail probabilities 0.10 and 0.05. Multiplying

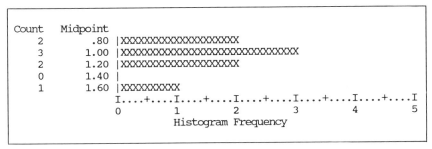

```
Count   Midpoint
  2        .80  |XXXXXXXXXXXXXXXXXXXX
  3       1.00  |XXXXXXXXXXXXXXXXXXXXXXXXXXXXXX
  2       1.20  |XXXXXXXXXXXXXXXXXXXX
  0       1.40  |
  1       1.60  |XXXXXXXXXX
               I....+....I....+....I....+....I....+....I....+....I
               0         1         2         3         4         5
                             Histogram Frequency
```

Figure 7.5 SPSS/PC histogram of mortality ratio for hospitals with nurse staffing problems

```
Count   Midpoint
  1        .55  |XXXXXXXXXX
  3        .85  |XXXXXXXXXXXXXXXXXXXXXXXXXXXXXX
  1       1.15  |XXXXXXXXXX
               I....+....I....+....I....+....I....+....I....+....I
               0         1         2         3         4         5
                             Histogram Frequency
```

Figure 7.6 SPSS/PC histogram of mortality ratio for hospitals without nurse staffing problems

TABLE 7.5 SURFACE LIGHT DOSE FOR PATIENTS WITH BRONCHOGENIC CARCINOMA

Patients with Complete Response		Patients with Less Than Complete Response	
PATIENT NO.	LIGHT DOSE (mW/cm^2)	PATIENT NO.	LIGHT DOSE (mW/cm^2)
1	450	14	250
2	300	15	300
3	300	16	400
4	300	17	300
5	200	18	200
6	300	19	500
7	200	20	200
8	200	21	200
9	200	22	300
10	150	23	500
11	200	24	170
12	300	25	250
13	300	26	200
		27	150
		28	200
		29	200
		30	300
		31	250
		32	100
		33	180
		34	64
		35	150
		36	250
		37	250
		38	250

by 2, we get 2(0.10) = 0.20 and 2(0.05) = 0.10, so

$$0.10 < \text{two-tailed } p\text{-value} < 0.20$$

Since the p-value is greater than 0.10, we cannot reject the hypothesis that the population means are equal. In fact, the p-value is so large that we cannot reject this hypothesis at any reasonable significance level. If the population means are equal, more than 10% of all possible samples will produce pooled-variance t statistics at least as extreme as 1.46. In other words, sample results like ours are not unlikely if the population means are equal. The data do not provide evidence against the hypothesis of equal population means.

Since we cannot reject the hypothesis that the population means are equal at the 0.10 significance level, 0 is in the 90% confidence interval for $\mu_1 - \mu_2$, which is (−0.04, 0.42).

Example 7.9

A study evaluated the use of phototherapy for localized bronchogenic carcinoma.[11] Table 7.5 shows the surface light dose during the first phototherapy treatment for 13 patients who had a complete response and 25 patients who had less than a complete response. Can we use a pooled-variance t test to test the hypothesis that the population light dose

means are the same for the complete-response and incomplete-response populations?

All of the light doses are based on different patients. Knowing the light dose for one patient gives no information about the light dose for another patient, so the observations are independent. The data appear to be extremely nonnormal, however. There are only four dose values for the 13 patients with a complete response, and data with such a limited range of values cannot have even an approximately normal distribution. We cannot use a pooled-variance t test to test the hypothesis that the population means are equal. The Mann-Whitney test described in Chapter 11 can be used instead to test the hypothesis that the complete-response and incomplete-response populations of light doses are identical.

Example 7.10

Suppose a new diuretic was tested on 15 healthy subjects. After subjects used the diuretic for three days, their serum potassium concentrations were measured. Four of these subjects then participated in a second study, in which another diuretic was tested. Six new subjects were also used in this study, for a total of 10 subjects. Again, serum potassium concentrations were measured after subjects used the diuretic for three days. Can a pooled-variance t test be used to test the hypothesis that the population potassium means are the same for the two diuretic populations?

Because four subjects used both diuretics, the between-samples independence assumption does not hold for all observations. The repeated measurements on these four subjects cannot be considered independent, and a pooled-variance t test cannot be done on all of the data. If the repeated measurements are excluded (leaving 11 subjects in the diuretic-1 group and six subjects in the diuretic-2 group), two independent samples result. A pooled-variance t test can be done on these samples if the normality and equal-variance assumptions are satisfied.*

7.6 THE SEPARATE-VARIANCE t TEST

If all of the assumptions for the pooled-variance t test are satisfied except the equal-variance assumption, a separate-variance t test can be done to test the null hypothesis (7.22).[†] This test requires the same assumptions as the separate-variance confidence interval for $\mu_1 - \mu_2$ described in Chapter 6.

---

*The paired t test discussed in Section 7.7 might be used to analyze the potassium concentrations for the subjects who used both diuretics.

[†]The separate-variance t test is also called *Welch's t test*.

1. Random Sampling. As long as the samples are not biased, random sampling is not necessary.

2. Independent Samples. The separate-variance t test cannot be done if the samples are not independent.

3. Independent Observations Within Each Sample. If this assumption is violated, the separate-variance t test cannot be done.

4. Sampling from Normal Populations. The separate-variance t test can be used to analyze nonnormal data if the sample is large enough to compensate for nonnormal populations. This test should not be done if the data are extremely nonnormal (e.g., if the data have only a few possible values). Consult a statistician if you are not sure whether your samples are large enough to compensate for nonnormality.

Like the separate-variance confidence interval, the separate-variance t test does not assume that the population variances are unequal. It simply does not *require* equal population variances. Using the separate-variance t test when the population variances are equal is not an error, but using the pooled-variance t test when the population variances are not equal is a serious mistake. If the ratio of the sample variances is greater than 2 or less than 0.5, the pooled-variance t test should not be used.

The separate-variance t statistic is given by

$$t = \frac{\bar{x}_1 - \bar{x}_2 - \Delta_0}{\sqrt{\dfrac{s_1^2}{n_1} + \dfrac{s_2^2}{n_2}}} \qquad (7.28)$$

It can be shown that the separate-variance t statistic has approximately a t distribution with f degrees of freedom if the null hypothesis (7.22) is true and the data are independent random samples from normal populations. The degrees of freedom f are given by the formula introduced in Chapter 6.

$$f = \frac{\left(\dfrac{s_1^2}{n_1} + \dfrac{s_2^2}{n_2}\right)^2}{\dfrac{\left(\dfrac{s_1^2}{n_1}\right)^2}{n_1 - 1} + \dfrac{\left(\dfrac{s_2^2}{n_2}\right)^2}{n_2 - 1}}$$

When a two-sided separate-variance t test is done, the p-value is the two-tailed probability

$$P\left(\begin{array}{c} t \text{ statistic} \leq -|t_{\text{calc}}| \quad \text{or} \\ t \text{ statistic} \geq |t_{\text{calc}}| \end{array} \right) \qquad (7.29)$$

where t_{calc} is the calculated value of the separate-variance t statistic. This p-value is the probability of getting a separate-variance t statistic at least as extreme as the calculated t statistic if the null hypothesis (7.22) is true. If the one-sided alternative hypothesis H_A: $\mu_1 - \mu_2 > \Delta_0$ is used, the p-value is $P(t \text{ statistic} \geq t_{\text{calc}})$. If the alternative hypothesis H_A: $\mu_1 - \mu_2 < \Delta_0$ is used, the p-value is $P(t \text{ statistic} \leq t_{\text{calc}})$. When the one-tailed p-value is less than or equal to $1/2$, the two-tailed p-value is twice the one-tailed p-value. Table E.4 is used to obtain approximate p-values.

Like all of the test statistics described in this chapter, the separate-variance t statistic is a ratio of the form

$$\frac{\text{difference between sample estimate and hypothesized value}}{\text{estimated standard deviation of sample estimate}}$$

Hence, a large absolute value of this t statistic provides evidence against the null hypothesis (7.22), and a small absolute value of this t statistic does not provide evidence against this hypothesis. When the p-value for the separate-variance t statistic is less than the previously selected significance level α, we reject the null hypothesis (7.22). When the p-value is greater than or equal to α, we cannot reject the null hypothesis (7.22) at this significance level.

As expected, the separate-variance t test and the separate-variance confidence interval for $\mu_1 - \mu_2$ are related. If the null hypothesis (7.22) is rejected at the significance level α, the number Δ_0 will not be included in the $100(1 - \alpha)\%$ separate-variance confidence interval for $\mu_1 - \mu_2$. If the null hypothesis (7.22) is not rejected at the significance level α, the $100(1 - \alpha)\%$ separate-variance confidence interval for $\mu_1 - \mu_2$ will include the number Δ_0. The hypothesis test and the confidence interval are consistent. If the null hypothesis (7.22) is rejected, a confidence interval is often obtained to estimate $\mu_1 - \mu_2$.

Example 7.11

In a study of linear scleroderma, serum IgG levels were reported for nine patients with inactive disease and 30 patients with active disease.[12] These values are shown in Table 7.6. Can a separate-variance t test be used to test the hypothesis that the difference between the population IgG means for the inactive-disease and active-disease populations is -230? In other words, can the separate-variance t test be used to test H_0: $\mu_1 - \mu_2 = -230$?

The independence assumptions seem reasonable, since the IgG for one patient does not tell us anything about the IgG for another patient. A histogram for the inactive-disease group (Figure 7.7) appears consistent with sampling from an approximately normal distribution. Although the histogram for the active-disease group (Figure 7.8) is skewed, the sample is large enough to compensate for a skewed population. From Table 7.6, the ratio of the sample variances is $(180.8)^2/(435.2)^2 = 0.2$, which is less than 0.5. The separate-variance t test seems appropriate.

We will use a 0.01 significance level to carry out a two-sided test of the null hypothesis

$$H_0: \mu_1 - \mu_2 = -230 \qquad (7.30)$$

Here Δ_0 is -230. The calculated separate-variance t statistic is

$$t = \frac{983.9 - 1285.5 - (-230)}{\sqrt{\dfrac{(180.8)^2}{9} + \dfrac{(435.2)^2}{30}}} = \frac{-71.6}{99.7} = -0.72$$

The degrees of freedom f are

$$f = \frac{\left(\dfrac{(180.8)^2}{9} + \dfrac{(435.2)^2}{30}\right)^2}{\dfrac{\left(\dfrac{(180.8)^2}{9}\right)^2}{9-1} + \dfrac{\left(\dfrac{(435.2)^2}{30}\right)^2}{30-1}}$$

$$= \frac{98910433}{3023399} = 32.7$$

Rounding *down* to the nearest integer, we get 32 df.

Table E.4 does not list 32 df, so we have to approximate. Looking in the row for 30 df in Table E.4, we find that 0.72 is between the adjacent numbers 0.530 and 0.854, which correspond to the upper-tail probabilities 0.30 and 0.20. Multiplying by 2, we get

$$0.40 < \text{two-tailed } p\text{-value} < 0.60$$

Since the p-value is greater than 0.01, we cannot reject the null hypothesis (7.30) at the significance level 0.01. In fact, the p-value is so large that we cannot reject this hypothesis at any reasonable significance level. More than 40% of all possible samples produce calculated separate-variance t statistics at least as extreme as -0.72 if the null hypothesis (7.30) is true. The data do not provide

evidence against this null hypothesis. If we compute a 99% confidence interval for $\mu_1 - \mu_2$, we get the interval estimate $(-575.8, -27.4)$, which includes the hypothesized value -230.

Example 7.12

Suppose a pediatric nurse wanted to determine whether mothers and fathers view the importance

TABLE 7.6   SERUM IgG FOR PATIENTS WITH LINEAR SCLERODERMA

Patients with Inactive Disease		Patients with Active Disease	
PATIENT NO.	IgG (mg/dl)	Patient No.	IgG (mg/dl)
1	680	10	1220
2	980	11	1150
3	1025	12	1300
4	950	13	1430
5	840	14	1300
6	1250	15	1475
7	950	16	740
8	1250	17	1250
9	930	18	1070
Mean ± SD	983.9 ± 180.8	19	800
		20	880
		21	1400
		22	1100
		23	1000
		24	1100
		25	1550
		26	660
		27	820
		28	1250
		29	1400
		30	1950
		31	1200
		32	1850
		33	930
		34	1700
		35	1250
		36	1150
		37	1140
		38	2900
		39	1600
		Mean ± SD	1285.5 ± 435.2

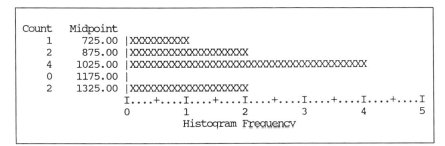

```
Count   Midpoint
    1     725.00 |XXXXXXXXXX
    2     875.00 |XXXXXXXXXXXXXXXXXXXX
    4    1025.00 |XXXXXXXXXXXXXXXXXXXXXXXXXXXXXXXXXXXXXXXXXX
    0    1175.00 |
    2    1325.00 |XXXXXXXXXXXXXXXXXXXX
           I....+....I....+....I....+....I....+....I....+....I
           0         1         2         3         4         5
                    Histogram Frequency
```

Figure 7.7   SPSS/PC histogram of serum IgG for patients with inactive linear scleroderma

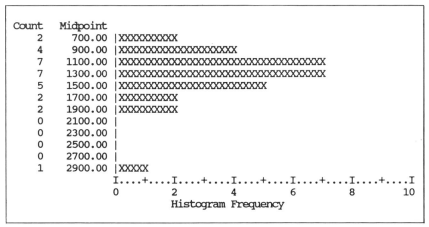

```
Count   Midpoint
   2     700.00  |XXXXXXXXXX
   4     900.00  |XXXXXXXXXXXXXXXXXXXX
   7    1100.00  |XXXXXXXXXXXXXXXXXXXXXXXXXXXXXXXXXXXXX
   7    1300.00  |XXXXXXXXXXXXXXXXXXXXXXXXXXXXXXXXXXXXX
   5    1500.00  |XXXXXXXXXXXXXXXXXXXXXXXXX
   2    1700.00  |XXXXXXXXXX
   2    1900.00  |XXXXXXXXXX
   0    2100.00  |
   0    2300.00  |
   0    2500.00  |
   0    2700.00  |
   1    2900.00  |XXXXX
            I....+....I....+....I....+....I....+....I....+....I
            0         2         4         6         8        10
                       Histogram Frequency
```

Figure 7.8 SPSS/PC histogram of serum IgG for patients with active linear scleroderma

of diptheria-tetanus-pertussis (DTP) vaccination differently. During three consecutive busy evenings, her clinic waiting room was crowded with at least 10 parents with their children. While these people were waiting, the nurse entered the waiting room and explained the purpose of DTP vaccination. She then went around the room and asked each parent to tell her how important DTP vaccination is, using the following scale.

1 = not at all important
2 = slightly important
3 = moderately important
4 = very important
5 = extremely important

For the 27 mothers interviewed, the mean rating is 4.1 and the standard deviation is 0.3. For the 11 fathers interviewed, the mean rating is 3.2 and the standard deviation is 0.7. Can a separate-variance t test be used to test the hypothesis that the population means are equal? Here the populations of interest to the nurse consist of all mothers and all fathers.

The separate-variance t test cannot be used because the data violate every assumption on which the test is based. First, the samples consist primarily of parents with sick children. Since the populations of interest are all mothers and fathers, these samples are extremely biased. Second, the nurse asked each parent about vaccination in the presence of other parents, so a parent's rating is likely to be influenced by the responses of other parents. If five parents in a row state emphatically that vaccination is extremely important, the sixth parent is unlikely to state that vaccination is not at all important. The ratings from the same evening cannot be considered independent, even though they were obtained from different parents, so both of the independence assumptions are violated. Finally, the ratings have an extremely nonnormal distribution, with only five

possible values. No statistical method allows us to use these data to test hypotheses about the population.

7.7 THE PAIRED t TEST

When we want to use paired samples to test the null hypothesis (7.22), we cannot use the pooled-variance t test or the separate-variance t test. Another t test, called the *paired t test*, must be considered. This test requires the same assumptions as the paired-samples confidence interval for $\mu_1 - \mu_2$ discussed in Chapter 6.

1. Random Sampling of Differences. The differences need not be a random sample if the sample is not biased.

2. Paired Samples. If the samples are not paired, the paired t test cannot be done.

3. Independent Differences. The paired t test cannot be done if the differences are not independent.

4. Sampling from a Normal Population of Differences. If the *differences* do not come from a normal population, the paired t test can still be done if the number of differences is large enough to compensate for nonnormality. This test should not be done if the differences are extremely nonnormal (e.g., if the differences have only a few possible values). If you are not sure whether the sample of differences is large enough to compensate for a nonnormal population, consult a statistician.

To carry out the paired t test, we first convert the two paired samples into one sample of differences, as described for the paired-samples confidence interval procedure. It can be shown that the population mean of the differences is equal to $\mu_1 - \mu_2$ and the sample mean of the differences is equal to $\bar{x}_1 - \bar{x}_2$. Thus, the sample mean of the differences is our estimate of $\mu_1 - \mu_2$. The paired t statistic is given by

$$t = \frac{\bar{d} - \Delta_0}{s_d / \sqrt{n}} \qquad (7.31)$$

where $\bar{d}$ is the sample mean of the differences, s_d is the sample standard deviation of the differences, and n is the number of differences. It can be shown that the paired t statistic has a t distribution with $n - 1$ degrees of freedom if the null hypothesis (7.22) is true and the differences are a random sample from a normal population. When a two-sided test is used, the p-value for the paired t statistic is the two-tailed probability

$$P\left(\begin{array}{c} t \text{ statistic} < -|t_{\text{calc}}| \quad \text{or} \\ t \text{ statistic} > |t_{\text{calc}}| \end{array} \right) \qquad (7.32)$$

where t_{calc} is the calculated value of the paired t statistic. This p-value is the probability of getting a paired t statistic at least as extreme as the calculated t statistic if the null hypothesis (7.22) is true. If the one-sided alternative hypothesis H_A: $\mu_1 - \mu_2 > \Delta_0$ is used, the p-value is $P(t \text{ statistic} \geq t_{\text{calc}})$. If the alternative hypothesis H_A: $\mu_1 - \mu_2 < \Delta_0$ is used, the p-value is $P(t \text{ statistic} \leq t_{\text{calc}})$. As expected, the two-tailed p-value is twice the one-tailed p-value when the one-tailed p-value is less than or equal to $1/2$. Approximate p-values can be obtained from Table E.4.

The paired t statistic has the usual test-statistic format. The top part measures the discrepancy between the sample estimate and the hypothesized value, and the bottom part measures the variability of the sample estimate. The same reasoning as before shows that a large absolute value of the paired t statistic provides evidence against the null hypothesis (7.22), and a small absolute value of the t statistic does not provide evidence against this hypothesis. Large t statistics have small p-values, and we reject the null hypothesis (7.22) if the p-value is less than the previously selected significance level α. We cannot reject the null hypothesis (7.22) at this

TABLE 7.7 PREINSTRUCTION AND POSTINSTRUCTION TEST SCORES (% CORRECT) FOR DIALYSIS PATIENTS

Patient No.	Before Instruction	After Instruction	Difference (Before − After)
1	65	85	− 20
2	81	69	12
3	69	92	− 23
4	42	69	− 27
5	77	88	− 11
6	69	88	− 19
7	69	92	− 23
8	69	77	− 8
9	77	88	− 11
10	58	96	− 38
Mean ± SD	67.6 ± 11.1	84.4 ± 9.5	− 16.8 ± 13.4

significance level if the p-value is greater than or equal to α.

The usual relationship between a test statistic and its corresponding confidence interval holds for the paired t test and the paired-samples confidence interval. If the null hypothesis (7.22) is rejected at the significance level α, the $100(1 - \alpha)\%$ confidence interval for $\mu_1 - \mu_2$ will not include the number Δ_0. If (7.22) is not rejected at the significance level α, the $100(1 - \alpha)\%$ confidence interval for $\mu_1 - \mu_2$ will include the number Δ_0. When we reject the null hypothesis (7.22), we usually want to estimate $\mu_1 - \mu_2$ with a confidence interval.

Example 7.13

In a study of dialysis patient education, 10 patients on dialysis were given programmed instruction about kidney function and renal failure.[13] Patients were tested on this information before and after instruction. The preinstruction and postinstruction test scores for these patients are shown in Table 7.7. Can a paired t test be used to test the hypothesis that the population test score mean before instruction is the same as the population test score mean after instruction? Here the population consists of all dialysis patients similar to those in the study.

The differences between the preinstruction and postinstruction test scores should be independent if

```
Count   Midpoint
   1     -37.50  |XXXXXXXXXX
   5     -22.50  |XXXXXXXXXXXXXXXXXXXXXXXXXXXXXXXXXXXXXXXXXXXXXXXXXXXX
   3      -7.50  |XXXXXXXXXXXXXXXXXXXXXXXXXXXXXX
   1       8.50  |XXXXXXXXXX
                 I....+....I....+....I....+....I....+....I....+....I
                 0         1         2         3         4         5
                          Histogram Frequency
```

Figure 7.9 SPSS/PC histogram of test score difference

none of the patients cheated. Knowing one patient's difference tells us nothing about another patient's difference. A histogram of the differences, shown in Figure 7.9, is consistent with sampling from a normal population. Only a histogram of the *differences* is obtained, since histograms for the paired samples tell us nothing about the distribution of the differences. A paired *t* test seems appropriate for these data.

Let us use a 0.05 significance level to test the null hypothesis that the population means are equal. The differences have a mean of -16.8 and a standard deviation of 13.4, so the calculated paired *t* statistic is

$$t = \frac{-16.8}{13.4/\sqrt{10}} = -3.96$$

Looking in the row for 9 df in Table E.4, we find that 3.96 is between the adjacent numbers 3.690 and 4.781, which correspond to the upper-tail probabilities 0.0025 and 0.0005. Multiplying by 2, we get

$$0.001 < \text{two-tailed } p\text{-value} < 0.005$$

We reject the hypothesis of equal population means at the 0.05 significance level. Less than 0.5% of all possible samples produce paired *t* statistics at least as extreme as -3.96, if the null hypothesis (7.23) is true. A 95% paired-samples confidence interval for $\mu_1 - \mu_2$ is given by the interval estimate $(-26.4, -7.2)$, which does not include 0.

Example 7.14

A study described the response of 22 dogs with hyposomatotropism to xylazine stimulation.[14] The data in Table 7.8 are the plasma growth hormone (GH) levels before and 30 minutes after xylazine stimulation. Can a paired *t* test be used to test the hypothesis that the pre-xylazine and post-xylazine population GH means are the same?

The samples are evidently paired, and the differences appear to be independent, since the difference for one dog gives no information about the difference for another dog. If the differences are calculated, all of them are 0 except the difference of 3.1 for the fourth dog. Because the distribution of the differences is extremely nonnormal, we cannot use the paired *t* test. The difficulty with these data stems from the lower detection limit of the GH assay, which is 0.39 ng/ml. Since all but one of the GH levels are equal to or below the detection limit, no statistical procedure allows us to use these censored data to determine whether xylazine affects GH levels.

Example 7.15

Six patients with interstitial lung disease (ILD) were studied to determine their responses to treatment with azathioprine or prednisone.[15] Table 7.9 shows

TABLE 7.8   PLASMA GH LEVELS IN DOGS WITH HYPOSOMATOTROPISM BEFORE AND AFTER XYLAZINE STIMULATION

Dog No.	Basal GH (ng/ml)	GH (ng/ml) 30 Minutes After Xylazine
1	0.39	0.39
2	0.39	0.39
3	0.39	0.39
4	8.1	5.0
5	0.39	0.39
6	0.39	0.39
7	0.39	0.39
8	0.39	0.39
9	0.39	0.39
10	0.39	0.39
11	0.39	0.39
12	0.39	0.39
13	0.39	0.39
14	0.39	0.39
15	0.39	0.39
16	0.39	0.39
17	0.39	0.39
18	0.39	0.39
19	0.39	0.39
20	0.39	0.39
21	0.39	0.39
22	0.39	0.39

preexercise and postexercise $PaCO_2$ values for three of these patients after a course of treatment with azathioprine and bronchodilators. Can a paired *t* test be used to test the hypothesis that the population preexercise mean is the same as the population postexercise mean? Here the population is the theoretical population that would result if all patients with ILD similar to those in the study were treated with azathioprine and bronchodilators.

Although the data are clearly paired, each patient has two differences. Since the differences for any given patient cannot be considered independent, the independence assumption is violated. A paired *t* test cannot be done on all six differences. The differences could be split into two samples, with one sample consisting of the first differences and the other consisting of the second differences. If the corresponding populations are normal or nearly

TABLE 7.9   PREEXERCISE AND POSTEXERCISE $PaCO_2$ FOR PATIENTS WITH INTERSTITIAL LUNG DISEASE

Patient No.	Date	PaCO₂ PRE	PaCO₂ POST	Difference
1	1/85	43	50	-7
	7/85	42	49	-7
2	3/85	38	37	1
	6/85	39	36	3
3	8/83	32	35	-3
	2/84	39	36	3

```
Group 1:  GROUP  EQ     1.00          Group 2:  GROUP  EQ     2.00


t-test for:  RATIO

                    Number            Standard   Standard
                    of Cases   Mean   Deviation    Error

          Group 1      8      1.0838     .244       .086
          Group 2      5       .8940     .187       .084


               | Pooled Variance Estimate | Separate Variance Estimate
               |                          |
     F   2-Tail|   t    Degrees of 2-Tail |   t    Degrees of 2-Tail
  Value  Prob. | Value  Freedom    Prob.  | Value  Freedom    Prob.
               |                          |
   1.70  .635  |  1.48    11       .167   |  1.58   10.35     .144
```

Figure 7.10   SPSS/PC *t*-test output for mortality-ratio data

```
Paired samples t-test:  PRETEST
                        POSTTEST

Variable     Number            Standard   Standard
             of Cases   Mean   Deviation    Error

PRETEST        10     67.6000   11.147      3.525
POSTTEST       10     84.4000    9.536      3.016


(Difference) Standard    Standard |    2-Tail   |   t    Degrees of 2-Tail
    Mean     Deviation     Error  | Corr. Prob. | Value  Freedom    Prob.
                                  |             |
  -16.8000    13.415      4.242   |  .166  .647 | -3.96     9        .003
```

Figure 7.11   SPSS/PC paired *t*-test output for test score data

normal, two paired *t* tests could be done, one for each sample of differences. A paired *t* test based on only three observations has a very small chance of detecting a difference between the population means unless this difference is very large. Such a test is said to have low *power*. Power is discussed further in Section 7.9 and Appendix A.

We have discussed three *t* tests for testing the null hypothesis (7.22), plus a one-sample *t* test for testing the null hypothesis (7.17). Because there are so many *t* tests, it is important to specify exactly which test was used. Medical and health care articles often include only vague descriptions, such as the statement that "a Student's *t* test was done." Since "Student's *t* test" could mean any of the four *t* tests described in this chapter, the reader has no way of determining whether the correct test was used.

7.8   COMPUTER OUTPUT FOR *t* TESTS

Computer packages can be used to carry out all of the *t* tests discussed here. The most widely available statistical software systems are SPSS (encountered in Chapter 2) and SAS.* Not only do computer programs eliminate tedious calculations, they also provide exact *p*-values. In SPSS, the T-TEST procedure is used to obtain *t* tests. In SAS, the TTEST and MEANS procedures are used.

Figures 7.10 and 7.11 show *t*-test output produced by the SPSS/PC package. The output in Figure 7.10 shows the pooled-variance and separate-variance *t* tests of the null hypothesis (7.23), using the mortality-ratio data of Example 7.8. The

---

*The operation of SAS is described in several manuals.[16–18]

calculated pooled-variance t statistic, listed under "t Value," is 1.48, which differs slightly from our calculated pooled-variance t statistic because of rounding error. The exact two-tailed p-value for the pooled-variance t test, listed under "2-Tail Prob.," is 0.167, which lies in the range we obtained for this p-value ($0.10 <$ two-tailed p-value < 0.20). The column labeled "Standard Error" contains the estimated standard deviations of the sample means ($s_1/\sqrt{n_1}$ and $s_2/\sqrt{n_2}$). The number listed under "F Value" is the ratio of the larger sample variance to the smaller sample variance. This value also agrees with our calculations, within rounding error. The "2-Tail Prob." given next to the F value concerns a test of the hypothesis that the population variances are equal. We will not describe this test, which relies so heavily on the normality assumption that it has little practical value. If the F value is greater than 2, the separate-variance t-test output should be used. If the F value is less than or equal to 2, the pooled-variance t-test output should be used, unless there is some reason to suspect that the population variances are not equal.

The output in Figure 7.11 shows the SPSS/PC paired t-test output for the test score data of Example 7.13. The calculated paired t statistic, listed under "t Value," is -3.96, which is the same as our calculated paired t statistic. The exact p-value for the two-sided paired t test, listed under "2-Tail Prob.," is 0.003, which lies in the range we obtained earlier ($0.001 <$ two-tailed p-value < 0.005. The value under "Corr." should be ignored for now. (This value is the Pearson correlation coefficient for the before-instruction test scores and the after-instruction test scores. The Pearson correlation co-

efficient is discussed in Chapter 12.) Sometimes the p-value given in SPSS output is .000. This does *not* mean that the p-value is 0, but that the p-value is less than or equal to 0.0005.

SAS t-test output for the same data sets is shown in Figures 7.12 and 7.13. Figure 7.12 shows the pooled-variance and separate-variance t tests for the mortality-ratio data. In this output, the calculated t statistics are listed under "T." The column labeled "VARIANCES" indicates which t test was done. "UNEQUAL" refers to the separate-variance t test and "EQUAL" refers to the pooled-variance t test. The pooled-variance t statistic has the value 1.4798, which rounds off to the SPSS/PC pooled-variance t value of 1.48. The degrees of freedom are listed under "DF," and the exact p-values for two-sided t tests are listed under "PROB > |T|." In the column labeled "STD ERROR," the estimated standard deviations of the sample means are printed. The F' value of 1.70 is the ratio of the larger sample variance to the smaller sample variance, and "PROB > F'" refers to the p-value for the F test for equal variances mentioned earlier. In Figure 7.13, the calculated paired t statistic for the test score data is shown under "T," and the p-value for the two-sided paired t test is shown under "PR>|T|."

A computer can do the calculations required for hypothesis testing, but it cannot determine whether assumptions hold or whether the correct test was selected. If a computer is asked to perform an inappropriate test, it will do so without protest as long as the calculations can be carried out. A computer will cheerfully perform a Z test on nonindependent data or a t test on grossly nonnormal data.

```
VARIABLE: RATIO

GROUP        N              MEAN            STD DEV          STD ERROR

   1         8          1.08375000       0.24395184        0.08625000
   2         5          0.89400000       0.18702941        0.08364209

VARIANCES        T        DF    PROB > |T|

UNEQUAL       1.5793     10.3      0.1444
EQUAL         1.4798     11.0      0.1670

FOR H0: VARIANCES ARE EQUAL, F'=    1.70 WITH 7 AND 4 DF
        PROB > F'= 0.6354
```

Figure 7.12 SAS t-test output for mortality-ratio data

VARIABLE	MEAN	STD ERROR OF MEAN	T	PR>|T|
DIFF	−16.80000000	4.24211687	−3.96	0.0033

Figure 7.13 SAS paired t-test output for test score data

The fact that a computer produced a test statistic does not mean that the statistic was appropriate. Computers eliminate tedious calculations, but they cannot take on the responsibility for selecting the correct test. Even in this age of high technology, there is no substitute for a statistically literate researcher.

7.9 TESTING PITFALLS

Certain aspects of testing are frequent sources of difficulty and warrant discussion here.

1. Violations of Independence Assumptions and Extreme Violations of Normality Assumptions. The same remarks as in Chapter 6 apply here.

2. P-Values. *P*-values are often interpreted incorrectly in the medical and health care literature. The most common misinterpretation is the notion that a *p*-value is the probability that the null hypothesis is true. This mistake arises when population parameters are viewed as random variables, an erroneous idea discussed in Chapter 6. Since population parameters are fixed numbers, a null hypothesis about a population parameter is either true or false. If it is true, the probability that the null hypothesis is true is 1. If it is false, the probability that the null hypothesis is true is 0.

Another common misinterpretation of *p*-values is the idea that a *p*-value is the probability that the sample results were due to chance, or sampling variability. To say that the sample results were due to sampling variability is to say that the null hypothesis is true, so this misinterpretation is a variation of the mistaken idea that the *p*-value is the probability that the null hypothesis is true.

A *p*-value is correctly interpreted as follows: *The p-value is the probability of getting a test statistic at least as extreme as the calculated test statistic if the null hypothesis is true.* If the *p*-value is 0.61, the probability of getting a test statistic at least as extreme as the calculated test statistic is 0.61, if the null hypothesis is true. In other words, 61% of all possible samples produce test statistics at least as extreme as the calculated test statistic if the null hypothesis is true.

Whenever possible, exact *p*-values should be calculated and reported. Many medical and health care articles only report whether the *p*-value is less than the significance level.* If an article states that the *p*-value is less than 0.05, we have no way of knowing whether the *p*-value is 0.049, say, or 0.000014, and there is a big difference between these *p*-values. A 0.05 significance level may be accepted by some researchers, but others may pre-

fer a different significance level. If the exact *p*-value is given, the reader can use whatever significance level she prefers to determine whether the null hypothesis should be rejected.

3. Statistical Significance Versus Practical Significance. When the null hypothesis is rejected, the hypothesis test is said to be *statistically significant.* Statistical significance is frequently confused with practical or clinical significance. A statistically significant test, no matter how small the *p*-value, does not guarantee that the results have any practical significance. Suppose a *p*-value of 0.0002 leads us to conclude that the population mean duration of pain relief for patients given a new analgesic is greater than the population mean duration of pain relief for patients given ibuprofen. If a 99% confidence interval for the difference between the population mean durations of pain relief is (0.2 minutes, 1.1 minutes), the new drug has no practical significance at all as far as increased duration of pain relief is concerned. If these results are reported by stating that the new drug significantly increases the mean duration of pain relief, readers will be misled into thinking that the drug causes a large increase in mean pain relief.

For this reason, researchers should avoid such statements as "the difference between the means was significant" or "the mean was significantly different from 0." Instead, results should be summarized with statements like the following.

> "We concluded that the population mean BUN for older patients does not equal the population mean BUN for younger patients (separate-variance *t* test, *p* = 0.036)."

> "We rejected the hypothesis that the population mean difference is 0 (paired *t* test, *p* = 0.0072)."

Further information about reporting statistical results can be found in Appendix B.

4. Nonsignificant Tests. A nonsignificant *p*-value does not imply that the null hypothesis is true. If extremely large samples are used, the test has a good chance of rejecting a false null hypothesis. In this case, a nonsignificant *p*-value provides evidence in favor of the null hypothesis. But if small samples are used, the test has little chance of rejecting a false null hypothesis. In this case, a nonsignificant *p*-value does *not* provide evidence in favor of the null hypothesis. When small samples are used, we have no way of knowing whether nonsignificant *p*-values result from a true null hypothesis or from a small chance of rejecting a false null hypothesis.

A common error in the medical and health care literature is the assumption that a failure to reject the null hypothesis constitutes proof that the null hypothesis is true. Even if the null hypothesis is false, a statistical test may have such a small chance of rejecting the null hypothesis that it would be surprising if a statistically significant *p*-value were obtained.

---

*In the medical and health care literature, *p*-values are usually abbreviated as *p* or *P* and reported with parenthetical statements like "($p < 0.01$)," "($P > 0.10$)," or "($p = 0.029$)."

Consider the debate over single-dose versus multiple-dose antibiotic treatment for uncomplicated urinary tract infections (UTIs). Two researchers examined 14 randomized controlled experiments on this subject.[19] Although 12 of these 14 studies failed to find a statistically significant difference between single-dose and multiple-dose treatment, none of them included enough patients to have a large chance of detecting a difference. When data from these studies were combined, the percentage cured with single-dose amoxicillin therapy was found to be 69% and the percentage cured with conventional multidose therapy was found to be 84%.* These sample proportions allow us to reject the hypothesis of equal population proportions. Many health professionals had assumed that the nonsignificant studies established the equivalent effectiveness of single-dose and multiple-dose therapy.

5. The Multiplicity Problem. When many hypothesis tests are done, we want to be fairly sure that *all* of them are correct. Suppose 100 paired *t* tests are carried out with the significance level 0.05, and the null hypothesis for each test is true. If only one paired *t* test is done at this significance level, the probability that we will reject the null hypothesis (if it is true) is 0.05. When 100 paired *t* tests are done at the 0.05 significance level, we expect about five of them to have *p*-values less than 0.05 if all the null hypotheses are true. We are virtually certain that about five of these tests will lead to the incorrect decision to reject a true null hypothesis. This is called the *multiplicity problem*, and it occurs whenever large numbers of hypothesis tests are carried out.

A medical analogy may help you see the problem more clearly. Suppose the probability of recovery from intervertebral disc disease is 0.11 if no treatment is given. If you see a patient with intervertebral disc disease who refuses treatment, you can be fairly certain (89% sure) that the patient will not recover. But if you see 100 patients with untreated intervertebral disc disease, you cannot be certain that *all* of these patients will not recover. In fact, you can be fairly sure that about 11 of them will recover. The same sort of situation produces the multiplicity problem in hypothesis testing.

How can we deal with the multiplicity problem? One method involves the use of smaller significance levels for each test when a large number of tests is done. Specifically, a *Bonferroni adjustment* can be made. If *k* tests are to be done, we adjust the significance level α by dividing it by *k*. The *p*-value for each test is compared with the adjusted significance level to determine whether the null hypothesis can be rejected. If this is done, the probability of mistakenly rejecting *any* of the null hypotheses when they are true is less than or equal to α. (This fact is not obvious and requires a proof that we will omit.)

The unadjusted significance level is the *overall significance level*, the significance level for *all* of the null hypotheses considered as a group. The overall significance level is an upper bound for the probability of rejecting any of the null hypotheses if all of them are true. If we plan to do 28 *t* tests and we want an overall significance level of 0.05, the significance level used for each test is $0.05/28 = 0.0018$. If we plan to do 35 *Z* tests and we want an overall significance level of 0.10, the significance level for each test is $0.10/35 = 0.0029$.

The Bonferroni adjustment has an important disadvantage. Its use reduces the probability of rejecting a null hypothesis when the null hypothesis is false. The probability of rejecting a false null hypothesis is called the *power* of a test. We want the power to be as large as possible. The power can be made equal to 1 only by examining the entire population or by always rejecting the null hypothesis. If the null hypothesis is always rejected and it happens to be true, the probability of mistakenly rejecting a true null hypothesis is 1. The only way to increase power without increasing the chance that you reject a true hypothesis is to obtain a larger sample.*

One way to reduce the loss of power caused by Bonferroni adjustments is to compromise when you select your overall significance level. Instead of using an overall significance level of 0.05, you may want to settle for a level of 0.10 or 0.20. Other methods for dealing with the multiplicity problem are described in Chapters 8 and 13.

SUMMARY

Hypothesis testing is done to determine whether data provide evidence against a null hypothesis. Hypotheses about a population proportion are tested with the one-sample *Z* test, which is based on the standard normal distribution. Hypotheses about a difference between population proportions are tested with the two-sample *Z* test, which is also based on the standard normal distribution. The one-sample *t* test is based on *t* distributions and is used to test hypotheses about a population mean. Three test procedures based on *t* distributions are used to test hypotheses about a difference between population means: the pooled-variance *t* test, the

---

*Data from different studies cannot be combined arbitrarily, and several criteria were used in this article to determine whether the UTI data should be pooled. These criteria are discussed in the article and elsewhere.[20]

---

*Appendix A includes a brief description of the relationship between power and sample size. Further information can be found in other texts.[21]

separate-variance t test, and the paired t test. These t tests require different assumptions.

Some of the assumptions required for hypothesis tests can be relaxed, whereas others cannot be. If the independence assumptions for a hypothesis test are not met, the test cannot be done. If the normality assumptions for a hypothesis test are not met, the test can be done if approximate normality holds. Hypothesis tests that assume normality cannot be done if the data are extremely nonnormal.

All hypothesis tests produce p-values. The p-value is the probability of getting a test statistic at least as extreme as the calculated test statistic if the null hypothesis is true. It is *not* the probability that the null hypothesis is true. A p-value is compared with the significance level selected by the researcher in order to decide whether to reject the null hypothesis. When a decision about the null hypothesis is made, two mistakes can result: a Type I error or a Type II error. It is not possible to determine whether these mistakes were made when a hypothesis test is done.

Common pitfalls in hypothesis testing are the violation of assumptions, the misinterpretation of p-values, the confusion of statistical significance with practical significance, the misinterpretation of nonsignificant tests, and the multiplicity problem.

FORMULAS FOR QUANTITIES NEEDED TO OBTAIN TEST STATISTICS

$$s_{prop} = \sqrt{\frac{\hat{p}(1 - \hat{p})}{n}}$$

$$s_{diff} = \sqrt{\frac{\hat{p}_1(1 - \hat{p}_1)}{n_1} + \frac{\hat{p}_2(1 - \hat{p}_2)}{n_2}}$$

$$s_{pool} = \sqrt{\frac{(n_1 - 1)s_1^2 + (n_2 - 1)s_2^2}{n_1 + n_2 - 2}}$$

$$s_d = \sqrt{\frac{\sum_{i=1}^{n}(d_i - \bar{d})^2}{n - 1}}$$

$$f = \frac{\left(\dfrac{s_1^2}{n_1} + \dfrac{s_2^2}{n_2}\right)^2}{\dfrac{\left(\dfrac{s_1^2}{n_1}\right)^2}{n_1 - 1} + \dfrac{\left(\dfrac{s_2^2}{n_2}\right)^2}{n_2 - 1}}$$

FORMULAS FOR TEST STATISTICS

Null Hypothesis	Test Statistic	Distribution of Test Statistic
$p = p_0$	$Z = \dfrac{\hat{p} - p_0}{s_{prop}}$	Approximately standard normal
$p_1 = p_2$	$Z = \dfrac{\hat{p}_1 - \hat{p}_2}{s_{diff}}$	Approximately standard normal
$\mu = \mu_0$	$t = \dfrac{\bar{x} - \mu_0}{s/\sqrt{n}}$	t distribution with $n - 1$ df
$\mu_1 - \mu_2 = \Delta_0$	For INDEPENDENT samples WITH equal-variance assumption: $t = \dfrac{\bar{x}_1 - \bar{x}_2 - \Delta_0}{s_{pool}\sqrt{\dfrac{1}{n_1} + \dfrac{1}{n_2}}}$	t distribution with $n_1 + n_2 - 2$ df
$\mu_1 - \mu_2 = \Delta_0$	For INDEPENDENT samples WITHOUT equal-variance assumption $t = \dfrac{\bar{x}_1 - \bar{x}_2 - \Delta_0}{\sqrt{\dfrac{s_1^2}{n_1} + \dfrac{s_2^2}{n_2}}}$	Approximate t distribution with f df
$\mu_1 - \mu_2 = \Delta_0$	For PAIRED samples $t = \dfrac{\bar{d} - \Delta_0}{s_d/\sqrt{n}}$	t distribution with $n - 1$ df

PROBLEMS

The following instructions apply to problems 2 through 25.

1. In each problem, data are presented and a question is asked. Determine whether any of the hypothesis tests described in this chapter are appropriate for answering the question. If no test is appropriate, state which assumptions are violated.

2. If a hypothesis test is appropriate, carry out the test. Specify the null and alternative hypotheses and find the most exact p-value that can be obtained from the tables in this text. Interpret the p-value and use the test results to answer the question in the problem.

3. Do not use one-sided tests unless the excluded possibility cannot occur or the excluded possibility is of no interest to anyone who might look up the test results.

Descriptive statistics and histograms are provided when necessary. Unnecessary statistics and histograms are given in some problems. Histograms for samples with less than five observations are not informative and are not given. Do not worry about slightly or moderately nonnormal histograms if the data have a large number of possible values. Unless the histogram is extremely nonnormal and the sample is very small, you can assume that the central limit theorem applies to the data.

1. Construct a flowchart that will help you determine which of the test statistics discussed in this chapter might be appropriate for particular data sets. This flowchart will closely resemble the confidence-interval flowchart obtained for problem 6.1. The flowchart should begin as follows:

TABLE 7.10 GRAVIDITY FOR WOMEN IN KETONURIA GROUPS

Ketonuria for < 3 Days	Ketonuria for ≥ 3 Days
2	1
3	1
1	2
2	
1	Mean $\pm$ SD 1.3 ± 0.6
1	
Mean $\pm$ SD 1.7 ± 0.8	

shown in Table 7.10. A histogram for the women with ketonuria for less than three days is shown in Figure 7.14. (A histogram for the women with ketonuria for at least three days cannot be used to check normality because the sample size is only 3.) Do the data provide evidence that the population gravidity mean for women with ketonuria for less than three days differs from the population gravidity mean for women with ketonuria for at least three days? Use a 0.01 significance level.

3. A study was conducted to determine whether the Valsalva response occurs during the tensing portion of progressive relaxation.[23] Forty-three per cent of 60 healthy adult volunteers exhibited the Valsalva response during progressive relaxation. A nurse believes that the population proportion of healthy adults who exhibit the Valsalva response during progressive relaxation is 0.40. Do the data provide evidence that the population proportion is not 0.40? Use a 0.05 significance level.

4. A study evaluated the success of surgical stabilization of the rheumatoid cervical spine for relief

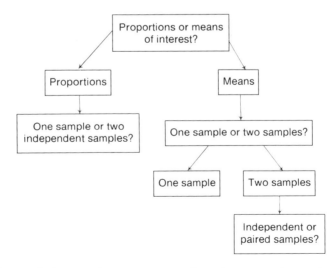

2. In a study of ketonuria in normal pregnancy, gravidity was reported for six women who had ketonuria for less than three days during pregnancy and for three women who had ketonuria for at least three days during pregnancy.[22] These data are

of cord compression and associated neurological impairment.[24] Thirty-two patients underwent a total of 40 operations, and 58% of these operations were successful. A surgeon believes that the population success rate for this surgery is 65%. Do the data

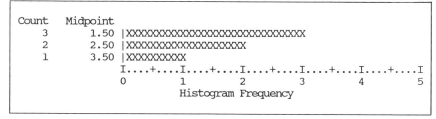

```
Count   Midpoint
   3      1.50   |XXXXXXXXXXXXXXXXXXXXXXXXXXXXXX
   2      2.50   |XXXXXXXXXXXXXXXXXXXX
   1      3.50   |XXXXXXXXXX
               I....+....I....+....I....+....I....+....I....+....I
               0         1         2         3         4         5
                         Histogram Frequency
```

Figure 7.14 SPSS/PC histogram of gravidity for women with ketonuria for less than three days

provide evidence that the population success rate is not 65%? Use a 0.05 significance level.

5. Thirty-six final-year medical students and 28 senior house officers answered a questionnaire about radiology.[25] The scores obtained are shown in Table 7.11. The lowest possible score is −37 and the highest possible score is 37. Histograms are shown in Figures 7.15 and 7.16. Do the data provide evidence that the population mean score for final-year medical students differs from the population mean score for senior house officers? Use a 0.001 significance level.

6. In a study designed to investigate the side effects of fenfluramine in autistic children, 42% of 11 autistic children exhibited listlessness before fenfluramine use and 66% exhibited listlessness during the last 14 weeks of fenfluramine use.[26] Do the data provide evidence that the population proportion of

TABLE 7.11   QUESTIONNAIRE SCORE FOR MEDICAL STUDENTS AND SENIOR HOUSE OFFICERS

Medical students

−2	11	8	6	10	12
6	8	−2	3	7	10
10	5	11	8	11	13
13	5	7	9	11	1
1	11	15	12	6	7
17	6	7	0	2	2

Mean ± SD   7.4 ± 4.6

House officers

21	14	11	9	17	5
5	9	12	14	16	22
17	13	10	24	5	16
7	15	13	16	19	
14	11	8	10	20	

Mean ± SD   13.3 ± 5.2

```
Count   Midpoint
   3      -.50   |XXXXXXXXXXXXXX
   5      2.50   |XXXXXXXXXXXXXXXXXXXXXXXXX
   6      5.50   |XXXXXXXXXXXXXXXXXXXXXXXXXXXXX
   8      8.50   |XXXXXXXXXXXXXXXXXXXXXXXXXXXXXXXXXXXXXX
  10     11.50   |XXXXXXXXXXXXXXXXXXXXXXXXXXXXXXXXXXXXXXXXXXXXXXXX
   3     14.50   |XXXXXXXXXXXXXX
   1     17.50   |XXXXX
               I....+....I....+....I....+....I....+....I....+....I
               0         2         4         6         8        10
                         Histogram Frequency
```

Figure 7.15 SPSS/PC histogram of medical students' scores

```
Count   Midpoint
   4      6.50   |XXXXXXXXXXXXXXXXXXX
   5      9.50   |XXXXXXXXXXXXXXXXXXXXXXXX
   5     12.50   |XXXXXXXXXXXXXXXXXXXXXXXX
   7     15.50   |XXXXXXXXXXXXXXXXXXXXXXXXXXXXXXXXXX
   3     18.50   |XXXXXXXXXXXXXX
   3     21.50   |XXXXXXXXXXXXXX
   1     24.50   |XXXXX
               I....+....I....+....I....+....I....+....I....+....I
               0         2         4         6         8        10
                         Histogram Frequency
```

Figure 7.16 SPSS/PC histogram of house officers' scores

TABLE 7.12 TISSUE OXYGEN TENSION (mm Hg) BEFORE AND AFTER HEATING

Patient No.	Before Heat	After Heat*	Difference (Before − After)
1	56	83	−27
	30	77	−47
	30	73	−43
2	32	79	−47
	33	56	−23
3	44	79	−35
4	90	100	−10
5	55	84	−29
	39	76	−37
6	43	103	−60
	43	119	−76
7	47	93	−46
8	78	112	−34
Mean ± SD	47.7 ± 18.4	87.2 ± 17.4	−39.5 ± 16.8

*Adjusted for temperature

autistic children who exhibit listlessness before fenfluramine use differs from the population proportion of autistic children who exhibit listlessness during fenfluramine use? Use a 0.05 significance level.

7. A study evaluated the effect of an infant development program (IDP) on the mental and physical development of low-birthweight infants.[27]

Low-birthweight infants were randomly assigned to an IDP group or a traditional-care group. At one year adjusted age, 4% of the 67 IDP infants and 18% of the 66 traditional-care infants showed developmental delay. Do the data provide evidence that the IDP population proportion of infants with developmental delay differs from the traditional-care population proportion of infants with developmental delay? Use a 0.01 significance level.

8. The effect of local heat on blood flow and oxygen tension in wounds was examined.[28] Table 7.12 shows the tissue oxygen tension ($Psqo_2$) before and after heating for eight patients. Histograms are shown in Figures 7.17 through 7.19. Do the data provide evidence that the population $Psqo_2$ mean after heating differs from the population $Psqo_2$ mean before heating? Use a 0.05 significance level.

9. In a study of rehabilitation outcomes in children with brain injury, the records of children with head trauma were examined.[29] Of the 109 children who were comatose on admission, 16% remained in a persistent vegetative state at discharge. A nurse believes that the population proportion of comatose children with head trauma who remain in a persistent vegetative state is 0.25. Do the data provide evidence that the population proportion is not 0.25? Use a 0.10 significance level.

10. A study of platelet aggregation in feline cardiomyopathy reported the platelet counts for 16

```
Count   Midpoint
  5       35.00  |XXXXXXXXXXXXXXXXXXXXXXXXXXXXXXXXXXXXXXXXXXXXXXXXXXX
  4       45.00  |XXXXXXXXXXXXXXXXXXXXXXXXXXXXXXXXXXXXXXXXX
  2       55.00  |XXXXXXXXXXXXXXXXXXXX
  0       65.00  |
  1       75.00  |XXXXXXXXXX
  0       85.00  |
  1       95.00  |XXXXXXXXXX
                 I....+....I....+....I....+....I....+....I....+....I....+....I
                 0         1         2         3         4         5
                          Histogram Frequency
```

Figure 7.17 SPSS/PC histogram of $Psqo_2$ before heating

```
Count   Midpoint
  1       55.00  |XXXXXXXXXX
  0       65.00  |
  5       75.00  |XXXXXXXXXXXXXXXXXXXXXXXXXXXXXXXXXXXXXXXXXXXXXXXXXXX
  2       85.00  |XXXXXXXXXXXXXXXXXXXX
  1       95.00  |XXXXXXXXXX
  2      105.00  |XXXXXXXXXXXXXXXXXXXX
  2      115.00  |XXXXXXXXXXXXXXXXXXXX
                 I....+....I....+....I....+....I....+....I....+....I....+....I
                 0         1         2         3         4         5
                          Histogram Frequency
```

Figure 7.18 SPSS/PC histogram of $Psqo_2$ after heating

```
Count   Midpoint
    1     -75.00  |XXXXXXXXXX
    0     -65.00  |
    1     -55.00  |XXXXXXXXXX
    4     -45.00  |XXXXXXXXXXXXXXXXXXXXXXXXXXXXXXXXXXXXXXXXXX
    3     -35.00  |XXXXXXXXXXXXXXXXXXXXXXXXXXXXXX
    3     -25.00  |XXXXXXXXXXXXXXXXXXXXXXXXXXXXXX
    1     -15.00  |XXXXXXXXXX
                  I....+....I....+....I....+....I....+....I....+....I
                  0         1         2         3         4         5
                            Histogram Frequency
```

Figure 7.19 SPSS/PC histogram of Psqo$_2$ difference

TABLE 7.13   PLATELET COUNT ($\times 10^5/mm^3$) FOR HEALTHY CATS AND CATS WITH CARDIOMYOPATHY

Healthy cats

2.24	2.10	6.30	2.40
2.54	2.98	2.70	2.70
3.04	2.78	3.76	2.10
2.12	4.01	2.55	3.11

Mean ± SD   2.96 ± 1.05

Cats with cardiomyopathy

2.42	3.12	2.18	4.69
3.61	5.50	4.27	
6.24	2.40	2.42	

Mean ± SD   3.68 ± 1.44

healthy cats and 10 cats with cardiomyopathy.[30] These counts are shown in Table 7.13. Histograms are shown in Figures 7.20 and 7.21. Do the data provide evidence that the population mean platelet count for healthy cats differs from the population mean platelet count for cats with cardiomyopathy? Use a 0.05 significance level.

11. In a study of depressive illness, eight inpatients with major depression were asked to rate their degree of depression on a visual analog scale upon entering the study and upon discharge.[31] The scale consisted of a 100-mm line with one end labeled "not at all depressed" and the other labeled "extremely depressed." Patients were asked to mark

```
Count   Midpoint
    4      1.90   |XXXXXXXXXXXXXXXXXXXX
    9      2.90   |XXXXXXXXXXXXXXXXXXXXXXXXXXXXXXXXXXXXXXXXXXXXXXX
    2      3.90   |XXXXXXXXXX
    0      4.90   |
    1      5.90   |XXXXX
                  I....+....I....+....I....+....I....+....I....+....I
                  0         2         4         6         8        10
                            Histogram Frequency
```

Figure 7.20 SPSS/PC histogram of platelet count for healthy cats

```
Count   Midpoint
    1      1.90   |XXXXXXXXXX
    4      2.90   |XXXXXXXXXXXXXXXXXXXXXXXXXXXXXXXXXXXXXXXXXX
    2      3.90   |XXXXXXXXXXXXXXXXXXXX
    1      4.90   |XXXXXXXXXX
    2      5.90   |XXXXXXXXXXXXXXXXXXXX
                  I....+....I....+....I....+....I....+....I....+....I
                  0         1         2         3         4         5
                            Histogram Frequency
```

Figure 7.21 SPSS/PC histogram of platelet count for cats with cardiomyopathy

**TABLE 7.14   DEPRESSION RATING DURING
HOSPITALIZATION AND UPON DISCHARGE**

	Depression Rating		
Patient No.	During Hospitalization	Upon Discharge	Difference (During − Discharge)
1	32	4	28
2	55	14	41
3	33	6	27
4	30	16	14
5	94	9	85
6	99	40	59
7	97	75	22
8	51	31	20
Mean ± SD	61.4 ± 30.6	24.4 ± 24.0	37.0 ± 24.0

```
Count   Midpoint
  3       40.00  |XXXXXXXXXXXXXXXXXXXXXXXXXXXXXX
  2       60.00  |XXXXXXXXXXXXXXXXXXX
  0       80.00  |
  3      100.00  |XXXXXXXXXXXXXXXXXXXXXXXXXXXXXX
                 I....+....I....+....I....+....I....+....I....+....I
                 0         1         2         3         4         5
                            Histogram Frequency
```

Figure 7.22   SPSS/PC histogram of depression rating during hospitalization

```
Count   Midpoint
  5       10.00  |XXXXXXXXXXXXXXXXXXXXXXXXXXXXXXXXXXXXXXXXXXXXXXXXXX
  1       30.00  |XXXXXXXXXX
  1       50.00  |XXXXXXXXXX
  1       70.00  |XXXXXXXXXX
                 I....+....I....+....I....+....I....+....I....+....I
                 0         1         2         3         4         5
                            Histogram Frequency
```

Figure 7.23   SPSS/PC histogram of depression rating upon discharge

```
Count   Midpoint
  1       10.00  |XXXXXXXXXX
  4       30.00  |XXXXXXXXXXXXXXXXXXXXXXXXXXXXXXXXXXXXXXXXXX
  2       50.00  |XXXXXXXXXXXXXXXXXXXXX
  0       70.00  |
  1       90.00  |XXXXXXXXXX
                 I....+....I....+....I....+....I....+....I....+....I
                 0         1         2         3         4         5
                            Histogram Frequency
```

Figure 7.24   SPSS/PC histogram of depression rating difference

the line at the point corresponding to their state of depression. The resulting depression ratings are shown in Table 7.14. Histograms are shown in Figures 7.22 through 7.24. A psychiatric nurse believes that the difference between the population depression rating mean during hospitalization and the population depression rating mean upon discharge is 35. Do the data provide evidence that the difference between the population means is not 35? Use a 0.05 significance level.

12. A study investigated the effects of milrinone in dogs with severe idiopathic myocardial failure.[32] Table 7.15 shows the pulmonary capillary wedge pressure (PCWP) before and after milrinone administration for 13 dogs with dilated cardiomyopathy. Histograms are shown in Figures 7.25 through 7.27. Do the data provide evidence that the population PCWP mean after milrinone administration differs from the population PCWP mean before milrinone administration? Use a 0.01 significance level.

13. In a study of patients with ectopic ACTH production, plasma ACTH values were reported for 10 patients with occult tumors and six patients with clinically evident tumors.[33] These values are shown in Table 7.16. Histograms are shown in Figures 7.28 and 7.29. An endocrinologist believes that the difference between the population ACTH mean for patients with occult tumors and the population ACTH mean for patients with evident tumors is

-1005. Do the data provide evidence that the difference between the population means is not -1005? Use a 0.005 significance level.

14. A study investigated the effect of splenectomy on the incidence of postoperative complications in patients with traumatic injuries.[34] Eighty patients underwent exploratory laparotomy for nonsplenic trauma and 80 patients underwent total

TABLE 7.15 PCWP (mm Hg) BEFORE AND AFTER MILRINONE ADMINISTRATION

Patient No.	Before	After	Difference (Before − After)
1	25	15	10
2	16	4	12
3	19	4	15
4	20	8	12
5	17	6	11
6	27	19	8
7	25	18	7
8	25	6	19
9	24	18	6
10	29	11	18
11	13	5	8
12	43	33	10
13	20	11	9
Mean ± SD	23.3 ± 7.5	12.2 ± 8.4	11.2 ± 4.0

```
Count    Midpoint
   1       12.50   |XXXXXXXXXX
   3       17.50   |XXXXXXXXXXXXXXXXXXXXXXXXXXXXXX
   3       22.50   |XXXXXXXXXXXXXXXXXXXXXXXXXXXXXX
   5       27.50   |XXXXXXXXXXXXXXXXXXXXXXXXXXXXXXXXXXXXXXXXXXXXXXXXXXX
   0       32.50   |
   0       37.50   |
   1       42.50   |XXXXXXXXXX
                   I....+....I....+....I....+....I....+....I....+....I
                   0         1         2         3         4         5
                             Histogram Frequency
```

Figure 7.25 SPSS/PC histogram of PCWP before milrinone administration

```
Count    Midpoint
   2        2.50   |XXXXXXXXXXXXXXXXXXXX
   4        7.50   |XXXXXXXXXXXXXXXXXXXXXXXXXXXXXXXXXXXXXXXXXX
   2       12.50   |XXXXXXXXXXXXXXXXXXXX
   4       17.50   |XXXXXXXXXXXXXXXXXXXXXXXXXXXXXXXXXXXXXXXXXX
   0       22.50   |
   0       27.50   |
   1       32.50   |XXXXXXXXXX
                   I....+....I....+....I....+....I....+....I....+....I
                   0         1         2         3         4         5
                             Histogram Frequency
```

Figure 7.26 SPSS/PC histogram of PCWP after milrinone administration

```
Count   Midpoint
   2      6.50   |XXXXXXXXXXXXXXXXXXX
   5      9.50   |XXXXXXXXXXXXXXXXXXXXXXXXXXXXXXXXXXXXXXXXXXXXXXXX
   3     12.50   |XXXXXXXXXXXXXXXXXXXXXXXXXXXXX
   1     15.50   |XXXXXXXXXX
   2     18.50   |XXXXXXXXXXXXXXXXXXX
                 I....+....I....+....I....+....I....+....I....+....I
                 0         1         2         3         4         5
                           Histogram Frequency
```

Figure 7.27 SPSS/PC histogram of PCWP difference

TABLE 7.16   PLASMA ACTH (ng/l) FOR PATIENTS WITH OCCULT OR EVIDENT TUMORS

Occult Tumors	Evident Tumors
165	1502
92	662
141	389
69	2340
244	907
121	1459
230	
82	Mean ± SD 1209.8 ± 705.7
123	
134	
Mean ± SD 140.1 ± 58.6	

splenectomy after traumatic injury. Thirty-six per cent of the non-splenic-trauma patients and 42% of the splenectomy patients had infectious postoperative complications. Do the data provide evidence that the non-splenic-trauma population proportion of patients with infectious postoperative complications differs from the splenectomy population proportion of patients with infectious postoperative complications? Use a 0.10 significance level.

15. A study compared the effectiveness of labetalol and hydralazine for managing severe hypertension complicating pregnancy.[35] Patients with hypertension during pregnancy were randomly assigned to receive either labetalol or hydralazine. Table 7.17 shows five-minute Apgar scores for infants of 13 women given labetalol and infants of six women given hydralazine. Histograms are shown in Figures 7.30 and 7.31. Do the data provide evidence that the population mean Apgar score for infants of mothers given labetalol differs from the population mean Apgar score for infants of mothers given hydralazine? Use a 0.05 significance level.

16. A study examined the level of school achievement for long-term survivors of childhood acute lymphocytic leukemia.[36] Table 7.18 shows the discrepancy between the achieved and expected reading-grade level for 18 children treated eight to

```
Count   Midpoint
   3     75.00   |XXXXXXXXXXXXXXXXXXXXXXXXXXXXXX
   4    125.00   |XXXXXXXXXXXXXXXXXXXXXXXXXXXXXXXXXXXXXX
   1    175.00   |XXXXXXXXXX
   2    225.00   |XXXXXXXXXXXXXXXXXXX
                 I....+....I....+....I....+....I....+....I....+....I
                 0         1         2         3         4         5
                           Histogram Frequency
```

Figure 7.28   SPSS/PC histogram of plasma ACTH for patients with occult tumors

```
Count   Midpoint
   2     450.00   |XXXXXXXXXXXXXXXXXXX
   3    1350.00   |XXXXXXXXXXXXXXXXXXXXXXXXXXXX
   1    2250.00   |XXXXXXXXXX
                  I....+....I....+....I....+....I....+....I....+....I
                  0         1         2         3         4         5
                            Histogram Frequency
```

Figure 7.29   SPSS/PC histogram of plasma ACTH for patients with evident tumors

TABLE 7.17 APGAR SCORE (5 MINUTES) FOR INFANTS OF MOTHERS GIVEN LABETALOL OR HYDRALAZINE

Labetalol			Hydralazine	
9	8	8	7	8
9	8	8	9	5
9	9	9	1	
9	9		9	
7	9		Mean ± SD 6.5 ± 3.1	
Mean ± SD 8.5 ± 0.7				

TABLE 7.18 DISCREPANCY BETWEEN ACHIEVED READING-GRADE LEVEL AND EXPECTED READING-GRADE LEVEL

Patient No.	Discrepancy
1	− 1.1
2	− 6.5
3	− 2.9
4	− 4.4
5	− 0.3
6	− 3.0
7	− 3.3
8	− 1.3
9	− 2.1
10	0.1
11	− 2.5
12	− 1.2
13	3.8
14	− 1.4
15	− 1.5
16	− 2.1
17	− 3.2
18	− 4.4
Mean ± SD	− 2.1 ± 2.2

10 years earlier for acute lymphocytic leukemia. A negative discrepancy means that the achieved level was less than the expected level and a positive discrepancy means that the achieved level was greater than the expected level. A histogram is shown in Figure 7.32. A pediatric nurse believes that the population mean discrepancy for long-term survivors of childhood acute lymphocytic leukemia is − 3. Do the data provide evidence that the population mean is not − 3? Use a 0.01 significance level.

17. In a study of elastic fibers in normal and sun-damaged skin, sun-exposed and sun-protected skin samples were obtained postmortem from 14 subjects.[37] Two skin samples, one sun-exposed and one sun-protected, were taken from each skin samples. The degree of elastosis for these skin samples is shown in Table 7.19. Histograms are shown in Figures 7.33 through 7.35. A dermatologist believes that the difference between the population mean elastosis for sun-exposed skin and the population mean elastosis for sun-protected skin is 2.5. Do the

data provide evidence that the population mean difference is not 2.5? Use a 0.001 significance level.

18. In a study of pancreactomized patients, blood glucose concentrations were reported for 12 pancreactomized subjects 120 minutes after ingesting 100 grams of glucose.[38] These concentrations are shown in Table 7.20. A histogram is shown in Figure 7.36. An internist believes that the population blood glucose mean is 440. Do the data provide evidence that the population mean is not 440? Use a 0.05 significance level.

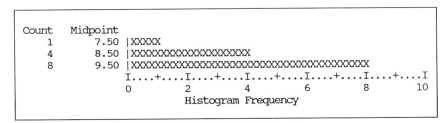

```
Count  Midpoint
   1      7.50  |XXXXX
   4      8.50  |XXXXXXXXXXXXXXXXXXXX
   8      9.50  |XXXXXXXXXXXXXXXXXXXXXXXXXXXXXXXXXXXXXXXXXX
                I....+....I....+....I....+....I....+....I....+....I
                0         2         4         6         8        10
                          Histogram Frequency
```

Figure 7.30 SPSS/PC histogram of Apgar score for infants of mothers given labetalol

```
Count  Midpoint
   1      2.50  |XXXXXXXXXX
   1      5.50  |XXXXXXXXXX
   4      8.50  |XXXXXXXXXXXXXXXXXXXXXXXXXXXXXXXXXXXXXXXXXX
                I....+....I....+....I....+....I....+....I....+....I
                0         1         2         3         4         5
                          Histogram Frequency
```

Figure 7.31 SPSS/PC histogram of Apgar score for infants of mothers given hydralazine

```
Count    Midpoint
   1       -6.00  |XXXXX
   4       -4.00  |XXXXXXXXXXXXXXXXXXXX
  10       -2.00  |XXXXXXXXXXXXXXXXXXXXXXXXXXXXXXXXXXXXXXXXXXXXXXXXXXXX
   2        0.0   |XXXXXXXXXX
   0        2.00  |
   1        4.00  |XXXXX
                  I....+....I....+....I....+....I....+....I....+....I
                  0         2         4         6         8        10
                              Histogram Frequency
```

Figure 7.32   SPSS/PC histogram of reading-grade discrepancy

TABLE 7.19   DEGREE OF ELASTOSIS* IN SUN-PROTECTED AND SUN-EXPOSED SKIN

Subject No.	Exposed	Protected	Difference (Exposed-Protected)
1	0	0	0
2	0	0	0
3	1	0	1
4	2	0	2
5	3	0	3
6	2	1	1
7	1	0	1
8	3	0	3
9	1	0	1
10	2	0	2
11	3	0	3
12	2	0	2
13	2	0	2
14	2	1	1
Mean ± SD	1.7 ± 1.0	0.1 ± 0.4	1.6 ± 1.0

*0 = none, 1 = mild, 2 = moderate, 3 = severe

TABLE 7.20   BLOOD GLUCOSE FOR PANCREACTOMIZED SUBJECTS

Patient No.	Blood Glucose (mg/dl)
1	215
2	388
3	576
4	346
5	380
6	265
7	508
8	404
9	352
10	639
11	414
12	404
Mean ± SD	407.6 ± 119.7

19. A study of the mutagenicity of antineoplastic agents investigated nurses who handle antineo-

```
Count    Midpoint
   2        .50   |XXXXXXXXXX
   3       1.50   |XXXXXXXXXXXXXXX
   6       2.50   |XXXXXXXXXXXXXXXXXXXXXXXXXXXXXX
   3       3.50   |XXXXXXXXXXXXXXX
                  I....+....I....+....I....+....I....+....I....+....I
                  0         2         4         6         8        10
                              Histogram Frequency
```

Figure 7.33   SPSS/PC histogram of degree of elastosis for exposed skin

```
Count    Midpoint
  12        .50   |XXXXXXXXXXXXXXXXXXXXXXXXXXXXXXXX
   2       1.50   |XXXXX
                  I....+....I....+....I....+....I....+....I....+....I
                  0         4         8        12        16        20
                              Histogram Frequency
```

Figure 7.34   SPSS/PC histogram of degree of elastosis for protected skin

```
Count    Midpoint
  2        .50  |XXXXXXXXXXXXXXXXXX
  5       1.50  |XXXXXXXXXXXXXXXXXXXXXXXXXXXXXXXXXXXXXXXXXXXXX
  4       2.50  |XXXXXXXXXXXXXXXXXXXXXXXXXXXXXXXXXXXX
  3       3.50  |XXXXXXXXXXXXXXXXXXXXXXXXXXX
               I....+....I....+....I....+....I....+....I....+....I
               0         1         2         3         4         5
                         Histogram Frequency
```

Figure 7.35 SPSS/PC histogram of elastosis difference

plastic agents.[39] Seventy-nine per cent of 28 nurses who prepared and administered antineoplastic agents had mutagenic urine activity and 45% of 31 nurses who only administered antineoplastic agents had mutagenic urine activity. Do the data provide evidence that the proportion of nurses with mutagenic urine activity in the population that prepares and administers antineoplastic agents differs from the proportion of nurses with mutagenic urine activity in the population that only administers antineoplastic agents? Use a 0.05 significance level.

20. A study reported the hearing gain in 22 ears from 19 patients after surgery for postinflammatory acquired atresia.[40] These values are shown in Table 7.21. A histogram is shown in Figure 7.37. An otologist believes that the population hearing gain mean is 2.9. Do the data provide evidence that the population mean is not 2.9? Use a 0.01 significance level.

21. The success of minimal arthroscopic surgery and rehabilitation was evaluated for 49 patients with a total of 51 chronic symptomatic anterior-cruciate deficient knees.[41] Table 7.22 shows the results for 37 knees with meniscal lesions and 14 knees

TABLE 7.21 HEARING GAIN IN 22 EARS AFTER SURGERY FOR ACQUIRED ATRESIA*

1	3	3	2	1
3	1	2	1	1
1	2	1	3	
2	3	3	2	
3	2	2	3	
	Mean ± SD	2.0 ± 0.8		

*1 = 11–20 dB, 2 = 21–30 dB, 3 = > 30 dB

without meniscal lesions. Histograms are shown in Figures 7.38 and 7.39. Do the data provide evidence that the population mean result score for knees with meniscal lesions differs from the population mean result score for knees without meniscal lesions? Use a 0.05 significance level.

22. In a study of electrocoagulation for the treatment of upper gastrointestinal (GI) tract hemorrhage, 44 patients with active upper GI bleeding were randomly assigned to receive either electrocoagulation or sham electrocoagulation.[42] Of the 23 patients who received sham electrocoagulation, 57%

```
Count    Midpoint
  2       250.00  |XXXXXXXXXXXXXXXXXX
  4       350.00  |XXXXXXXXXXXXXXXXXXXXXXXXXXXXXXXXXXXXXX
  3       450.00  |XXXXXXXXXXXXXXXXXXXXXXXXXXXX
  2       550.00  |XXXXXXXXXXXXXXXXXX
  1       650.00  |XXXXXXXXXX
               I....+....I....+....I....+....I....+....I....+....I
               0         1         2         3         4         5
                         Histogram Frequency
```

Figure 7.36 SPSS/PC histogram of blood glucose

```
Count    Midpoint
  7       1.50  |XXXXXXXXXXXXXXXXXXXXXXXXXXXXXXXXXXXX
  7       2.50  |XXXXXXXXXXXXXXXXXXXXXXXXXXXXXXXXXXXX
  8       3.50  |XXXXXXXXXXXXXXXXXXXXXXXXXXXXXXXXXXXXXXXX
               I....+....I....+....I....+....I....+....I....+...I
               0         2         4         6         8        10
                         Histogram Frequency
```

Figure 7.37 SPSS/PC histogram of hearing gain

TABLE 7.22 RESULTS FOR KNEES WITH LESIONS AND KNEES WITHOUT LESIONS*

Knees with lesions

4	1	1	3	1
1	3	2	1	4
2	1	2	3	1
3	4	1	1	2
1	2	3	3	4
2	4	3	4	
1	2	2	4	
4	3	3	1	

Mean ± SD   2.4 ± 1.2

Knees without lesions

4	1	2	1	1
1	2	3	2	1
2	1	2	3	

Mean ± SD   1.9 ± 0.9

*1 = poor, 2 = fair, 3 = good, 4 = excellent

required emergency intervention. Of the 21 patients who received electrocoagulation, 14% required emergency intervention. Do the data provide evidence that the sham electrocoagulation population proportion of patients who require emergency intervention differs from the electrocoagulation population proportion of patients who require emergency intervention? Use a 0.005 significance level.

23. A study of osteoporosis in men with hyperprolactinemic hypogonadism reported the serum testosterone for six men before and after treatment with surgery or bromocriptine.[43] These testosterone levels are shown in Table 7.23. Histograms are shown in Figures 7.40 through 7.42. Do the data provide evidence that the population testosterone mean before treatment differs from the population testosterone mean after treatment? Use a 0.05 significance level.

```
Count   Midpoint
   12     1.50   |XXXXXXXXXXXXXXXXXXXXXXXXXXXXXXX
    8     2.50   |XXXXXXXXXXXXXXXXXXXX
    9     3.50   |XXXXXXXXXXXXXXXXXXXXXXX
    8     4.50   |XXXXXXXXXXXXXXXXXXXX
              I....+....I....+....I....+....I....+....I....+....I
              0        4        8       12       16       20
                        Histogram Frequency
```

Figure 7.38   SPSS/PC histogram of result for knees with lesions

```
Count   Midpoint
    6     1.50   |XXXXXXXXXXXXXXXXXXXXXXXXXXXXXXXXX
    5     2.50   |XXXXXXXXXXXXXXXXXXXXXXXXXXX
    2     3.50   |XXXXXXXXXX
    1     4.50   |XXXXX
              I....+....I....+....I....+....I....+....I....+....I
              0        2        4        6        8       10
                        Histogram Frequency
```

Figure 7.39   SPSS/PC histogram of result for knees without lesions

TABLE 7.23 PRETREATMENT AND POSTTREATMENT SERUM TESTOSTERONE (ng/dl) FOR MEN WITH HYPERPROLACTINEMIC HYPOGONADISM

Patient No.	Before Treatment	After Treatment	Difference (Before − After)
1	127	501	− 374
2	58	250	− 192
3	171	357	− 186
4	87	80	7
5	186	140	46
6	379	460	− 81
Mean ± SD	168.0 ± 114.2	298.0 ± 170.7	− 130.0 ± 154.1

```
Count   Midpoint
   3     75.00   |XXXXXXXXXXXXXXXXXXXXXXXXXXXXXXX
   2    225.00   |XXXXXXXXXXXXXXXXXXXX
   1    375.00   |XXXXXXXXXX
                 I....+....I....+....I....+....I....+....I....+....I
                 0        1        2        3        4        5
                         Histogram Frequency
```

Figure 7.40 SPSS/PC histogram of before-treatment testosterone

```
Count   Midpoint
   2    100.00   |XXXXXXXXXXXXXXXXXXXX
   2    300.00   |XXXXXXXXXXXXXXXXXXXX
   2    500.00   |XXXXXXXXXXXXXXXXXXXX
                 I....+....I....+....I....+....I....+....I....+....I
                 0        1        2        3        4        5
                         Histogram Frequency
```

Figure 7.41 SPSS/PC histogram of after-treatment testosterone

```
Count   Midpoint
   1   -330.00   |XXXXXXXXXX
   2   -190.00   |XXXXXXXXXXXXXXXXXXXX
   2    -50.00   |XXXXXXXXXXXXXXXXXXXX
   1     90.00   |XXXXXXXXXX
                 I....+....I....+....I....+....I....+....I....+....I
                 0        1        2        3        4        5
                         Histogram Frequency
```

Figure 7.42 SPSS/PC histogram of testosterone difference

24. In a study of urinary incontinence in mares, the average maximal urethral closure pressure (MUCP) was reported for 12 normal mares and three incontinent mares.[44] These pressures are shown in Table 7.24. A histogram for the normal mares is shown in Figure 7.43. (A histogram for the incontinent mares cannot be used to check normality because the sample size is only 3.) Do the data provide evidence that the population mean mare–average MUCP for normal mares differs from the population mean mare–average MUCP for incontinent mares? Use a 0.10 significance level.

25. A study of group education for high blood pressure control reported that 62% of 66 hypertensive patients showed positive changes related to exercise, smoking, weight, or blood pressure after group education.[45] A nurse believes that the population proportion of hypertensive patients who would show positive changes after group education is 0.50. Do the data provide evidence that the population proportion is not 0.50? Use a 0.05 significance level.

26. Find an article in a medical or health care journal in which a t test was incorrectly used to analyze nonindependent or extremely nonnormal data, or a Z test was incorrectly used to analyze nonindependent data. Photocopy the article and write a letter to the journal editor that clearly describes the statistical error.

TABLE 7.24   MARE–AVERAGE MUCP (cm H$_2$O) FOR NORMAL AND INCONTINENT MARES

Normal	Incontinent
50.0	35.1
85.4	34.5
131.2	15.3
109.5	
67.3	Mean ± SD 28.3 ± 11.3
57.2	
73.9	
64.7	
96.1	
60.1	
84.9	
91.1	

Mean ± SD   81.0 ± 23.7

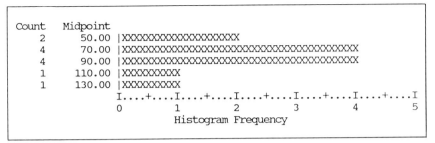

```
Count  Midpoint
   2     50.00 |XXXXXXXXXXXXXXXXXXX
   4     70.00 |XXXXXXXXXXXXXXXXXXXXXXXXXXXXXXXXXXXXXX
   4     90.00 |XXXXXXXXXXXXXXXXXXXXXXXXXXXXXXXXXXXXXX
   1    110.00 |XXXXXXXXX
   1    130.00 |XXXXXXXXX
              I....+....I....+....I....+....I....+....I....+....I
              0         1         2         3         4         5
                          Histogram Frequency
```

Figure 7.43 SPSS/PC histogram of mare–average MUCP for normal mares

REFERENCES

1. Daly RC, Pairolero PC, Piehler JM, et al: Pulmonary aspergilloma: Results of surgical treatment. J Thorac Cardiovasc Surg 92:981–988, 1986.
2. Smeak DD, DeHoff WD: Total ear canal ablation: Clinical results in the dog and cat. Vet Surg 15:161–170, 1986.
3. Schlesselman JJ: Case-Control Studies. New York: Oxford, 1982.
4. Eberly TW, Miles MS, Carter MC, et al: Parental stress after the unexpected admission of a child to the intensive care unit. Crit Care Q 8:57–65, 1985.
5. Hayden FG, Albrecht JK, Kaiser DL, et al: Prevention of natural colds by contact prophylaxis with intranasal alpha$_2$-interferon. N Engl J Med 314:71–75, 1986.
6. Sorbi M, Tellegen B: Differential effects of training in relaxation and stress-coping in patients with migraine. Headache 26:473–481, 1986.
7. Raskova J, Ghobrial I, Czerwinski DK, et al: B-cell activation and immunoregulation in end-stage renal disease patients receiving hemodialysis. Arch Intern Med 147:89–93, 1987.
8. Goodnough SK: The effects of oxygen and hyperinflation on arterial oxygen tension after endotracheal suctioning. Heart Lung 14:11–17, 1985.
9. Bannister P, Sheridan P, Dibble J, et al: Benign hypercalcemia and "benign hypocalcemia" in the same family. Ann Intern Med 105:217–219, 1986.
10. Knaus WA, Draper EA, Wagner DP, et al: An evaluation of outcome from intensive care in major medical centers. Ann Intern Med 104:410–418, 1986.
11. Edell ES, Cortese DA: Bronchoscopic phototherapy with hematoporhyrin derivative for treatment of localized bronchogenic carcinoma: A 5-year experience. Mayo Clin Proc 62:8–14, 1987.
12. Falanga V, Medsger TA, Reichlin M, et al: Linear scleroderma. Clinical spectrum, prognosis, and laboratory abnormalities. Ann Intern Med 104:849–857, 1986.
13. Watchous SM, Thurston HI, Carter MC: The nurse educator and the adult dialysis patient. Nurs Forum 19:69–84, 1980.
14. Scott DW, Walton DK: Hyposomatotropism in the mature dog: A discussion of 22 cases. J Am Anim Hosp Assoc 22:467–473, 1986.
15. Demeter SL: Interstitial vasculitis-interstitial lung disease: Case studies. Angiology 37:325–338, 1986.
16. SAS Introductory Guide. 3rd ed. Cary: SAS Institute, 1985.
17. SAS User's Guide: Basics, Version 5 Edition. Cary: SAS Institute, 1985.
18. SAS User's Guide: Statistics, Version 5 Edition. Cary: SAS Institute, 1985.
19. Philbrick JT, Bracikowski JP: Single-dose antibiotic treatment for uncomplicated urinary tract infections: Less for less? Arch Intern Med 145:1672–1678, 1985.
20. Goldman L, Feinstein AR: Anticoagulants and myocardial infarction. The problems of pooling, drowning, and floating. Ann Intern Med 90:92–94, 1979.
21. Cohen J: Statistical Power Analysis for the Behavioral Sciences. 2nd ed. Hillsdale: Erlbaum, 1988.
22. Chez RA, Curcio FD: Ketonuria in normal pregnancy. Obstet Gynecol 69:272–274, 1987.
23. Herman J: The effect of progressive relaxation on Valsalva response in healthy adults. Res Nurs Health 10:171–176, 1987.
24. Zoma A, Sturrock RD, Fisher WD, et al: Surgical stabilization of the rheumatoid cervical spine. A review of indications and results. J Bone Joint Surg 69B:8–12, 1987.
25. Cozens NJA: Are we taught how to use a radiology department as medical students? Clin Radiol 38:137–139, 1987.
26. Realmuto GM, Jensen J, Klykylo W, et al: Untoward effects of fenfluramine in autistic children. J Clin Psychopharmacol 6:350–355, 1986.
27. Resnick MB, Eyler FD, Nelson RM, et al: Developmental intervention for low birth weight infants: Improved early developmental outcome. Pediatrics 80:68–74, 1987.
28. Rabkin JM, Hunt TK. Local heat increases blood flow and oxygen tension in wounds. Arch Surg 122:221–225, 1987.
29. Edwards PA: Rehabilitation outcomes in children with brain injury. Rehab Nurs 12:125–127, 1987.
30. Helenski CA, Ross JN: Platelet aggregation in feline cardiomyopathy. J Vet Intern Med 1:24–28, 1987.
31. Blackburn IM, Whalley LJ, Christie JE, et al: Mood, cognition and cortisol: Their temporal relationships during recovery from depressive illness. J Affect Disord 13:31–43, 1987.
32. Kittleson MD, Johnson LE, Pion PD: The acute hemodynamic effects of milrinone in dogs with severe idiopathic myocardial failure. J Vet Intern Med 1:121–127, 1987.
33. Howlett TA, Drury PL, Perry L, et al: Diagnosis and management of ACTH-dependent Cushing's syndrome: Comparison of the features in ectopic and pituitary ACTH production. Clin Endocrinol 24:699–713, 1986.
34. Willis BK, Deitch EA, McDonald JC: The influence of trauma to the spleen on postoperative complications and mortality. J Trauma 26:1073–1076, 1986.

35. Mabie WC, Gonzalez AR, Sibai BM, et al: A comparative trial of labetalol and hydralazine in the acute management of severe hypertension complicating pregnancy. Obstet Gynecol *70*:328–333, 1987.

36. Peckham VC, Meadows AT, Bartel N, et al: Educational late effects in long-term survivors of childhood acute lymphocytic leukemia. Pediatrics *81*:127–133, 1988.

37. Mera SL, Lovell CR, Jones RR, et al: Elastic fibres in normal and sun-damaged skin: An immunohistochemical study. Br J Dermatol *117*:21–27, 1987.

38. Bajorunas DR, Fortner JG, Jaspan JB: Glucagon immunoreactivity and chromatographic profiles in pancreactomized humans: Paradoxical response to oral glucose. Diabetes *35*:886–893, 1986.

39. Rogers B: Work practices of nurses who handle antineoplastic agents. AAOHN J *35*:24–31, 1987.

40. Tos M, Balle V: Postinflammatory acquired atresia of the external auditory canal: Late results of surgery. Am J Otol *7*:365–370, 1986.

41. Fowler PJ, Regan WD: The patient with symptomatic chronic anterior cruciate ligament insufficiency. Results of minimal arthroscopic surgery and rehabilitation. Am J Sports Med *15*:321–325, 1987.

42. Laine L: Multipolar electrocoagulation in the treatment of active upper gastrointestinal tract hemorrhage. A prospective controlled trial. N Engl J Med *316*:1613–1617, 1987.

43. Greenspan SL, Neer RM, Ridgway EC, et al: Osteoporosis in men with hyperprolactinemic hypogonadism. Ann Intern Med *104*:777–782, 1986.

44. Kay AD, Lavoie J: Urethral pressure profilometry in mares. J Am Vet Med Assoc *191*:212–216, 1987.

45. Wyka-Fitzgerald C, Levesque P, Panciera T, et al: Long-term evaluation of group education for high blood pressure control. Cardiovasc Nurs *20*:13–18, 1984.

8

ONE-WAY ANALYSIS OF VARIANCE

CHAPTER OBJECTIVES

After studying this chapter and working the problems, you should be able to:

1. Explain how one-way analysis of variance results are calculated

2. Interpret one-way analysis of variance results

3. Explain the rationale for data transformation

4. Recognize data that violate assumptions required for one-way analysis of variance

5. Interpret SPSS and SAS one-way analysis of variance output

6. Calculate and interpret Tukey and Bonferroni confidence intervals for one-way analysis of variance

7. Determine whether one-way analyses of variance reported in the medical and health care literature are appropriate

---

Methods described in the previous chapter can be used to compare two population means, but we often want to compare three or more population means. Such comparisons could be done with t tests. If we wanted to compare three population means by testing the hypothesis that all three population means are equal, we could carry out three t tests: a test of the hypothesis H_0: $\mu_1 = \mu_2$, a test of the hypothesis H_0: $\mu_1 = \mu_3$, and a test of the hypothesis H_0: $\mu_2 = \mu_3$. This approach is inefficient, however, and suffers from the multiplicity problem described in Chapter 7.

In this chapter, and in Chapters 9 and 13, we will examine better methods for comparing three or more means. One-way analysis of variance (ANOVA), described in this chapter, requires inde-

pendent samples and is a generalization of the pooled-variance t test. One-factor repeated-measures analysis of variance, described in Chapter 9, requires repeated measurements and is a generalization of the paired t test.

8.1 HYPOTHESIS TESTS

In a study of burned patients more than 60 years of age, three groups of elderly burned patients were examined: 11 patients who died within three days (Group 1), 20 patients who died within five to 48 days (Group 2), and 11 patients who survived (Group 3).[1] Table 8.1 shows the percentage of total body surface area that was burned (% TBSA) for these

TABLE 8.1   % TBSA AND SQUARE ROOT OF % TBSA

Patient No.	% TBSA	Square Root of % TBSA
Group 1: Died within three days		
1	65	8.06
2	53	7.28
3	48	6.93
4	71	8.43
5	50	7.07
6	36	6.00
7	60	7.75
8	30	5.48
9	50	7.07
10	74	8.60
11	80	8.94
Mean ± SD	56.1 ± 15.6	7.42 ± 1.07
Group 2: Died within five to 48 days		
12	10	3.16
13	17	4.12
14	20	4.47
15	35	5.92
16	23	4.80
17	38	6.16
18	36	6.00
19	36	6.00
20	30	5.48
21	42	6.48
22	35	5.92
23	15	3.87
24	17	4.12
25	38	6.16
26	25	5.00
27	56	7.48
28	50	7.07
29	30	5.48
30	11	3.32
31	60	7.75
Mean ± SD	31.2 ± 14.2	5.44 ± 1.31
Group 3: Survived		
32	30	5.48
33	18	4.24
34	17	4.12
35	17	4.12
36	41	6.40
37	15	3.87
38	24	4.90
39	22	4.69
40	20	4.47
41	19	4.36
42	34	5.83
Mean ± SD	23.4 ± 8.2	4.77 ± 0.81

42 patients. This table also shows the square roots of these percentages, the purpose of which will be explained shortly. An obvious question of interest concerns whether % TBSA is related to survival, as we would expect it to be. If μ_1, μ_2, and μ_3 are the population % TBSA means corresponding to

Groups 1, 2, and 3, we would like to test the null hypothesis

$$H_0: \mu_1 = \mu_2 = \mu_3 \qquad (8.1)$$

In general, we want to compare k means (where $k \geq 3$) by testing the null hypothesis

$$H_0: \mu_1 = \mu_2 = \mu_3 = \cdots = \mu_k \qquad (8.2)$$

The alternative hypothesis is always

H_A: At least one population mean does not equal another population mean $\qquad (8.3)$

We cannot carry out a one-way ANOVA test of the null hypothesis (8.2) using any sort of one-sided alternative hypothesis. Alternative hypotheses such as $H_A: \mu_1 < \mu_2 < \mu_3 < \cdots < \mu_k$ cannot be used.

If we reject the null hypothesis (8.2), we cannot conclude that all of the population means are different. We can conclude only that at least one population mean does not equal another population mean. Other methods are needed to determine which population means are different. Some of these methods are discussed in Sections 8.3 through 8.5.

Assume that we have k independent samples, which we want to use to test the null hypothesis (8.2). Let $\bar{x}_1$ be the mean of the first sample, let $\bar{x}_2$ be the mean of the second sample, and so on. If we combine all of the samples into one sample, we can also calculate the mean of the combined sample. This mean, called the *overall mean* or *grand mean*, is denoted by $\bar{x}$. The sample sizes are denoted by n_1, n_2, n_3, and so on, and need not be equal. The sample standard deviations are denoted by s_1, s_2, s_3, and so forth.

A one-way ANOVA test of the null hypothesis (8.2) requires calculation of the following quantities.

Between-Groups Sum of Squares (SSB). This quantity is calculated according to the formula

$$SSB = \sum_{i=1}^{k} n_i (\bar{x}_i - \bar{x})^2 \qquad (8.4)$$

We can translate this formula into steps for calculation.

STEP 1.   Calculate each sample mean and the overall mean for the combined sample.

STEP 2.   Subtract the overall mean from each sample mean to get k differences.

STEP 3.   Square each of the differences obtained in step 2.

STEP 4.   Multiply each of the squared differences obtained in step 3 by the corresponding sample size. For example, $(\bar{x}_3 - \bar{x})^2$ is multiplied by n_3. This produces k *weighted* squared differences.

STEP 5.   Add all of the weighted squared differences obtained in step 4.

Within-Groups Sum of Squares (SSW). This quantity is calculated according to the formula

$$SSW = \sum_{i=1}^{k} (n_i - 1)s_i^2 \qquad (8.5)$$

We can translate this formula into steps for calculation.

STEP 1. Calculate the variance for each sample.

STEP 2. Multiply each sample variance by the corresponding sample size minus 1. For example, s_2^2 is multiplied by $(n_2 - 1)$. This produces k *weighted sample variances.*

STEP 3. Add all of the weighted sample variances obtained in step 2.

Between-Groups Degrees of Freedom. This is simply $k - 1$.

Within-Groups Degrees of Freedom. Let n_T denote the size of the combined sample: $n_T = n_1 + n_2 + n_3 + \cdots + n_k$. The within-groups degrees of freedom are $n_T - k$.

Between-Groups Mean Square (MSB). This is the between-groups sum of squares divided by the between-groups degrees of freedom.

$$MSB = \frac{SSB}{k - 1} \qquad (8.6)$$

Within-Groups Mean Square (MSW). This is the within-groups sum of squares divided by the within-groups degrees of freedom.*

$$MSW = \frac{SSW}{n_T - k} \qquad (8.7)$$

Our statistic for testing the null hypothesis (8.2) is an *F statistic* based on the mean squares:

$$F = \frac{MSB}{MSW} \qquad (8.8)$$

The F statistic cannot be negative, since both its numerator (top part) and denominator (bottom part) are sums of squares divided by positive numbers.

Why does the F statistic make sense as a test of the null hypothesis (8.2)? To answer this, we need to reexamine the formulas for sums of squares. SSB is the sum of the weighted squared differences between the sample means and the overall mean. If

all of the population means are the same, the sample means will usually be close to each other. As a result, the sample means will usually be close to the overall mean and the weighted squared differences will usually be small. Thus, SSB and MSB will usually be small when all of the population means are the same. If some of the population means are quite different, the corresponding sample means will usually be quite different, so some of the sample means will usually be quite different from the overall mean. Some of the weighted squared differences between the sample means and the overall mean will then be large, making SSB and MSB large. A large MSB, therefore, provides evidence against the null hypothesis (8.2), and a small MSB does not provide evidence against this hypothesis.

We also need to take into account the variability of the data. This is what MSW does. As a weighted combination of the sample variances, MSW measures the estimated variability of the data. If the data are highly variable, MSW will be large. If the data are only slightly variable, MSW will be small. Since MSW is on the bottom of the F statistic, a large MSW makes the F statistic small. A small MSW makes the F statistic large.

The F statistic is large when some of the differences between the sample means and the overall mean are large relative to the variability of the data. The F statistic is small when the differences between the sample means and the overall mean are small relative to the variability of the data. A large F statistic, therefore, provides evidence against the null hypothesis (8.2) and a small F statistic does not provide evidence against this hypothesis.

How large does an F statistic have to be to warrant rejection of the null hypothesis (8.2)? As you might expect, this is determined by the p-value associated with the calculated F statistic. If an F statistic is so large that it has a small p-value, we reject the null hypothesis (8.2). To obtain p-values, we need to know the distribution of the F statistic. It can be shown that this statistic has an F *distribution with $k - 1$ numerator degrees of freedom and $n_T - k$ denominator degrees of freedom* if the null hypothesis (8.2) is true and independent random samples are taken from normal populations with equal variances. The F distribution is a skewed distribution with a frequency curve determined by two sets of degrees of freedom (df), the *numerator degrees of freedom* (d_1) and the *denominator degrees of freedom* (d_2). Random variables with F distributions cannot have negative values. The frequency curve for the F distribution with 6 and 12 degrees of freedom is shown in Figure 8.1.

The p-value for the F statistic (8.8) is given by the upper-tail probability

$$P(F \text{ statistic} \geq F_{\text{calc}})$$

where F_{calc} is the calculated F statistic. Approxi-

---

*The within-groups mean square is also called the *error mean square* (MSE); the within-groups degrees of freedom are also called the *error degrees of freedom*; and the within-groups sum of squares is also called the *error sum of squares* (SSE).

mate p-values can be obtained from Table E.5 in Appendix E. This table is based on upper percentage points of F distributions. If F_{d_1, d_2} is a random variable having an F distribution with d_1 and d_2 degrees of freedom, the α upper percentage point of this distribution is the number F_{α, d_1, d_2} such that

$$P\left(F_{d_1, d_2} \geq F_{\alpha, d_1, d_2}\right) = \alpha$$

Since Table E.5 lists upper percentage points for only a few tail probabilities, we cannot obtain exact p-values from this table.

To obtain approximate p-values from Table E.5, we first locate the column for our numerator degrees of freedom and the rows for our denominator degrees of freedom. We then find two adjacent numbers in the appropriate column and rows such that F_{calc} lies between these numbers, if possible. These numbers are upper percentage points, and the p-value lies between the probabilities to which they correspond. If F_{calc} is very large, it will be larger than any of the appropriate upper percentage points given in the table. When this happens, we find the largest upper percentage point in the appropriate column and rows. The p-value is *less* than the corresponding probability. If F_{calc} is very small, it will be smaller than any of the appropriate upper percentage points listed. In this case, we find the smallest upper percentage point in the appropriate column and rows. The p-value is *greater* than the corresponding probability. These possibilities are illustrated in the following example.

Example 8.1

What are the p-values for the following calculated F statistics?

1. $F_{calc} = 4.77$, four samples, $n_1 = 3$, $n_2 = 8$, $n_3 = 8$, $n_4 = 5$. The numerator degrees of freedom are $k - 1 = 4 - 1 = 3$, and the denominator degrees of freedom are $n_T - k = (3 + 8 + 8 + 5) - 4 = 20$. Locating the column and rows for these degrees of freedom in Table E.5, we find that 4.77 lies between the numbers 3.86 and 4.94. Since these numbers are the 0.025 and 0.01 upper percentage

points of the F distribution with 3 and 20 df,

$$0.01 < p\text{-value} < 0.025$$

2. $F_{calc} = 22.59$, three samples, $n_1 = n_2 = n_3 = 10$. The numerator degrees of freedom are $k - 1 = 3 - 1 = 2$, and the denominator degrees of freedom are $n_T - k = (10 + 10 + 10) - 3 = 27$. Since 27 is not listed under the denominator degrees of freedom, we have to approximate. The closest listed degrees of freedom are 24 and 30, and 27 lies midway between them. Choosing the smaller degrees of freedom, we examine the rows for 24 df and the column for 2 df. There is no number larger than 22.59 in this column and these rows. The largest number is 9.34, which is the 0.001 upper percentage point. Hence,

$$p\text{-value} < 0.001$$

3. $F_{calc} = 0.62$, five samples, $n_1 = n_2 = n_3 = 5$, $n_4 = n_5 = 10$. The numerator degrees of freedom are $k - 1 = 5 - 1 = 4$, and the denominator degrees of freedom are $n_T - k = (5 + 5 + 5 + 10 + 10) - 5 = 30$. In the column for 4 numerator degrees of freedom and the rows for 30 denominator degrees of freedom, there is no number smaller than 0.62. The smallest number, 0.858, is the 0.50 upper percentage point, so

$$p\text{-value} > 0.50$$

4. $F_{calc} = 2.91$, six samples, $n_1 = n_2 = 3$, $n_3 = 4$, $n_4 = 5$, $n_5 = n_6 = 3$. The numerator degrees of freedom are $k - 1 = 6 - 1 = 5$, and the denominator degrees of freedom are $(3 + 3 + 4 + 5 + 3 + 3) - 6 = 15$. In the column for 5 numerator degrees of freedom and the rows for 15 denominator degrees of freedom, we find the number 2.90, which is almost equal to F_{calc}. Since this number corresponds to the 0.05 upper percentage point,

$$p\text{-value} \cong 0.05$$

As always, the p-value determines whether the null hypothesis is rejected. Before carrying out an F test, the researcher selects a significance level α. If the p-value is less than α, the null hypothesis (8.2) is rejected. If the p-value is greater than or equal to α, the null hypothesis (8.2) cannot be rejected at this significance level. The p-value is interpreted in the usual way: it is the probability of getting an F statistic at least as extreme as the calculated F statistic if the null hypothesis (8.2) is true.

One-way ANOVA F tests are always two-sided in the sense that one-sided alternative hypotheses cannot be used. But the p-values for these F tests are always *one-tailed*, involving only the upper tail of the F distribution. This is not inconsistent, because it makes sense to reject the null hypothesis (8.2) only when the F statistic is large. A small F statistic does not provide evidence against this hypothesis. The p-values for two-sided t tests and Z tests are two-tailed because extreme positive *or*

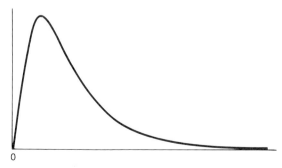

Figure 8.1 F distribution with $d_1 = 6$ df and $d_2 = 12$ df

extreme negative statistics provide evidence against the null hypothesis.

One-way ANOVA requires the following assumptions about the data.

1. Random Samples. Random sampling is not essential as long as the samples are not biased.

2. Independent Samples. This assumption is crucial and must not be violated.[2] If the data consist of repeated measurements on the same patients, one-way ANOVA cannot be used to test the null hypothesis (8.2). Instead, repeated-measures analysis of variance should be considered. The use of one-way ANOVA to analyze repeated measurements is a common mistake in the medical and health care literature.

3. Independent Observations Within Each Sample. If the observations within each sample are not independent, one-way ANOVA cannot be done.

4. Normal Populations. If the samples are large enough, one-way ANOVA can be done when the populations are not exactly normal, thanks to the central limit theorem. One-way ANOVA cannot be done when any of the populations are extremely nonnormal (e.g., when the data have only a few possible values). Consult a statistician if you are not sure whether your samples are large enough to compensate for nonnormal populations.

5. Equal Variances. All of the population variances should be equal or similar. Examination of the sample variances gives us some idea of whether this assumption is reasonable, but there is no simple rule for deciding whether the population variances are equal.* If in doubt, consult a statistician.

Let us determine whether these assumptions are reasonable for the burn survival data. The data are not a random sample, but this is not important. The samples appear to be independent and the observations within each sample seem to be independent, since the % TBSA for one patient tells us nothing about the % TBSA for another patient. Quick histograms of the % TBSA values for the three groups are shown in Figures 8.2 through 8.4. Although the histogram for Group 1 suggests an approximately normal population, the histograms for Groups 2 and 3 indicate skewed populations. From Table 8.1, we obtain the sample variances: $s_1^2 = (15.6)^2 = 243.4$, $s_2^2 = (14.2)^2 = 201.6$, and $s_3^2 = (8.2)^2 = 67.2$. The ratio of the largest variance to the smallest variance is $243.4/67.2 = 3.6$. A discrepancy of this size is possible if the population variances are equal, but it seems unlikely. The equal-variance and normality assumptions are both questionable for these data.

---

*Neter, Wasserman, and Kutner describe statistics for testing the null hypothesis that the population variances are equal.[3] These tests rely so heavily on the assumption of normality that their practical value is quite limited.

```
30 – 39 | XX
40 – 49 | X
50 – 59 | XXX
60 – 69 | XX
70 – 79 | XX
80 – 89 | X
```

Figure 8.2   Quick histogram of % TBSA for Group 1

```
10 – 19 | XXXXX
20 – 29 | XXX
30 – 39 | XXXXXXXX
40 – 49 | X
50 – 59 | XX
60 – 69 | X
```

Figure 8.3   Quick histogram of % TBSA for Group 2

```
10 – 15 | X
16 – 21 | XXXXX
22 – 27 | XX
28 – 33 | X
34 – 39 | X
40 – 45 | X
```

Figure 8.4   Quick histogram of % TBSA for Group 3

Although one-way ANOVA is not ruled out, it would produce only an approximate p-value.

We can obtain better one-way ANOVA results if we *transform* the data. In other words, we will analyze the data in units other than the original units. Instead of analyzing the % TBSA values, we will analyze the *square roots* of the % TBSA values. Why would we want to do this? Let us examine the histograms (Figures 8.5 through 8.7) and the sample variances of the square-root % TBSA data. The histogram for the square-root Group 2 data appears much more normal than the histogram for the original Group 2 data. The Group 1 histogram also seems fairly normal, although the Group 3 histogram is still skewed. The discrepancy between the sample variances is smaller, since the ratio of the largest variance to the smallest variance is $(1.31)^2/(0.81)^2 = 2.6$, from Table 8.1. The square-root data do not satisfy the one-way ANOVA assumptions exactly, but they are more consistent with these assumptions than the original data. For this reason, we will analyze the square-root data. The resulting p-value will still be approximate, but it will be more accurate than a p-value based on the original data. Our populations consist of the square-root % TBSA values for all elderly burned patients similar to those in the study.

```
5.40 – 6.19 |XX
6.20 – 6.99 |X
7.00 – 7.79 |XXXX
7.80 – 8.59 |XX
8.60 – 9.39 |XX
```

Figure 8.5   Quick histogram of square-root % TBSA for Group 1

```
3.00 – 3.99 |XXX
4.00 – 4.99 |XXXX
5.00 – 5.99 |XXXXX
6.00 – 6.99 |XXXXX
7.00 – 7.99 |XXX
```

Figure 8.6   Quick histogram of square-root % TBSA for Group 2

```
3.50 – 3.99 |X
4.00 – 4.49 |XXXXX
4.50 – 4.99 |XX
5.00 – 5.49 |X
5.50 – 5.99 |X
6.00 – 6.49 |X
```

Figure 8.7   Quick histogram of square-root % TBSA for Group 3

Data transformations of this sort are often used to correct violations of normality and equal-variance assumptions. Positively skewed data can often be made less skewed by taking square roots, logarithms, or reciprocals $(1/x_i)$. Negatively skewed data can sometimes be made less skewed by squaring the data. Although data transformation may seem like a sleazy statistical trick, it involves nothing more than changing the *units* of the data. Just as it is reasonable to analyze weights in kilograms rather than pounds, it is reasonable to analyze the square roots of % TBSA values rather than the % TBSA values. If you are not accustomed to thinking in square-root units or logarithm units, data transformation may strike you as rather strange. At this point, you need not feel comfortable with transformed units. It is more important for you to remember that data transformations often make the use of powerful statistical methods possible.*

Let us calculate an *F* statistic to test the null hypothesis that the population square-root % TBSA means are equal, using a 0.01 significance level. The

---

*Further discussion of data transformation can be found in Chapter 12 and in other texts.[3]

sample means and standard deviations for the square-root data are given in Table 8.1. The overall mean can be calculated from the combined sample:

$$\bar{x} = \frac{8.06 + \cdots + 3.16 + \cdots + 5.83}{42} = 5.78$$

Using this overall mean and the sample means, sample standard deviations, and sample sizes, we can apply formulas (8.4) through (8.7) to get the following sums of squares, degrees of freedom, and mean squares.

$$
\begin{aligned}
\text{SSB} &= 11(7.42 - 5.78)^2 + 20(5.44 - 5.78)^2 \\
&\quad + 11(4.77 - 5.78)^2 \\
&= 11(2.69) + 20(0.12) + 11(1.02) \\
&= 29.59 + 2.40 + 11.22 = 43.21
\end{aligned}
$$

$$
\begin{aligned}
\text{SSW} &= (11 - 1)(1.07)^2 + (20 - 1)(1.31)^2 \\
&\quad + (11 - 1)(0.81)^2 \\
&= 10(1.14) + 19(1.72) + 10(0.66) \\
&= 11.40 + 32.68 + 6.60 = 50.68
\end{aligned}
$$

Between-groups df = $3 - 1 = 2$

Within-groups df = $(11 + 20 + 11) - 3 = 39$

$$\text{MSB} = \frac{43.21}{2} = 21.60$$

$$\text{MSW} = \frac{50.68}{39} = 1.30$$

On the basis of these results, the calculated *F* statistic is

$$F = \frac{21.60}{1.30} = 16.62$$

This *F* statistic has 2 and 39 df. Since Table E.5 has no rows for 39 df, we have to approximate. Using the column for 2 df and the rows for 30 df, we find that 16.62 is larger than the 0.001 upper percentage point, which is 8.77. Hence,

p-value < 0.001

We reject the null hypothesis (8.2) at any significance level greater than or equal to 0.001. Since our significance level is 0.01, we reject this hypothesis and conclude that at least some of the population means are different. Without further analysis (discussed in Sections 8.4 and 8.5), we cannot say which population means are different.

Example 8.2

In a study of the effect of verapamil on portal hypertension, the wedged hepatic venous pressure (WHVP) values shown in Table 8.2 were reported.[4] These pressures were determined for six patients with postnecrotic cirrhosis before intravenous (IV)

TABLE 8.2 WEDGED HEPATIC VENOUS PRESSURE BEFORE AND AFTER IV AND ORAL ADMINISTRATION OF VERAPAMIL

Patient No.	Basal Value	1 hr Post IV Verapamil	1 mo Post Oral Verapamil	3 mo Post Oral Verapamil
1	35	34	26	27
2	23	20	13	11
3	21	20	15	21
4	19	17	11	16
5	25	21	17	27
6	27	21	17	17

administration of verapamil, one hour after IV administration of verapamil, one month after continuous oral administration of verapamil, and three months after continuous oral administration of verapamil. Can we use one-way ANOVA to test the hypothesis that the population baseline and post-verapamil WHVP means are equal?

Although the WHVP values within each sample are independent, the samples are not independent. Repeated WHVP measurements were obtained for each patient, so one-way ANOVA cannot be done. One-factor repeated-measures ANOVA should be considered instead.

Example 8.3

In a study of activities of daily living for women before and after myocardial infarction (MI), the level of physical activity was rated as follows[5]:

1 = no limitation of physical activity
2 = slight limitation of physical activity
3 = marked limitation of physical activity
4 = inability to carry out any physical activity without discomfort

Three women who sustained an anterior or anterior-lateral MI had a mean post-MI activity score of 1.3 ($s = 0.6$). Twelve women who sustained an inferior or inferior-lateral MI had a mean post-MI activity score of 1.7 ($s = 0.8$). Six women who sustained a subendocardial MI had a mean post-MI activity score of 2.0 ($s = 0.6$). Can one-way ANOVA be used to test the hypothesis that the three population post-MI mean scores are equal?

Since the data have only four possible values, the populations are so nonnormal that one-way ANOVA is not appropriate. This type of nonnormality cannot be corrected by transforming the data. No matter what transformation is used, the transformed data will still have only four possible values. The Kruskal-Wallis test described in Chapter 11 could be used to test the hypothesis that the three populations of post-MI scores are identical.

8.2 COMPUTER OUTPUT

Because one-way ANOVA calculations are extremely tedious, it is easy to make mistakes when

Source	Degrees of Freedom	Sum of Squares	Mean Square
Between groups	$k - 1$	SSB	MSB
Within groups	$n_T - k$	SSW	MSW
Total	$n_T - 1$	SST	

Figure 8.8 One-way analysis-of-variance table format

doing them by hand. The unpleasant task of grinding out one-way ANOVA results is best left to a computer, which has nothing better to do. If SPSS or SAS software is used, an exact p-value for the F statistic is given. In SPSS, one-way ANOVA is done by the ONEWAY program, and in SAS, by the ANOVA and GLM programs. Both SPSS and SAS present the one-way ANOVA results in an *analysis-of-variance table*. This table has the format shown in Figure 8.8 and is the customary way of presenting one-way ANOVA results.

The one-way ANOVA table includes a *total sum of squares* (SST) and *total degrees of freedom*. If the overall variance s^2 is calculated for the combined sample consisting of all k samples, the total sum of squares is given by

$$total\ sum\ of\ squares = (n_T - 1)s^2$$

The total degrees of freedom are $n_T - 1$. A total mean square is usually not computed. It can be shown that

$$SST = SSB + SSW$$

and

$$total\ df = between\text{-}groups\ df + within\text{-}groups\ df$$

The degrees of freedom for the one-way ANOVA F statistic can be obtained from the one-way ANOVA table. The numerator degrees of freedom are the between-groups degrees of freedom and the denominator degrees of freedom are the within-groups degrees of freedom.

Figures 8.9 and 8.10 show the SPSS/PC ONEWAY and SAS ANOVA output for the burn square-root data. The results in the SPSS/PC and

Source	D.F.	Sum of Squares	Mean Squares	F Ratio	F Prob.
Between Groups	2	43.0592	21.5296	16.6017	.0000
Within Groups	39	50.5762	1.2968		
Total	41	93.6354			

Figure 8.9 SPSS/PC one-way ANOVA output for square-root % TBSA

SOURCE	DF	SUM OF SQUARES	MEAN SQUARE
MODEL	2	43.05915956	21.52957978
ERROR	39	50.57622074	1.29682617
CORRECTED TOTAL	41	93.63538030	
MODEL F =	16.60		PR > F = 0.0001

Figure 8.10 SAS one-way ANOVA output for square-root % TBSA

SAS output agree with our computations except for slight differences due to rounding error. The calculated F statistic is given under "F Ratio" in the SPSS/PC output and after "MODEL F = " in the SAS output. The p-value given under "F Prob." in the SPSS/PC output is 0.0000. This does not mean that the p-value is 0, but that it is less than or equal to 0.00005. This p-value is given as 0.0001 after "PR > F = " in the SAS output, which means that the p-value rounds off to 0.0001. In the SAS output, the MODEL sum of squares is the between-groups sum of squares, the ERROR sum of squares is the within-groups sum of squares, and the COR-RECTED TOTAL sum of squares is the total sum of squares.

Although a computer can perform one-way ANOVA calculations, it cannot determine whether independence or normality assumptions hold. This is entirely the responsibility of the researcher. If a computer is given data that violate assumptions, it will carry out the analysis anyway. When important assumptions are violated, the output can be danger-ously misleading.

8.3 MULTIPLE COMPARISONS

If we cannot reject the hypothesis that all of the population means are equal, the analysis is finished. If we reject this hypothesis, the analysis has just started. We then want to determine which popula-

tion means are different. This usually involves more than one comparison between population means, so we have to contend with the multiplicity problem. We can compare population means by obtaining confidence intervals for differences between popula-tion means, but we want to be fairly sure that *all* of our confidence intervals include the differences be-tween the population means.

Suppose we obtain 100 confidence intervals for differences between population means. We want to be 95% sure that *all* of these confidence intervals include the differences between the population means. If we use one of the procedures described in Chapter 6 to obtain 100 95% confidence intervals, we cannot be 95% sure that *all* of these confidence intervals include the differences between the popu-lation means. Since 95% confidence intervals do *not* include the population parameter 5% of the time, we are fairly sure that about five of our confidence intervals do not include the differences between the population means.

What we need are *multiple-comparison proce-dures*, which guarantee an *overall confidence level*. An overall confidence level allows us to be fairly sure that *all* of the confidence intervals include the differences between the population means. When we use a multiple-comparison procedure with a $100(1 - \alpha)\%$ overall confidence level, we can be $100(1 - \alpha)\%$ sure that *all* of the confidence intervals we calculate include the differences be-tween the population means. We will describe two multiple-comparison procedures, the Tukey method and the Bonferroni method.* *The Tukey and Bonferroni procedures described in this chapter require independent samples and cannot be used when repeated measurements are obtained.* These procedures are sometimes mistakenly used in medical and health care research to analyze repeated measurements. Errors like this can produce extremely misleading results.

8.4 THE TUKEY METHOD FOR MULTIPLE COMPARISONS

The Tukey method for obtaining confidence intervals is based on *studentized range distributions*. The nature of these distributions will not be described here. We need only be familiar with the use of Table E.6 in Appendix E. This table lists 0.10, 0.05, and 0.01 upper percentage points of selected studentized range distributions. Like F distributions, studentized range distributions have numerator and denominator degrees of freedom. Let $q_{\alpha, k, n_T - k}$ be the α upper percentage point of the studentized range distribution with k numerator degrees of freedom and $n_T - k$ denominator degrees of freedom. Note that the numerator degrees of freedom are *not* $k - 1$.

The Tukey procedure requires estimated variances of the sample means. It can be shown that the estimated variance of the ith sample mean is given by the formula

$$\text{var}(\bar{x}_i) = \frac{\text{MSW}}{n_i} \qquad (8.9)$$

The sample size n_i is the number of observations in the ith sample (the sample from which the mean $\bar{x}_i$ was obtained). Using the MSW for the square-root % TBSA data, we obtain the following estimated variances for the square-root % TBSA sample means.

$$\text{var}(\bar{x}_1) = \frac{1.30}{11} = 0.12$$

$$\text{var}(\bar{x}_2) = \frac{1.30}{20} = 0.06$$

$$\text{var}(\bar{x}_3) = \frac{1.30}{11} = 0.12$$

The $100(1 - \alpha)\%$ Tukey confidence intervals for differences between the population means are given

by

$$\left((\bar{x}_i - \bar{x}_j) - \frac{(q_{\alpha, k, n_T - k})}{\sqrt{2}} \sqrt{\widetilde{\text{var}(\bar{x}_i) + \text{var}(\bar{x}_j)}} \, , \right.$$
$$\left. (\bar{x}_i - \bar{x}_j) + \frac{(q_{\alpha, k, n_T - k})}{\sqrt{2}} \sqrt{\text{var}(\bar{x}_i) + \text{var}(\bar{x}_j)} \right) \qquad (8.10)$$

where $\bar{x}_i$ and $\bar{x}_j$ are the means for the ith and jth samples. When formula (8.10) is used to obtain confidence intervals for the differences $\mu_i - \mu_j$, we can be $100(1 - \alpha)\%$ sure that all of the Tukey confidence intervals include the differences between the population means. In other words, the overall confidence level is $100(1 - \alpha)\%$.

Let us obtain 90% Tukey confidence intervals for the square-root burn data. Because we rejected the hypothesis that all of the population square-root % TBSA means are equal, we want to determine which population means are different. Our studentized range upper percentage point is $q_{.10, 3, 39}$. The numerator degrees of freedom are listed in the first row of Table E.6, and the denominator degrees of freedom are listed in the first column. Since 39 df are not listed, we have to approximate. Looking up 3 in the top row and 40 in the first column, we find the number in the column headed by 3 and in the row beginning with 40. This number, 2.99, is approximately equal to $q_{.10, 3, 39}$. Using the estimated variances on this page and the sample means in Table 8.1, we can apply formula (8.10) to calculate our Tukey confidence intervals as follows.

Confidence Interval for $\mu_1 - \mu_2$ (Died Within Three Days Versus Died Within Five to 48 Days).

$$\left((7.42 - 5.44) - \frac{2.99}{\sqrt{2}} \sqrt{0.12 + 0.06} \, , \right.$$
$$\left. (7.42 - 5.44) + \frac{2.99}{\sqrt{2}} \sqrt{0.12 + 0.06} \right)$$

$$(1.98 - 0.90, \, 1.98 + 0.90)$$

$$(1.08, 2.88)$$

Confidence Interval for $\mu_1 - \mu_3$ (Died Within Three Days Versus Survived).

$$\left((7.42 - 4.77) - \frac{2.99}{\sqrt{2}} \sqrt{0.12 + 0.12} \, , \right.$$
$$\left. (7.42 - 4.77) + \frac{2.99}{\sqrt{2}} \sqrt{0.12 + 0.12} \right)$$

$$(2.65 - 1.04, \, 2.65 + 1.04)$$

$$(1.61, 3.69)$$

---

*Other multiple-comparison methods for one-way ANOVA are described elsewhere.[3, 6]

Confidence Interval for $\mu_2 - \mu_3$ (Died Within Five to 48 Days Versus Survived).

$$\left((5.44 - 4.77) - \frac{2.99}{\sqrt{2}} \sqrt{0.06 + 0.12} \, , \right.$$

$$\left. (5.44 - 4.77) + \frac{2.99}{\sqrt{2}} \sqrt{0.06 + 0.12} \right)$$

$$(0.67 - 0.90, \, 0.67 + 0.90)$$

$$(-0.23, \, 1.57)$$

How do we interpret these Tukey confidence intervals? We are 90% sure that the following is true.

1. The population mean square-root % TBSA for patients who died within three days is larger than the population mean square-root % TBSA for patients who died within five to 48 days. The difference between the population means might be moderate (no less than 1.08) or large (as high as 2.88).

2. The population mean square-root % TBSA for patients who died within three days is larger than the population mean square-root % TBSA for patients who survived. The difference between the population means might be moderate (no less than 1.61) or large (as high as 3.69).

3. We cannot say that the population mean square-root % TBSA for patients who died within five to 48 days differs from the population mean square-root % TBSA for patients who survived. (The confidence interval includes 0.)

Because the *overall* confidence level is 90%, we can be 90% sure that *all* of these conclusions are correct. We can be fairly sure that (1) the population mean square-root % TBSA for elderly burn patients who die within three days is larger than the population mean square-root % TBSA for elderly burn patients who die within five to 48 days; (2) the population mean square-root % TBSA for elderly burn patients who die within three days is larger than the population mean square-root % TBSA for elderly burn patients who survive; and (3) we cannot say that the population mean square-root % TBSA for elderly burn patients who die within five to 48 days differs from the population mean square-root % TBSA for elderly burn patients who survive.

For the square-root burn data, we made all possible comparisons between the means. Suppose we had examined the sample means and then selected one comparison of interest. Would we still need to use a multiple-comparison procedure, given that only one confidence interval would be calculated? The answer is an emphatic *yes*. Because we selected the comparison after examining the sample means, we informally made several comparisons of sample means. We sorted through the sample means to decide which confidence interval to obtain. These informal comparisons must be taken into account

when the confidence interval is obtained, so a multiple-comparison procedure must be used.

When a researcher examines sample means to determine which population means to compare, she usually obtains confidence intervals for population mean differences corresponding to differences between large sample means and small sample means. The distributions of such differences as

largest sample mean − smallest sample mean

are not accurately reflected in the confidence-interval procedures described in Chapter 6. They *are* accurately reflected in the Tukey procedure and other multiple-comparison procedures. For this reason, a multiple-comparison procedure must be used whenever a comparison is selected after examining the sample means.

8.5 THE BONFERRONI METHOD FOR MULTIPLE COMPARISONS

The Bonferroni method increases the confidence level for each confidence interval in order to ensure a specified overall confidence level. Suppose that the comparisons to be made are selected *before* examining the sample means, and define the number c by

$$c = \text{number of comparisons to be made}$$

If the comparisons are selected *after* examining the sample means, we define c differently:

$$c = \text{total number of } \textit{possible} \text{ comparisons}$$

In the second case, c is the number of comparisons that *could* be made, whether or not we actually make them. If there are four population means and we select three comparisons *after* examining the sample means, c is not 3. There are six possible comparisons (μ_1 versus μ_2, μ_1 versus μ_3, μ_1 versus μ_4, μ_2 versus μ_3, μ_2 versus μ_4, and μ_3 versus μ_4), so c is 6. If we had selected three comparisons *before* examining the sample means, c would be 3.

Bonferroni confidence intervals are based on adjusted upper percentage points of the t distribution with $n_T - k$ degrees of freedom. Instead of using the $\alpha/2$ upper percentage point, we use the $\alpha/2c$ upper percentage point. The $100(1 - \alpha)\%$ Bonferroni confidence intervals for differences between the population means are given by the formula

$$\left((\bar{x}_i - \bar{x}_j) - (t_{\alpha/2c, \, n_T-k}) \sqrt{\text{var}(\bar{x}_i) + \text{var}(\bar{x}_j)} \, , \right.$$

$$\left. (\bar{x}_i - \bar{x}_j) + (t_{\alpha/2c, \, n_T-k}) \sqrt{\text{var}(\bar{x}_i) + \text{var}(\bar{x}_j)} \right) \tag{8.11}$$

The estimated variances in this formula are given by formula (8.9). If formula (8.11) is used to obtain confidence intervals for the differences $\mu_i - \mu_j$, we can be $100(1 - \alpha)\%$ sure that all of the Bonferroni confidence intervals include the differences between the population means. The overall confidence level is $100(1 - \alpha)\%$.

Let us obtain 90% Bonferroni confidence intervals for the square-root burn data. Suppose we decided, *before* examining the sample means, that we wanted only the confidence intervals for $\mu_1 - \mu_2$ and $\mu_1 - \mu_3$. Then $c = 2$, so $\alpha/2c = 0.10/4 = 0.025$, and $t_{.025, 39} \cong t_{.025, 40} = 2.021$. The 90% Bonferroni confidence intervals are calculated as follows.

Confidence Interval for $\mu_1 - \mu_2$ (Died Within Three Days Versus Died Within Five to 48 Days).

$$\big((7.42 - 5.44) - (2.021)\sqrt{0.12 + 0.06}\,,$$
$$(7.42 - 5.44) + (2.021)\sqrt{0.12 + 0.06}\,\big)$$
$$(1.98 - 0.86, 1.98 + 0.86)$$
$$(1.12, 2.84)$$

Confidence Interval for $\mu_1 - \mu_3$ (Died Within Three Days Versus Survived).

$$\big((7.42 - 4.77) - (2.021)\sqrt{0.12 + 0.12}\,,$$
$$(7.42 - 4.77) + (2.021)\sqrt{0.12 + 0.12}\,\big)$$
$$(2.65 - 0.99, 2.65 + 0.99)$$
$$(1.66, 3.64)$$

We can be 90% sure that *both* of these confidence intervals include the differences between the population means. The interpretation of these confidence intervals is similar to the interpretation of the Tukey confidence intervals on p. 154.

The 90% Bonferroni confidence intervals are preferable to the 90% Tukey confidence intervals because the Bonferroni confidence intervals are slightly narrower (more precise). But suppose we decide to obtain 90% Bonferroni confidence intervals for the differences $\mu_1 - \mu_2$ and $\mu_1 - \mu_3$ *after* examining the sample means. Then we need to take into account the informal comparisons made by sorting through the sample means, so c is equal to 3, the number of possible comparisons. We have $\alpha/2c = 0.10/6 = 0.017$, and $t_{.017, 39} \cong t_{.015, 40} = 2.250$. If we calculate the 90% Bonferroni confidence intervals using this upper percentage point, we get the confidence intervals (1.03, 2.93) for $\mu_1 - \mu_2$ and (1.55, 3.75) for $\mu_1 - \mu_3$. These confidence intervals are wider (less precise) than the Tukey confidence intervals.

For the square-root burn data, the 90% Tukey confidence intervals are preferable if the comparisons are selected after examining the sample means or if all possible comparisons are made. The 90% Bonferroni confidence intervals are preferable if the comparisons μ_1 versus μ_2 and μ_1 versus μ_3 are selected before examining the sample means.

In general, the Tukey procedure tends to produce narrower confidence intervals than the Bonferroni procedure when all of the possible comparisons are of interest or when comparisons are selected *after* looking at the sample means. The Bonferroni procedure tends to produce narrower confidence intervals than the Tukey procedure when there is a large number of possible comparisons and a few comparisons are selected *before* looking at the sample means.

To determine which procedure will produce the narrowest confidence intervals, we obtain both the Tukey studentized range upper percentage point and the Bonferroni t upper percentage point. If the studentized range value divided by $\sqrt{2}$ is less than the t value, the Tukey confidence intervals will be narrower. If the studentized range value divided by $\sqrt{2}$ is greater than the t value, the Bonferroni confidence intervals will be narrower. If the studentized range value divided by $\sqrt{2}$ is equal to the t value, the Tukey and Bonferroni confidence intervals will be the same. For the square-root burn data, we obtain $q_{.10, 3, 39}/\sqrt{2} \cong 2.99/\sqrt{2} = 2.114$ and $t_{.017, 39} \cong t_{.015, 40} = 2.250$ when all possible comparisons are taken into account. Since 2.114 is less than 2.250, we would choose the Tukey procedure for making all possible comparisons.

Unlike the test statistics and confidence intervals discussed in Chapters 6 and 7, the F statistic and the corresponding multiple-comparison confidence intervals can be inconsistent. All of the $100(1 - \alpha)\%$ multiple-comparison confidence intervals can include 0 even when the hypothesis of equal population means is rejected at the significance level α. Such inconsistencies are quite irritating, since the confidence intervals do not allow us to decide which population means are different. Fortunately, such discrepancies are the exception rather than the rule. One way of resolving this problem is to reduce the overall confidence level until at least one of the confidence intervals does not include 0.

SUMMARY

One-way analysis of variance is used to test the hypothesis that three or more population means are equal. Independent samples, normal or approximately normal populations, and equal or similar population variances are required for one-way ANOVA. Sometimes data must be transformed before using one-way ANOVA in order to reduce skewness or to obtain more similar variances. An F statistic based on mean squares is used to test the hypothesis of equal population means. If the hypothesis of equal population means is rejected, a multiple-comparison procedure is used to determine which population means are different. Two commonly used multiple-comparison procedures are the Tukey method and the Bonferroni method. The multiple-comparison procedure that produces the narrowest confidence intervals should be used.

FREQUENTLY USED ONE-WAY ANOVA FORMULAS

F statistic for testing H_0: $\mu_1 = \mu_2 = \cdots = \mu_k$:

$$F = \frac{\text{MSB}}{\text{MSW}}$$

Estimated variance of sample mean:

$$\text{var}(\bar{x}_i) = \frac{\text{MSW}}{n_i}$$

$100(1 - \alpha)\%$ Tukey confidence interval:

$$\left((\bar{x}_i - \bar{x}_j) - \frac{(q_{\alpha, k, n_T - k})}{\sqrt{2}} \sqrt{\text{var}(\bar{x}_i) + \text{var}(\bar{x}_j)}, \right.$$
$$\left. (\bar{x}_i - \bar{x}_j) + \frac{(q_{\alpha, k, n_T - k})}{\sqrt{2}} \sqrt{\text{var}(\bar{x}_i) + \text{var}(\bar{x}_j)} \right)$$

$100(1 - \alpha)\%$ Bonferroni confidence interval:

$$\left((\bar{x}_i - \bar{x}_j) - (t_{\alpha/2c, n_T - k}) \sqrt{\text{var}(\bar{x}_i) + \text{var}(\bar{x}_j)}, \right.$$
$$\left. (\bar{x}_i - \bar{x}_j) + (t_{\alpha/2c, n_T - k}) \sqrt{\text{var}(\bar{x}_i) + \text{var}(\bar{x}_j)} \right)$$

PROBLEMS

The following instructions apply to problems 1 through 17.

1. In each problem, data are described, SPSS/PC one-way ANOVA output is presented, and a question about the data is asked. Determine whether one-way ANOVA is appropriate for analyzing the data. If one-way ANOVA is not appropriate, state which assumptions are violated.

2. If the one-way ANOVA assumptions are satisfied, carry out an F test. State the null and alternative hypotheses and find the most exact p-value that can be obtained from Table E.5. Interpret the p-value.

3. If the hypothesis of equal population means is rejected, carry out an appropriate multiple-comparison procedure. Use the confidence intervals and the p-value to answer the question in the problem.

You may want to obtain quick histograms for each sample. Do not worry about slightly or moderately nonnormal histograms if the data have a large number of possible values. Unless the data are extremely nonnormal and the sample is very small, you can assume that the central limit theorem applies to the data.

1. A study evaluated the effect of three drugs on the duration of succinylcholine-induced muscle relaxation.[7] Twenty patients were randomly assigned to four groups of five patients each. Patients in each group either received no drug or received Innovar, droperidol, or fentanyl before induction of anesthesia. Table 8.3 shows the duration of succinylcholine-induced muscle relaxation for these patients. Do the data provide evidence that some of the population duration means for different drugs are different? Use a 0.10 significance level for testing the hypothesis of equal population means and a multiple-comparison overall confidence level of 90%. If the hypothesis of equal population means is re-

---

TABLE 8.3 DURATION (min) OF SUCCINYLCHOLINE-INDUCED MUSCLE RELAXATION WITH SAMPLE MEANS AND STANDARD DEVIATIONS

No-Drug Group	Innovar Group	Droperidol Group	Fentanyl Group
5.9	16.1	10.3	7.2
8.0	11.2	6.8	10.5
11.5	9.0	5.3	8.5
6.0	8.8	3.2	4.2
9.2	10.2	6.5	6.5
8.1 ± 2.3	11.1 ± 3.0	6.4 ± 2.6	7.4 ± 2.3

Source	D.F.	Sum of Squares	Mean Squares
Between Groups	3	60.0935	20.0312
Within Groups	16	106.2760	6.6423
Total	19	166.3695	

Figure 8.11 SPSS/PC one-way ANOVA output for duration of muscle relaxation

jected, assume that the only comparisons of interest are those between the Innovar group and the other groups. Also assume that these comparisons were selected before examining the sample means.

2. A study of glomerulonephritis in the dog reported the albumin values in Table 8.4 for 40 dogs with naturally developing glomerulonephritis.[8] Three types of disease were studied: membranous glomerulonephritis, mesangioproliferative glomeru-

lonephritis, and membranoproliferative glomerulonephritis. Do the data provide evidence that some of the population albumin means for different types of glomerulonephritis are different? Use a 0.01 significance level for testing the hypothesis of equal population means and a 95% multiple-comparison overall confidence level.

3. In a study of taste function in patients with anorexia nervosa and bulimia nervosa, taste recog-

TABLE 8.4 ALBUMIN (g/dl) FOR DOGS WITH GLOMERULONEPHRITIS WITH SAMPLE MEANS AND STANDARD DEVIATIONS

Membranous Glomerulonephritis			Mesangioproliferative Glomerulonephritis			Membranoproliferative Glomerulonephritis		
1.3	2.0	0.9	2.1	2.4	1.6	2.9	2.4	3.0
2.2	2.4	1.2	2.5	1.4	2.8	2.7	2.7	2.5
2.9	2.6		3.6	2.5	2.9	1.9	2.1	2.2
3.1	3.7		1.7	1.2	2.4	2.0	1.8	
2.4	1.0		1.3	2.1	2.9	2.3	3.7	
	2.14 ± 0.89			2.23 ± 0.69			2.48 ± 0.53	

Figure 8.12 SPSS/PC one-way ANOVA output for albumin

Source	D.F.	Sum of Squares	Mean Squares
Between Groups	2	.7762	.3881
Within Groups	37	18.6816	.5049
Total	39	19.4578	

TABLE 8.5 TASTE RECOGNITION SCORE FOR ANOREXIC PATIENTS AFTER TREATMENT WITH SAMPLE MEANS AND STANDARD DEVIATIONS

Patient No.	Recognition Score			
	SWEET	SALTY	SOUR	BITTER
1	4	2	3	4
2	3	4	4	2
3	3	4	0	5
4	4	4	4	4
5	4	5	6	4
6	1	3	3	3
7	3	5	4	3
	3.1 ± 1.1	3.9 ± 1.1	3.4 ± 1.8	3.6 ± 1.0

Figure 8.13 SPSS/PC one-way ANOVA output for recognition score

Source	D.F.	Sum of Squares	Mean Squares
Between Groups	3	1.8571	.6190
Within Groups	24	39.1429	1.6310
Total	27	41.0000	

nition scores were reported for seven anorexic patients after treatment.[9] These data are shown in Table 8.5. The higher the score, the better the taste recognition. Do the data provide evidence that some of the population recognition score means for sweet, salty, sour, and bitter substances are different? Use a 0.05 significance level for testing the hypothesis of equal population means and a 95% overall confidence level for multiple comparisons.

4. In a study of drug-induced occupational allergy, the response to bacampicillin was measured by a sensitivity index (SI).[10] Table 8.6 shows the logarithms of the SI values for various groups of 35 workers and work applicants. (The data were transformed by taking logarithms in order to reduce skewness and obtain more similar variances.) The larger the log SI value, the greater the proliferative response. Do the data provide evidence that some of the population log SI means for different group classifications are different? Use a 0.001 significance level for testing the hypothesis of equal population means and a 99% overall confidence level for multiple comparisons. If the hypothesis of equal population means is rejected, assume that the only comparisons of interest are those between Group 4 and the other groups. Also assume that these comparisons were selected before examining the sample means.

5. A study of chronic lung disease reported the forced expiratory volumes in one second (FEV_1s) shown in Table 8.7 for three groups of patients: nine patients with a tracheostomy and lung disease, 10 patients with parenchymal lung disease but no tracheostomy, and five patients with a tracheostomy

TABLE 8.6   LOG SI FOR WORKERS AND WORK APPLICANTS WITH GROUP MEANS AND STANDARD DEVIATIONS

Group 1: Allergic Workers Employed in Bacampicillin Production		Group 2: Allergic Workers with Negative Skin Tests Employed in Bacampicillin Production		Group 3: Healthy Workers Handling Drugs for Several Years		Group 4: Work Applicants	
1.81	0.64	0.74	1.16	0.10	0.00	0.26	0.74
0.79	1.28	1.13		−0.11	0.59	−0.36	0.18
1.61		0.53		−0.51	0.59	0.10	1.19
2.19		1.74		0.47		0.59	0.34
1.63		1.48		−0.51		0.18	0.53
1.16		0.88		−0.36		−0.22	
1.39 ± 0.52		1.10 ± 0.42		0.03 ± 0.44		0.32 ± 0.44	

Source	D.F.	Sum of Squares	Mean Squares
Between Groups	3	10.4117	3.4706
Within Groups	31	6.4389	0.2077
Total	34	16.8506	

Figure 8.14 SPSS/PC one-way ANOVA output for log SI

TABLE 8.7 FEV_1 (% PREDICTED) WITH SAMPLE MEANS AND STANDARD DEVIATIONS

Group 1: Tracheostomy and Lung Disease		Group 2: Lung Disease and No Tracheostomy		Group 3: Tracheostomy and No Lung Disease
63	57	54	39	77
60	55	47	53	91
62	55	74	62	81
31	35	67	45	86
73		66	53	110
54.6 ± 13.4		56.0 ± 11.0		89.0 ± 12.9

Figure 8.15 SPSS/PC one-way ANOVA output for FEV$_1$

Source	D.F.	Sum of Squares	Mean Squares
Between Groups	2	4501.1111	2250.5556
Within Groups	21	3196.2222	152.2011
Total	23	7697.3333	

but no clinically obvious lung disease.[11] Do the data provide evidence that some of the population FEV$_1$ means for different group classifications are different? Use a 0.01 significance level for testing the hypothesis of equal population means and a 95% overall confidence level for multiple comparisons.

6. In a study of blood protein binding of cyclosporine in transplant patients, the ratio of the cyclosporine concentration in whole blood to the cyclosporine concentration in plasma (WB/P ratio) was reported for three groups of subjects: eight kidney-transplant patients, five liver-transplant patients, and four healthy subjects.[12] These data are shown in Table 8.8. Do the data provide evidence that some of the population WB/P ratio means for different group classifications are different? Use a 0.05 significance level for testing the hypothesis of equal population means and a 90% overall confidence level for multiple comparisons. If the hypothesis of equal population means is rejected, assume that the only comparisons of interest are those between healthy subjects and transplant patients. Also assume that these comparisons were selected before examining the sample means.

7. A study of the frequency with which physicians prescribe drugs reported the rates of prescribing shown in Table 8.9 for 65 physicians in three specialties.[13] Do the data provide evidence that some of the population prescribing rate means for different physician specialties are different? Use a 0.05 significance level for testing the hypothesis of equal population means and a 95% overall confidence level for multiple comparisons.

8. In a study of an acuity system, patient–average acuity points were reported for 23 patients in three categories: cerebrovascular accident (nine pa-

TABLE 8.8 WB/P RATIO FOR TRANSPLANT PATIENTS AND HEALTHY SUBJECTS WITH SAMPLE MEANS AND STANDARD DEVIATIONS

Kidney Transplant	Liver Transplant	Healthy Subjects
1.35	1.59	1.69
1.02	1.36	2.06
0.85	1.27	2.05
1.15	1.29	1.93
0.94	1.12	
0.93		1.93 ± 0.17
0.91	1.33 ± 0.17	
1.21		
1.04 ± 0.17		

tients), gastrointestinal (GI) bleeding (nine patients), and drug overdose (five patients).[14] These acuity points are shown in Table 8.10. Do the data provide evidence that some of the population acuity point means for different categories are different? Use a 0.05 significance level for testing the hypothesis of equal population means and a 95% overall confidence level for multiple comparisons.

9. A study of antipsychotic drugs reported the length of hospital stay (LOS) for 28 chronic schizophrenic inpatients treated with chlorpromazine, haloperidol, or fluphenazine.[15] The square roots of these data are shown in Table 8.11. (The data were transformed by taking square roots in order to make the distributions more normal.) Do the data provide evidence that some of the population square-root LOS means for different drug treatments are different? Use a 0.01 significance level for testing the hypothesis of equal population

Figure 8.16 SPSS/PC one-way ANOVA output for WB/P ratio

Source	D.F.	Sum of Squares	Mean Squares
Between Groups	2	2.1012	1.0506
Within Groups	14	.4190	.0299
Total	16	2.5202	

TABLE 8.9 PRESCRIBING RATE FOR PHYSICIANS IN THREE SPECIALTIES WITH SAMPLE MEANS AND STANDARD DEVIATIONS*

Internal Medicine				Obstetrics/ Gynecology		Pediatrics		
3	1	1	3	1	2	1	2	3
2	3	2	2	2	3	1	3	2
2	1	3	1	2	3	2	2	2
1	1	2	1	3	2	3	1	3
3	2	2	3	1	3	3	2	2
1	3	1	3	1	1	1	3	
2	1	3	3			3	1	
2	3	1		2.0 ± 0.9				
3	2	2				2.1 ± 0.8		
2.0 ± 0.8								

*1 = low, 2 = intermediate, 3 = high

TABLE 8.10 PATIENT–AVERAGE ACUITY POINTS WITH SAMPLE MEANS AND STANDARD DEVIATIONS

Cerebrovascular Accident	GI Bleeding	Overdose
555	663	480
897	662	734
469	717	367
676	804	504
777	771	531
565	687	
791	397	523.2 ± 133.4
397	976	
773	377	
655.6 ± 167.9	672.7 ± 188.7	

Source	D.F.	Sum of Squares	Mean Squares
Between Groups	2	.1015	.0507
Within Groups	62	42.7601	.6897
Total	64	42.8615	

Figure 8.17 SPSS/PC one-way ANOVA output for prescribing rate

Source	D.F.	Sum of Squares	Mean Squares
Between Groups	2	79014.7169	39507.3585
Within Groups	20	581415.0222	29070.7511
Total	22	660429.7391	

Figure 8.18 SPSS/PC one-way ANOVA output for acuity points

means and a 95% overall confidence level for multiple comparisons.

10. A study evaluated the efficacy of different types of aerobic exercise for weight loss.[16] Moderately obese women were randomly assigned to one of three exercise programs without dietary restriction: walking, cycling, or swimming. Table 8.12 shows the weight changes (before-program weight − after-program weight) for 29 of these women. Do the data provide evidence that some of the population weight-change means for different exercise programs are different? Use a 0.05 significance level for testing the hypothesis of equal population means and a 95% overall confidence level for multiple comparisons.

11. In a study of walking gait in dogs, the weight distribution among limbs shown in Table 8.13 was reported for 17 healthy dogs.[17] Do the data provide

TABLE 8.11 SQUARE ROOT OF LENGTH OF HOSPITALIZATION (SQUARE-ROOT DAYS) FOR CHRONIC SCHIZOPHRENIC INPATIENTS WITH SAMPLE MEANS AND STANDARD DEVIATIONS

Chlorpromazine	Haloperidol	Fluphenazine
4.90	5.29	5.83
1.41	4.47	2.83
5.57	4.47	1.00
5.66	2.65	1.00
5.39	5.39	5.10
3.74	1.00	3.16
1.00	5.29	6.08
2.00	1.00	
6.56	4.80	3.57 ± 2.15
4.24	2.45	
	5.29	
4.05 ± 1.95		
	3.83 ± 1.73	

Figure 8.19 SPSS/PC one-way ANOVA output for square root of length of hospitalization

Source	D.F.	Sum of Squares	Mean Squares
Between Groups	2	.9312	.4656
Within Groups	25	91.8604	3.6744
Total	27	92.7916	

TABLE 8.12 WEIGHT CHANGE (POUNDS) FOR EXERCISE GROUPS WITH SAMPLE MEANS AND STANDARD DEVIATIONS

Walking		Cycling		Swimming	
17	7	16	20	0	−4
18	15	24	23	−11	2
15	16	16	13	−8	
18	34	16	17	1	
17	13	21		−6	
18		20		−6	
17.1 ± 6.5		18.6 ± 3.5		-4.0 ± 4.6	

TABLE 8.13 WEIGHT DISTRIBUTION AMONG LIMBS WITH SAMPLE MEANS AND STANDARD DEVIATIONS

Dog No.	Weight Distribution (%)			
	LEFT FORELIMB	RIGHT FORELIMB	LEFT HINDLIMB	RIGHT HINDLIMB
1	28.7	27.6	21.8	21.9
2	29.7	30.3	20.5	19.5
3	32.4	30.5	18.2	18.9
4	30.1	28.7	20.8	20.4
5	27.6	27.3	22.2	22.9
6	28.6	28.7	21.9	20.8
7	30.1	28.6	20.9	20.4
8	28.2	29.1	20.9	21.8
9	30.8	28.5	21.2	19.5
10	28.4	30.7	20.9	20.0
11	26.6	28.1	21.7	23.4
12	31.0	39.0	20.0	20.0
13	28.3	26.4	23.8	21.5
14	29.7	30.4	19.6	20.3
15	33.1	31.8	17.9	17.2
16	28.7	29.9	21.4	20.0
17	31.6	32.4	18.4	17.6
	29.6 ± 1.7	29.9 ± 2.8	20.7 ± 1.5	20.4 ± 1.6

evidence that some of the population weight distribution percentage means for different limbs are different? Use a 0.01 significance level for testing the hypothesis of equal population means and a 95% overall confidence level for multiple comparisons.

12. In a study of multiple myeloma and renal failure, the calcium levels at admission were reported for 33 patients with multiple myeloma and

Figure 8.20 SPSS/PC one-way ANOVA output for weight change

Source	D.F.	Sum of Squares	Mean Squares
Between Groups	2	2767.4495	1383.7248
Within Groups	26	679.3091	26.1273
Total	28	3446.7586	

Figure 8.21 SPSS/PC one-way ANOVA output for weight distribution percentage

Source	D.F.	Sum of Squares	Mean Squares
Between Groups	3	1446.0335	482.0112
Within Groups	64	258.2341	4.0349
Total	67	1704.2676	

TABLE 8.14 SQUARE-ROOT CALCIUM (SQUARE-ROOT mM/l) AT ADMISSION FOR PATIENTS WITH MULTIPLE MYELOMA AND RENAL FAILURE WITH SAMPLE MEANS AND STANDARD DEVIATIONS

Completely Reversible RF	Partially Reversible RF	Nonreversible RF With Dialysis	Nonreversible RF Without Dialysis
1.64	1.58	1.55	1.75
1.55	1.73	1.82	1.57
1.92	2.02	1.42	1.58
1.58	1.70	1.75	1.45
1.87	1.58	1.69	1.64
1.61	1.61	1.54	1.60
1.76	1.41	1.47	1.59
1.71 ± 0.15	1.53	1.87	1.56
	1.55	1.64 ± 0.17	1.55
	1.64 ± 0.17		1.59 ± 0.08

```
                           Sum of      Mean
      Source        D.F.   Squares    Squares

Between Groups        3     .0552      .0184

Within Groups        29     .6135      .0212

Total                32     .6688
```

Figure 8.22 SPSS/PC one-way ANOVA output for square-root calcium

severe renal failure (RF).[18] Table 8.14 shows the square roots of these calcium levels. (The data were transformed by taking square roots in order to reduce skewness and obtain more similar variances.) Patients were classified into four groups according to RF outcome: seven patients with completely reversible RF, nine patients with partially reversible RF, eight patients with nonreversible RF who had to undergo chronic dialysis, and nine patients with nonreversible RF who did not undergo chronic dialysis. Do the data provide evidence that some of the population square-root calcium means at admission for different RF outcomes are different? Use a 0.10 significance level for testing the hypothesis of equal population means and a 90% overall confidence level for multiple comparisons.

13. A study examined respiratory muscle function in patients with unilateral diaphragmatic paralysis (UDP).[19] Table 8.15 shows the maximal inspiratory pressure (PI_{max}) for three groups of subjects: eight patients with UDP, seven patients with UDP and cardiopulmonary disease, and 11 normal subjects. Do the data provide evidence that some of the population PI_{max} means for different group classifications are different? Use a 0.01 significance level for testing the hypothesis of equal population means and a 95% overall confidence level for multiple comparisons.

14. A study evaluated the accuracy of a primer-dependent polymerase labeling index (PDP-LI) as a measure of the proliferative activity of human solid

TABLE 8.15 PI_{max} (cm H_2O) WITH SAMPLE MEANS AND STANDARD DEVIATIONS

UDP Only	UDP and Cardiopulmonary Disease	Normal	
99	44	116	161
64	70	140	116
82	40	140	152
66	27	70	140
59	37	116	124
66	18	123	
43	37	127.1 ± 24.3	
92	39.0 ± 16.2		
71.4 ± 18.4			

tumors.[20] Table 8.16 shows the logarithms of the PDP-LI values for 16 patients with metastatic breast carcinoma, 25 patients with nonmetastatic breast carcinoma, 13 patients with epithelial carcinoma of the ovary, and eight patients with head and neck squamous-cell carcinoma. (The data were transformed by taking logarithms in order to reduce skewness and obtain more similar variances.) The higher the log PDP-LI value, the greater the proliferative activity. Do the data provide evidence that some of the population log PDP-LI means for different tumor types are different? Use a 0.05 significance level for testing the hypothesis of equal population means and a 90% overall confidence level for multiple comparisons. If the hypothesis of equal population means is rejected, assume that the only comparisons of interest are nonmetastatic breast carcinoma versus metastatic breast carcinoma, nonmetastatic breast carcinoma versus ovarian carcinoma, head and neck carcinoma versus metastatic breast carcinoma, and head and neck carcinoma versus ovarian carcinoma. Also assume that these comparisons were selected before examining the sample means.

15. A study evaluated the effectiveness of cimetidine as a preoperative medication in decreasing the volume of gastric contents in obese patients.[21] Table 8.17 shows the square-root gastric volume for three groups of patients: 20 patients given 300 mg cimetidine orally every six hours starting at 6:00 p.m. the evening before surgery; 19 patients given 300 mg cimetidine orally every six hours starting at

12:00 a.m. the night before surgery; and 22 patients given a placebo capsule orally every six hours starting at 12:00 a.m. the night before surgery. (The data were transformed by taking square roots in order to reduce skewness and obtain more similar variances.) Do the data provide evidence that some of the population square-root gastric volume means for different drug regimens are different? Use a 0.01 significance level for testing the hypothesis of equal population means and a 90% multiple-comparison overall confidence level.

16. A study investigated the relationship between sulphoxidation capacity and sodium aurothiomalate (SA) toxicity in patients with rheumatoid arthritis (RA).[22] Table 8.18 shows the sulphoxidation score for three groups of RA patients: 24 patients without major adverse reactions to SA, 11 patients with major adverse renal reactions to SA,

Source	D.F.	Sum of Squares	Mean Squares
Between Groups	2	35745.8313	17872.9156
Within Groups	23	9876.7841	429.4254
Total	25	45622.6154	

Figure 8.23 SPSS/PC one-way ANOVA output for PI_{max}

TABLE 8.16   LOGARITHM OF PDP-LI WITH SAMPLE MEANS AND STANDARD DEVIATIONS

Metastatic Breast Carcinoma		Nonmetastatic Breast Carcinoma			Ovarian Carcinoma		Head and Neck Carcinoma
2.09	2.22	0.69	1.16	1.61	1.77	2.09	2.58
0.53	1.50	1.10	1.39	1.76	1.53	2.67	0.34
0.69	1.77	−0.22	0.69	2.42	2.34	1.10	1.74
2.04	3.13	1.39	1.76	2.08	2.58	1.61	1.99
2.56	2.83	1.41	0.69	1.84	2.46		1.36
3.11	0.26	1.25	0.00	2.82	1.87		1.65
1.50	1.39	1.57	1.76	1.34	3.02		1.99
2.26		1.34	1.44		2.35		2.35
1.97		1.70	2.01		3.66		1.75 ± 0.69
1.87 ± 0.86		1.40 ± 0.67			2.23 ± 0.68		

Source	D.F.	Sum of Squares	Mean Squares
Between Groups	3	6.3431	2.1144
Within Groups	58	30.9443	.5335
Total	61	37.2874	

Figure 8.24 SPSS/PC one-way ANOVA output for log PDP-LI

**TABLE 8.17 SQUARE-ROOT GASTRIC VOLUME (SQUARE-ROOT ml)
FOR PATIENTS GIVEN CIMETIDINE OR PLACEBO
WITH SAMPLE MEANS AND STANDARD DEVIATIONS**

Cimetidine Starting at 6 p.m.		Cimetidine Starting at 12 a.m.		Placebo	
6.63	3.87	8.66	1.73	3.87	3.00
2.83	3.32	4.00	6.32	1.41	5.74
3.00	7.28	2.24	2.24	3.61	3.61
2.00	3.61	3.32	2.83	4.12	5.66
6.00	3.00	3.00	7.81	0.00	3.16
5.00	3.16	6.32	2.24	4.36	5.29
5.10	0.00	6.86	4.47	5.29	2.24
2.83	6.93	5.83	2.45	5.83	2.24
3.16	3.16	3.46		3.16	4.24
0.00		4.24		1.73	3.32
2.00		3.00		7.35	3.00
3.64 ± 2.02		4.26 ± 2.09		3.74 ± 1.70	

Source	D.F.	Sum of Squares	Mean Squares
Between Groups	2	4.3586	2.1793
Within Groups	58	216.5746	3.7340
Total	60	220.9332	

Figure 8.25 SPSS/PC one-way ANOVA output for square-root gastric volume

**TABLE 8.18 SULPHOXIDATION SCORE FOR RA
PATIENTS WITH SAMPLE MEANS AND STANDARD
DEVIATIONS**

No Major Adverse Reactions		Major Adverse Renal Reactions	Major Adverse Dermatological Reactions
0.00	0.43	0.83	1.32
0.73	0.77	1.12	1.66
0.77	0.80	1.60	1.68
0.43	1.11	1.64	0.83
1.26	0.83	2.03	1.60
1.01	1.01	2.04	1.68
1.11	1.16	0.83	1.68
1.16	1.20	1.37	1.76
0.91	1.30	1.62	
1.33	1.35	1.76	1.52 ± 0.31
1.58	1.71	2.04	
1.96	2.06		
		1.54 ± 0.45	
1.08 ± 0.47			

and eight patients with major adverse dermatological reactions to SA. (This score is the square root of the logarithm of the sulphoxidation index score reported in the study. The data were transformed in this way to reduce skewness and obtain more similar variances.) The higher the score, the *worse* the sulphoxidation capacity. Do the data provide evidence that some of the population sulphoxidation score means for different reaction groups are different? Use a 0.05 significance level for testing the hypothesis of equal population means and a 90% overall confidence level for multiple comparisons.

17. A study examined factors related to the pharmacokinetics of valproic acid (VPA) in epileptics.[23] Table 8.19 shows the square root of the VPA clearance for four groups of children with seizure disorders: 13 children taking no concurrent anticonvulsants, seven children taking phenytoin, six children taking phenobarbital, and 12 children taking

Source	D.F.	Sum of Squares	Mean Squares
Between Groups	2	2.1395	1.0698
Within Groups	40	7.8361	.1959
Total	42	9.9756	

Figure 8.26 SPSS/PC one-way ANOVA output for sulphoxidation score

**TABLE 8.19   SQUARE-ROOT VPA CLEARANCE (SQUARE-ROOT ml/min/kg)
FOR CHILDREN WITH SEIZURE DISORDERS
WITH SAMPLE MEANS AND STANDARD DEVIATIONS**

No Concurrent Anticonvulsants		Phenytoin	Phenobarbital	Phenytoin and Phenobarbital	
0.47	0.44	0.62	0.86	0.57	0.73
0.41	0.51	0.53	0.60	0.65	0.62
0.64	0.53	0.54	0.55	0.42	0.71
0.45	0.51	0.41	0.65	0.64	0.82
0.41	0.69	0.56	0.84	0.82	0.73
0.37	0.62	0.52	0.94	0.65	
0.61		0.58		0.72	
0.51 ± 0.10		0.54 ± 0.07	0.74 ± 0.16	0.67 ± 0.11	

Figure 8.27 SPSS/PC one-way ANOVA output for square-root VPA clearance

Source	D.F.	Sum of Squares	Mean Squares
Between Groups	3	.3092	.1031
Within Groups	34	.4101	.0121
Total	37	.7193	

phenytoin and phenobarbital. (The data were transformed by taking square roots in order to reduce skewness and obtain more similar variances.) Do the data provide evidence that some of the population square-root VPA clearance means for different drugs are different? Use a 0.01 significance level for testing the hypothesis of equal population means and a 95% overall confidence level for multiple comparisons. If the hypothesis of equal population means is rejected, assume that the only comparisons of interest are those between the children taking no concurrent anticonvulsants and the other groups of children. Also assume that these comparisons were selected before examining the sample means.

18. Find an article in a medical or health care journal in which one-way ANOVA was incorrectly used to analyze nonindependent or extremely nonnormal data. Photocopy the article and write a letter to the journal editor that clearly describes the statistical error.

REFERENCES

1. Anous MM, Heimbach DM: Causes of death and predictors in burned patients more than 60 years of age. J Trauma 26:135–139, 1986.
2. Scariano SM, Davenport JM: The effects of violations of independence assumptions in the one-way ANOVA. Am Statistician 41:123–129, 1987.
3. Neter J, Wasserman W, Kutner MH: Applied Linear Statistical Models: Regression, Analysis of Variance, and Experimental Designs. 2nd ed. Homewood: Irwin, 1985.
4. Kong C, Lay C, Tsai Y, et al: The hemodynamic effect of verapamil on portal hypertension in patients with postnecrotic cirrhosis. Hepatology 6:423–426, 1986.
5. Mickus D: Activities of daily living in women after myocardial infarction. Heart Lung 15:376–381, 1986.
6. Winer BJ: Statistical Principles in Experimental Design. 2nd ed. New York: McGraw-Hill, 1971.
7. Moore GB, Ciresi S, Kallar S: The effect of Innovar versus droperidol or fentanyl on the duration of action of succinylcholine. AANA J 54:130–136, 1986.
8. Center SA, Smith CA, Wilkinson E, et al: Clinicopathologic, renal immunofluorescent, and light microscopic features of glomerulonephritis in the dog: 41 cases (1975–1985). J Am Vet Med Assoc 190:81–90, 1987.
9. Nakai Y, Kinoshita F, Koh T, et al: Taste function in patients with anorexia nervosa and bulimia nervosa. Int J Eating Disord 6:257–265, 1987.
10. Stejskal VDM, Olin RG, Forsbeck M: The lymphocyte transformation test for diagnosis of drug-induced occupational allergy. J Allergy Clin Immunol 77:411–426, 1986.
11. Fletcher EC, Schaaf JW, Miller J, et al: Long-term cardiopulmonary sequelae in patients with sleep apnea and chronic lung disease. Am Rev Respir Dis 135:525–533, 1987.
12. Zaghloul I, Ptachcinski RJ, Burckart GJ, et al: Blood protein binding of cyclosporine in transplant patients. J Clin Pharmacol 27:240–242, 1987.
13. Johnson P.E, Arevedo DJ, Kleburtz KD: Variation in individual physicians' prescribing. J Ambul Care Manag 9:25–37, 1986.

14. Adams R, Johnson B: Acuity and staffing under prospective payment. J Nurs Admin *16*:21–25, 1986.

15. Bamrah JS, Kumar V, Krska J, et al: Interactions between procyclidine and neuroleptic drugs. Some pharmacological and clinical aspects. Br J Psychiatry *149*:726–733, 1986.

16. Gwinup G: Weight loss without dietary restriction: Efficacy of different forms of aerobic exercise. Am J Sports Med *15*:275–279, 1987.

17. Budsberg SC, Verstraete MC, Soutas-Little RW: Force plate analysis of the walking gait in healthy dogs. Am J Vet Res *48*:915–918, 1987.

18. Rota S, Mougenot B, Baudouin B, et al: Multiple myeloma and severe renal failure: A clinicopathologic study of outcome and prognosis in 34 patients. Medicine *66*:126–137, 1987.

19. Lisboa C, Pare PD, Pertuze J, et al: Inspiratory muscle function in unilateral diaphragmatic paralysis. Am Rev Respir Dis *134*:488–492, 1986.

20. Alama A, Conte PF, Di Marco E, et al: Proliferative activity of human solid tumors evaluated by thymidine labeling index and primer-dependent α-DNA polymerase. Oncology *43*:385–389, 1986.

21. Stull DL, Zinn M, Fales JT, et al: The effectiveness of cimetidine as a preoperative medication in increasing gastric pH and decreasing gastric volume in obese patients. AANA J *51*:385–394, 1983.

22. Ayesh R, Mitchell SC, Waring RH, et al: Sodium aurothiomalate toxicity and sulphoxidation capacity in rheumatoid arthritic patients. Br J Rheumatol *26*:197–201, 1987.

23. Hall K, Otten N, Johnston B, et al: A multivariable analysis of factors governing the steady-state pharmacokinetics of valproic acid in 52 young epileptics. J Clin Pharmacol *25*:261–268, 1985.

ONE-FACTOR
REPEATED-MEASURES
ANALYSIS OF VARIANCE

CHAPTER OBJECTIVES

After studying this chapter and working the problems,
you should be able to:

1. Explain how univariate one-factor repeated-measures analysis-of-variance results are calculated

2. Determine whether the univariate approach to one-factor repeated-measures analysis of variance is appropriate

3. Interpret univariate, multivariate, and adjusted univariate results for one-factor repeated-measures analysis of variance

4. Recognize data that violate assumptions required for one-factor repeated-measures analysis of variance

5. Interpret SPSS and SAS one-factor repeated-measures analysis-of-variance output

6. Calculate and interpret paired Bonferroni confidence intervals for one-factor repeated-measures analysis of variance

Repeated measurements are often obtained in medical and health care research. AIDS patients may be followed over time to determine changes in hematological components. Subjects may be given different doses of a drug at different times in order to evaluate the effect of dose. Multiple sclerosis patients may be studied for several years to determine changes in self-sufficiency. Because repeated measurements are not independent, one-way analysis of variance (ANOVA) cannot be used to test the hypothesis that three or more population means are equal. Instead, repeated-measures analysis of variance should be considered for testing this hypothesis. In this chapter, we will describe methods for analyzing repeated-measures designs with one *factor*.

A factor is a characteristic used to classify observations into different groups. For the burn data in Chapter 8, the factor is the survival outcome, since survival outcome is used to classify patients into three different groups. Other examples of factors include race, length of hospital stay, type of surgery, stage of illness, location of tumor, and weeks of treatment. The *levels* of a factor are the possible categories of the factor. The survival outcome factor in Chapter 8 has three levels: 1 = death within three days, 2 = death within five to 48 days, and 3 = survival. We often evaluate the effects of a factor by testing the hypothesis that the means of the populations corresponding to different factor levels are equal. When the data consist of samples of repeated measurements, repeated-measures ANOVA is frequently appropriate for testing this hypothesis.

Why are repeated measurements obtained? Convenience is often a reason and not always a good one. When repeated measurements are obtained, fewer subjects are needed. But the primary advantage of repeated measurements is a possible increase in precision. The responses of different subjects to the same treatment can be quite dissimilar. Use of repeated measurements allows us to separate out the variability attributable to differences among subjects. This may reduce the error variability, resulting in more precise estimates of factor effects.

Repeated-measures designs can have serious drawbacks, all involving the interference of previous treatments with the effects of later treatments. *Carryover effects* occur when a new treatment is given while the effects of previous treatments are still present. For example, subjects may be given a second anesthetic before fully recovering from the first anesthetic. Long recovery times after the second anesthetic may be due to carryover effects from the first anesthetic. Failure to realize this will lead to the mistaken conclusion that the second anesthetic has long recovery times. *Latent effects* arise when the effects of previous treatments appear to have worn off but are activated when later treatments are given. For example, a dog may show no obvious effects from a megadose dexamethasone suppression test done three weeks earlier, but the previous testing may affect later adrenal-function tests.

Learning effects occur when the mere repetition of a treatment or activity changes subjects' responses. Patients may become accustomed to a medical procedure or intolerant of it after undergoing the procedure several times. For example, patients may become increasingly nauseated during successive chemotherapy sessions because of nausea experienced during previous chemotherapy.

Two steps should be taken to minimize the risk of treatment interference when repeated measurements are obtained. First, sufficient time should elapse between treatments to ensure that the chance of carryover effects is small. Second, the order in which treatments are given should be determined by randomization for each subject, so that some subjects receive treatments in different orders. If these steps cannot be carried out, or substantial interference between treatments is expected, the risk of confounded effects is quite high. In this case, repeated measurements should not be obtained.

9.1 HYPOTHESIS TESTS

A study with repeated measurements investigated the effect of acebutolol and propranolol therapy for ventricular arrhythmias.[1] Patients with frequent premature ventricular contractions (PVCs) were given either propranolol or acebutolol for several weeks, then switched to the other drug after a one-week placebo washout period. Table 9.1 shows the heart rates for nine of these patients during the no-drug, placebo, and drug periods. Because heart rates for the same patient cannot be considered independent, one-way ANOVA cannot be used to test the null hypothesis that the four population heart rate means are equal:

$$H_0: \mu_1 = \mu_2 = \mu_3 = \mu_4 \qquad (9.1)$$

One-factor repeated-measures ANOVA will be used instead to test this hypothesis.

TABLE 9.1 BASELINE AND TREATMENT HEART RATE FOR PATIENTS WITH FREQUENT PREMATURE VENTRICULAR CONTRACTIONS

Patient No.	Drug			
	NONE (BASELINE)	PROPRANOLOL	PLACEBO	ACEBUTOLOL
1	94	67	90	67
2	57	52	69	55
3	81	74	69	73
4	82	59	71	72
5	67	65	74	72
6	78	72	80	72
7	87	75	106	74
8	82	68	76	59
9	90	74	82	80
Mean ± SD	79.8 ± 11.5	67.3 ± 7.7	79.7 ± 12.0	69.3 ± 7.8

In general, we often want to test the null hypothesis that three or more population means are equal:

$$H_0: \mu_1 = \mu_2 = \mu_3 = \cdots = \mu_k \qquad (9.2)$$

If one-factor repeated-measures ANOVA is appropriate for testing this hypothesis, all of the population means μ_i are based on observations from the same population of subjects. The alternative hypothesis is

$$H_A: \text{At least one population mean does} \atop \text{not equal another population mean} \qquad (9.3)$$

If we reject the null hypothesis (9.2), we cannot conclude that all of the population means are different. Multiple comparisons must be done to determine which population means are different. A method for obtaining multiple comparisons is described in Section 9.3.

There are several methods for testing the null hypothesis (9.2): the *univariate approach*, the *multivariate approach*, and the *adjusted univariate approaches*. The univariate and adjusted univariate approaches are based on sums of squares involving sample means and standard deviations. Calculation of these sums of squares can be done with a calculator. The multivariate approach is not carried out with a calculator; it requires a computer and a statistical software package.

All of these approaches are based on the assumption that the repeated measurements come from a multivariate normal distribution.* When the univariate approach is used, additional assumptions concerning variances and covariances are also required.† These variance-covariance assumptions involve matrix algebra and will not be described here. Further information can be found in other texts.[3] If the variance-covariance assumptions hold, the univariate approach should be used. When the assumptions of the univariate approach hold, the univariate approach is usually more powerful than the multivariate approach and always more powerful than the adjusted univariate approach. If the variance-

covariance assumptions do not hold, the univariate approach cannot be used. The multivariate approach or an adjusted univariate approach must be used instead.

To determine whether the univariate approach should be used, we use a statistical test called *Mauchly's test of sphericity*. This is a test of the hypothesis that the variance-covariance assumptions needed for the univariate approach are met. Mauchly's test is not calculated by hand. Instead, it can be obtained from SPSS or SAS software. *If the p-value for Mauchly's test is greater than or equal to the significance level α selected by the researcher, the univariate approach can be used. If the p-value is less than α, the multivariate approach or an adjusted univariate approach should be used.* Because Mauchly's test is not very powerful when the sample size is small, a large significance level (such as 0.10) is appropriate when the test is used for small samples.

Figure 9.1 shows the results of Mauchly's test of sphericity for the heart-rate data. The p-value, listed after "Significance = ," is 0.589. Since this p-value is greater than any reasonable significance level, we should use the univariate approach to test the hypothesis of equal population means.

Because we have not described the calculation of Mauchly's test, this test may seem rather mysterious. Unfortunately, nothing can be done to dispel the mystery unless you are well acquainted with matrix algebra. The formula for Mauchly's test involves esoteric functions of matrices that would make no sense at all to most readers of this text.* The *use* of Mauchly's test is straightforward, however. A *nonsignificant p*-value for Mauchly's test indicates that the univariate approach should be used. A *significant p*-value for Mauchly's test indicates that the univariate approach cannot be used and that the multivariate approach or an adjusted univariate approach must be used instead. The formula for Mauchly's test can be found in other texts.[2]

Like one-way ANOVA, univariate one-factor repeated-measures ANOVA requires the calculation of sample means, which we will call *factor means*. The sample factor mean for factor level i, denoted by $\bar{x}_i$, is the mean of all the observations for factor level i. The sample factor mean $\bar{x}_i$ is the sample estimate of the population factor mean μ_i for factor level i. For the heart-rate data, the factor of interest

---

*The assumption of multivariate normality implies that the observations for each factor level have a normal distribution. We will not describe this assumption further, since a complete definition involves matrix algebra. Further information about multivariate normality can be found in other texts.[2]

†The covariance of two random variables is a measure of the degree to which they are associated in a linear way.

---

*A concise introduction to matrix algebra is provided by Strang.[4]

Figure 9.1 SPSS/PC output for Mauchly's test of sphericity for heart-rate data

```
Mauchly sphericity test, W =        .57398
Chi-square approx. =              3.73187 with 5 D. F.
Significance =                      .589
```

is drug, with four levels: 1 = no drug, 2 = propranolol, 3 = placebo, and 4 = acebutolol. The sample factor means for these data can be obtained from Table 9.1.

$$\text{no drug mean } \bar{x}_1 = 79.8$$

$$\text{propranolol mean } \bar{x}_2 = 67.3$$

$$\text{placebo mean } \bar{x}_3 = 79.7$$

$$\text{acebutolol mean } \bar{x}_4 = 69.3$$

An *overall mean* (also called the *grand mean*) and an *overall standard deviation* are also calculated. These are the mean and standard deviation of all the observations and are denoted by $\bar{x}$ and s. For the heart-rate data, the overall mean and standard deviation are

$$\bar{x} = 74.0 \qquad s = 11.2$$

The *overall variance* is the square of the overall standard deviation.

Subject means and *subject standard deviations* must also be obtained. The mean and standard deviation for a subject are the mean and standard deviation of all the observations for that subject. We will denote the mean and standard deviation for the jth subject by $\bar{x}_{\text{subject}j}$ and $s_{\text{subject}j}$. For the first patient in the drug study, the subject mean and subject standard deviation are

$$\bar{x}_{\text{subject}1} = \frac{(94 + 67 + 90 + 67)}{4} = 79.5$$

$$s_{\text{subject}1} = 14.5$$

For the second subject, the subject mean and subject standard deviation are

$$\bar{x}_{\text{subject}2} = \frac{(57 + 52 + 69 + 55)}{4} = 58.2$$

$$s_{\text{subject}2} = 7.5$$

The *subject variance* is the square of the subject standard deviation. Table 9.2 shows the subject means and subject standard deviations for the heart-rate data.

TABLE 9.2 SUBJECT MEANS AND SUBJECT STANDARD DEVIATIONS FOR HEART-RATE DATA

Patient No.	$\bar{x}_{\text{subject}j}$	$s_{\text{subject}j}$
1	79.5	14.5
2	58.2	7.5
3	74.2	5.0
4	71.0	9.4
5	69.5	4.2
6	75.5	4.1
7	85.5	14.9
8	71.2	10.0
9	81.5	6.6

After the means and standard deviations have been obtained, sums of squares are calculated. Let n denote the number of subjects and let k denote the number of factor levels. The total number of observations is $n \times k$. For the heart-rate data, $n = 9$ and $k = 4$, for a total of $9 \times 4 = 36$ observations. The following sums of squares, degrees of freedom, and mean squares are calculated in univariate one-factor repeated-measures ANOVA.

Total Sum of Squares (SST). This quantity is calculated according to the formula

$$\text{SST} = [(nk) - 1]s^2 \qquad (9.4)$$

Factor Sum of Squares (SSF). This quantity is calculated according to the formula

$$\text{SSF} = n \times \sum_{i=1}^{k} (\bar{x}_i - \bar{x})^2 \qquad (9.5)$$

We can translate this formula into steps for calculation.

STEP 1.   Calculate each sample factor mean and the overall mean.

STEP 2.   Subtract the overall mean from each sample factor mean to get k differences.

STEP 3.   Square each of the differences obtained in step 2.

STEP 4.   Add all of the squared differences obtained in step 3.

STEP 5.   Multiply the sum of the squared differences obtained in step 4 by n.

Between-Subjects Sum of Squares (SSBS). This quantity is calculated according to the formula

$$\text{SSBS} = k \times \sum_{j=1}^{n} (\bar{x}_{\text{subject}j} - \bar{x})^2 \qquad (9.6)$$

We can translate this formula into steps for calculation.

STEP 1.   Calculate each subject mean and the overall mean.

STEP 2.   Subtract the overall mean from each subject mean to get n differences.

STEP 3.   Square each of the differences obtained in step 2.

STEP 4.   Add all of the squared differences obtained in step 3.

STEP 5.   Multiply the sum of the squared differences obtained in step 4 by k.

Within-Subjects Sum of Squares (SSWS). This quantity is calculated according to the formula

$$\text{SSWS} = (k - 1) \times \sum_{j=1}^{n} s_{\text{subject}j}^2 \qquad (9.7)$$

We can translate this formula into steps for calculation.

Source	Degrees of Freedom	Sum of Squares	Mean Square
Between subjects	$n - 1$	SSBS	MSBS
Within subjects	$n(k - 1)$	SSWS	MSWS
Factor	$k - 1$	SSF	MSF
Error	$(n - 1)(k - 1)$	SSE	MSE
Total	$(nk) - 1$	SST	

Figure 9.2 Univariate one-factor repeated-measures analysis of variance table

STEP 1. Calculate all of the subject variances.

STEP 2. Add all of the subject variances.

STEP 3. Multiply the sum of the subject variances obtained in step 2 by $k - 1$.

Error Sum of Squares (SSE). This quantity can be calculated by subtraction according to the formula

$$SSE = SST - SSF - SSBS \qquad (9.8)$$

Total Degrees of Freedom. This is $(nk) - 1$.

Factor Degrees of Freedom. This is $k - 1$.

Between-Subjects Degrees of Freedom. This is $n - 1$.

Within-Subjects Degrees of Freedom. This is $n(k - 1)$.

Error Degrees of Freedom. This is $(n - 1) \times (k - 1)$.

Factor Mean Square (MSF). This is the factor sum of squares divided by the factor degrees of freedom:*

$$MSF = \frac{SSF}{k - 1} \qquad (9.9)$$

Between-Subjects Mean Square (MSBS). This is the between-subjects sum of squares divided by the between-subjects degrees of freedom:

$$MSBS = \frac{SSBS}{n - 1} \qquad (9.10)$$

Within-Subjects Mean Square (MSWS). This is the within-subjects sum of squares divided by the within-subjects degrees of freedom:

$$MSWS = \frac{SSWS}{n(k - 1)} \qquad (9.11)$$

Error Mean Square (MSE). This is the error sum of squares divided by the error degrees of freedom:*

$$MSE = \frac{SSE}{(n - 1)(k - 1)} \qquad (9.12)$$

The sums of squares, degrees of freedom, and mean squares are usually presented in a one-factor repeated-measures analysis of variance table, which has the format shown in Figure 9.2. An F statistic is used to test the null hypothesis (9.2) and is calculated according to the formula

$$F = \frac{MSF}{MSE} \qquad (9.13)$$

If the null hypothesis (9.2) is true and the assumptions of the univariate approach are met, the F statistic (9.13) has an F distribution with $k - 1$ numerator degrees of freedom and $(n - 1)(k - 1)$ denominator degrees of freedom. The numerator degrees of freedom are the factor degrees of freedom and the denominator degrees of freedom are the error degrees of freedom. These degrees of freedom can be obtained from the repeated-measures ANOVA table.

The p-value for the F statistic is

$$P(F \text{ statistic} \geq F_{calc})$$

where F_{calc} is the calculated value of the F statistic. We reject the null hypothesis (9.2) if the calculated F statistic is so large that its p-value is less than the significance level α chosen by the researcher before carrying out the analysis. If the p-value is greater than or equal to α, we cannot reject the null hypothesis (9.2). Approximate p-values for F statistics can be obtained from Table E.5, as described in Chapter 8. The p-value is interpreted in the usual way: it is the probability of getting an F statistic at least as extreme as the calculated F statistic if the null hypothesis (9.2) is true.

---

*The factor mean square is also called the *treatment mean square* and the factor sum of squares is also called the *treatment sum of squares*.

*The error mean square is also called the *residual mean square* and the error sum of squares is also called the *residual sum of squares*.

Univariate one-factor repeated-measures ANOVA is based on the following assumptions.

1. Random Sample of Subjects. If the sample is not biased, random sampling is not crucial.

2. Repeated Measurements on a Group of Subjects. One-factor repeated-measures ANOVA cannot be done if repeated measurements are not obtained.

3. Independence of Observations Within Each Factor Level. All of the observations within factor level 1 must be independent, all of the observations within factor level 2 must be independent, and so on. The observations for *different* factor levels are not necessarily independent, since repeated measurements were obtained. If this assumption is violated, one-factor repeated-measures ANOVA cannot be done.

4. Multivariate Normality. Multivariate normality implies that the observations for each factor level come from normal populations. This assumption can be checked in part by examining histograms of the observations for each factor level. If the histograms suggest nonnormal populations, the assumption of multivariate normality may not be reasonable for the data. If the histograms are consistent with normal populations, multivariate normality may or may not hold. Repeated-measures ANOVA can be done when the data have an approximate multivariate normal distribution if the sample is large enough. Repeated-measures ANOVA cannot be done when any of the populations are extremely nonnormal (e.g., when the data have only a few possible values). Consult a statistician if you are not sure whether your sample is large enough to compensate for nonnormality.

5. Variance-Covariance Assumptions. If the p-value for Mauchly's test is less than the significance level α, we cannot assume that the variance-covariance assumptions needed for the univariate approach are reasonable for the data. If the p-value for Mauchly's test is greater than or equal to α, we assume that the variance-covariance assumptions are reasonable for the data.

Let us evaluate these assumptions for the heart-rate data. The sample of patients is not random, but this is not important. Repeated measurements were obviously obtained. The observations within any drug period are based on different patients and appear to be independent. Quick histograms of the observations for the four drug periods are shown in Figures 9.3 through 9.6. Although the histogram of the acebutolol heart rate is consistent with sampling from a normal population, the other histograms suggest skewed populations. The sample size is large enough to compensate for moderately skewed populations, however. Mauchly's test (Figure 9.1) indicates that the variance-covariance assumptions needed for the univariate approach are satisfied.

```
55 – 64  |X
65 – 74  |X
75 – 84  |XXXX
85 – 94  |XXX
```

Figure 9.3 Quick histogram of no-drug heart rate

```
50 – 57  |X
58 – 65  |XX
66 – 73  |XXX
74 – 81  |XXX
```

Figure 9.4 Quick histogram of propranolol heart rate

We will carry out a univariate one-factor repeated-measures ANOVA with a 0.01 significance level.

The sums of squares for the heart rates are calculated as follows, using the means and standard deviations on p. 170 and in Table 9.2.

$$\text{SST} = [(9 \times 4) - 1] \times (11.2)^2 = 4390.4$$

$$\text{SSF} = 9 \times [(79.8 - 74.0)^2 + (67.3 - 74.0)^2$$
$$+ (79.7 - 74.0)^2 + (69.3 - 74.0)^2]$$
$$= 9 \times 133.1 = 1197.9$$

$$\text{SSBS} = 4 \times [(79.5 - 74.0)^2 + (58.2 - 74.0)^2$$
$$+ \cdots + (81.5 - 74.0)^2]$$
$$= 4 \times 507.8 = 2031.2$$

$$\text{SSWS} = (4 - 1) \times [(14.5)^2 + (7.5)^2 + \cdots + (6.6)^2]$$
$$= 3 \times 779.9 = 2339.7$$

$$\text{SSE} = 4390.4 - 1197.9 - 2031.2 = 1161.3$$

Total df = $(9 \times 4) - 1 = 35$

Factor df = $4 - 1 = 3$

Between-subjects df = $9 - 1 = 8$

Within-subjects df = $9(4 - 1) = 27$

Error df = $(9 - 1)(4 - 1) = 24$

$$\text{MSF} = \frac{1197.9}{3} = 399.3$$

$$\text{MSBS} = \frac{2031.2}{8} = 253.9$$

$$\text{MSWS} = \frac{2339.7}{27} = 86.7$$

$$\text{MSE} = \frac{1161.3}{24} = 48.4$$

```
61 – 70 | XX
71 – 80 | XXXX
81 – 90 | XX
91 – 100 |
101 – 110 | X
```

Figure 9.5   Quick histogram of placebo heart rate

```
55 – 63 | XX
64 – 72 | XXXX
73 – 81 | XXX
```

Figure 9.6   Quick histogram of acebutolol heart rate

The results of these calculations are displayed in the one-factor repeated-measures ANOVA table shown in Table 9.3. The calculated F statistic is

$$F = \frac{399.3}{48.4} = 8.25$$

From Table 9.3, we see that this F statistic has 3 and 24 df. We can use Table E.5 to find an approximate p-value for our F statistic:

$$p\text{-value} < 0.001$$

We reject the hypothesis that all of the four population means are equal at the 0.01 significance level and conclude that at least one population mean

TABLE 9.3   UNIVARIATE ONE-FACTOR REPEATED-MEASURES ANOVA TABLE FOR HEART-RATE DATA

Source	Degrees of Freedom	Sum of Squares	Mean Square
Between subjects	8	2031.2	253.9
Within subjects	27	2339.7	86.7
Drug factor	3	1197.9	399.3
Error	24	1161.3	48.4
Total	35	4390.4	

does not equal another population mean. Without appropriate multiple comparisons (described in Section 9.3), we cannot determine which population means are different.

Suppose we had mistakenly analyzed the heart-rate data with one-way ANOVA, an inappropriate procedure because of the non-independent samples. Would this error affect our conclusions? Figure 9.7 shows the one-way ANOVA results for the heart-rate data. The p-value given for testing the null hypothesis (9.1) is 0.0162. This p-value is much larger than the repeated-measures p-value, which is less than 0.001. If we use one-way ANOVA to analyze the heart-rate data, we cannot reject the null hypothesis (9.1) at the 0.01 significance level. If we use one-factor repeated-measures ANOVA to analyze the data, we can reject this hypothesis at the 0.01 significance level. The incorrect statistical results are quite different from the correct statistical results, as is often the case when the wrong procedure is used.

Let us consider data that cannot be analyzed with the univariate approach. Table 9.4 shows the square root of the serum ALT before, during, and after spontaneous reactivation of chronic hepatitis B for eight patients.[5] The data were transformed by taking square roots in order to reduce skewness. We would like to use repeated-measures ANOVA to test the null hypothesis that the population baseline, reactivation, and resolution population square-root ALT means are equal:

$$H_0: \mu_1 = \mu_2 = \mu_3$$

The factor of interest is disease state, with three levels: 1 = before reactivation, 2 = reactivation, 3 = resolution. Mauchly's test of sphericity for these data, shown in Figure 9.8, has a p-value less than or equal to 0.0005. We reject the hypothesis that the univariate variance-covariance assumptions are met at any reasonable significance level and conclude that the univariate approach cannot be used to analyze the square-root ALT data. The multivariate approach or an adjusted univariate approach must be used. We will use a 0.05 significance level for our multivariate and adjusted univariate analyses.

The multivariate and adjusted univariate approaches to repeated-measures ANOVA are based

```
                                Sum of        Mean           F        F
         Source        D.F.     Squares       Squares       Ratio    Prob.

Between Groups           3      1185.4167     395.1389      3.9793   .0162

Within Groups           32      3177.5556      99.2986

Total                   35      4362.9722
```

Figure 9.7   SPSS/PC output for inappropriate one-way ANOVA for heart-rate data

**TABLE 9.4 SQUARE-ROOT ALT (SQUARE-ROOT UNITS/LITER)
FOR PATIENTS WITH CHRONIC ACTIVE HEPATITIS**

Patient No.	Disease State		
	BEFORE REACTIVATION	REACTIVATION	RESOLUTION
1	3.87	29.33	4.58
2	8.89	57.40	5.00
3	7.42	14.70	8.19
4	5.66	34.93	5.00
5	5.00	17.09	5.00
6	13.04	34.54	7.21
7	8.12	29.83	4.90
8	7.35	19.36	6.16
Mean ± SD	7.42 ± 2.82	29.65 ± 13.68	5.76 ± 1.31

```
Mauchly sphericity test, W =        .06540
Chi-square approx. =          16.36324 with 2 D. F.
Significance =                 .000
```

Figure 9.8 SPSS/PC output for Mauchly's test of sphericity for square-root ALT data

on the same assumptions as the univariate approach, with one important exception. The variance-covariance assumptions needed for the univariate approach are not required for the multivariate and adjusted univariate approaches. The assumptions needed for the multivariate and adjusted univariate approaches are random sampling, repeated measurements, independence of the observations within any factor level, and multivariate normality. The remarks made earlier about these assumptions (p. 172) also apply to the multivariate and adjusted univariate approaches.

Let us check these assumptions for the square-root ALT values. The subjects were not a random sample, but this is not essential. The data obviously consist of repeated measurements, and the square-root ALT values for a given disease state were obtained for different subjects and appear to be independent. Histograms of the data for the three factor levels (Figures 9.9 through 9.11) are consistent with sampling from normal or approximately normal populations. The multivariate and adjusted univariate approaches to one-factor repeated-measures ANOVA seem appropriate for these data.

How does the multivariate approach differ from the univariate approach? The multivariate approach

```
5.00 – 15.99 | X
16.00 – 26.99 | XX
27.00 – 37.99 | XXXX
38.00 – 48.99 |
49.00 – 59.99 | X
```

Figure 9.10 Quick histogram of reactivation square-root ALT

```
3.00 – 4.99 | XX
5.00 – 6.99 | XXXX
7.00 – 8.99 | XX
```

Figure 9.11 Quick histogram of resolution square-root ALT

is a more general method in which linear combinations of the differences between observations for different factor levels are analyzed. Multivariate statistics, such as Pillai's trace, Hotelling's trace, Wilks' lambda, and Roy's largest root, are used instead of F statistics to test the hypothesis that all of the population factor means are equal. We will not describe the calculation of these multivariate test statistics or the mechanics of the multivariate approach. Both topics involve rather technical aspects of matrix algebra. Further information can be found in other texts.[2, 6]

Although multivariate and univariate p-values are based on different statistics, they are used in the same way. If the multivariate p-value is less than

```
1.00 – 3.99 | X
4.00 – 6.99 | XX
7.00 – 9.99 | XXXX
10.00 – 12.99 |
13.00 – 15.99 | X
```

Figure 9.9 Quick histogram of baseline square-root ALT

```
EFFECT .. STATE
Multivariate Tests of Significance (S = 1, M = 0, N = 2 )

Test Name        Value   Approx. F Hypoth. DF   Error DF  Sig. of F

Pillais         .77021   10.05518      2.00       6.00      .012
Hotellings     3.35173   10.05518      2.00       6.00      .012
Wilks           .22979   10.05518      2.00       6.00      .012
Roys            .77021
```

Figure 9.12 SPSS/PC multivariate one-factor repeated-measures ANOVA output for square-root ALT

the significance level α, the hypothesis that all of the population factor means are equal is rejected. If the multivariate p-value is greater than or equal to α, the hypothesis of equal population means cannot be rejected. The multivariate p-value is interpreted in the usual way: it is the probability of getting a multivariate test statistic at least as extreme as the calculated multivariate test statistic if the null hypothesis (9.2) is true.

Figure 9.12 shows the SPSS/PC multivariate one-factor repeated-measures ANOVA output for the square-root ALT data. The only parts of this output that concern us are the p-values for the multivariate test statistics, listed under "Sig. of F." These p-values are all 0.012, so we reject the hypothesis of equal population factor means at the 0.05 significance level. We could not reject this hypothesis at the 0.01 significance level.

Adjusted univariate approaches can also be used when the univariate method is not appropriate. When adjusted univariate approaches are used, univariate results are obtained, but the degrees of freedom for the univariate F statistic are adjusted by making them smaller. SPSS/PC and SAS output include two numbers that can be used to adjust the degrees of freedom. The first number, called the *Greenhouse-Geisser (GG) epsilon*, tends to make the degrees of freedom too small, especially when the sample size is small. The second number, called the *Huynh-Feldt (HF) epsilon*, does not overadjust in this way.

The use of either of these adjustment epsilons is simple. Both the numerator and denominator degrees of freedom for the univariate F statistic are multiplied by the Greenhouse-Geisser epsilon or the Huynh-Feldt epsilon and then rounded off to the nearest integer. The numbers that result are the adjusted degrees of freedom for the F statistic. The adjusted univariate p-value for the univariate F statistic is based on the adjusted degrees of freedom. We will not describe methods for calculating the HF and GG epsilons. Further information is provided by Huynh and Feldt[7] and Greenhouse and Geisser.[8]

Table 9.5 shows the univariate repeated-measures F statistic, the unadjusted univariate degrees of freedom for this F statistic, and the HF and GG epsilons for the square-root ALT data. Multiplying

TABLE 9.5 UNIVARIATE REPEATED-MEASURES ANOVA *F* STATISTIC AND ADJUSTMENT EPSILONS FOR SQUARE-ROOT ALT DATA

$F = 22.64$, 2 and 14 df

Huynh-Feldt epsilon = 0.5255
Greenhouse-Geisser epsilon = 0.5169

the degrees of freedom by the HF epsilon, we get $2 \times 0.5255 = 1.05$ and $14 \times 0.5255 = 7.36$. Rounding off, we obtain 1 and 7 as the adjusted degrees of freedom. The GG epsilon also produces 1 and 7 as the adjusted degrees of freedom: $2 \times 0.5169 = 1.03$ and $14 \times 0.5169 = 7.24$. From Table E.5, the p-value for an F statistic of 22.64 with 1 and 7 df is between 0.001 and 0.005. This is the Huynh-Feldt and Greenhouse-Geisser adjusted univariate p-value for testing the null hypothesis that the three population square-root ALT means are equal. Both the Huynh-Feldt approach and the Greenhouse-Geisser approach allow us to reject this hypothesis at any significance level less than or equal to 0.005. Although the HF and GG adjusted univariate p-values are the same for the square-root ALT data, they are often different.

As the results for the square-root ALT data indicate, the adjusted univariate approaches and the multivariate approach can produce different p-values. Further discussion of the adjusted univariate approaches can be found in other texts.[2]

Example 9.1

A study evaluated the antibiotic resistance of *Streptococcus pneumoniae*, using isolates obtained from patients in a pneumococcal vaccine study.[9] Table 9.6 shows the minimal inhibitory concentrations (MICs) of various antibiotics for the 10 *S. pneumoniae* isolates that were resistant to penicillin. Can one-factor repeated-measures ANOVA be used to test the hypothesis that the population MIC means are the same for the four antibiotics?

The 10 MICs for each antibiotic type have only two or three values, suggesting extremely nonnormal distributions. The assumption of multivariate normality is not reasonable, and one-factor repeated-measures ANOVA cannot be used to test the hypothesis that all four population means are

TABLE 9.6 MINIMAL INHIBITORY CONCENTRATION (μg/ml) FOR ANTIBIOTIC-RESISTANT *S. pneumoniae*

Patient No.	Drug			
	OXACILLIN	AMPICILLIN	MEZLOCILLIN	CHLORAMPHENICOL
1	2.0	0.5	0.5	2.0
2	16.0	8.0	4.0	16.0
3	16.0	8.0	4.0	16.0
4	16.0	8.0	4.0	16.0
5	16.0	8.0	4.0	16.0
6	16.0	8.0	4.0	16.0
7	16.0	8.0	4.0	16.0
8	16.0	4.0	4.0	16.0
9	16.0	4.0	4.0	16.0
10	16.0	8.0	4.0	16.0
Mean $\pm$ SD	14.6 $\pm$ 4.4	6.4 $\pm$ 2.7	3.6 $\pm$ 1.1	14.6 $\pm$ 4.4

TABLE 9.7 IFN-GAMMA PRODUCTION IN BLOOD CULTURES FROM TUBERCULOSIS PATIENTS

Patient No.	Mitogen		
	PHA	CON A	PWM
1	44.3	14.1	18.7
2	63.1	12.2	38.9
3	75.4	24.9	20.9
4	40.6	12.5	25.6
5	91.3	6.3	16.1
6	58.1	10.8	6.5
7	24.3	3.2	3.4
8 (8/8/84)	12.4	2.5	3.9
(10/3/84)	24.0	7.1	4.1
9	26.5	5.5	12.5
10	13.9	2.3	2.1
11	5.5	0.9	1.4
12	3.2	1.2	4.5
13	5.4	1.6	0.7
14 (8/8/84)	4.9	1.0	2.2
(1/14/85)	3.4	0.5	0.8
Mean $\pm$ SD	31.0 $\pm$ 28.2	6.7 $\pm$ 6.7	10.1 $\pm$ 11.1

Although the data consist of repeated measurements, the assumption of independence within factor levels does not hold for all of the yields. Two cultures were taken from each of two patients, resulting in two sets of nonindependent observations within each mitogen type. If only the first yield from each patient is used, the independence assumption should hold. One-factor repeated-measures ANOVA could be used to analyze the resulting 14 independent observations if the multivariate normality assumption is reasonable.

9.2 COMPUTER OUTPUT

Calculations for multivariate one-factor repeated-measures ANOVA are carried out by a computer. Even the calculations for univariate one-factor repeated-measures ANOVA are painful enough to warrant leaving them to a computer. In SPSS, repeated-measures ANOVA calculations are done by the MANOVA procedure. In SAS, they are done by the ANOVA and GLM procedures. Part of the SPSS/PC and SAS repeated-measures output for the heart-rate data is shown in Figures 9.13 and 9.14. The usual warnings about the computer's inability to check assumptions still apply.

In the SPSS/PC output, the univariate error sum of squares is the WITHIN CELLS sum of squares listed under "AVERAGED Tests of Significance," and the univariate factor sum of squares is the DRUG sum of squares. The between-subjects sum of squares is the WITHIN CELLS sum of squares listed under "Tests of Between-Subjects Effects." The CONSTANT sum of squares is of no interest to us. The within-subjects sum of squares and the total sum of squares are not given. The SPSS/PC sums of squares differ from those we calculated because of differences in rounding. The univariate p-value for testing the null hypothesis (9.1) is given as .001 under "Sig of F" in the output for "AVERAGED Tests of Significance." The lower-bound epsilon given after the Greenhouse-Geisser and Huynh-

equal. The Friedman test described in Chapter 11 could be used instead to test the hypothesis that all possible rankings of the four MICs for any subject are equally likely.

Example 9.2

In a study of defective interferon gamma (IFN-gamma) production in patients with acute tuberculosis, the production of IFN-gamma was measured in blood cultures exposed to one of three mitogens: phytohemaglutinin (PHA), concanavalin A (Con A), or pokeweed mitogen (PWM).[10] Table 9.7 shows the IFN-gamma yield for 16 blood cultures from 14 tuberculosis patients. Can one-factor repeated-measures ANOVA be used to test the hypothesis that the population mean IFN-gamma yields are the same for cultures exposed to PHA, Con A, or PWM?

```
Tests of Between-Subjects Effects.

Tests of Significance for T1 using UNIQUE sums of squares
Source of Variation          SS       DF       MS         F  Sig of F

WITHIN CELLS            2023.72        8   252.97
CONSTANT             197284.03        1 197284.03    779.89     .000


- - - - - - - - - -


Tests involving 'DRUG' Within-Subject Effect.


Mauchly sphericity test, W =       .57398
Chi-square approx. =          3.73187 with 5 D. F.
Significance =                 .589

Greenhouse-Geisser Epsilon =      .77745
Huynh-Feldt Epsilon =            1.00000
Lower-bound Epsilon =             .33333


- - - - - - - - - -


EFFECT .. DRUG
Multivariate Tests of Significance (S = 1, M = 1/2, N = 2 )

Test Name        Value  Approx. F Hypoth. DF   Error DF  Sig. of F

Pillais         .75355   6.11537      3.00       6.00      .030
Hotellings     3.05769   6.11537      3.00       6.00      .030
Wilks           .24645   6.11537      3.00       6.00      .030
Roys            .75355


- - - - - - - - - -


Tests involving 'DRUG' Within-Subject Effect.

AVERAGED Tests of Significance for MEAS.1 using UNIQUE sums of squares
Source of Variation          SS       DF       MS         F  Sig of F

WITHIN CELLS            1153.83       24    48.08
DRUG                   1185.42        3   395.14      8.22     .001
```

Figure 9.13 SPSS/PC repeated-measures ANOVA output for heart-rate data

Feldt epsilons is the smallest epsilon that can be used for adjusting the univariate F degrees of freedom. This number should not be used to adjust the degrees of freedom, since it overcorrects even more than the Greenhouse-Geisser epsilon.*

In the SAS output, the univariate factor sum of squares is the DRUG sum of squares, and the univariate error sum of squares is the ERROR (DRUG) sum of squares. The p-value for the univariate F statistic, listed below "PR > F" under "UNIVARIATE TESTS OF HYPOTHESES FOR WITHIN SUBJECT EFFECTS," is 0.0006. The adjusted univariate p-values are listed under "ADJ PR > F." The p-value when the Greenhouse-Geisser epsilon is used is listed under "G - G" as 0.0020, and the p-value when the Huynh-Feldt epsilon is used is listed under "H - F" as 0.0007. Two versions of Mauchly's test are given. The test we use is the one under "APPLIED TO ORTHOGONAL COMPONENTS:."

9.3 MULTIPLE COMPARISONS

Use of one-factor repeated-measures ANOVA for the heart-rate data led to the conclusion that at least one population mean does not equal another population mean. To determine which population means are different, we need a multiple-comparison

---

*The terminology used in MANOVA output is so esoteric that sorting out the relevant sums of squares and p-values can be quite a challenge for the uninitiated researcher. An excellent guide through the MANOVA-output maze is provided by Norusis and SPSS Inc.[6]

```
        TEST FOR SPHERICITY: MAUCHLY'S CRITERIA =    0.30953696
           CHISQUARE APPROXIMATION =   7.88300055 WITH 5 DF
                  PROB > CHISQUARE = 0.1628


        APPLIED TO ORTHOGONAL COMPONENTS:


        TEST FOR SPHERICITY: MAUCHLY'S CRITERIA =    0.57398363
           CHISQUARE APPROXIMATION =   3.73187122 WITH 5 DF
                  PROB > CHISQUARE = 0.5886



           MANOVA TEST CRITERIA AND EXACT F STATISTICS FOR
                THE HYPOTHESIS OF NO DRUG EFFECT
         H = ANOVA SS&CP MATRIX FOR: DRUG    E = ERROR SS&CP MATRIX

                    S=1      M=0.5     N=2.5

  STATISTIC                  VALUE       F     NUM DF    DEN DF  PR > F

  WILKS' LAMBDA             0.246446    6.115      3        6    0.0295
  PILLAI'S TRACE            0.753554    6.115      3        6    0.0295
  HOTELLING-LAWLEY TRACE    3.05769     6.115      3        6    0.0295
  ROY'S GREATEST ROOT       3.05769     6.115      3        6    0.0295


        UNIVARIATE TESTS OF HYPOTHESES FOR WITHIN SUBJECT EFFECTS

  SOURCE: DRUG

                                                     ADJ  PR > F
      DF      ANOVA SS     MEAN SQUARE  F VALUE  PR > F   G - G    H - F
       3    1185.416667    395.138889     8.22   0.0006  0.0020   0.0007

  SOURCE: ERROR(DRUG)

      DF      ANOVA SS     MEAN SQUARE
      24    1153.833333    48.076389

              GREENHOUSE-GEISSER EPSILON = 0.7774
                  HUYNH-FELDT EPSILON = 0.9798
```

Figure 9.14 SAS repeated-measures ANOVA output for heart-rate data

procedure. We cannot use the Tukey or Bonferroni procedures described in Chapter 8. These methods require factor means based on independent samples, and samples of repeated measurements are not independent.*

Another Bonferroni procedure can be used for multiple comparisons when repeated measurements are obtained. This method is based on Bonferroni-adjusted paired-samples confidence intervals. If the comparisons to be made are selected *before* examining the sample means, define the number c by

$$c = \text{number of comparisons to be made}$$

If the comparisons are selected *after* examining the

sample means, define c by

$$c = \text{total number of } \textit{possible} \text{ comparisons}$$

Paired-samples Bonferroni confidence intervals are based on adjusted upper percentage points of the t distribution with $n - 1$ degrees of freedom. Specifically, $100(1 - \alpha)\%$ paired-samples Bonferroni confidence intervals for differences between factor population means are given by the formula

$$\left((\bar{x}_i - \bar{x}_j) - (t_{\alpha/2c, n-1}) \frac{s_d}{\sqrt{n}}, \right.$$
$$\left. (\bar{x}_i - \bar{x}_j) + (t_{\alpha/2c, n-1}) \frac{s_d}{\sqrt{n}} \right) \quad (9.14)$$

where n is the number of subjects and s_d is the standard deviation of the differences between the factor level i observations and the factor level j observations. The difference $\bar{x}_i - \bar{x}_j$ is always equal

---

*The misuse of multiple-comparison procedures that require independent samples is a common error in medical and health care research.

TABLE 9.8   HEART-RATE DIFFERENCES

Patient No.	No Drug − Propranolol	No Drug − Placebo	No Drug − Acebutolol	Propranolol − Acebutolol
1	27	4	27	0
2	5	−12	2	−3
3	7	12	8	1
4	23	11	10	−13
5	2	−7	−5	−7
6	6	−2	6	0
7	12	−19	13	1
8	14	6	23	9
9	16	8	10	−6
Mean ± SD	12.4 ± 8.5	0.1 ± 10.8	10.4 ± 9.8	−2.0 ± 6.2

to the mean of the differences between the factor level i observations and the factor level j observations, subject to rounding error. If formula (9.14) is used to obtain confidence intervals for the differences $\mu_i - \mu_j$, we can be $100(1 - \alpha)\%$ sure that all of the paired-samples Bonferroni confidence intervals include the differences between the population means. Our overall confidence level is $100(1 - \alpha)\%$.

The paired-samples Bonferroni confidence interval (9.14) is the same as the paired-samples confidence interval described in Chapter 6, except for the adjusted upper percentage points. Both confidence intervals require the same assumptions: random sampling, paired samples, independence of the differences, and sampling from a normal or approximately normal population of differences. The remarks made in Chapter 6 about these assumptions apply to the paired-samples Bonferroni confidence interval.

Let us obtain paired-samples Bonferroni confidence intervals for the heart-rate data, using an overall confidence level of 90%. We will assume that the following comparisons were selected before examining the sample means.

No drug versus propranolol: $\mu_1 - \mu_2$
No drug versus placebo: $\mu_1 - \mu_3$
No drug versus acebutolol: $\mu_1 - \mu_4$
Propranolol versus acebutolol: $\mu_2 - \mu_4$

Table 9.8 shows the heart-rate differences for these comparisons. Histograms of these differences are shown in Figures 9.15 through 9.18. The sample size is large enough to compensate for the skewed population suggested by the histogram in Figure 9.15, and the other histograms are consistent with

```
0 - 9 | XXXX
10 - 19 | XXX
20 - 29 | XX
```

Figure 9.15   Quick histogram of no-drug minus propranolol difference

```
-19 - -10 | XX
 -9 - 0 | XX
  1 - 10 | XXX
 11 - 20 | XX
```

Figure 9.16   Quick histogram of no-drug minus placebo difference

```
-10 - -1 | X
  0 - 9 | XXX
 10 - 19 | XXX
 20 - 29 | XX
```

Figure 9.17   Quick histogram of no-drug minus acebutolol difference

```
-13 - -8 | X
 -7 - -2 | XXX
 -1 - 4 | XXXX
  5 - 10 | X
```

Figure 9.18   Quick histogram of propranolol minus acebutolol difference

normal or approximately normal populations. Independence appears to hold for each of the four sets of differences in Table 9.8. The assumptions required for paired-samples Bonferroni confidence intervals seem reasonable, except for the random sampling assumption.

Since our four comparisons were selected before examining the sample means, $c = 4$. We have $\alpha = 0.10$, $\alpha/2c = 0.10/8 = 0.0125$, and $t_{.0125, 8} \cong t_{.01, 8} = 2.896$. Using this upper percentage point, the sample means in Table 9.1, and the standard deviations in Table 9.8, we obtain the following paired-samples Bonferroni confidence intervals.

Confidence Interval for $\mu_1 - \mu_2$ (No Drug Versus Propranolol).

$$\left((79.8 - 67.3) - (2.896)\frac{8.5}{\sqrt{9}}, \right.$$

$$\left. (79.8 - 67.3) + (2.896)\frac{8.5}{\sqrt{9}} \right)$$

$$(12.5 - 8.2, 12.5 + 8.2)$$

$$(4.3, 20.7)$$

Confidence Interval for $\mu_1 - \mu_3$ (No Drug Versus Placebo).

$$\left((79.8 - 79.7) - (2.896)\frac{10.8}{\sqrt{9}}, \right.$$

$$\left. (79.8 - 79.7) + (2.896)\frac{10.8}{\sqrt{9}} \right)$$

$$(0.1 - 10.4, 0.1 + 10.4)$$

$$(-10.3, 10.5)$$

Confidence Interval for $\mu_1 - \mu_4$ (No Drug Versus Acebutolol).

$$\left((79.8 - 69.3) - (2.896)\frac{9.8}{\sqrt{9}}, \right.$$

$$\left. (79.8 - 69.3) + (2.896)\frac{9.8}{\sqrt{9}} \right)$$

$$(10.5 - 9.5, 10.5 + 9.5)$$

$$(1.0, 20.0)$$

Confidence Interval for $\mu_2 - \mu_4$ (Propranolol Versus Acebutolol).

$$\left((67.3 - 69.3) - (2.896)\frac{6.2}{\sqrt{9}}, \right.$$

$$\left. (67.3 - 69.3) + (2.896)\frac{6.2}{\sqrt{9}} \right),$$

$$(-2.0 - 6.0, -2.0 + 6.0)$$

$$(-8.0, 4.0)$$

We are 90% sure that the following is true.

1. The no-drug population heart-rate mean is larger than the propranolol population heart-rate mean. The difference could be small (as low as 4.3), large (as high as 20.7), or moderate.
2. We cannot say that the no-drug population heart-rate mean differs from the placebo population heart-rate mean.
3. The no-drug population heart-rate mean is larger than the acebutolol population heart-rate

mean. The difference could be quite small (as low as 1.0), large (as high as 20.0), or somewhere in between.
4. We cannot say that the propranolol population heart-rate mean differs from the acebutolol population heart-rate mean.

The results indicate that lower heart rates occur during use of propranolol or acebutolol use than during use of no drug, on average. The data do not provide evidence for a difference between the propranolol population heart-rate mean and the acebutolol population heart-rate mean. Since we did not obtain confidence intervals for $\mu_2 - \mu_3$ or $\mu_3 - \mu_4$, we cannot make inferences comparing the placebo population heart-rate mean with the propranolol population heart-rate mean or with the acebutolol population heart-rate mean.

Like most multiple-comparison procedures, the paired-samples Bonferroni procedure can produce results that are inconsistent with the test of the hypothesis of equal population means. It is possible to reject the null hypothesis (9.2) at the significance level α and then obtain $100(1 - \alpha)\%$ paired-samples Bonferroni confidence intervals that all contain 0. Fortunately, such inconsistencies do not occur very often. As in one-way ANOVA, the solution to this problem is to reduce the overall confidence level until at least one of the confidence intervals does not contain 0.

Other multiple-comparison procedures for one-factor repeated-measures ANOVA have been described by Morrison.[2, 11] These methods will not be discussed here.

Sometimes more than one factor is of interest when repeated measurements are obtained. If two factors are used and one or both involve repeated measurements, hypotheses about population means can often be tested with *two-factor repeated-measures analysis of variance*. This procedure is an extension of one-factor repeated-measures analysis of variance. A discussion of two-factor repeated-measures ANOVA can be found in more advanced texts.[3, 6]

SUMMARY

When three or more samples of repeated measurements are obtained, one-factor repeated-measures analysis of variance is often used to test the hypothesis that the population means are equal. Repeated measurements should not be obtained if previous treatments can interfere with later treatments. Several approaches to one-factor repeated-measures ANOVA are available: the univariate approach, the multivariate approach, and the Huynh-Feldt and Greenhouse-Geisser adjusted univariate approaches. All of these approaches assume multivariate normality, and the univariate approach requires additional variance-covariance assumptions.

In the univariate approach, an F statistic based on mean squares is used to test the hypothesis of equal population means. In the adjusted univariate approaches, the univariate F statistic with adjusted degrees of freedom is used to test this hypothesis. In the multivariate approach, multivariate test statistics are used to test this hypothesis. Mauchly's test is done to determine whether the variance-covariance assumptions required for the univariate approach are reasonable for the data. If the hypothesis of equal population means is rejected, a paired-samples Bonferroni multiple-comparison procedure can be used to determine which population means are different.

FREQUENTLY USED ONE-FACTOR REPEATED-MEASURES ANOVA FORMULAS

Univariate F statistic for testing H_0: $\mu_1 = \mu_2 = \cdots = \mu_k$:

$$F = \frac{MSF}{MSE}$$

$100(1 - \alpha)\%$ paired-samples Bonferroni confidence interval:

$$\left((\bar{x}_i - \bar{x}_j) - \left(t_{\alpha/2c, n-1}\right)\frac{s_d}{\sqrt{n}}, \right.$$
$$\left. (\bar{x}_i - \bar{x}_j) + \left(t_{\alpha/2c, n-1}\right)\frac{s_d}{\sqrt{n}} \right)$$

PROBLEMS

The following instructions apply to all of the problems.

1. In each problem, data are described, SPSS/PC one-factor repeated-measures ANOVA output is presented, and a question is asked about the data. Determine whether one-factor repeated-measures ANOVA is appropriate for analyzing the data. If it is not appropriate, state which assumptions are violated.

2. If the one-factor repeated-measures ANOVA assumptions are satisfied, determine whether the univariate method is appropriate, using a 0.10 significance level for Mauchly's test. If the univariate method is appropriate, use the p-value for the univariate F test. If the univariate method is not appropriate, use the p-value for the multivariate method and the p-value for the Huynh-Feldt adjusted univariate method. Interpret the p-values.

3. If the hypothesis of equal population means is rejected, calculate paired-samples Bonferroni confidence intervals. Use the p-values and confidence intervals to answer the question in the problem.

You may want to obtain quick histograms for each factor level. Do not worry about slightly or moderately nonnormal histograms if the data have a large number of possible values. Unless the data are extremely nonnormal and the sample is very small, you can assume that the central limit theorem applies to the data.

1. A study evaluated the effect of testosterone therapy for autoimmune diseases associated with Klinefelter's syndrome (KS).[12] Table 9.9 shows the number of T helper cells per mm^3 for five KS patients with active autoimmune disease before treatment, after placebo treatment, and after testosterone treatment. Do the data provide evidence that some of the population mean numbers of T helper cells before treatment, after placebo treatment, and after testosterone treatment are different? Use a 0.10 significance level for testing the hypothesis of equal population means and a 90% overall confidence level for multiple comparisons.

2. A study evaluated the efficacy of a new aminodiphosphonate for treating patients with osteolytic lesions from metastases or myelomatosis.[13] Table 9.10 shows the logarithm of the urinary calcium/creatinine ratio for 16 patients before treatment and seven and 28 days after treatment. (The data were transformed by taking logarithms in order to reduce skewness and obtain more similar variances.) Do the data provide evidence that some of the population log ratio means before and after treatment are different? Use a 0.05 significance

TABLE 9.9 T HELPER CELLS (CELLS PER mm³) FOR KS PATIENTS WITH ACTIVE AUTOIMMUNE DISEASE

Patient No.	Before Treatment	After Placebo	After Testosterone
1	1000	1100	1067
2	1250	900	1126
3	1290	870	1232
4	915	1212	808
5	840	1200	960
Mean ± SD	1059.0 ± 201.3	1056.4 ± 162.7	1038.6 ± 162.2

```
Tests of Between-Subjects Effects.

Tests of Significance for T1 using UNIQUE sums of squares
Source of Variation          SS       DF       MS         F   Sig of F

WITHIN CELLS            47791.33      4   11947.83
CONSTANT             16579526.67      1   16579527   1387.66     .000


- - - - - - - - -


Tests involving 'DRUG' Within-Subject Effect.


Mauchly sphericity test, W =      .21942
Chi-square approx. =           4.55025 with 2 D. F.
Significance =                    .103

Greenhouse-Geisser Epsilon =     .56162
Huynh-Feldt Epsilon =            .62851
Lower-bound Epsilon =            .50000


- - - - - - - - -


EFFECT .. DRUG
Multivariate Tests of Significance (S = 1, M = 0, N = 1/2)

Test Name       Value  Approx. F Hypoth. DF   Error DF  Sig. of F

Pillais        .05695    .09058      2.00        3.00      .916
Hotellings     .06039    .09058      2.00        3.00      .916
Wilks          .94305    .09058      2.00        3.00      .916
Roys           .05695


- - - - - - - - - -


Tests involving 'DRUG' Within-Subject Effect.

AVERAGED Tests of Significance for MEAS.1 using UNIQUE sums of squares
Source of Variation          SS       DF       MS         F   Sig of F

WITHIN CELLS           325371.07      8   40671.38
DRUG                     1232.93      2     616.47    .02      .985
```

Figure 9.19 SPSS/PC one-factor repeated-measures ANOVA output for T helper cells

**TABLE 9.10 LOGARITHM OF URINARY CALCIUM/CREATININE
RATIO (LOG mg/g) BEFORE AND AFTER TREATMENT**

Patient No.	Before	7 Days After	28 Days After
1	4.19	2.64	3.04
2	4.97	4.55	4.85
3	5.54	4.50	4.62
4	5.42	5.26	5.01
5	5.83	5.42	5.13
6	6.10	5.39	5.34
7	6.30	6.12	5.80
8	4.61	3.61	3.83
9	4.80	4.51	3.81
10	5.32	4.19	4.60
11	5.61	5.51	5.12
12	4.26	4.28	3.47
13	4.84	4.63	4.84
14	4.66	4.20	4.42
15	5.92	5.03	5.00
16	5.04	3.85	3.99
Mean $\pm$ SD	5.21 $\pm$ 0.64	4.61 $\pm$ 0.85	4.55 $\pm$ 0.74

TABLE 9.11   LOG URINARY CALCIUM/CREATININE RATIO DIFFERENCES

Patient No.	Before − 7 Days After	Before − 28 Days After	7 Days After − 28 Days After
1	1.55	1.15	−0.40
2	0.42	0.12	−0.30
3	1.04	0.92	−0.12
4	0.16	0.41	0.25
5	0.41	0.70	0.29
6	0.71	0.76	0.05
7	0.18	0.50	0.32
8	1.00	0.78	−0.22
9	0.29	0.99	0.70
10	1.13	0.72	−0.41
11	0.10	0.49	0.39
12	−0.02	0.79	0.81
13	0.21	0.00	−0.21
14	0.46	0.24	−0.22
15	0.89	0.92	0.03
16	1.19	1.05	−0.14
Mean ± SD	0.61 ± 0.47	0.66 ± 0.34	0.05 ± 0.37

```
Tests of Between-Subjects Effects.

Tests of Significance for T1 using UNIQUE sums of squares
Source of Variation        SS       DF      MS        F   Sig of F

WITHIN CELLS             22.98      15     1.53
CONSTANT              1101.60       1  1101.60     719.21     .000


- - - - - - - - -


Tests involving 'DAY' Within-Subject Effect.


Mauchly sphericity test, W =       .83394
Chi-square approx. =              2.54237 with 2 D. F.
Significance =                     .280

Greenhouse-Geisser Epsilon =       .85759
Huynh-Feldt Epsilon =              .95759
Lower-bound Epsilon =              .50000


- - - - - - - - -


EFFECT .. DAY
Multivariate Tests of Significance (S = 1, M = 0, N = 6 )

Test Name       Value   Approx. F Hypoth. DF   Error DF  Sig. of F

Pillais        .80333   28.59172    2.00        14.00      .000
Hotellings    4.08453   28.59172    2.00        14.00      .000
Wilks          .19667   28.59172    2.00        14.00      .000
Roys           .80333


- - - - - - - - -


Tests involving 'DAY' Within-Subject Effect.

AVERAGED Tests of Significance for MEAS.1 using UNIQUE sums of squares
Source of Variation        SS       DF      MS        F   Sig of F

WITHIN CELLS             2.37       30     .08
DAY                      4.30        2    2.15      27.22     .000
```

Figure 9.20 SPSS/PC one-factor repeated-measures ANOVA output for log urinary calcium/creatinine ratio

TABLE 9.12 PERIPHERAL, ADRENAL, AND OVARIAN VEIN PLASMA SQUARE-ROOT TESTOSTERONE (SQUARE-ROOT ng/ml)

Patient No.	Peripheral Vein	Adrenal Vein	Ovarian Vein
1	1.06	1.69	1.12
2	0.90	1.79	0.99
3	0.57	1.41	0.59
4	0.99	1.56	0.77
5	0.92	1.24	4.06
6	0.49	0.58	1.88
7	0.85	1.13	2.70
8	1.04	1.23	4.99
9	1.10	1.74	1.52
10	1.03	2.25	1.70
11	0.62	1.30	1.80
12	1.80	3.41	3.05
Mean ± SD	0.95 ± 0.34	1.61 ± 0.70	2.10 ± 1.36

TABLE 9.13 SQUARE-ROOT TESTOSTERONE DIFFERENCES WITH MEANS AND STANDARD DEVIATIONS

Patient No.	Peripheral − Adrenal	Peripheral − Ovarian	Adrenal − Ovarian
1	−0.63	−0.06	0.57
2	−0.89	−0.09	0.80
3	−0.84	−0.02	0.82
4	−0.57	0.22	0.79
5	−0.32	−3.14	−2.82
6	−0.09	−1.39	−1.30
7	−0.28	−1.85	−1.57
8	−0.19	−3.95	−3.76
9	−0.64	−0.42	0.22
10	−1.22	−0.67	0.55
11	−0.68	−1.18	−0.50
12	−1.61	−1.25	0.36
Mean ± SD	−0.66 ± 0.44	−1.15 ± 1.30	−0.49 ± 1.55

level for testing the hypothesis of equal population means and a 95% overall confidence level for multiple comparisons.

3. A study examined sources of excessive androgen production in women with polycystic ovary syndrome (PCOS).[14] Table 9.12 shows the square roots of the testosterone concentrations for peripheral, adrenal, and ovarian vein plasma from 12 hirsute women with PCOS. (The data were transformed by taking square roots in order to reduce skewness and obtain more similar variances.) Do the data provide evidence that some of the population square-root testosterone means for different tissues are different? Use a 0.01 significance level for testing the hypothesis of equal population means and a 95% overall confidence level for multiple comparisons.

4. A study evaluated the effect of a program of nutritional and exercise instruction and behavioral techniques on weight loss in overweight children with myelomeningocele.[15] Table 9.14 shows the

percentage overweight for five children with myelomeningocele at the beginning of the program, four months after the program, and six months after the program. Do the data provide evidence that some of the population percentage overweight means before and after the program are different? Use a 0.05 significance level for testing the hypothesis of equal population means and a 90% overall confidence level for multiple comparisons.

5. In a study of diabetic renal hypouricemia, the urate clearance/creatinine clearance ratio was reported for seven diabetic patients with persistent hypouricemia.[16] Table 9.15 shows the logarithm of this ratio before and after administration of pyrazinamide or probenicid. (The data were transformed by taking logarithms in order to reduce skewness and obtain more similar variances.) Do the data provide evidence that some of the population log ratio means before and after drug administration are different? Use a 0.01 significance level for testing the hypothesis of equal population means

TABLE 9.14 PERCENTAGE OVERWEIGHT AT THE BEGINNING OF PROGRAM AND AFTER PROGRAM

Patient No.	Beginning of Program	Four Months After Program	Six Months After Program
1	28	6	4
2	50	29	31
3	56	54	49
4	50	42	49
5	76	86	97
Mean ± SD	52.0 ± 17.1	43.4 ± 29.7	46.0 ± 33.9

and a 90% overall confidence level for multiple comparisons.

6. In a study of African swine fever (ASF), pregnant sows were innoculated oronasally with ASF virus.[17] Samples of fetal tissue were then obtained and tested for the presence of ASF virus. Table 9.17 shows the percentage of sampled tissues that were positive for 13 sows. Do the data provide evidence that some of the population percentage means for different fetal tissues are different? Use a 0.01 significance level for testing the hypothesis of equal population means and a 95% overall confidence level for multiple comparisons.

7. In a study of HLA-B27–related arthritis, the response of arthritic HLA-B27 positive patients to sulfasalazine was investigated.[18] Table 9.18 shows the square root of the erythrocyte sedimentation rate (ESR) for eight of these patients before and after treatment. (The data were transformed by taking square roots in order to reduce skewness and obtain more similar variances.) Do the data provide evidence that some of the population square-root

```
Tests of Between-Subjects Effects.

Tests of Significance for T1 using UNIQUE sums of squares
Source of Variation          SS        DF        MS          F  Sig of F

WITHIN CELLS              11.30        11      1.03
CONSTANT                  86.73         1     86.73       84.45      .000


- - - - - - - - -


Tests involving 'TISSUE' Within-Subject Effect.


Mauchly sphericity test, W =        .16717
Chi-square approx. =         17.88749 with 2 D. F.
Significance =                       .000

Greenhouse-Geisser Epsilon =        .54560
Huynh-Feldt Epsilon =               .55983
Lower-bound Epsilon =               .50000


- - - - - - - - -


EFFECT .. TISSUE
Multivariate Tests of Significance (S = 1, M = 0, N = 4 )

Test Name        Value  Approx. F Hypoth. DF   Error DF  Sig. of F

Pillais         .85688  29.93484       2.00      10.00      .000
Hotellings     5.98697  29.93484       2.00      10.00      .000
Wilks           .14312  29.93484       2.00      10.00      .000
Roys            .85688


- - - - - - - - -


Tests involving 'TISSUE' Within-Subject Effect.

AVERAGED Tests of Significance for MEAS.1 using UNIQUE sums of squares
Source of Variation          SS        DF        MS          F  Sig of F

WITHIN CELLS              15.66        22       .71
TISSUE                     8.01         2      4.00        5.62      .011
```

Figure 9.21 SPSS/PC one-factor repeated-measures ANOVA output for square-root testosterone

```
Tests of Between-Subjects Effects.

Tests of Significance for T1 using UNIQUE sums of squares
Source of Variation         SS      DF       MS        F  Sig of F

WITHIN CELLS             8605.73     4   2151.43
CONSTANT                33323.27     1  33323.27    15.49     .017

- - - - - - - - -


Tests involving 'PROGRAM' Within-Subject Effect.


   Mauchly sphericity test, W =       .23771
   Chi-square approx. =        4.31009 with 2 D. F.
   Significance =                 .116

   Greenhouse-Geisser Epsilon =    .56744
   Huynh-Feldt Epsilon =           .64124
   Lower-bound Epsilon =           .50000

- - - - - - - - -


EFFECT .. PROGRAM
Multivariate Tests of Significance (S = 1, M = 0, N = 1/2)

Test Name        Value  Approx. F Hypoth. DF   Error DF  Sig. of F

Pillais         .58279   2.09532      2.00       3.00      .269
Hotellings     1.39688   2.09532      2.00       3.00      .269
Wilks           .41721   2.09532      2.00       3.00      .269
Roys            .58279

- - - - - - - - -


Tests involving 'PROGRAM' Within-Subject Effect.

AVERAGED Tests of Significance for MEAS.1 using UNIQUE sums of squares
Source of Variation         SS      DF       MS        F  Sig of F

WITHIN CELLS              713.47     8     89.18
PROGRAM                   194.53     2     97.27     1.09     .381
```

Figure 9.22 SPSS/PC one-factor repeated-measures ANOVA output for percentage overweight

**TABLE 9.15   LOGARITHM OF URATE CLEARANCE /
CREATININE CLEARANCE RATIO (LOG %)**

Patient No.	Control	After Pyrazinamide	After Probenecid
1	3.73	1.70	4.79
2	3.61	1.50	4.29
3	3.28	1.25	4.30
4	3.59	−0.22	3.94
5	2.98	−0.51	4.20
6	2.75	0.53	3.95
7	2.91	−0.36	4.40
Mean ± SD	3.26 ± 0.39	0.56 ± 0.94	4.27 ± 0.29

**TABLE 9.16   LOG URATE CLEARANCE / CREATININE
CLEARANCE RATIO DIFFERENCES**

Patient No.	Control − Pyrazinamide	Control − Probenecid	Pyrazinamide − Probenecid
1	2.03	−1.06	−3.09
2	2.11	−0.68	−2.79
3	2.03	−1.02	−3.05
4	3.81	−0.35	−4.16
5	3.49	−1.22	−4.71
6	2.22	−1.20	−3.42
7	3.27	−1.49	−4.76
Mean ± SD	2.71 ± 0.78	−1.00 ± 0.38	−3.71 ± 0.82

```
Tests of Between-Subjects Effects.

Tests of Significance for T1 using UNIQUE sums of squares
Source of Variation          SS       DF      MS          F   Sig of F

WITHIN CELLS                3.84       6      .64
CONSTANT                  152.65       1   152.65     238.33      .000

- - - - - - - - -

Tests involving 'DRUG' Within-Subject Effect.


Mauchly sphericity test, W =       .49937
Chi-square approx. =           3.47205 with 2 D. F.
Significance =                     .176

Greenhouse-Geisser Epsilon =       .66639
Huynh-Feldt Epsilon =              .78520
Lower-bound Epsilon =              .50000

- - - - - - - - -

EFFECT .. DRUG
Multivariate Tests of Significance (S = 1, M = 0, N = 1 1/2)

Test Name        Value  Approx. F Hypoth. DF   Error DF  Sig. of F

Pillais         .96226  63.73887      2.00       5.00      .000
Hotellings    25.49555  63.73887      2.00       5.00      .000
Wilks           .03774  63.73887      2.00       5.00      .000
Roys            .96226

- - - - - - - - -

Tests involving 'DRUG' Within-Subject Effect.

AVERAGED Tests of Significance for MEAS.1 using UNIQUE sums of squares
Source of Variation          SS       DF      MS          F   Sig of F

WITHIN CELLS                2.86      12      .24
DRUG                       51.55       2    25.78     108.29      .000
```

Figure 9.23 SPSS/PC one-factor repeated-measures ANOVA output for log urate clearance/creatinine clearance ratio

ESR means before and after treatment are different? Use a 0.05 significance level for testing the hypothesis of equal population means and a 90% overall confidence level for multiple comparisons. If the hypothesis of equal population means is rejected, assume that the only comparisons of interest are those between the before-treatment population mean and the after-treatment population means. Also assume that these comparisons were selected before examining the sample means.

8. In a study of growth hormone (GH) response to clonidine, the responses of normal GH secretors to clonidine were reported.[19] Table 9.20 shows the reciprocal of the GH level [1/(GH level)] for 11 of these subjects before and after clonidine. (The data were transformed by taking reciprocals in order to reduce skewness and obtain more similar variances.)

The smaller the reciprocal GH, the larger the GH. Do the data provide evidence that some of the population reciprocal GH means before and after clonidine administration are different? Use a 0.05 significance level for testing the hypothesis of equal population means and a 90% overall confidence level for multiple comparisons. If the hypothesis of equal population means is rejected, assume that the only comparisons of interest are those between the before-clonidine population mean and the after-clonidine population means. Also assume that these comparisons were selected before examining the sample means.

9. A study evaluated the effect of dietary protein restriction on renal function in patients with diabetic nephropathy.[20] Table 9.21 shows the reciprocal of the serum creatinine [1/(serum creatinine)]

**TABLE 9.17 PERCENTAGE OF FETAL TISSUE SAMPLES
TESTING POSITIVE FOR ASF VIRUS**

	Fetal Tissue			
Sow No.	PLACENTA	AMNIOTIC FLUID	UMBILICUS	LIVER
1	12.5	0.0	0.0	0.0
2	0.0	0.0	0.0	0.0
3	90.0	36.4	0.0	0.0
4	0.0	0.0	0.0	0.0
5	11.1	20.0	0.0	0.0
6	64.3	57.1	0.0	0.0
7	0.0	14.3	0.0	0.0
8	18.2	36.4	0.0	9.1
9	87.5	66.7	75.0	60.0
10	100.0	25.0	100.0	87.5
11	100.0	30.0	100.0	0.0
12	37.5	10.0	0.0	10.0
13	20.0	11.1	0.0	0.0
Mean ± SD	41.6 ± 40.6	23.6 ± 21.3	21.2 ± 40.6	12.8 ± 27.8

```
Tests of Between-Subjects Effects.

Tests of Significance for T1 using UNIQUE sums of squares
Source of Variation          SS        DF       MS          F   Sig of F

WITHIN CELLS              36654.69     12   3054.56
CONSTANT                  31987.04      1  31987.04      10.47      .007


 - - - - - - - -


Tests involving 'TISSUE' Within-Subject Effect.


Mauchly sphericity test, W =        .61423
Chi-square approx. =            5.22583 with 5 D. F.
Significance =                      .389

Greenhouse-Geisser Epsilon =       .81591
Huynh-Feldt Epsilon =             1.00000
Lower-bound Epsilon =              .33333


 - - - - - - - - -


EFFECT .. TISSUE
Multivariate Tests of Significance (S = 1, M = 1/2, N = 4 )

Test Name       Value  Approx. F Hypoth. DF   Error DF  Sig. of F

Pillais         .47323   2.99458      3.00     10.00      .082
Hotellings      .89838   2.99458      3.00     10.00      .082
Wilks           .52677   2.99458      3.00     10.00      .082
Roys            .47323


 - - - - - - - - -


Tests involving 'TISSUE' Within-Subject Effect.

AVERAGED Tests of Significance for MEAS.1 using UNIQUE sums of squares
Source of Variation          SS        DF       MS          F  Sig of F

WITHIN CELLS              17704.46     36    491.79
TISSUE                     5737.48      3   1912.49       3.89     .017
```

Figure 9.24 SPSS/PC one-factor repeated-measures ANOVA output for tissue percentage

TABLE 9.18 SQUARE-ROOT ESR (SQUARE-ROOT mm/h) FOR ARTHRITIC PATIENTS BEFORE AND AFTER SULFASALAZINE TREATMENT

Patient No.	0 Months	3 Months	6 Months	12 Months
1	8.83	3.74	3.16	2.83
2	6.63	2.24	2.00	3.00
3	5.57	4.24	2.24	2.45
4	5.00	3.32	1.41	2.00
5	9.06	3.16	2.00	1.41
6	6.93	4.24	2.00	1.73
7	7.07	5.74	5.10	3.16
8	3.87	3.46	4.00	3.74
Mean ± SD	6.62 ± 1.79	3.77 ± 1.02	2.74 ± 1.25	2.54 ± 0.79

for eight diabetic patients with progressive renal dysfunction 12 months before protein restriction, at the start of protein restriction, and 12 months after protein restriction. (The data were transformed by taking reciprocals in order to reduce skewness and obtain more similar variances.) The smaller the reciprocal serum creatinine, the larger the serum creatinine. Do the data provide evidence that some of the population reciprocal serum creatinine means at different times are different? Use a 0.10 significance level for testing the hypothesis of equal population means and a 90% overall confidence level for multiple comparisons.

10. In a study of the effect of diet on urinary oxalate, urinary oxalate excretion was reported for two subjects after four diets.[21] These values are shown in Table 9.23. Do the data provide evidence that some of the population urinary oxalate excretion means for different diets are different? Use a 0.05 significance level for testing the hypothesis of equal population means and a 90% overall confidence level for multiple comparisons. If the hypothesis of equal population means is rejected, assume that the only comparisons of interest are those between the low purine diet and the other diets. Also assume that these comparisons were selected before examining the sample means.

11. A study investigated the effect of procainamide on ventricular tachycardia (VT).[22] Table 9.24 shows the logarithm of the cycle length of VT

for 15 patients in whom induction of VT was not suppressed by procainamide. (The data were transformed by taking logarithms in order to reduce skewness and obtain more similar variances.) The log VT cycle lengths were obtained before and after increasing doses of procainamide. Do the data provide evidence that some of the population log VT cycle length means before and after procainamide administration are different? Use a 0.01 significance level for testing the hypothesis of equal population means and a 90% overall confidence level for multiple comparisons. If the hypothesis of equal population means is rejected, assume that the only comparisons of interest are those between the no-procainamide population mean and the procainamide population means. Also assume that these comparisons were selected before examining the sample means.

12. A study evaluated the effectiveness of sodium cromoglycate and verapamil in increasing the provocation dose of methacholine that produced a 20% fall in forced expiratory volume in one second (FEV_1) in children with asthma.[23] The logarithm of the provocation dose for 15 children with asthma is shown in Table 9.26. (The data were transformed by taking logarithms in order to reduce skewness and obtain more similar variances.) Do the data provide evidence that some of the population log provocation dose means before and after administration of sodium cromoglycate, verapamil, or saline are different? Use a 0.05 significance level for testing the hypothesis of equal population means and a 95% overall confidence level for multiple comparisons. If the hypothesis of equal population means is rejected, assume that the only comparisons of interest are those between the baseline population mean and the saline, verapamil, and sodium cromoglycate population means. Also assume that these comparisons were selected after examining the sample means.

13. In a study of lead in breast milk, the lead concentration in breast milk from women who were not occupationally exposed to lead was reported.[24] The lead concentrations for eight women are shown in Table 9.28. Do the data provide evidence that some of the population lead concentration means at

TABLE 9.19 SQUARE-ROOT ESR DIFFERENCES

Patient No.	0 Months − 3 Months	0 Months − 6 Months	0 Months − 12 Months
1	5.09	5.67	6.00
2	4.39	4.63	3.63
3	1.33	3.33	3.12
4	1.68	3.59	3.00
5	5.90	7.06	7.65
6	2.69	4.93	5.20
7	1.33	1.97	3.91
8	0.41	−0.13	0.13
Mean ± SD	2.85 ± 2.02	3.88 ± 2.24	4.08 ± 2.26

```
Tests of Between-Subjects Effects.

Tests of Significance for T1 using UNIQUE sums of squares
Source of Variation          SS      DF        MS        F  Sig of F

WITHIN CELLS              14.67       7      2.10
CONSTANT                 491.02       1    491.02   234.27      .000


- - - - - - - - - -


Tests involving 'TIME' Within-Subject Effect.


  Mauchly sphericity test, W =        .23803
  Chi-square approx. =        8.21335 with 5 D. F.
  Significance =                 .145

  Greenhouse-Geisser Epsilon =    .53812
  Huynh-Feldt Epsilon =           .67555
  Lower-bound Epsilon =           .33333


- - - - - - - - - -


EFFECT .. TIME
Multivariate Tests of Significance (S = 1, M = 1/2, N = 1 1/2)

Test Name       Value  Approx. F Hypoth. DF   Error DF  Sig. of F

Pillais        .79798   6.58351      3.00       5.00      .035
Hotellings    3.95011   6.58351      3.00       5.00      .035
Wilks          .20202   6.58351      3.00       5.00      .035
Roys           .79798


- - - - - - - - - -


Tests involving 'TIME' Within-Subject Effect.

AVERAGED Tests of Significance for MEAS.1 using UNIQUE sums of squares
Source of Variation          SS      DF        MS        F  Sig of F

WITHIN CELLS              30.43      21      1.45
TIME                     84.88       3     28.29    19.53      .000
```

Figure 9.25 SPSS/PC one-factor repeated-measures ANOVA output for square-root ESR

**TABLE 9.20 RECIPROCAL OF GROWTH HORMONE [1/(ng/ml)]
BEFORE AND AFTER CLONIDINE**

Patient No.	0 Minutes	30 Minutes	60 Minutes	90 Minutes	120 Minutes
1	0.17	0.50	0.67	0.83	0.37
2	1.25	1.67	1.00	0.29	0.48
3	0.05	0.10	0.21	0.36	0.63
4	2.00	2.00	0.11	0.19	0.16
5	0.12	0.42	0.71	0.91	0.83
6	0.28	0.83	0.67	0.91	1.43
7	0.53	0.83	0.83	0.53	1.00
8	2.00	0.77	0.05	0.07	0.29
9	0.83	1.67	2.00	1.43	1.00
10	1.00	1.43	0.83	0.19	0.16
11	0.59	0.91	1.11	1.11	0.71
Mean ± SD	0.80 ± 0.70	1.01 ± 0.60	0.74 ± 0.55	0.62 ± 0.44	0.64 ± 0.40

```
Tests of Between-Subjects Effects.

Tests of Significance for T1 using UNIQUE sums of squares
Source of Variation          SS       DF       MS       F  Sig of F

WITHIN CELLS               4.04      10      .40
CONSTANT                  32.11       1    32.11    79.47     .000

- - - - - - - - -


Tests involving 'TIME' Within-Subject Effect.


Mauchly sphericity test, W =         .04419
Chi-square approx. =            26.25333 with 9 D. F.
Significance =                   .002

Greenhouse-Geisser Epsilon =     .41498
Huynh-Feldt Epsilon =            .48738
Lower-bound Epsilon =            .25000


- - - - - - - - -


EFFECT .. TIME
Multivariate Tests of Significance (S = 1, M = 1 , N = 2 1/2)

Test Name         Value  Approx. F Hypoth. DF   Error DF  Sig. of F

Pillais          .37105   1.03243      4.00       7.00      .454
Hotellings       .58996   1.03243      4.00       7.00      .454
Wilks            .62895   1.03243      4.00       7.00      .454
Roys             .37105


- - - - - - - - -


Tests involving 'TIME' Within-Subject Effect.

AVERAGED Tests of Significance for MEAS.1 using UNIQUE sums of squares
Source of Variation          SS       DF       MS       F  Sig of F

WITHIN CELLS              11.02      40      .28
TIME                      1.08        4      .27      .98     .428
```

Figure 9.26 SPSS/PC one-factor repeated-measures ANOVA output for reciprocal growth hormone

TABLE 9.21   RECIPROCAL OF SERUM CREATININE BEFORE AND AFTER
PROTEIN RESTRICTION AND AT START OF PROTEIN RESTRICTION

Patient No.	12 Months Before Restriction	At Start of Restriction	12 Months After Restriction
1	0.834	0.714	0.745
2	0.610	0.588	0.826
3	0.554	0.454	0.453
4	0.613	0.435	0.511
5	0.833	0.714	0.523
6	0.885	0.833	0.817
7	0.502	0.303	0.327
8	0.548	0.476	0.770
Mean ± SD	0.672 ± 0.153	0.565 ± 0.178	0.622 ± 0.191

TABLE 9.22   RECIPROCAL SERUM CREATININE DIFFERENCES

Patient No.	12 Months Before − Start	12 Months Before − 12 Months After	Start − 12 Months After
1	0.120	0.089	−0.031
2	0.022	−0.216	−0.238
3	0.100	0.101	0.001
4	0.178	0.102	−0.076
5	0.119	0.310	0.191
6	0.052	0.068	0.016
7	0.199	0.175	−0.024
8	0.072	−0.222	−0.294
Mean ± SD	0.108 ± 0.060	0.051 ± 0.183	−0.057 ± 0.152

```
Tests of Between-Subjects Effects.

Tests of Significance for T1 using UNIQUE sums of squares
Source of Variation        SS      DF       MS        F  Sig of F

WITHIN CELLS              .50       7      .07
CONSTANT                 9.21       1     9.21    129.10      .000

- - - - - - - - - -


Tests involving 'TIME' Within-Subject Effect.


Mauchly sphericity test, W =      .23599
Chi-square approx. =          8.66371 with 2 D. F.
Significance =                    .013

Greenhouse-Geisser Epsilon =      .56689
Huynh-Feldt Epsilon =             .60263
Lower-bound Epsilon =             .50000

- - - - - - - - - -


EFFECT .. TIME
Multivariate Tests of Significance (S = 1, M = 0, N = 2 )

Test Name       Value  Approx. F Hypoth. DF   Error DF  Sig. of F

Pillais        .83740  15.45075      2.00       6.00      .004
Hotellings    5.15025  15.45075      2.00       6.00      .004
Wilks          .16260  15.45075      2.00       6.00      .004
Roys           .83740

- - - - - - - - - -


Tests involving 'TIME' Within-Subject Effect.

AVERAGED Tests of Significance for MEAS.1 using UNIQUE sums of squares
Source of Variation        SS      DF       MS        F  Sig of F

WITHIN CELLS              .14      14      .01
TIME                     .05       2      .02     2.32      .135
```

Figure 9.27   SPSS/PC one-factor repeated-measures ANOVA output for reciprocal serum creatinine

**TABLE 9.23   URINARY OXALATE EXCRETION (mmol / 24 h)
AFTER DIFFERENT DIETS**

	Diet			
Subject No.	Low Purine	Low Purine + Guanosine	Low Purine + Guanosine + Allopurinol	Low Purine + Allopurinol
1, 1st assay	0.416	0.336	0.369	0.364
1, 2nd assay	0.319	0.408	0.348	0.363
1, 3rd assay	0.375	0.313	0.318	0.353
2, 1st assay	0.241	0.223	0.241	0.308
2, 2nd assay	0.220	0.225	0.240	0.280
2, 3rd assay	0.260	0.225	0.250	0.290
Mean ± SD	0.305 ± 0.078	0.288 ± 0.077	0.294 ± 0.058	0.326 ± 0.038

```
Tests of Between-Subjects Effects.

Tests of Significance for T1 using UNIQUE sums of squares
Source of Variation        SS      DF      MS          F  Sig of F

WITHIN CELLS              .07       5     .01
CONSTANT                 2.21       1    2.21      156.41     .000


- - - - - - - - -


Tests involving 'DIET' Within-Subject Effect.


Mauchly sphericity test, W =        .15515
Chi-square approx. =         6.93592 with 5 D. F.
Significance =              .225

Greenhouse-Geisser Epsilon =      .62119
Huynh-Feldt Epsilon =             .97579
Lower-bound Epsilon =             .33333


- - - - - - - - -


EFFECT .. DIET
Multivariate Tests of Significance (S = 1, M = 1/2, N = 1/2)

Test Name        Value  Approx. F Hypoth. DF   Error DF  Sig. of F

Pillais         .75346   3.05611      3.00         3.00      .192
Hotellings     3.05611   3.05611      3.00         3.00      .192
Wilks           .24654   3.05611      3.00         3.00      .192
Roys            .75346


- - - - - - - - -


Tests involving 'DIET' Within-Subject Effect.

AVERAGED Tests of Significance for MEAS.1 using UNIQUE sums of squares
Source of Variation        SS      DF      MS          F  Sig of F

WITHIN CELLS              .01      15     .00
DIET                      .01       3     .00       1.85      .182
```

Figure 9.28   SPSS/PC one factor repeated measures ANOVA output for urinary oxalate excretion

different times are different? Use a 0.10 significance level for testing the hypothesis of equal population means and a 90% overall confidence level for multiple comparisons. If the hypothesis of equal population means is rejected, assume that the only comparisons of interest are those between the postpartum day 20 mean and the other postpartum means. Also assume that these comparisons were selected before examining the sample means.

14. A study investigated the effect of propranolol and nifedipine on exercise-induced attacks of chest pain in patients with variant angina.[25] Patients with variant angina were asked to exercise on a bicycle ergometer until persistent angina or ST-segment elevation occurred. Table 9.29 shows the exercise duration while taking a placebo, propranolol, or nifedipine for 15 patients with exercise-induced attack. Do the data provide evidence that some of the population exercise duration means for different drugs are different? Use a 0.01 significance level for testing the hypothesis of equal population means and a 90% overall confidence level for multiple comparisons.

15. In a study of thiopentone levels during cardiopulmonary bypass, the percentage of thiopentone not bound to plasma protein was reported for seven patients before bypass, at the cessation of bypass, and after bypass.[26] These percentages are shown in Table 9.31. Do the data provide evidence that some of the population unbound percentage means at different stages of bypass are different? Use a 0.05 significance level for testing the hypothe-

TABLE 9.24 LOGARITHM OF VT CYCLE LENGTH (log msec) FOR PATIENTS IN WHOM INDUCTION OF VT WAS NOT SUPPRESSED

| Patient No. | Procainamide Dose (mg/kg) | | | | |
	0	7.5	15	22.5	30
1	5.67	5.74	5.80	6.04	6.04
2	5.67	5.94	6.06	6.09	6.15
3	5.56	5.77	5.89	5.91	5.91
4	5.83	6.04	6.06	6.13	6.17
5	5.56	5.70	5.80	5.83	5.86
6	5.74	5.83	5.94	6.09	6.09
7	5.63	5.94	6.04	6.11	6.17
8	5.80	5.91	5.74	6.17	6.17
9	5.80	6.02	6.15	6.17	6.19
10	5.77	6.09	6.25	6.31	6.36
11	5.56	5.70	5.83	5.86	5.89
12	5.52	5.70	5.83	5.93	6.02
13	5.91	6.15	5.91	5.97	5.99
14	5.97	6.19	6.35	5.60	5.60
15	5.63	5.77	5.89	5.91	5.91
Mean ± SD	5.71 ± 0.14	5.90 ± 0.17	5.97 ± 0.18	6.01 ± 0.18	6.03 ± 0.18

TABLE 9.25 LOG VT CYCLE LENGTH DIFFERENCES

Patient No.	7.5 − 0	15 − 0	22.5 − 0	30 − 0
1	0.07	0.13	0.37	0.37
2	0.27	0.39	0.42	0.48
3	0.21	0.33	0.35	0.35
4	0.21	0.23	0.30	0.34
5	0.14	0.24	0.27	0.30
6	0.09	0.20	0.35	0.35
7	0.31	0.41	0.48	0.54
8	0.11	−0.06	0.37	0.37
9	0.22	0.35	0.37	0.39
10	0.32	0.48	0.54	0.59
11	0.14	0.27	0.30	0.33
12	0.18	0.31	0.41	0.50
13	0.24	0.00	0.06	0.08
14	0.22	0.38	−0.37	−0.37
15	0.14	0.26	0.28	0.28
Mean ± SD	0.19 ± 0.08	0.26 ± 0.15	0.30 ± 0.21	0.33 ± 0.23

```
Tests of Between-Subjects Effects.

Tests of Significance for T1 using UNIQUE sums of squares
Source of Variation           SS       DF       MS         F  Sig of F

WITHIN CELLS                 1.00      14       .07
CONSTANT                  2632.19       1   2632.19  36805.28      .000


- - - - - - - - -


Tests involving 'DOSE' Within-Subject Effect.


  Mauchly sphericity test, W =       .00272
  Chi-square approx. =          73.32498 with 9 D. F.
  Significance =                     .000

  Greenhouse-Geisser Epsilon =       .36905
  Huynh-Feldt Epsilon =              .40209
  Lower-bound Epsilon =              .25000


- - - - - - - - -


EFFECT .. DOSE
Multivariate Tests of Significance (S = 1, M = 1 , N = 4 1/2)

Test Name        Value  Approx. F Hypoth. DF   Error DF  Sig. of F

Pillais         .91687  30.33179      4.00      11.00      .000
Hotellings    11.02974  30.33179      4.00      11.00      .000
Wilks           .08313  30.33179      4.00      11.00      .000
Roys            .91687


- - - - - - - - -


Tests involving 'DOSE' Within-Subject Effect.

AVERAGED Tests of Significance for MEAS.1 using UNIQUE sums of squares
Source of Variation           SS       DF       MS         F  Sig of F

WITHIN CELLS                 1.03      56       .02
DOSE                         1.03       4       .26     14.05      .000
```

Figure 9.29 SPSS/PC one-factor repeated-measures ANOVA output for log VT cycle length

**TABLE 9.26 LOG PROVOCATION DOSE OF METHACHOLINE (LOG μg)
THAT PRODUCED A 20% FALL IN FEV_1**

Patient No.	Drug			
	BASELINE	SALINE	VERAPAMIL	SODIUM CROMOGLYCATE
1	4.09	4.17	5.35	5.01
2	4.38	4.79	4.41	3.76
3	2.89	4.20	5.04	4.87
4	4.28	4.57	4.44	3.47
5	4.01	5.44	5.19	4.91
6	3.22	3.85	4.04	4.25
7	3.81	4.09	5.50	4.06
8	2.77	3.14	3.40	2.64
9	4.44	4.41	4.96	4.72
10	4.44	4.62	5.78	6.06
11	4.55	4.87	5.39	6.23
12	4.42	4.91	5.01	4.98
13	3.74	5.46	5.75	2.83
14	2.71	3.91	5.14	5.62
15	2.89	5.58	5.70	4.44
Mean $\pm$ SD	3.78 $\pm$ 0.69	4.53 $\pm$ 0.67	5.01 $\pm$ 0.68	4.52 $\pm$ 1.06

TABLE 9.27 LOG PROVOCATION DOSE DIFFERENCES

Patient No.	Baseline − Saline	Baseline − Verapamil	Baseline − Sodium Cromoglycate
1	−0.08	−1.26	−0.92
2	−0.41	−0.03	0.62
3	−1.31	−2.15	−1.98
4	−0.29	−0.16	0.81
5	−1.43	−1.18	−0.90
6	−0.63	−0.82	−1.03
7	−0.28	−1.69	−0.25
8	−0.37	−0.63	0.13
9	0.03	−0.52	−0.28
10	−0.18	−1.34	−1.62
11	−0.32	−0.84	−1.68
12	−0.49	−0.59	−0.56
13	−1.72	−2.01	0.91
14	−1.20	−2.43	−2.91
15	−2.69	−2.81	−1.55
Mean ± SD	−0.76 ± 0.76	−1.23 ± 0.84	−0.75 ± 1.10

```
Tests of Between-Subjects Effects.

Tests of Significance for T1 using UNIQUE sums of squares
Source of Variation          SS       DF       MS         F  Sig of F

WITHIN CELLS               17.47     14      1.25
CONSTANT                 1193.71      1   1193.71    956.85     .000

- - - - - - - - -

Tests involving 'DRUG' Within-Subject Effect.


Mauchly sphericity test, W =        .42976
Chi-square approx. =          10.74430 with 5 D. F.
Significance =                   .057

Greenhouse-Geisser Epsilon =      .70234
Huynh-Feldt Epsilon =             .82977
Lower-bound Epsilon =             .33333

- - - - - - - - -


EFFECT .. DRUG
Multivariate Tests of Significance (S = 1, M = 1/2, N = 5 )

Test Name       Value  Approx. F Hypoth. DF   Error DF  Sig. of F

Pillais        .70761   9.68028     3.00       12.00      .002
Hotellings    2.42007   9.68028     3.00       12.00      .002
Wilks          .29329   9.68028     3.00       12.00      .002
Roys           .70761

- - - - - - - -


Tests involving 'DRUG' Within-Subject Effect.

AVERAGED Tests of Significance for MEAS.1 using UNIQUE sums of squares
Source of Variation          SS       DF       MS         F  Sig of F

WITHIN CELLS               17.63     42       .42
DRUG                       11.66      3      3.89       9.26     .000
```

Figure 9.30 SPSS/PC one-factor repeated-measures ANOVA output for log provocation dose

TABLE 9.28   LEAD CONCENTRATION (μmol/l) IN BREAST MILK

Subject No.	Postpartum Day				
	3	7	10	14	20
1	0.15	0.13	0.18	0.12	0.17
2	0.21	0.18	0.25	0.23	0.24
3	0.21	0.23	0.18	0.19	0.22
4	0.25	0.23	0.19	0.22	0.23
5	0.26	0.25	0.24	0.23	0.21
6	0.22	0.30	0.21	0.31	0.26
7	0.21	0.23	0.21	0.16	0.18
8	0.18	0.18	0.22	0.21	0.24
Mean ± SD	0.21 ± 0.04	0.22 ± 0.05	0.21 ± 0.03	0.21 ± 0.06	0.22 ± 0.03

```
Tests of Between-Subjects Effects.

Tests of Significance for T1 using UNIQUE sums of squares
Source of Variation      SS       DF       MS        F   Sig of F

WITHIN CELLS            .04        7       .01
CONSTANT              1.81        1      1.81    346.71      .000

- - - - - - - - -

Tests involving 'DAY' Within-Subject Effect.


Mauchly sphericity test, W =        .23187
Chi-square approx. =            7.91681 with 9 D. F.
Significance =                      .543

Greenhouse-Geisser Epsilon =       .64126
Huynh-Feldt Epsilon =             1.00000
Lower-bound Epsilon =              .25000

- - - - - - - - -

EFFECT .. DAY
Multivariate Tests of Significance (S = 1, M = 1 , N = 1 )

Test Name      Value   Approx. F Hypoth. DF   Error DF  Sig. of F

Pillais       .26176    .35457      4.00        4.00       .830
Hotellings    .35457    .35457      4.00        4.00       .830
Wilks         .73824    .35457      4.00        4.00       .830
Roys          .26176

- - - - - - - - -

Tests involving 'DAY' Within-Subject Effect.

AVERAGED Tests of Significance for MEAS.1 using UNIQUE sums of squares
Source of Variation      SS       DF       MS        F   Sig of F

WITHIN CELLS            .02       28       .00
DAY                    .00        4       .00       .17      .952
```

Figure 9.31 SPSS/PC one-factor repeated-measures ANOVA output for lead concentration

TABLE 9.29   EXERCISE DURATION (MINUTES) FOR 15 PATIENTS WITH EXERCISE-INDUCED ATTACK

| Patient No. | Drug | | |
	PLACEBO	PROPRANOLOL	NIFEDIPINE
1	2.4	3.1	8.0
2	8.6	3.0	7.3
3	4.8	2.7	10.5
4	4.2	1.8	6.4
5	7.2	1.9	9.2
6	6.4	3.8	7.6
7	5.5	5.2	7.1
8	9.8	5.3	9.2
9	1.8	3.2	5.0
10	7.5	4.1	7.9
11	7.7	4.8	5.9
12	7.8	5.3	7.9
13	4.5	3.0	5.7
14	3.9	7.5	9.6
15	4.6	6.8	7.2
Mean ± SD	5.8 ± 2.3	4.1 ± 1.7	7.6 ± 1.5

sis of equal population means and a 95% overall confidence level for multiple comparisons. If the hypothesis of equal population means is rejected, assume that the only comparisons of interest are those between the before-bypass population mean and the cessation-of-bypass and after-bypass population means. Also assume that these comparisons were selected before examining the sample means.

16. A study examined the disposition of platinum in ovarian cancer patients receiving cisplatin.[27] Table 9.33 shows the square root of the renal clearance of total plasma platinum for four consecutive six-hour intervals. These clearance values were obtained for nine ovarian cancer patients. (The data were transformed by taking square roots in order to reduce skewness and obtain more similar variances.) Do the data provide evidence that some of the population square-root clearance means for successive six-hour intervals are different? Use a 0.01 significance level for testing the hypothesis of equal population means and a 95% overall confidence level for multiple comparisons. If the hypothesis of equal population means is rejected, assume that the only comparisons of interest are those between the 0–6-hour population mean and the other population means. Also assume that these comparisons were selected before examining the sample means.

17. In a study of urinary dysfunction associated with stroke, urination control ratings were reported for 13 stroke patients on the first, 12th, and 24th

TABLE 9.30   EXERCISE DURATION DIFFERENCES

Patient No.	Placebo − Propranolol	Placebo − Nifedipine	Propranolol − Nifedipine
1	−0.7	−5.6	−4.9
2	5.6	1.3	−4.3
3	2.1	−5.7	−7.8
4	2.4	−2.2	−4.6
5	5.3	−2.0	−7.3
6	2.6	−1.2	−3.8
7	0.3	−1.6	−1.9
8	4.5	0.6	−3.9
9	−1.4	−3.2	−1.8
10	3.4	−0.4	−3.8
11	2.9	1.8	−1.1
12	2.5	−0.1	−2.6
13	1.5	−1.2	−2.7
14	−3.6	−5.7	−2.1
15	−2.2	−2.6	−0.4
Mean ± SD	1.7 ± 2.7	−1.9 ± 2.4	−3.5 ± 2.1

```
Tests of Between-Subjects Effects.

Tests of Significance for T1 using UNIQUE sums of squares
Source of Variation          SS      DF      MS          F  Sig of F

WITHIN CELLS               65.51     14    4.68
CONSTANT                 1533.58      1 1533.58      327.73     .000


- - - - - - - - -


Tests involving 'DRUG' Within-Subject Effect.


Mauchly sphericity test, W =        .91328
Chi-square approx. =               1.17927 with 2 D. F.
Significance =                      .555

Greenhouse-Geisser Epsilon =        .92020
Huynh-Feldt Epsilon =              1.00000
Lower-bound Epsilon =               .50000


- - - - - - - - -


EFFECT .. DRUG
Multivariate Tests of Significance (S = 1, M = 0, N = 5 1/2)

Test Name        Value   Approx. F Hypoth. DF   Error DF  Sig. of F

Pillais          .75934  20.50927      2.00       13.00     .000
Hotellings      3.15527  20.50927      2.00       13.00     .000
Wilks            .24066  20.50927      2.00       13.00     .000
Roys             .75934


- - - - - - - - -


Tests involving 'DRUG' Within-Subject Effect.

AVERAGED Tests of Significance for MEAS.1 using UNIQUE sums of squares
Source of Variation          SS      DF      MS          F  Sig of F

WITHIN CELLS               81.98     28    2.93
DRUG                       93.71      2   46.85       16.00     .000
```

Figure 9.32 SPSS/PC one-factor repeated-measures ANOVA output for exercise duration

TABLE 9.31 UNBOUND PERCENTAGE OF THIOPENTONE

Patient No.	Before Bypass	At Cessation of Bypass	After Bypass
1	15.1	23.3	21.3
2	17.2	21.3	21.4
3	16.7	27.7	23.3
4	19.4	22.2	22.5
5	13.3	17.1	16.3
6	17.6	25.4	20.6
7	16.8	23.0	17.8
Mean ± SD	16.6 ± 1.9	22.9 ± 3.3	20.5 ± 2.5

TABLE 9.32 UNBOUND THIOPENTONE PERCENTAGE DIFFERENCES

Patient No.	Before − At Cessation	Before − After
1	−8.2	−6.2
2	−4.1	−4.2
3	−11.0	−6.6
4	−2.8	−3.1
5	−3.8	−3.0
6	−7.8	−3.0
7	−6.2	−1.0
Mean ± SD	−6.3 ± 2.9	−3.9 ± 2.0

```
Tests of Between-Subjects Effects.

Tests of Significance for T1 using UNIQUE sums of squares
Source of Variation          SS       DF       MS          F  Sig of F

WITHIN CELLS                90.58      6      15.10
CONSTANT                  8372.02      1    8372.02     554.56    .000


- - - - - - - - -


Tests involving 'TIME' Within-Subject Effect.


Mauchly sphericity test, W =         .79668
Chi-square approx. =                1.13650 with 2 D. F.
Significance =                       .567

Greenhouse-Geisser Epsilon =         .83104
Huynh-Feldt Epsilon =               1.00000
Lower-bound Epsilon =                .50000


- - - - - - - - -


EFFECT .. TIME
Multivariate Tests of Significance (S = 1, M = 0, N = 1 1/2)

Test Name       Value  Approx. F Hypoth. DF   Error DF  Sig. of F

Pillais         .86191  15.60355      2.00       5.00      .007
Hotellings     6.24142  15.60355      2.00       5.00      .007
Wilks           .13809  15.60355      2.00       5.00      .007
Roys            .86191


- - - - - - - - -


Tests involving 'TIME' Within-Subject Effect.

AVERAGED Tests of Significance for MEAS.1 using UNIQUE sums of squares
Source of Variation          SS       DF       MS          F  Sig of F

WITHIN CELLS                36.16     12       3.01
TIME                       140.18      2      70.09      23.26    .000
```

Figure 9.33 SPSS/PC one-factor repeated-measures ANOVA output for unbound thiopentone percentage

TABLE 9.33 SQUARE-ROOT RENAL CLEARANCE (SQUARE-ROOT ml · min^{-1} · m^2) OF TOTAL PLASMA PLATINUM FOR SIX-HOUR INTERVALS

Patient No.	0–6 Hours	6–12 Hours	12–18 Hours	18–24 Hours
1	3.87	4.49	5.20	3.27
2	4.08	3.15	3.70	3.39
3	4.69	2.21	1.45	1.08
4	5.13	2.45	1.71	1.54
5	3.56	1.34	1.01	0.94
6	2.59	2.98	1.40	0.85
7	5.59	2.02	1.67	1.67
8	4.56	2.72	1.13	1.32
9	5.62	3.23	2.18	1.65
Mean ± SD	4.41 ± 0.99	2.73 ± 0.89	2.16 ± 1.39	1.75 ± 0.95

TABLE 9.34   SQUARE-ROOT RENAL CLEARANCE DIFFERENCES

Patient No.	0–6 Hours – 6–12 Hours	0–6 Hours – 12–18 Hours	0–6 Hours – 18–24 Hours
1	−0.62	−1.33	0.60
2	0.93	0.38	0.69
3	2.48	3.24	3.61
4	2.68	3.42	3.59
5	2.22	2.55	2.62
6	−0.39	1.19	1.74
7	3.57	3.92	3.92
8	1.84	3.43	3.24
9	2.39	3.44	3.97
Mean ± SD	1.68 ± 1.42	2.25 ± 1.78	2.66 ± 1.34

```
Tests of Between-Subjects Effects.

Tests of Significance for T1 using UNIQUE sums of squares
Source of Variation        SS       DF       MS        F  Sig of F

WITHIN CELLS            19.81        8     2.48
CONSTANT              274.61        1   274.61    110.90      .000

- - - - - - - - - -

Tests involving 'TIME' Within-Subject Effect.


Mauchly sphericity test, W =        .11991
Chi-square approx. =             14.25781 with 5 D. F.
Significance =                      .014

Greenhouse-Geisser Epsilon =        .48109
Huynh-Feldt Epsilon =               .55868
Lower-bound Epsilon =               .33333

- - - - - - - - - -


EFFECT .. TIME
Multivariate Tests of Significance (S = 1, M = 1/2, N = 2 )

Test Name      Value   Approx. F Hypoth. DF   Error DF  Sig. of F

Pillais        .91451  21.39547     3.00       6.00       .001
Hotellings   10.69774  21.39547     3.00       6.00       .001
Wilks          .08549  21.39547     3.00       6.00       .001
Roys           .91451

- - - - - - - - - -

Tests involving 'TIME' Within-Subject Effect.

AVERAGED Tests of Significance for MEAS.1 using UNIQUE sums of squares
Source of Variation        SS       DF       MS        F  Sig of F

WITHIN CELLS           17.11       24      .71
TIME                   36.97        3    12.32     17.28      000
```

Figure 9.34   SPSS/PC one-factor repeated-measures ANOVA output for square-root renal clearance

TABLE 9.35 URINATION CONTROL RATING FOR STROKE PATIENTS DURING HOSPITALIZATION*

Patient No.	Day 1	Day 12	Day 24
1	4	4	2
2	4	4	3
3	3	2	1
4	1	1	1
5	1	1	1
6	4	3	1
7	4	1	1
8	4	1	1
9	1	1	1
10	1	1	1
11	2	1	1
12	4	3	3
13	4	2	1
Mean ± SD	2.8 ± 1.4	1.9 ± 1.2	1.4 ± 0.8

*1 = completely in control, 2 = occasional accident, 3 = frequent accidents, 4 = never in control

day of hospitalization.[28] These ratings are shown in Table 9.35. Do the data provide evidence that some of the population mean urination control ratings for different days of hospitalization are different? Use a 0.05 significance level for testing the hypothesis of equal population means and a 90% overall confidence level for multiple comparisons.

REFERENCES

1. Platia EV, Berdoff R, Stone G, et al: Comparison of acebutolol and propranolol therapy for ventricular arrhythmias. J Clin Pharmacol 25:130–137, 1985.
2. Morrison DF: Multivariate Statistical Methods. 2nd ed. New York: McGraw-Hill, 1976.
3. Winer BJ: Statistical Principles in Experimental Design. 2nd ed. New York: McGraw-Hill, 1971.
4. Strang GW: Linear Algebra and Its Applications. 2nd ed. New York: Academic, 1980.

```
Tests of Between-Subjects Effects.

Tests of Significance for T1 using UNIQUE sums of squares
Source of Variation          SS        DF       MS        F   Sig of F

WITHIN CELLS               33.90       12      2.82
CONSTANT                  164.10        1    164.10     58.09      .000

- - - - - - - - -


Tests involving 'DAY' Within-Subject Effect.


Mauchly sphericity test, W =       .74108
Chi-square approx. =             3.29617 with 2 D. F.
Significance =                     .192

Greenhouse-Geisser Epsilon =      .79433
Huynh-Feldt Epsilon =             .89578
Lower-bound Epsilon =             .50000


- - - - - - - - - -


EFFECT .. DAY
Multivariate Tests of Significance (S = 1, M = 0, N = 4 1/2)

Test Name       Value   Approx. F Hypoth. DF   Error DF  Sig. of F

Pillais         .59475   8.07200      2.00      11.00      .007
Hotellings     1.46764   8.07200      2.00      11.00      .007
Wilks           .40525   8.07200      2.00      11.00      .007
Roys            .59475


- - - - - - - - - -


Tests involving 'DAY' Within-Subject Effect.

AVERAGED Tests of Significance for MEAS.1 using UNIQUE sums of squares
Source of Variation      .   SS        DF       MS        F  Sig of F

WITHIN CELLS               13.79       24       .57
DAY                        14.21        2      7.10     12.36      .000
```

Figure 9.35 SPSS/PC one-factor repeated-measures ANOVA output for urination control rating

5. Tong MJ, Sampliner RE, Govindarajan S, et al: Spontaneous reactivation of hepatitis B in Chinese patients with HBsAg-positive chronic active hepatitis. Hepatology 7:713–718, 1987.

6. Norusis MJ, SPSS Inc: SPSS/PC+ Advanced Statistics V3.0 for the IBM PC/XT/AT and PS/2. Chicago: SPSS, 1989.

7. Huynh H, Feldt LS: Estimation of the Box correction for degrees of freedom from sample data in randomized block and split-plot designs. J Educ Stat 1:69–82, 1976.

8. Greenhouse SW, Geisser S: On methods in the analysis of profile data. Psychometrika 24:95–112, 1959.

9. Simberkoff MS, Lukaszewski M, Cross A, et al: Antibiotic-resistant isolates of Streptococcus pneumoniae from clinical specimens: A cluster of serotype 19A organisms in Brooklyn, New York. J Infect Dis 153:78–82, 1986.

10. Vilcek J, Klion A, Henriksen-DeStefano D, et al: Defective gamma-interferon production in peripheral blood leukocytes of patients with acute tuberculosis. J Clin Immunol 6:146–151, 1986.

11. Morrison DF: The analysis of a single sample of repeated measurements. Biometrics 28:55–71, 1972.

12. Bizzarro A, Valentini G, Di Martino G, et al: Influence of testosterone therapy on clinical and immunological features of autoimmune diseases associated with Klinefelter's syndrome. J Clin Endocrinol Metab 64:32–36, 1987.

13. Attardo-Parrinello G, Merlini G, Pavesi F, et al: Effects of a new aminodiphosphonate (aminohydroxybutylidene diphosphonate) in patients with osteolytic lesions from metastases and myelomatosis. Comparison with dichloromethylene diphosphonate. Arch Intern Med 147:1629–1633, 1987.

14. Wajchenberg BL, Achando SS, Okada H, et al: Determination of the source(s) of androgen overproduction in hirsutism associated with polycystic ovary syndrome by simultaneous adrenal and ovarian venous catheterization. Comparison with the dexamethasone suppression test. J Clin Endocrinol Metab 63:1204–1210, 1986.

15. Killam PE, Apodaca L, Manella KJ, et al: Behavioral pediatric weight rehabilitation for children with myelomeningocele. MCN 8:280–286, 1983.

16. Shichiri M, Iwamoto H, Shiigai T: Diabetic renal hypouricemia. Arch Intern Med 147:225–228, 1987.

17. Schlafer DH, Mebus CA: Abortion in sows experimentally infected with African swine fever virus: Pathogenesis studies. Am J Vet Res 48:246–254, 1987.

18. Mielants H, Veys EM: HLA-B27 related arthritis and bowel inflammation. Part 1. Sulfasalazine (salazopyrin) in HLA-B27 related reactive arthritis. J Rheumatol 12:287–293, 1985.

19. Englehart J, Jensen J, Garfinkel B, et al: Clonidine and growth hormone response (correspondence). Am J Dis Child 140:186–187, 1986.

20. Evanoff GV, Thompson CS, Brown J, et al: The effect of dietary protein restriction on the progression of diabetic nephropathy. A 12-month follow-up. Arch Intern Med 147:492–495, 1987.

21. Morris GS, Simmonds HA, Toseland PA, et al: Urinary oxalate levels are not affected by dietary purine intake or allopurinol. Br J Urol 60:292–300, 1987.

22. Morady F, DiCarlo LA, de Buitleir M, et al: Effects of incremental doses of procainamide on ventricular refractoriness, intraventricular conduction, and induction of ventricular tachycardia. Circulation 74:1355–1364, 1986.

23. Boner AL, Vallone G, Andreoli A, et al: Nebulised sodium cromoglycate and verapamil in methacholine induced asthma. Arch Dis Child 62:264–268, 1987.

24. Ong CN, Phoon WO, Law HY, et al: Concentrations of lead in maternal blood, cord blood, and breast milk. Arch Dis Child 60:756–759, 1985.

25. Kugiyama K, Yasue H, Horio Y, et al: Effects of propranolol and nifedipine on exercise-induced attack in patients with variant angina: Assessment by exercise thallium-201 myocardial scintigraphy with quantitative rotational tomography. Circulation 74:374–380, 1986.

26. Morgan DJ, Crankshaw DP, Prideaux PR, et al: Thiopentone levels during cardiopulmonary bypass. Changes in plasma protein binding during continuous infusion. Anaesthesia 41:4–10, 1986.

27. Griffiths H, Shelley MD, Fish RG: A modified pharmacokinetic model for platinum disposition in ovarian cancer patients receiving cisplatin. Eur J Clin Pharmacol 33:67–72, 1987.

28. Rottcamp BC: A holistic approach to identifying factors associated with an altered pattern of urinary elimination in stroke patients. J Neurosurg Nurs 17:37–44, 1985.

10

ANALYSIS OF FREQUENCY DATA

CHAPTER OBJECTIVES

After studying this chapter and working the problems, you should be able to:

1. Carry out and interpret hypothesis tests concerning two or more population proportions, association between two variables, and differences between paired population proportions

2. Recognize data that violate assumptions required for the chi-square test of hypothesized proportions, the chi-square test of association, and the McNemar test for paired proportions

3. Interpret SPSS and SAS chi-square test output and SPSS McNemar test output

4. Determine whether chi-square tests reported in the medical and health care literature are appropriate

---

Some medical and health care data have such a small number of possible values that the normality assumption does not hold even approximately. Statistical procedures that require normality or approximate normality cannot be used to analyze such data. This rules out t tests (Chapter 7), analysis of variance (Chapters 8 and 13), repeated-measures analysis of variance (Chapter 9), and correlation and regression (Chapter 12). Other methods are needed to analyze data with only a few possible values.

Such data are usually reported by listing the number or percentage of subjects that have each value. Let us consider data from a study of pain in hospitalized cancer patients. Sixty-nine cancer patients who experienced pain at some point during hospitalization were asked to rate the severity of

their current pain according to the Present Pain Intensity Index (PPI)[1]:

0 = no pain
1 = mild pain
2 = discomforting pain
3 = distressing pain
4 = horrible pain
5 = excruciating pain

The results of this study can be summarized by listing the number or percentage of patients who reported no current pain (PPI = 0), the number or percentage of patients who reported mild current pain (PPI = 1), and so on. When the number of times each possible value occurs is reported, the resulting data are called *frequency data*. A *frequency* is the number of times a particular value or

TABLE 10.1 DISTRIBUTION OF PAIN RATING

Rating	Frequency
0	34
1	10
2	17
3	6
4	1
5	1

range of values occurs. The frequencies for the cancer pain ratings are shown in Table 10.1. From this table, we see that 34 patients had a PPI rating of 0 (no current pain), 10 patients had a PPI rating of 1 (mild current pain), and so on.

We often want to use frequency data to test hypotheses, and appropriate methods are available. The most frequently tested hypotheses concern the following.

1. Two or more population proportions
2. Association between two variables
3. Differences between paired population proportions

We will describe three methods for using frequency data to test hypotheses: the chi-square test of hypothesized proportions, the chi-square test of association, and the McNemar test for paired proportions.

10.1 HYPOTHESES ABOUT TWO OR MORE POPULATION PROPORTIONS

Suppose an oncology nurse believes that half of cancer patients with pain at some point during hospitalization would have PPI ratings equal to 0. She also believes that one-tenth of cancer patients would have each of the other PPI ratings. How can we determine whether the data in Table 10.1 provide evidence against her view?

Let us begin by stating the nurse's view about cancer pain more formally. She believes that the following proportions hold for the population of cancer patients with pain at some point during hospitalization.

Population proportion with PPI 0 rating = 0.50
Population proportion with PPI 1 rating = 0.10
Population proportion with PPI 2 rating = 0.10
Population proportion with PPI 3 rating = 0.10
Population proportion with PPI 4 rating = 0.10
Population proportion with PPI 5 rating = 0.10

Let us abbreviate these population proportions as follows: p_1 = population proportion with PPI 0 rating, p_2 = population proportion with PPI 1 rating, and so on. We want to test the null hypothesis

$$H_0: p_1 = 0.50, \; p_2 = 0.10, \; p_3 = 0.10, \qquad (10.1)$$
$$p_4 = 0.10, \; p_5 = 0.10, \; p_6 = 0.10$$

The alternative hypothesis is

H_A: At least one of the hypothesized population proportions is wrong $\qquad (10.2)$

None of the statistical procedures described in the previous chapters can be used to test the null hypothesis (10.1). The appropriate method for testing this hypothesis is the *chi-square test of hypothesized proportions*. ("Chi-square" is pronounced "kī square.") The chi-square test of hypothesized proportions is used to test hypotheses like (10.1) when frequencies have been obtained for two or more mutually exclusive categories that include all of the data. When we say that categories are mutually exclusive, we mean that no observation can be classified into more than one category. The categories "female" and "male" are mutually exclusive, since a subject cannot be both female and male. The categories "renal disease," "hepatic disease," and "cardiac disease" are not mutually exclusive, since a patient can have more than one type of disease.

If p_i is the population proportion for category i, and p_{i0} (pronounced "p sub i nought") is the *hypothesized* population proportion for category i, the general null hypothesis tested is

$$H_0: p_1 = p_{10}, \; p_2 = p_{20}, \; \ldots, \; p_k = p_{k0} \qquad (10.3)$$

where k is greater than or equal to 2. The alternative hypothesis is (10.2).

The hypothesized population proportions p_{i0} are numbers specified by the researcher. They are not derived by any statistical method. For the cancer-pain data, p_{10} is 0.50 and all of the other hypothesized population proportions are 0.10. Hypothesized population proportions are sometimes obtained from a theoretical model, such as a genetic model of inheritance. The sum of all the hypothesized proportions must equal 1 ($p_{10} + p_{20} + \cdots + p_{k0} = 1$), since the categories are mutually exclusive and include all of the data. None of the hypothesized population proportions can equal 0.

To test the null hypothesis (10.3), we need to calculate *expected frequencies*, the frequencies we would expect if all of the hypothesized population proportions were correct. Let n denote the total number of observations. The expected frequency for category i is denoted by E_i and is calculated according to the formula

$$E_i = n \times p_{i0} \qquad (10.4)$$

For the cancer-pain data, the expected frequencies are

$$E_1 = 69 \times 0.50 = 34.5$$
$$E_2 = E_3 = E_4 = E_5 = E_6 = 69 \times 0.1 = 6.9$$

The sum of the expected frequencies is always equal to n, subject to rounding error. The proof of this will be omitted. For the cancer-pain data, the sum of the expected frequencies is 34.5 + 6.9 + 6.9 + 6.9 + 6.9 + 6.9 = 69.

The *observed frequencies* are the actual frequencies obtained from the data and are denoted by O_i. For the cancer-pain data, the observed frequencies can be obtained from Table 10.1:

$$O_1 = 34 \qquad O_2 = 10 \qquad O_3 = 17$$
$$O_4 = 6 \qquad O_5 = 1 \qquad O_6 = 1$$

To test the null hypothesis (10.3), we use a χ^2 statistic (pronounced "ki square statistic") that measures the discrepancies between the observed and expected frequencies. This χ^2 statistic is calculated according to the formula

$$\chi^2 = \sum_{i=1}^{k} \frac{(O_i - E_i)^2}{E_i} \qquad (10.5)$$

We can translate this formula into steps for calculation.

STEP 1. Calculate the k expected frequencies.

STEP 2. Subtract each expected frequency from its corresponding observed frequency to get k differences. For example, E_1 is subtracted from O_1.

STEP 3. Square each of the differences obtained in step 2.

STEP 4. Divide each of the squared differences obtained in step 3 by the corresponding expected frequency. For example, $(O_3 - E_3)^2$ is divided by E_3. This produces k adjusted squared differences.

STEP 5. Add all of the adjusted squared differences obtained in step 4.

The resulting χ^2 statistic cannot be negative, since it is a sum of squares divided by positive numbers.

A calculation formula can also be used to obtain the χ^2 statistic. This formula is easier to use and always produces the same χ^2 statistic as formula (10.5), subject to rounding error. It is not obvious that both formulas give the same result, and we will omit the proof. The calculation formula is

$$\chi^2 = \left(\sum_{i=1}^{k} \frac{O_i^2}{E_i} \right) - n \qquad (10.6)$$

We can translate this formula into steps for calculation.

STEP 1. Calculate the k expected frequencies.

STEP 2. Square each observed frequency.

STEP 3. Divide each squared observed frequency by its corresponding expected frequency to obtain k adjusted squared frequencies. For example, O_2^2 is divided by E_2.

STEP 4. Add all of the adjusted squared frequencies obtained in step 3.

STEP 5. Subtract the total sample size from the sum of the adjusted squared frequencies obtained in step 4.

Why does the χ^2 statistic make sense as a test of the null hypothesis (10.3)? Let us examine formula (10.5) more closely. The differences $O_i - E_i$ measure the discrepancies between the observed frequencies and the expected frequencies. By squaring these differences, we prevent positive and negative differences from canceling each other. When we divide each squared difference by the corresponding expected frequency, we take the size of the expected frequencies into account and thereby standardize the squared differences. A difference $O_i - E_i$ of 141 is large if the expected frequency is equal to 180, but the same difference is small if the expected frequency is equal to 8100. Dividing by E_i takes this into account.

A large χ^2 statistic indicates large discrepancies between the observed and expected frequencies. A small χ^2 statistic indicates small discrepancies between the observed and expected frequencies. Thus, a large χ^2 statistic provides evidence against the null hypothesis (10.3). A small χ^2 statistic does not provide evidence against this hypothesis.

How large does a χ^2 statistic have to be to justify rejection of the null hypothesis (10.3)? As usual, this is determined by the p-value associated with the statistic. If the χ^2 statistic is so large that its p-value is less than the significance level α, we reject the null hypothesis (10.3). If the p-value is greater than or equal to α, we cannot reject this hypothesis. The p-value is interpreted in the usual way: it is the probability of getting a χ^2 statistic at least as extreme as the calculated χ^2 statistic if the null hypothesis (10.3) is true.

To obtain p-values, we need to know the distribution of the χ^2 statistic. It can be shown that this statistic has an approximate chi-square distribution with $k - 1$ degrees of freedom (df) if the null hypothesis (10.3) is true and certain assumptions are satisfied. Chi-square distributions are skewed distributions with frequency curves determined by their degrees of freedom. Random variables with chi-square distributions cannot have negative values. The frequency curves for three chi-square distributions are shown in Figure 10.1.

The p-value for the χ^2 statistic (10.5) is given by the probability

$$P\left(\chi^2 \text{ statistic} \geq \chi^2_{\text{calc}} \right)$$

where χ^2_{calc} is the calculated χ^2 statistic. Approximate p-values can be obtained from Table E.7 in Appendix E. This table is based on upper percentage points of chi-square distributions. If χ^2_d is a random variable having a chi-square distribution with d degrees of freedom, the α upper percentage point of this distribution is the number $\chi^2_{\alpha, d}$ such that

$$P\left(\chi^2_d \geq \chi^2_{\alpha, d} \right) = \alpha$$

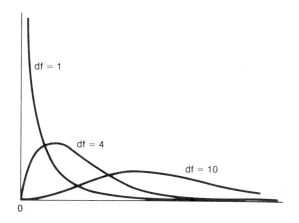

Figure 10.1 Chi-square distributions with 1, 4, and 10 degrees of freedom.

Since Table E.7 only lists upper percentage points for selected probabilities, we cannot get exact p-values from this table.

To obtain approximate p-values from Table E.7, we first locate the row for our degrees of freedom. We then find two adjacent numbers in this row such that χ^2_{calc} lies between them, if possible. These numbers are upper percentage points, and the p-value lies between the probabilities to which they correspond. If χ^2_{calc} is very large, it will be larger than any of the appropriate upper percentage points given in the table. When this happens, we find the largest upper percentage point in the appropriate row. The p-value is *less* than the corresponding probability. If χ^2_{calc} is very small, it will be smaller than any of the appropriate upper percentage points listed. In this case, we find the smallest upper percentage point in the appropriate row. The p-value is *greater* than the corresponding probability. These possibilities are illustrated in the following example.

Example 10.1

What are the p-values for the following calculated χ^2 statistics?

1. $\chi^2_{calc} = 9.87$, three categories. The degrees of freedom are $3 - 1 = 2$. In the row for 2 df, 9.87 lies between 9.210 and 10.597. Since these values are the 0.01 and 0.005 upper percentage points of the chi-square distribution with 2 df,

$$0.005 < p\text{-value} < 0.01$$

2. $\chi^2_{calc} = 38.71$, four categories. The degrees of freedom are $4 - 1 = 3$. The largest value in the row for 3 df is 17.730. Since this value is the 0.0005 upper percentage point and 38.71 is greater than 17.730,

$$p\text{-value} < 0.0005$$

3. $\chi^2_{calc} = 0.11$, six categories. The degrees of freedom are $6 - 1 = 5$. The smallest value in the row for 5 df is 0.158. Since this value is the 0.9995

upper percentage point and 0.11 is less than 0.158,

$$p\text{-value} > 0.9995$$

4. $\chi^2_{calc} = 2.71$, two categories. The degrees of freedom are $2 - 1 = 1$. In the row for 1 df, the value 2.706 is quite close to 2.71. Since 2.706 is the 0.10 upper percentage point,

$$p\text{-value} \cong 0.10$$

Chi-square tests of hypothesized proportions are always two-sided, in the sense that one-sided alternative hypotheses cannot be used. But the p-values are always one-tailed, involving only the upper tail of the chi-square distribution. The test is performed in this way because it makes sense to reject the null hypothesis (10.3) only when the χ^2 statistic is large. A small χ^2 statistic does not provide evidence against this hypothesis. When two-sided t tests or Z tests are done, two-tailed p-values are obtained because extreme positive *or* extreme negative statistics provide evidence against the null hypothesis.

The chi-square test of hypothesized proportions requires the following assumptions about the data.

1. Random Sampling. If the sample is not biased, random sampling is not crucial.

2. Independent Observations. The chi-square test of hypothesized proportions cannot be done if independence does not hold.

3. Mutually Exclusive Categories That Include All Observations. If categories overlap or fail to include all of the data, the chi-square test of hypothesized proportions cannot be done.

4. Sufficiently Large Expected Frequencies. The chi-square test of hypothesized proportions is based on an approximation that works best when the *expected* frequencies are fairly large. A rough guide is given by the following rule: No expected frequency should be less than 1, and no more than 20% of the expected frequencies should be less than 5. If this does not hold, categories can sometimes be combined to make the expected frequencies larger. No assumptions are made about the size of the *observed* frequencies.

Let us evaluate these assumptions for the cancer-pain data. Random sampling was not done, but this is not essential. The independence assumption is reasonable, since one patient's PPI rating tells us nothing about another patient's PPI rating. The PPI categories are mutually exclusive and include all of the patient ratings. All of the expected frequencies given on p. 206 are greater than 5. The chi-square test is appropriate for testing the null hypothesis (10.1). We will use a 0.01 significance level.

Only one formula is needed to obtain the χ^2 statistic, but we will apply both formulas to illustrate their use. Using formula (10.5), the observed frequencies in Table 10.1, and the expected frequencies on p. 206, we get

$$\chi^2 = \frac{(34 - 34.5)^2}{34.5} + \frac{(10 - 6.9)^2}{6.9} + \frac{(17 - 6.9)^2}{6.9}$$
$$+ \frac{(6 - 6.9)^2}{6.9} + \frac{(1 - 6.9)^2}{6.9} + \frac{(1 - 6.9)^2}{6.9}$$
$$= \frac{0.25}{34.5} + \frac{9.61}{6.9} + \frac{102.01}{6.9} + \frac{0.81}{6.9}$$
$$+ \frac{34.81}{6.9} + \frac{34.81}{6.9}$$
$$= 0.007 + 1.393 + 14.784 + 0.117$$
$$+ 5.045 + 5.045$$
$$= 26.391$$

Using formula (10.6) and the same observed and expected frequencies, we get

$$\chi^2 = \left(\frac{34^2}{34.5} + \frac{10^2}{6.9} + \frac{17^2}{6.9} + \frac{6^2}{6.9} + \frac{1^2}{6.9} + \frac{1^2}{6.9} \right) - 69$$
$$= (33.507 + 14.493 + 41.884 + 5.217$$
$$+ 0.145 + 0.145) - 69$$
$$= 95.391 - 69 = 26.391$$

Since there are six categories, the degrees of freedom are $6 - 1 = 5$. In the row for 5 df in Table E.7, the largest value is 22.105. Since this value is the 0.0005 upper percentage point and 26.391 is larger than 22.105, the approximate *p*-value is

$$p\text{-value} < 0.0005$$

We reject the null hypothesis (10.1) at the 0.01 significance level and conclude that at least one of the hypothesized population proportions is wrong.

Example 10.2

A study of pediatric eye injuries reported the frequency of eye injuries for each season, based on a sample of 278 children with eye injuries.[2] These

TABLE 10.2 DISTRIBUTION OF SEASON DURING WHICH EYE INJURY OCCURRED

Season	Frequency
Winter (December–February)	55
Spring (March–May)	86
Summer (June–August)	70
Fall (September–November)	67

frequencies are shown in Table 10.2. Can the chi-square test of hypothesized proportions be used to test the hypothesis that the chance of pediatric eye injuries is the same for all four seasons? Let p_1 be the population proportion of eye injuries occurring during the winter, p_2 the population proportion of eye injuries occurring during the spring, p_3 the population proportion of eye injuries occurring during the summer, and p_4 the population proportion of eye injuries occurring during the fall. We want to test the null hypothesis

$$H_0: p_1 = 0.25, \; p_2 = 0.25, \\ p_3 = 0.25, \; p_4 = 0.25 \qquad (10.7)$$

The alternative hypothesis is (10.2).

Let us determine whether the required assumptions hold. The data are not a random sample, but this is not essential. Independence appears to hold, since the seasonal classification of one child provides no information about the seasonal classification of another child. The categories are mutually exclusive and include all of the data. The expected frequencies are large enough, since all are equal to $278 \times 0.25 = 69.5$. The chi-square test of hypothesized proportions is appropriate. We will use a 0.05 significance level.

Using formula (10.5), the observed frequencies in Table 10.2, and the expected frequencies of 69.5, we get

$$\chi^2 = \frac{(55 - 69.5)^2}{69.5} + \frac{(86 - 69.5)^2}{69.5}$$
$$+ \frac{(70 - 69.5)^2}{69.5} + \frac{(67 - 69.5)^2}{69.5}$$
$$= \frac{210.25}{69.5} + \frac{272.25}{69.5} + \frac{0.25}{69.5} + \frac{6.25}{69.5}$$
$$= 3.025 + 3.917 + 0.004 + 0.090$$
$$= 7.036$$

Using formula (10.6), we get

$$\chi^2 = \left(\frac{55^2}{69.5} + \frac{86^2}{69.5} + \frac{70^2}{69.5} + \frac{67^2}{69.5} \right) - 278$$
$$= (43.525 + 106.417 + 70.504 + 64.590) - 278$$
$$= 285.036 - 278 = 7.036$$

TABLE 10.3   DISTRIBUTION OF VACCINATION RESPONSES

Reaction	Frequency
No reaction	754
Type I reactions	141
Type II reactions	160
Type III reactions	21

There are four categories, so the degrees of freedom are $4 - 1 = 3$. In the row for 3 df in Table E.7, 7.036 lies between the numbers 6.251 and 7.815. Since these are the 0.10 and 0.05 upper percentage points, the approximate p-value is

$$0.05 < p\text{-value} < 0.10$$

We cannot reject the null hypothesis (10.7) at the 0.05 significance level. The data do not provide evidence that pediatric eye injuries are more likely in some seasons than in others.

Example 10.3

In a study of adverse reactions to feline leukemia vaccination, responses to 1029 vaccinations in 679 cats were monitored.[3] There were 322 vaccination reactions, classified as follows:

Type I reactions: discomfort or pain on injection
Type II reactions: systemic reactions, including depression, lethargy, inappetence, and pyrexia
Type III reactions: hypersensitivity, usually expressed as vomiting, edema, erythema, and cyanosis

The frequencies for vaccination responses are shown in Table 10.3.

Suppose a vaccine manufacturer reported the following proportions of vaccination responses.

No reaction: 0.935
Type I reactions: 0.090
Type II reactions: 0.031
Type III reactions: 0.004

Can we use the frequencies in Table 10.3 to test the hypothesis that the population proportions of vaccination responses are equal to the manufacturer's proportions? Since there are more vaccinations than cats, some of the cats were vaccinated more than once. A cat's responses to several vaccinations cannot be considered independent, so the independence assumption is not reasonable for these data. In addition, a cat can have more than one type of reaction, so the reaction type categories are not mutually exclusive.* The chi-square test of hypothe-

sized proportions cannot be used to analyze these data.

If more information were available, we could divide the data into first vaccination responses, second vaccination responses, and third vaccination responses. We could then carry out one-sample Z tests if the resulting samples were large enough. For each set of vaccination responses, we could use the one-sample Z test to test the hypothesis that the population proportion of cats with no reaction to first vaccination is 0.935, then use the one-sample Z test again to test the hypothesis that the population proportion of cats with Type I reactions to first vaccination is 0.090, and so on. This would result in a total of 12 one-sample Z tests, so a Bonferroni adjustment of the significance level would be needed. This adjustment could be obtained by dividing the desired overall significance level by 12.

Example 10.4

A study investigated 14 cases of hemolytic-uremic syndrome.[4] Of the 14 patients, one was black, one was Hispanic, and 12 were white. A physician believes that the racial proportions of hemolytic-uremic syndrome cases for the population of blacks, Hispanics, and whites are black, 0.05; Hispanic, 0.05; and white, 0.90. Can the chi-square test of hypothesized proportions be used to determine whether the data provide evidence against her view?

The independence assumption is reasonable, but the expected frequencies are too small. Blacks and Hispanics have the same expected frequency of 0.7 (14×0.05), which is less than 1. Only the expected frequency for whites is at least 5 ($14 \times 0.90 = 12.6$), so 67% of the expected frequencies are less than 5. If the black and Hispanic categories are combined into one black-or-Hispanic category, the hypothesized proportion for the combined category is 0.05 + 0.05 = 0.10. The expected frequency for the combined category is $14 \times 0.10 = 1.4$, which is still too small. Fifty percent of the expected frequencies are less than 5, so combining categories does not help. The chi-square test of hypothesized proportions cannot be used to analyze these data. More data need to be obtained to increase the expected frequencies.

10.2   HYPOTHESES ABOUT ASSOCIATION BETWEEN TWO VARIABLES

Medical and health care research frequently concerns the question of whether two variables are related. When one or both variables are continuous, regression analysis and correlation coefficients (Chapter 12) can often be used to measure certain types of association. When one variable is continuous and the other is a discrete variable that represents group membership or time period, methods for comparing means (Chapters 7, 8, 9, and 13) are

---

*Overlapping categories account for the fact that the total number of responses in Table 10.3 (1076) is greater than the total number of vaccinations (1029). They also account for the fact that the sum of the manufacturer's proportions (1.060) is greater than 1.

TABLE 10.4 DISTRIBUTION OF WOMEN ACCORDING TO POSITION AND DIFFICULTY OF BEARING-DOWN EFFORTS

Position	Bearing-Down Efforts		
	EASY	AVERAGE	DIFFICULT
Sitting	19	10	8
Supine	6	5	12

often appropriate. When both variables are discrete, with only a few possible values, none of these methods is appropriate. Instead, the *chi-square test of association* can often be used to test the hypothesis that the variables are not related.

Suppose a study investigates whether presurgery anxiety scores are related to sex. If anxiety is measured as a continuous variable (e.g., with a visual analog scale), methods for comparing means might be used to determine whether the population anxiety score means differ for women and men. If anxiety is measured with discrete ratings having only a few possible values (e.g., 1 = not anxious, 2 = slightly anxious, 3 = moderately anxious, 4 = extremely anxious), methods for comparing means cannot be used. In this case, the chi-square test of association should be considered for testing the hypothesis that anxiety rating and sex are not related.

Like the chi-square test of hypothesized proportions, the chi-square test of association is based on a χ^2 statistic that compares observed and expected frequencies. The observed frequencies are obtained from a *contingency table*, a table obtained by cross-classifying the data according to the variables of interest. We have already worked with contingency tables in Chapter 3, although we did not use this term.

Table 10.4 shows a contingency table that cross-classifies 60 nulliparous women in labor according to position during labor (sitting, supine) and the woman's rating of the difficulty of bearing-down efforts in the second stage of labor (easy, average, difficult).[5] From this table, we see that 19 women in the sitting position found bearing-down efforts easy, six women in the supine position found bearing-down efforts easy, 10 women in the sitting position found bearing-down efforts average, and so on.

We would like to test the null hypothesis that there is no association between position and difficulty of bearing-down efforts.

H_0: There is no association between position and difficulty of bearing-down efforts (10.8)

The alternative hypothesis states that position and difficulty of bearing-down efforts are associated.

H_A: There is an association between position and difficulty of bearing-down efforts (10.9)

The variable whose categories are listed in the rows of a contingency table is called the *row variable*. The variable whose categories are listed in the columns of a contingency table is called the *column variable*. In Table 10.4, position is the row variable and difficulty of bearing-down efforts is the column variable. The terms "row variable" and "column variable" are merely convenient tags for distinguishing between the variables. The choice of row and column variables is irrelevant as far as statistics is concerned; it affects only the format of the table. We will denote the number of row variable categories by r and the number of column variable categories by c.

The general null hypothesis tested by the chi-square test of association is the hypothesis of no association between the row variable and the column variable.

H_0: There is no association between the row variable and the column variable (10.10)

The general alternative hypothesis states that association between the row variable and the column variable is present.

H_A: There is an association between the row variable and the column variable (10.11)

To calculate the χ^2 statistic for testing the null hypothesis (10.10), we need to calculate *row totals* and *column totals* for the contingency table. The row total for a row in a contingency table is obtained by adding all of the frequencies in that row. For Table 10.4, the row totals are

$$\text{row 1 total} = 19 + 10 + 8 = 37$$
$$\text{row 2 total} = 6 + 5 + 12 = 23$$

The column total for a column in a contingency table is obtained by adding all of the frequencies in that column. For Table 10.4, the column totals are

$$\text{column 1 total} = 19 + 6 = 25$$
$$\text{column 2 total} = 10 + 5 = 15$$
$$\text{column 3 total} = 8 + 12 = 20$$

The sum of all the row totals is always equal to the sample size n, and the sum of all the column totals is always equal to n.

Row and column totals are used to calculate expected frequencies under the assumption that the hypothesis of no association is true. The expected frequency for the ith category of the row variable and the jth category of the column variable is denoted by E_{ij} and is calculated as follows:

$$E_{ij} = \frac{(\text{row } i \text{ total})(\text{row } j \text{ total})}{n} \quad (10.12)$$

It is not obvious why this formula gives the frequencies expected when the null hypothesis (10.10) is true, and the proof will be omitted. The sum of all the expected frequencies is always equal to n, subject to rounding error. Again, the proof will be omitted. The total number of expected frequencies is $r \times c$.

For the labor data, the expected frequencies are

$$E_{11} = \frac{(\text{row 1 total})(\text{column 1 total})}{60}$$
$$= \frac{(37)(25)}{60} = 15.4$$

$$E_{12} = \frac{(\text{row 1 total})(\text{column 2 total})}{60}$$
$$= \frac{(37)(15)}{60} = 9.2$$

$$E_{13} = \frac{(\text{row 1 total})(\text{column 3 total})}{60}$$
$$= \frac{(37)(20)}{60} = 12.3$$

$$E_{21} = \frac{(\text{row 2 total})(\text{column 1 total})}{60}$$
$$= \frac{(23)(25)}{60} = 9.6$$

$$E_{22} = \frac{(\text{row 2 total})(\text{column 2 total})}{60}$$
$$= \frac{(23)(15)}{60} = 5.8$$

$$E_{23} = \frac{(\text{row 2 total})(\text{column 3 total})}{60}$$
$$= \frac{(23)(20)}{60} = 7.7$$

The observed frequencies are the actual frequencies in the contingency table. The observed frequency for the ith category of the row variable and the jth category of the column variable is denoted by O_{ij}. For the labor data, the observed frequencies are

$$O_{11} = 19 \qquad O_{12} = 10 \qquad O_{13} = 8$$
$$O_{21} = 6 \qquad O_{22} = 5 \qquad O_{23} = 12$$

The χ^2 statistic for testing the null hypothesis (10.10) can be calculated according to the formula

$$\chi^2 = \sum_{\text{all } i,\, j} \frac{(O_{ij} - E_{ij})^2}{E_{ij}} \qquad (10.13)$$

We can translate this formula into steps for calculation.

STEP 1.   Calculate all of the expected frequencies.

STEP 2.   Subtract each expected frequency from its corresponding observed frequency to get $r \times c$ differences. For example, E_{11} is subtracted from O_{11}.

STEP 3.   Square each of the differences obtained in step 2.

STEP 4.   Divide each of the squared differences obtained in step 3 by the corresponding expected frequency. For example, $(O_{21} - E_{21})^2$ is divided by E_{21}. This produces $r \times c$ adjusted squared differences.

STEP 5.   Add all of the adjusted squared differences obtained in step 4.

The resulting χ^2 statistic cannot be negative, since it is a sum of squares divided by positive numbers.*

A calculation formula can also be used to obtain the χ^2 statistic. This formula is easier to use and always produces the same χ^2 statistic as formula (10.13), subject to rounding error. It is not obvious that both formulas give the same results, and we will omit the proof. The calculation formula is given by

$$\chi^2 = \left(\sum_{\text{all } i,\, j} \frac{O_{ij}^2}{E_{ij}} \right) - n \qquad (10.14)$$

We can translate this formula into steps for calculation.

STEP 1.   Calculate the $r \times c$ expected frequencies.

STEP 2.   Square each observed frequency.

STEP 3.   Divide each squared observed frequency by its corresponding expected frequency to obtain $r \times c$ adjusted squared frequencies. For example, O_{22}^2 is divided by E_{22}.

STEP 4.   Add all of the adjusted squared frequencies obtained in step 3.

STEP 5.   Subtract the total sample size from the sum of the adjusted squared frequencies obtained in step 4.

Since the χ^2 statistic (10.13) is large when some of the discrepancies between the observed and expected frequencies are large, we reject the null hypothesis (10.10) when the χ^2 statistic is large. A small χ^2 statistic does not provide evidence against this hypothesis.

---

*When both the row and column variables have only two categories, a χ^2 statistic called the *Yates-corrected χ^2 statistic* is sometimes used instead of the χ^2 statistic (10.13). The Yates-corrected χ^2 statistic tends to produce p-values that are too large,[6] and we do not recommend its use. Further information about the Yates-corrected χ^2 statistic can be found in other texts.[7]

The p-value for the χ^2 statistic (10.13) is given by the probability

$$P\left(\chi^2 \text{ statistic} \geq \chi^2_{\text{calc}}\right)$$

where χ^2_{calc} is the calculated χ^2 statistic. We use this p-value to determine whether the χ^2 statistic is large enough to warrant rejection of the null hypothesis (10.10). If the p-value is less than the significance level α, we reject this hypothesis. If the p-value is greater than or equal to α, we cannot reject this hypothesis. The p-value is interpreted in the usual way: it is the probability of getting a χ^2 statistic at least as extreme as the calculated χ^2 statistic if the null hypothesis (10.10) is true.

It can be shown that the χ^2 statistic (10.13) has an approximate chi-square distribution with $(r - 1)(c - 1)$ degrees of freedom if the null hypothesis (10.10) is true and certain assumptions are met. Approximate p-values for the χ^2 statistic are obtained from Table E.7 in essentially the same way as described in Section 10.1. Only the degrees of freedom are different.

The chi-square test of association requires the following assumptions about the data.

1. Random Sampling. As usual, random sampling is not required if the sample is not biased.

2. Independent Observations. If the observations are not all independent, the chi-square test of association cannot be done. Misuse of the chi-square test of association to analyze frequencies from non-independent data is a common error in the medical and health care literature.

3. Mutually Exclusive Row and Column Variable Categories That Include All Observations. The chi-square test of association cannot be done when categories overlap or fail to include all of the data.

4. Sufficiently Large Expected Frequencies. The chi-square test of association is based on an approximation that works best when the *expected* frequencies are fairly large. A rough guide is given by the following rule: No expected frequency should be less than 1, and no more than 20% of the expected frequencies should be less than 5. If this does not hold, row or column variable categories can sometimes be combined to make the expected frequencies larger. No assumptions are made about the size of the *observed* frequencies.*

Let us evaluate these assumptions for the labor data. Random sampling was not done, but this is

---

*Another test, called *Fisher's exact test*, is sometimes used when the expected frequencies are small and both variables have only two categories. Unfortunately, Fisher's exact test works only if the row and column totals never change when the sample changes.[8] Because the assumption of constant row and column totals almost never holds in practice, we do not recommend the use of this test.

not essential. The independence assumption is reasonable, since one woman's response tells us nothing about another woman's response. The categories for difficulty of bearing-down efforts are mutually exclusive and include all of the women's responses. The position categories are also mutually exclusive and include all of the responses. None of the expected frequencies on p. 212 are less than 5. The chi-square test of association is appropriate for testing the null hypothesis (10.8). We will use a 0.05 significance level.

Only one formula is needed to calculate our χ^2 statistic, but we will use both formulas to illustrate their use. Applying formula (10.13), with the observed frequencies in Table 10.4 and the expected frequencies on p. 212, we get

$$
\begin{aligned}
\chi^2 &= \frac{(19 - 15.4)^2}{15.4} + \frac{(10 - 9.2)^2}{9.2} + \frac{(8 - 12.3)^2}{12.3} \\
&\quad + \frac{(6 - 9.6)^2}{9.6} + \frac{(5 - 5.8)^2}{5.8} + \frac{(12 - 7.7)^2}{7.7} \\
&= \frac{12.96}{15.4} + \frac{0.64}{9.2} + \frac{18.49}{12.3} + \frac{12.96}{9.6} \\
&\quad + \frac{0.64}{5.8} + \frac{18.49}{7.7} \\
&= 0.842 + 0.070 + 1.503 + 1.350 \\
&\quad + 0.110 + 2.401 \\
&= 6.276
\end{aligned}
$$

Applying formula (10.14), we get

$$
\begin{aligned}
\chi^2 &= \left(\frac{19^2}{15.4} + \frac{10^2}{9.2} + \frac{8^2}{12.3} + \frac{6^2}{9.6} + \frac{5^2}{5.8} + \frac{12^2}{7.7} \right) - 60 \\
&= (23.442 + 10.870 + 5.203 + 3.750 \\
&\quad + 4.310 + 18.701) - 60 \\
&= 66.276 - 60 = 6.276
\end{aligned}
$$

The position variable has two categories ($r = 2$) and the variable representing difficulty of bearing-down efforts has three categories ($c = 3$), so the degrees of freedom are $(2 - 1)(3 - 1) = 2$. In the row for 2 df in Table E.7, 6.276 lies between the numbers 5.991 and 7.378. Since these values are the 0.05 and 0.025 upper percentage points, the approximate p-value is

$$0.025 < p\text{-value} < 0.05$$

We reject the null hypothesis (10.8) at the 0.05 significance level and conclude that position and ease of bearing-down efforts are associated. We will discuss methods for determining the nature of the association shortly.

Example 10.5 _____

A study investigated the efficacy of high-voltage shock for the treatment of venomous snakebites.[9] Table 10.5 cross-classifies 41 snakebite patients ac-

TABLE 10.5 DISTRIBUTION OF PATIENTS ACCORDING TO OUTCOME AND SHOCK TREATMENT

Outcome	Shock Treatment	
	GIVEN	REFUSED
Snakebite complications	0	7
No snakebite complications	34	0

cording to two variables: shock treatment (given, refused) and outcome (snakebite complications, no snakebite complications). Can the chi-square test of association be used to test the hypothesis that there is no association between shock treatment and outcome?

The independence assumption is reasonable, and both variables have mutually exclusive categories that include all of the data. One of the expected frequencies is much less than 5, however: $E_{12} = (7 \times 7)/41 = 1.20$. Since there are only four expected frequencies, 25% of the expected frequencies are less than 5. The chi-square test of association should not be used to analyze these data. More data are needed to increase the size of the expected frequencies.

Example 10.6

In a study of phlebitis at intravenous (IV) catheter sites, 7134 IVs were started and evaluated.[10] Table 10.6 cross-classifies IV catheterizations according to two variables: type of catheter and phlebitis rating. The higher the phlebitis rating, the more severe the phlebitis. A phlebitis rating of 0 indicates that phlebitis was not present. Can the chi-square test of association be used to test the hypothesis that there is no association between the type of catheter and the phlebitis rating?

Because the data are based on IV catheterizations and not patients, the independence assumption is questionable. It seems likely that some patients were catheterized several times, and the phlebitis ratings for the same patient cannot be considered independent. Unless one catheterization was done per patient, the chi-square test of association cannot be used to analyze these data. If we

TABLE 10.6 DISTRIBUTION OF IV CATHETERIZATIONS ACCORDING TO TYPE OF CATHETER AND PHLEBITIS RATING

Type of Catheter	Phlebitis Rating					
	0	1	2	3	4	5
Abbott thick-wall	1090	113	159	11	3	0
Terumo thin-wall	1241	108	161	11	3	0
Deseret thick-wall	1199	101	99	7	0	0
Critikon thin-wall	1130	125	162	9	4	1
Becton-Dickinson thick-wall	1109	131	142	9	6	0

knew which ratings belonged to each patient, we could split the data according to first catheterization, second catheterization, and so on. All of the ratings for a given catheterization would be independent. Separate chi-square tests of association could then be done for each set of ratings for a catheterization if the expected frequencies were large enough.

If the hypothesis of no association cannot be rejected, the analysis is finished. If this hypothesis is rejected, further analysis is needed to determine the nature of the association. This is done by examining *row percentages* or *column percentages*. The row percentage for category i of the row variable and category j of the column variable is denoted by row pct_{ij} and is calculated as follows:

$$\text{row pct}_{ij} = \frac{O_{ij}}{\text{row } i \text{ total}} \times 100 \qquad (10.15)$$

The column percentage for category i of the row variable and category j of the column variable is denoted by column pct_{ij} and is calculated as follows:

$$\text{column pct}_{ij} = \frac{O_{ij}}{\text{column } j \text{ total}} \times 100 \qquad (10.16)$$

For the labor data, we can use the observed frequencies in Table 10.4 and the row totals on p. 211 to obtain the row percentages.

$$\text{row pct}_{11} = \frac{19}{37} \times 100 = 51.4\%$$

$$\text{row pct}_{12} = \frac{10}{37} \times 100 = 27.0\%$$

$$\text{row pct}_{13} = \frac{8}{37} \times 100 = 21.6\%$$

$$\text{row pct}_{21} = \frac{6}{23} \times 100 = 26.1\%$$

$$\text{row pct}_{22} = \frac{5}{23} \times 100 = 21.7\%$$

$$\text{row pct}_{23} = \frac{12}{23} \times 100 = 52.2\%$$

The column percentages for the labor data can be obtained from the observed frequencies in Table 10.4 and the column totals on p. 211.

$$\text{column pct}_{11} = \frac{19}{25} \times 100 = 76.0\%$$

$$\text{column pct}_{12} = \frac{10}{15} \times 100 = 66.7\%$$

$$\text{column pct}_{13} = \frac{8}{20} \times 100 = 40.0\%$$

$$\text{column pct}_{21} = \frac{6}{25} \times 100 = 24.0\%$$

$$\text{column pct}_{22} = \frac{5}{15} \times 100 = 33.3\%$$

$$\text{column pct}_{23} = \frac{12}{20} \times 10 = 60.0\%$$

Which percentages do we look at to determine the nature of the association? In many studies, one of the classification variables is an *independent variable*, a variable controlled by the researcher. For the labor data, the position variable is the independent variable. The researchers determined which position each woman used. They could not control the difficulty of bearing-down efforts. If the independent variable is the row variable, row percentages are examined to determine the nature of the association. If the independent variable is the column variable, column percentages are examined to determine the nature of the association.

In some studies, neither variable is controlled by the researcher and there is no independent variable. Suppose that the relationship between sex and smoking status is examined. Neither sex nor smoking status is an independent variable, since neither can be controlled by the researcher. But if sex is the row variable, it usually makes sense to examine row percentages rather than column percentages. Smoking status can be considered a response, whereas sex is not a response. By looking at row percentages, we are examining the estimated probability of smoking, given that a person is female, the estimated probability of smoking, given that a person is male, and so on. This makes more sense than examining the estimated probability of being female, given that a person smokes, the estimated probability of being female, given that a person does not smoke, and so on.

When one variable can be considered a response and the other variable cannot be considered a response, we usually base our percentages on the nonresponse variable. If the nonresponse variable is the row variable, row percentages are examined to determine the nature of the association. If the non-response variable is the column variable, column percentages are examined to determine the nature of the association.

Sometimes neither variable is a response variable or both variables are response variables. For data such as these, the choice of row or column percentages is often a matter of personal taste. A study might investigate whether agreement with one questionnaire statement is related to agreement with another questionnaire statement. Both of the agreement variables are responses, so row or column percentages cannot be selected in terms of the nonresponse variable. In this study, the choice of row or column percentages might be completely arbitrary.

TABLE 10.7   ROW PERCENTAGES FOR TABLE 10.4

Position	Bearing-Down Efforts		
	EASY	AVERAGE	DIFFICULT
Sitting	51.4%	27.0%	21.6%
Supine	26.1%	21.7%	52.2%

Let us examine the row percentages for the labor data to determine the nature of the association between position and difficulty of bearing-down efforts. These percentages are shown in Table 10.7. The row percentages indicate that women in the sitting position are more likely than women in the supine position to find bearing-down efforts easy and less likely to find bearing-down efforts difficult. There is little difference between the two positions for the average difficulty rating. Thus, the data suggest that bearing-down efforts tend to be easier in the sitting position than in the supine position.

When the hypothesis of no association is rejected, we cannot conclude that a causal relationship exists between the variables. *Association never implies causation.* Although association is necessary to show causation, it is not sufficient. When interpreting the labor study, we can say only that the sitting position is associated with easier bearing-down efforts; we cannot say that it is responsible for easier bearing-down efforts. It is possible that some other variable associated with the sitting position is responsible for easier bearing-down efforts. For example, women who used the sitting position might have had more homelike surroundings than women who used the supine position. The women's surroundings and not their positions might be responsible for the difference in difficulty of bearing-down efforts.

10.3   HYPOTHESES ABOUT DIFFERENCES BETWEEN PAIRED POPULATION PROPORTIONS

In a double-blind study of aspartame and headaches, 40 subjects were given aspartame and a placebo at different times.[11] All of these subjects had reported that headaches occurred after consuming products containing aspartame. Table 10.8 shows the number of subjects who reported headaches after consuming aspartame during the

TABLE 10.8   NUMBERS OF SUBJECTS REPORTING HEADACHES AFTER INGESTING PLACEBO OR ASPARTAME

Substance	Headache	
	PRESENT	NOT PRESENT
Placebo	18	22
Aspartame	14	26

TABLE 10.9   DISTRIBUTION OF SUBJECTS ACCORDING TO HEADACHE STATUS AFTER PLACEBO OR ASPARTAME

	Aspartame	
Placebo	HEADACHE	NO HEADACHE
Headache	6	12
No headache	8	14

TABLE 10.10   DISTRIBUTION OF SUBJECTS ACCORDING TO OCCURRENCE OF EVENT FOR SAMPLE 1 AND SAMPLE 2

	Sample 1	
Sample 2	EVENT OCCURS	EVENT DOES NOT OCCUR
Event occurs	O_{11}	O_{12}
Event does not occur	O_{21}	O_{22}

study and the number of subjects who reported headaches after consuming the placebo. If p_1 is the population proportion of people who have headaches after ingesting the placebo and p_2 is the population proportion of people who have headaches after ingesting aspartame, we would like to test the null hypothesis that the two population proportions are equal:

$$H_0: p_1 = p_2 \qquad (10.17)$$

The two-sided alternative hypothesis states that the two population proportions are not equal.

$$H_A: p_1 \neq p_2 \qquad (10.18)$$

From Table 10.8 we obtain sample estimates of the population proportions: $\hat{p}_1 = 18/40 = 0.45$ and $\hat{p}_2 - 14/40 = 0.35$. We cannot use the two-sample Z statistic described in Chapter 7 to test the hypothesis of equal population proportions because the independent-samples assumption is violated.* Since each subject was given both aspartame and the placebo, the frequencies in Table 10.8 are based on paired samples. The corresponding populations are also paired, and the population proportions p_1 and p_2 are *paired population proportions*.

The appropriate test for testing the hypothesis of equal paired population proportions is called the *McNemar test*. To carry out the McNemar test for the aspartame data, we need additional information. The study also reported that eight subjects had headaches after aspartame but not after the placebo, 12 subjects had headaches after the placebo but not after aspartame, six subjects had headaches after both aspartame and the placebo, and 14 subjects did not have headaches after aspartame or the placebo. This information *cannot* be obtained from Table 10.8. These additional results are shown in Table 10.9.

A table like Table 10.9 is required whenever the McNemar test is done. In general, if paired samples

are used to test the hypothesis of equal population proportions for some event, a table with the format of Table 10.10 must be obtained.

Since we want to test the hypothesis that the two paired population proportions are the same, we are interested in subjects who are inconsistent in their responses. For the aspartame data, we are interested in subjects with headaches after aspartame but not after the placebo and subjects with headaches after the placebo but not after aspartame.

When the frequencies are tabulated as in Table 10.10, the frequencies for the consistent responses are the frequencies O_{11} and O_{22}. The frequencies for the inconsistent responses are the frequencies O_{12} and O_{21}. Only one of the frequencies for the inconsistent responses is used to obtain the McNemar test statistic. The test statistic M for the McNemar test is simply O_{12}:

$$M = O_{12} \qquad (10.19)$$

The rationale for the McNemar M statistic is not obvious. A description of the reasoning behind formula (10.19) requires a rather technical discussion of probability and the binomial distribution. We will omit the rationale for the McNemar test and concentrate on the use of this test.*

If the test statistic M is used, the hypothesis of equal paired population proportions is rejected when M is too large or too small. When M is extremely large or small, its p-value is small. If the p-value for the M statistic is less than the significance level α, the null hypothesis (10.17) is rejected. If the p-value for the M statistic is greater than or

---

*Lack of independence also rules out the chi-square test of association for determining whether the substance ingested and headache status are associated. Misuse of the chi-square test of association to analyze frequencies from paired samples is a common error in the medical and health care literature.

---

*If $O_{12} + O_{21}$ is greater than 20, an approximate statistic for the two-sided McNemar test of the null hypothesis (10.17) is given by

$$\frac{(O_{12} - O_{21})^2}{O_{12} + O_{21}}$$

It can be shown that this statistic has an approximate chi-square distribution with 1 degree of freedom if the null hypothesis (10.17) is true and the McNemar test assumptions are satisfied. Further information about the approximate McNemar test can be found in other texts.[12]

equal to α, this hypothesis cannot be rejected. The p-value is interpreted in the usual way: it is the probability of getting an M statistic at least as extreme as the calculated M statistic if the null hypothesis (10.17) is true.

Table E.8 in Appendix E is used to obtain approximate two-tailed p-values for the M statistic. Let n_D equal the sum $O_{12} + O_{21}$. In other words, n_D is the number of subjects with discrepant responses. Let M_{calc} be the calculated value of the M statistic. To use Table E.8, we first calculate n_D. We then proceed as follows to obtain approximate p-values for M when the two-sided alternative hypothesis (10.18) is used.

STEP 1. Check to see whether M_{calc} is one of the numbers listed in the column headed by the probability 0.10 and in the row for your n_D value. If so, the p-value is less than 0.10. If not, the p-value is greater than 0.10.

STEP 2. If the p-value is greater than 0.10, no further information can be obtained from the table. If the p-value is less than 0.10, check to see whether M_{calc} is one of the numbers listed in the 0.05 column and in the row for your n_D value. If so, the p-value is less than 0.05. If not, the p-value is between 0.05 and 0.10.

STEP 3. If the p-value is between 0.05 and 0.10, no further information can be obtained from the table. If the p-value is less than 0.05, check to see whether M_{calc} is one of the numbers listed in the 0.02 column and in the row for your n_D value. If so, the p-value is less than 0.02. If not, the p-value is between 0.02 and 0.05.

STEP 4. If the p-value is between 0.02 and 0.05, no further information can be obtained from the table. If the p-value is less than 0.02, check to see whether M_{calc} is one of the numbers listed in the 0.01 column and in the row for your n_D value. If so, the p-value is less than 0.01. If not, the p-value is between 0.01 and 0.02.

When "none" is listed in a row and column in Table E.8, no M_{calc} has a p-value less than the probability for that column. Whatever the value of the M statistic, its p-value is greater than the probability for the column.

The use of Table E.8 is illustrated in the following example.

Example 10.7

What are the approximate p-values for the following calculated M statistics?

1. $M_{calc} = 11$, $O_{12} = 11$, $O_{21} = 5$. Since $n_D = 16$, we use the row that begins with 16. In the 0.10 column, we find " ≤ 4 or ≥ 12." Since 11 is *not* less than or equal to 4 or greater than or equal to 12, the approximate p-value is

$$p\text{-value} > 0.10$$

2. $M_{calc} = 1$, $O_{12} = 1$, $O_{21} = 11$. Since $n_D = 12$, we use the row that begins with 12. In the 0.10 column, we find " ≤ 2 or ≥ 10." Since 1 is less than 2, the p-value is less than 0.10. In the 0.05 column, we find " ≤ 2 or ≥ 10" again. Since 1 is less than 2, the p-value is less than 0.05. In the 0.02 column, we find " ≤ 1 or ≥ 11." Since 1 is equal to 1, the p-value is less than 0.02. In the 0.01 column, we find " ≤ 1 or ≥ 11" again. Since 1 is equal to 1, the approximate p-value is

$$p\text{-value} < 0.01$$

3. $M_{calc} = 22$, $O_{12} = 22$, $O_{21} = 8$. Since $n_D = 30$, we use the row that begins with 30. In the 0.10 column, we find " ≤ 10 or ≥ 20." Since 22 is greater than 20, the p-value is less than 0.10. In the 0.05 column, we find " ≤ 9 or ≥ 21." Since 22 is greater than 21, the p-value is less than 0.05. In the 0.02 column, we find " ≤ 8 or ≥ 22." Since 22 is equal to 22, the p-value is less than 0.02. In the 0.01 column, we find " ≤ 7 or ≥ 23." Since 22 is *not* less than or equal to 7 or greater than or equal to 23, the p-value is greater than 0.01. The approximate p-value is

$$0.01 < p\text{-value} < 0.02$$

4. $M_{calc} = 0$, $O_{12} = 0$, $O_{21} = 6$. Since $n_D = 6$, we use the row that begins with 6. In the 0.10 column, we find "0 or 6." Since 0 is equal to 0, the p-value is less than 0.10. In the 0.05 column, we find "0 or 6" again. Since 0 is equal to 0, the p-value is less than 0.05. In the 0.02 column, we find "none." No M_{calc} has a p-value less than 0.02 when $n_D = 6$, so the p-value is greater than 0.02. The approximate p-value is

$$0.02 < p\text{-value} < 0.05$$

5. $M_{calc} = 0$, $O_{12} = 0$, $O_{21} = 3$. Since $n_D = 3$, we use the row that begins with 3. In the 0.10 column, we find "none." No M_{calc} has a p-value less than 0.10 when $n_D = 3$, so the approximate p-value is

$$p\text{-value} > 0.10$$

One-sided McNemar tests have the alternative hypotheses H_A: $p_1 < p_2$ or H_A: $p_1 > p_2$. In general, one-sided tests are not recommended, for the same reasons discussed in Chapter 7. If you wish to carry out one-sided McNemar tests, a statistician should be consulted to obtain one-tailed p-values.

The McNemar test is based on the following assumptions.

1. Random Sampling. Random sampling is not essential as long as the samples are not biased.

2. Paired Samples. If paired samples are not obtained, the McNemar test cannot be done.

3. Independence Within Each Sample. All of the observations within the first sample must be independent and all of the observations within the second sample must be independent. Observations from different samples are not necessarily independent, since the samples are paired. If this assumption is violated, the McNemar test cannot be done.

Let us evaluate these assumptions for the aspartame data. Random sampling was not done, but this is not essential. The samples of observations indicating headache status are paired, since each subject took both aspartame and the placebo. Because the headache status of one subject tells us nothing about the headache status of another subject, independence within each sample seems to hold. The McNemar test is appropriate for testing the hypothesis of equal population aspartame and placebo headache proportions. We will use a 0.10 significance level.

From Table 10.9, we get $M = 12$ and $n_D = 12 + 8 = 20$. In the row beginning with 20 and the 0.10 column in Table E.8, we find " ≤ 5 or ≥ 15." Since 12 is *not* less than or equal to 5 or greater than or equal to 15, the approximate p-value is

$$p\text{-value} > 0.10$$

Using any reasonable significance level, we cannot reject the hypothesis that the population aspartame headache proportion is equal to the population placebo headache proportion.

Example 10.8 _____

A study evaluated oral tube holders and conventional taping for stabilizing oral endotracheal tubes.[13] Data were obtained for 30 patients who used both systems. Fifty-nine observations were obtained while patients were using the tube holder and 56 observations were obtained while patients were using adhesive tape. Table 10.11 shows the numbers of times lip excoriation was observed. Can we use these data to test the hypothesis that the population proportion of times lip excoriation occurs is the same during tube holder use and adhesive tape use?

Since there are 59 tube holder observations and 56 adhesive tape observations for 30 patients, repeated measurements were obtained for some patients during the use of each method. The within-samples independence assumption does not hold. In addition, the information needed to construct a table having the format of Table 10.10 is not given. Even if this information were available, the lack of within-samples independence would rule out the McNemar test. If we had the data for each patient, we could obtain the proportion of patients who experienced lip excoriation during the first use of the tube holder and the proportion who experienced lip excoriation during the first use of adhesive tape. The McNemar test could then be used to test the hypothesis that the corresponding paired population proportions are equal. The patients, and not the instances of tube holder use, would be the unit of analysis.

10.4 COMPUTER OUTPUT FOR ANALYSES OF FREQUENCY DATA

In SPSS, the NPAR TESTS procedure is used to carry out the chi-square test of hypothesized proportions. Both SPSS and SAS can be used to calculate the chi-square test of association. The CROSSTABS procedure in SPSS and the FREQ procedure in SAS are used to obtain this test. The McNemar test can be obtained in SPSS with the NPAR TESTS procedure. The usual warnings about the computer's inability to check assumptions still apply.

Figure 10.2 shows the SPSS/PC output for the

TABLE 10.11 NUMBERS OF TIMES LIP EXCORIATION OCCURRED DURING TUBE HOLDER OR ADHESIVE TAPE USE

Stabilization Method	Lip Excoriation	
	PRESENT	NOT PRESENT
Tube holder	5	54
Adhesive tape	18	38

```
            Cases
Category  Observed  Expected  Residual

    0.0        34     34.50      -.50
    1.00       10      6.90      3.10
    2.00       17      6.90     10.10
    3.00        6      6.90      -.90
    4.00        1      6.90     -5.90
    5.00        1      6.90     -5.90
               --
   Total       69

   Chi-Square           D.F.      Significance
     26.391               5              .000
```

Figure 10.2 SPSS/PC output for chi-square test of hypothesized proportions for cancer-pain data

chi-square test of expected frequencies for the cancer-pain data. The PPI ratings are listed under "Category," the observed frequencies are listed under "Cases Observed," and the expected frequencies are listed under "Expected." The numbers under "Residual" are the differences between the observed and expected frequencies (observed frequency minus expected frequency). The p-value for the χ^2 statistic is given under "Significance." The p-value listed is .000, which means that the p-value is less than or equal to 0.0005. It does not mean that the p-value is 0.

Figure 10.3 shows the SPSS/PC output for the chi-square test of association for the labor data. The contingency table gives the row percentages as well as the observed frequencies. The p-value is listed under "Significance" and is consistent with our approximate p-value, since 0.0428 is between 0.025 and 0.05. The smallest expected frequency is given under "Min E.F.," and the number of expected frequencies less than 5 is given under "Cells with E.F. < 5." The SAS output for the same chi-square test of association is shown in Figure 10.4. Observed frequencies and row percentages are given in the contingency table. Row and column totals are labeled "TOTAL." The p-value is given after "PROB =."

SPSS/PC McNemar test output for the aspartame data is shown in Figure 10.5. The two-tailed p-value listed after "2-tailed P" is consistent with

```
Crosstabulation:      POSITION
                  By EFFORTS

EFFORTS->    Count  |                              |  Row
             Row Pct |   1.00|   2.00|   3.00| Total
POSITION     --------+-------+-------+-------+
             1.00    |   19  |   10  |    8  |   37
                     |  51.4 |  27.0 |  21.6 |  61.7
                     +-------+-------+-------+
             2.00    |    6  |    5  |   12  |   23
                     |  26.1 |  21.7 |  52.2 |  38.3
                     +-------+-------+-------+
             Column      25      15      20      60
             Total      41.7    25.0    33.3   100.0


Chi-Square    D.F.    Significance     Min E.F.    Cells with E.F. < 5
----------    ----    ------------     --------    -------------------

  6.30317      2         .0428           5.750           None
```

Figure 10.3 SPSS/PC output for chi-square test of association for labor data

Figure 10.4 SAS output for chi-square test of association for labor data

```
               TABLE OF POSITION BY EFFORTS
       POSITION        EFFORTS

       FREQUENCY|
       ROW PCT  |    1 |    2 |    3 | TOTAL
       ---------+------+------+------+
              1 |  19  |  10  |   8  |   37
                | 51.35| 27.03| 21.62|
       ---------+------+------+------+
              2 |   6  |   5  |  12  |   23
                | 26.09| 21.74| 52.17|
       ---------+------+------+------+
       TOTAL       25     15     20     60
            STATISTICS FOR 2-WAY TABLES
CHI-SQUARE                        6.303   DF=   2   PROB=0.0428
```

```
                   ASPARTME
                2.00     1.00           Cases        40
              |--------|--------|
       1.00   |   12   |    6   |
PLACEBO       |--------|--------|     (Binomial)
       2.00   |   14   |    8   |     2-tailed P    .5034
              |--------|--------|
```

Figure 10.5 SPSS/PC output for McNemar test for aspartame data

our approximate p-value, since 0.5034 is greater than 0.10. The format of the table in the output differs from that of Table 10.9. In the SPSS/PC table, the columns are reversed so that the upper-left-hand frequency is equal to the M statistic.

SUMMARY

Data with only a few possible values cannot be analyzed with statistical methods that require normality or approximate normality. When such data are reported by listing the number or percentage of times each value occurs, they are called frequency data. To test hypotheses about frequency data, three methods are commonly used. The chi-square test of hypothesized proportions is used to test the hypothesis that two or more population proportions are equal to hypothesized values. The chi-square test of association is used to test the hypothesis that two variables are not associated. The McNemar test is used to test the hypothesis that two paired population proportions are equal. If the chi-square test of association leads to rejection of the hypothesis of no association, we cannot conclude that a causal relationship exists.

FREQUENTLY USED FORMULAS FOR ANALYZING FREQUENCY DATA

Expected frequencies for chi-square test of hypothesized proportions:

$E_i = n \times p_{i0}$

Chi-square statistic for chi-square test of hypothesized proportions:

$$\chi^2 = \left(\sum_{i=1}^{k} \frac{O_i^2}{E_i} \right) - n$$

Expected frequencies for chi-square test of association:

$$E_{ij} = \frac{(\text{row } i \text{ total})(\text{row } j \text{ total})}{n}$$

Chi-square statistic for chi-square test of association:

$$\chi^2 = \left(\sum_{\text{all } i, j} \frac{O_{ij}^2}{E_{ij}} \right) - n$$

Row percentage:

$$\text{row pct}_{ij} = \frac{O_{ij}}{\text{row } i \text{ total}} \times 100$$

Column percentage:

$$\text{column pct}_{ij} = \frac{O_{ij}}{\text{column } j \text{ total}} \times 100$$

M statistic for McNemar test:

$M = O_{12}$

TABLE 10.12   DISTRIBUTION OF CHILDREN ACCORDING TO TENDERNESS AND NEEDLE STRATEGY

	Needle Strategy	
Tenderness	ONE NEEDLE	TWO NEEDLES
Present	114	124
Not present	51	47

PROBLEMS

The following instructions apply to problems 1 through 28.

1. In each problem, data are presented and a question is asked about the data. Determine whether any of the tests described in this chapter are appropriate for answering this question. If no test is appropriate, state which assumptions are violated.

2. If a statistical test is appropriate, carry out the test. Specify the null and alternative hypotheses and find the most exact p-value that can be obtained from the tables in this text. Interpret the p-value and use the test results to answer the question in the problem.

1. A study investigated whether changing the syringe needle after drawing up diptheria-pertussis-tetanus (DPT) vaccine and before injecting the vaccine reduces the risk of local complications.[14] Children received either a two-needle vaccination or a one-needle vaccination. Table 10.12 shows the distribution of 336 children according to needle strategy and tenderness at the injection site. Do the data provide evidence that needle strategy and tenderness are associated? If so, describe the nature of the association. Use a 0.10 significance level.

2. A study evaluated the effectiveness of nurse teaching of patients.[15] Nurses selected information concerning disease processes or medications to teach patients, and patients were then interviewed to determine whether they had learned the information. Table 10.13 shows the frequencies for the differences between the number of items taught and the number of items learned for 53 hospitalized patients. A physician believes that all of the differences are equally likely. Do the data provide evi-

TABLE 10.13   DISTRIBUTION OF DIFFERENCE BETWEEN NUMBER OF ITEMS TAUGHT AND NUMBER OF ITEMS LEARNED

Difference	Frequency
0	26
1	11
2	5
3	6
4	3
5	2

TABLE 10.14 DISTRIBUTION OF WOMEN ACCORDING TO RETINOPATHY STATUS DURING AND AFTER PREGNANCY

During Pregnancy	After Pregnancy	
	RETINOPATHY	NO RETINOPATHY
Retinopathy	20	0
No retinopathy	3	10

TABLE 10.16 DISTRIBUTION OF DMSO TREATMENT RESULTS

Result	Frequency
Good	12
Fair	8
Poor	5

TABLE 10.15 DISTRIBUTION OF CHILDREN ACCORDING TO PRURITIS AND TYPE OF ANALGESIC

Pruritis	Analgesic		
	IV MORPHINE	CAUDAL MORPHINE	CAUDAL BUPIVACAINE
Present	0	2	1
Not present	15	13	12

TABLE 10.17 DISTRIBUTION OF SUBJECTS ACCORDING TO ROLE AND LENGTH OF RESPONSE TIME CONSIDERED REASONABLE

Role	Response Time (minutes)		
	5	10	15–20
Patient	18	12	7
Nurse	3	5	14

dence against her view? Use a 0.001 significance level.

3. In a study of changes in diabetic retinopathy during pregnancy, 33 pregnant women with insulin-dependent diabetes were monitored for changes in diabetic retinopathy.[16] Sixty-one percent of the women had retinopathy during pregnancy and 70% had retinopathy after delivery. Table 10.14 shows the distribution of women according to retinopathy status during and after pregnancy. Do the data provide evidence that the population proportion of pregnant diabetic women with retinopathy before delivery differs from the population proportion of diabetic women with retinopathy after delivery? Use a 0.05 significance level.

4. A double-blind study compared morphine and caudal bupivacaine for postoperative analgesia in children.[17] Children were randomly assigned to receive intravenous (IV) morphine, caudal morphine, or caudal bupivacaine for relief of postoperative pain. Table 10.15 shows the distribution of 43 children according to type of analgesic and occurrence of pruritis as a postoperative complication. Do the data provide evidence that type of analgesic and pruritis are associated? If so, describe the nature of the association. Use a 0.01 significance level.

5. In a study of intravesical dimethyl sulphoxide (DMSO) in the treatment of chronic inflammatory

bladder disease, the results of DMSO treatment shown in Table 10.16 were reported for 25 patients.[18] An internist believes that good, fair, and poor responses to DMSO treatment are equally likely for patients with chronic inflammatory bladder disease. Do the data provide evidence against her view? Use a 0.05 significance level.

6. A study examined patient and nurse perceptions of a reasonable length of time between a request for postoperative analgesia and the administration of analgesia.[19] Table 10.17 shows the distribution of 59 subjects according to role (patient or nurse) and length of response time considered reasonable. Do the data provide evidence that role and length of response time considered reasonable are associated? If so, describe the nature of the association. Use a 0.01 significance level.

7. In a study of factors associated with aspiration in adults with tracheal tubes, 907 observations were obtained for 31 critically ill intubated patients.[20] Table 10.18 shows the distribution of 904 of the observations according to route of intubation and occurrence of aspiration. Do the data provide evidence that route of intubation and aspiration are associated? If so, describe the nature of the association. Use a 0.01 significance level.

TABLE 10.18 DISTRIBUTION OF INTUBATIONS ACCORDING TO ASPIRATION AND ROUTE OF INTUBATION

Aspiration	Route of Intubation		
	OROTRACHEAL	NASOTRACHEAL	TRACHEOSTOMY
Occurred	137	24	86
Did not occur	411	116	130

TABLE 10.19 DISTRIBUTION OF DIABETIC PATIENTS ACCORDING TO ACC OCCURRENCE BEFORE AND AFTER DISINFECTANT USE

Before Disinfectant	After Disinfectant	
	ACCs	No ACCs
ACCs	10	18
No ACCs	2	10

TABLE 10.20 DISTRIBUTION OF CLAMBAKE PARTICIPANTS ACCORDING TO NUMBER OF CLAMS EATEN AND ILLNESS

Number of Clams Eaten	Illness	
	PRESENT	NOT PRESENT
0	1	44
1–6	8	30
7–12	15	9
13–24	19	7
25–36	12	3
37–102	17	3

TABLE 10.21 DISTRIBUTION OF PATIENTS ACCORDING TO MRI DIAGNOSIS AND X-RAY CT DIAGNOSIS

MRI Diagnosis	X-ray CT Diagnosis	
	NORMAL	NOT NORMAL
Normal	3	0
Not normal	7	12

TABLE 10.22 DISTRIBUTION OF DOGS ACCORDING TO LAMENESS AND ANTIBODY TITER RESULT

Lameness	Titer Result	
	SEROPOSITIVE	SERONEGATIVE
Present	165	78
Not present	16	7

8. A study examined the effect of disinfectant use on acute cutaneous complications (ACCs) during insulin-pump treatment.[21] At the time of the initial exam, 70% of 40 diabetic patients with insulin pumps had ACCs at the needle insertion site. After use of a disinfectant on the skin before needle insertion for two to four weeks, 30% of the patients had ACCs at the needle insertion site. Table 10.19 shows the distribution of patients according to ACC occurrence before and after disinfectant use. Do the data provide evidence that the population proportion of diabetic patients with ACCs before using the disinfectant differs from the population proportion of diabetic patients with ACCs after using the disinfectant? Use a 0.05 significance level.

9. In a study of Snow Mountain agent gastroenteritis from clams, two clambake-related gastroenteritis outbreaks were investigated.[22] Table 10.20 shows the distribution of 168 clambake participants according to the number of clams eaten and occurrence of illness. Do the data provide evidence that the number of clams eaten and illness are associated? If so, describe the nature of the association. Use a 0.01 significance level.

10. A study reported the results of X-ray computed tomography (CT) scans and magnetic resonance imaging (MRI) of the pituitary gland in 22 patients with various pituitary diseases.[23] The X-ray CT diagnosis was normal for 45% of the patients and the MRI diagnosis was normal for 14% of the patients. The distribution of patients according to the X-ray CT diagnosis and the MRI diagnosis is shown in Table 10.21. Do the data provide evidence that the population proportion of normal X-ray CT diagnoses differs from the population proportion of normal MRI diagnoses? Use a 0.10 significance level.

11. In a study of Lyme disease in the dog (canine borreliosis), clinical features of dogs suspected of having borreliosis were reported.[24] Table 10.22 shows the distribution of 266 dogs suspected of having borreliosis according to lameness and *Borrelia burgdorferi* antibody titer result. Do the data provide evidence that lameness and titer result are associated? If so, describe the nature of the association. Use a 0.01 significance level.

12. A study investigated the relationship between type of health insurance and tooth extraction in adults.[25] Patients were randomly assigned to receive different types of medical and dental insurance, which were classified into three categories: free (all dental care covered), intermediate (25% or 50% coinsurance rate), and stingy (95% coinsurance rate). Table 10.23 shows the distribution of 1210 patients according to tooth extraction and insurance type. Do the data provide evidence that type of insurance and tooth extraction are associated? If so, describe the nature of the association. Use a 0.05 significance level.

13. A study evaluated oral complications in 36 pediatric cancer patients.[26] Table 10.24 shows the distribution of patients according to history of rou-

TABLE 10.23 DISTRIBUTION OF PATIENTS ACCORDING TO TOOTH EXTRACTION AND TYPE OF INSURANCE

Tooth Extraction	Type of Insurance		
	FREE	INTERMEDIATE	STINGY
One or more	149	83	137
None	275	193	373

TABLE 10.24 DISTRIBUTION OF PEDIATRIC CANCER PATIENTS ACCORDING TO HISTORY OF ROUTINE DENTAL CARE AND ORAL COMPLICATIONS

History of Dental Care	Oral Complications	
	PRESENT	NOT PRESENT
Provided	4	13
Not provided	12	7

tine dental care and occurrence of oral complications. Do the data provide evidence that dental care history and oral complications are associated? If so, describe the nature of the association. Use a 0.05 significance level.

14. In a study of miliary dermatitis in cats, the results of intradermal skin testing were reported for 13 cats.[27] Seventy-seven percent of the cats had a skin-test reaction to fleas and 8% had a skin-test reaction to house-dust mites. Table 10.25 shows the distribution of cats according to skin-test reactions to fleas and house-dust mites. Do the data provide evidence that the population proportion of cats with miliary dermatitis that react to fleas differs from the population proportion of cats with miliary dermatitis that react to house-dust mites? Use a 0.01 significance level.

TABLE 10.25 DISTRIBUTION OF CATS ACCORDING TO SKIN-TEST REACTIONS TO FLEAS AND HOUSE-DUST MITES

Reaction to Fleas	Reaction to House-Dust Mites	
	PRESENT	NOT PRESENT
Present	1	9
Not present	0	3

TABLE 10.26 DISTRIBUTION OF CHILDHOOD CAUSES OF DEATH

Cause of Death	Frequency
Natural	312
Miscellaneous accident	186
Traffic accident	113
Homicide	62
Suicide	8

15. A study of childhood homicide reported the causes of death for 681 children.[28] These frequencies are shown in Table 10.26. A pediatric nurse believes that the following population proportions for causes of death in childhood hold.

$p_1 = P(\text{Natural death}) = 0.40$
$p_2 = P(\text{Miscellaneous accident}) = 0.30$
$p_3 = P(\text{Traffic accident}) = 0.20$
$p_4 = P(\text{Homicide}) = 0.08$
$p_5 = P(\text{Suicide}) = 0.02$

Do the data provide evidence against his view? Use a 0.10 significance level.

16. In a study of back injuries in nursing personnel, the specialty areas of 123 nurses and nurse aides with back injuries and 536 nurses and nurse aides without back injuries were reported.[29] Table 10.27 shows the distribution of subjects according to specialty and back injury status. Do the data provide evidence that specialty and back injury status are associated? If so, describe the nature of the association. Use a 0.01 significance level.

17. A study evaluated the use of resection arthroplasty as a salvage procedure for knees with infection after total arthroplasty.[30] Sixty-nine percent of 26 patients were able to walk with moderate, mild, or no restriction before surgery and 77% were able to walk with moderate, mild, or no restriction after surgery. Table 10.28 shows the distribution of patients according to walking ability before and after surgery. Do the data provide evidence that the population proportion of patients able to walk with moderate to no restriction before surgery differs from the population proportion of patients able to walk with moderate to no restriction after surgery? Use a 0.05 significance level.

18. In a study of the quality of life for heart-transplant patients, the frequency of bruises was recorded for 31 heart-transplant recipients on azathioprine-based protocols and 44 heart-transplant recipients on cyclosporine-based protocols.[31] Table 10.29 shows the distribution of recipients according to protocol and frequency of bruises. Do the data provide evidence that protocol and frequency of bruises are associated? If so, describe the nature of the association. Use a 0.01 significance level.

19. A study evaluated nurses' ability to detect nodules in silicone breast models.[32] Seventy-eight nurses were asked to determine the number of nodules present in a two-nodule breast model. Sev-

TABLE 10.27 DISTRIBUTION OF SUBJECTS ACCORDING TO BACK INJURY STATUS AND SPECIALTY

Back Injury Status	Specialty			
	MEDICINE	SURGERY	PSYCHIATRY	LONG-TERM CARE
Injured	67	15	23	18
Not injured	216	47	152	121

TABLE 10.28 DISTRIBUTION OF PATIENTS ACCORDING TO WALKING ABILITY BEFORE AND AFTER SURGERY

Before Surgery	After Surgery	
	MODERATE TO NO RESTRICTION	UNABLE TO WALK OR SEVERE RESTRICTION
Moderate to no restriction	17	1
Unable to walk or severe restriction	3	5

TABLE 10.29 DISTRIBUTION OF RECIPIENTS ACCORDING TO PROTOCOL AND FREQUENCY OF BRUISES

Protocol	Frequency of Bruises		
	NEVER	RARELY OR SOMETIMES	OFTEN OR ALWAYS
Azathioprine	4	8	19
Cyclosporine	10	23	11

TABLE 10.31 DISTRIBUTION OF BAL SPECIMENS ACCORDING TO CYTOLOGICAL EXAMINATION RESULT AND IF ASSAY RESULT

Cytological Examination Result	IF Assay Result	
	POSITIVE	NEGATIVE
Positive	14	0
Negative	1	26

TABLE 10.32 DISTRIBUTION OF RESPIRATORY STATUS IN HIGH-RISE SYNDROME

Respiratory Status	Frequency
Eupneic	53
Tachypneic	57
Dyspneic	14
Agonal	2
Apneic (DOA)*	3

*DOA = dead on arrival

enty-two of these nurses were then asked to examine the two-nodule model again and determine the number of nodules present. Table 10.30 shows the distribution of nurses according to examination number (first or second) and number of nodules detected. Do the data provide evidence that examination number and number of nodules detected are associated? If so, describe the nature of the association. Use a 0.10 significance level.

20. A study of methods for detecting cytomegalovirus (CMV) reported the results of different assays on 41 bronchoalveolar lavage (BAL) specimens from 30 bone-marrow-transplant recipients with pneumonia.[33] Cytological examination was positive for CMV for 34% of the BAL specimens, and immunofluorescence (IF) assays were positive for CMV for 37% of the BAL specimens. Table 10.31 shows the distribution of the BAL specimens according to cytological examination result and IF assay result. Do the data provide evidence that the population proportion of BAL specimens with positive cytological examination results differs from the population proportion of BAL specimens with positive IF assay results? Use a 0.05 significance level.

21. In a study of high-rise syndrome in cats, 132 cats that had fallen from a substantial height were examined.[34] Table 10.32 shows the respiratory status for 129 of these cats. A veterinarian believes that the following population proportions for respiratory status hold.

P(Eupnea) = 0.40
P(Tachypnea) = 0.40
P(Dyspnea) = 0.15
P(Agonal respiration) = 0.025
P(Apnea) = 0.025

Do the data provide evidence against her view? Use a 0.01 significance level.

22. A study evaluated the results of operative repair of the torn rotator cuff in 20 patients.[35] Sixty-five percent of the patients reported night and rest pain before surgery, and 5% reported night and rest pain after surgery. Table 10.33 shows the distribution of patients according to night and rest pain before and after surgery. Do the data provide evi-

TABLE 10.30 DISTRIBUTION OF NURSES ACCORDING TO EXAMINATION NUMBER AND NUMBER OF NODULES DETECTED

Examination Number	Number of Nodules Detected		
	0	1	2
First	14	30	34
Second	9	30	33

TABLE 10.33 DISTRIBUTION OF PATIENTS ACCORDING TO NIGHT AND REST PAIN BEFORE AND AFTER SURGERY

Before Surgery	After Surgery	
	REST / NIGHT PAIN PRESENT	REST / NIGHT PAIN ABSENT
Rest/night pain present	1	12
Rest/night pain absent	0	7

TABLE 10.34   DISTRIBUTION OF LIVER INJURY SEVERITY SCORE

Score	Frequency
I	10
II	23
III	18
IV	12
V	6

dence that the population proportion of patients with night and rest pain before surgery differs from the population proportion of patients with night and rest pain after surgery? Use a 0.05 significance level.

23. In a study of hepatic trauma management, the frequencies of liver injury severity scores (ISSs) shown in Table 10.34 were reported for 69 patients with hepatic injuries.[36] The higher the score, the more severe the injury. A surgeon believes that the following population proportions for ISSs hold.

P(ISS of I) = 0.1
P(ISS of II) = 0.6
P(ISS of III) = 0.1
P(ISS of IV) = 0.1
P(ISS of V) = 0.1

Do the data provide evidence against his view? Use a 0.005 significance level.

24. A study investigated the importance of coagulase-negative staphylococci in the development of peritonitis in patients undergoing peritoneal dialysis.[37] During a nine-month period, 182 cultures of pericatheter skin and anterior nares were obtained from 30 patients undergoing chronic outpatient peritoneal dialysis. Table 10.35 shows the distribution of these cultures according to culture site and type of organism cultured. Do the data provide evidence that the culture site and the type of organism cultured are associated? If so, describe the nature of the association. Use a 0.01 significance level.

25. A study examined the adjustment patterns of 24 chronic obstructive pulmonary disease (COPD) patients and 30 peripheral vascular disease (PVD) patients.[38] Table 10.36 shows the distribution of

TABLE 10.35   DISTRIBUTION OF CULTURES ACCORDING TO ORGANISM CULTURED AND CULTURE SITE

Organism	Culture Site	
	SKIN	NARES
Coagulase-negative staphylococci	25	77
Staphylococcus aureus	14	20
Miscellaneous	4	4
No growth	45	8

TABLE 10.36   DISTRIBUTION OF PATIENTS ACCORDING TO FATIGUE ON AWAKENING AND DISEASE

Fatigue on Awakening	Disease	
	COPD	PVD
Present	16	10
Not present	8	20

TABLE 10.37   DISTRIBUTION OF TWO-MONTH PERIOD DURING WHICH DOG BITES OCCURRED

Two-Month Period	Frequency
December–January	6
February–March	27
April–May	50
June–July	50
August–September	43
October–November	23

patients according to disease and fatigue on awakening. Do these data provide evidence that disease and fatigue on awakening are associated? If so, describe the nature of the association. Use a 0.05 significance level.

26. In a study of dog bites in children, the time period frequencies shown in Table 10.37 were reported for 199 pediatric dog-bite victims.[39] A pediatrician believes that dog bites in children are equally likely to occur during each of the two-month periods shown in Table 10.37. Do the data provide evidence against her belief? Use a 0.001 significance level.

27. A study examined the use of serum creatine kinase MB isoenzyme (CK-MB) screening for the assessment of possible cardiac injury in blunt trauma victims.[40] Ninety-seven percent of 29 patients with cardiac concussion had identifiable CK-MB present on the first day after injury and 45% had identifiable CK-MB present on the second day after injury. Table 10.38 shows the distribution of patients according to CK-MB presence on the first and second days. Do the data provide evidence that the population proportion of patients with CK-MB present on the first day differs from the population proportion

TABLE 10.38   DISTRIBUTION OF PATIENTS ACCORDING TO CK-MB PRESENCE ON DAYS 1 AND 2

Day 1	Day 2	
	PRESENT	NOT PRESENT
Present	12	16
Not present	1	0

TABLE 10.39   DISTRIBUTION OF SKIN GRAFT RESULTS

Results	Frequency
Excellent	94
Good	31
Fair	23
Poor	25

of patients with CK-MB present on the second day? Use a 0.05 significance level.

28. In a study of hypertrophic skin grafts in burned patients, 70 burned patients had 173 separate anatomic sites grafted.[41] Table 10.39 shows the results of these skin grafts. A surgical nurse believes that the following population proportions of skin graft results hold.

P(Excellent results) = 0.60
P(Good results) = 0.20
P(Fair results) = 0.15
P(Poor results) = 0.05

Do the data provide evidence against his belief? Use a 0.01 significance level.

29. Find an article in a medical or health care journal in which the chi-square test of hypothesized proportions or the chi-square test of association was incorrectly used to analyze nonindependent data. Photocopy the article and write a letter to the journal editor that clearly describes the statistical error.

REFERENCES

1. Donovan MI, Dillon P: Incidence and characteristics of pain in a sample of hospitalized cancer patients. Canc Nurs 10:85–92, 1987.
2. Grin TR, Nelson LB, Jeffers JB: Eye injuries in childhood. Pediatrics 80:13–17, 1987.
3. Rosenthal RC, Dworkis AS: Adverse reactions to Leukocell. J Am Anim Hosp Assoc 23:515–518, 1987.
4. Rogers MF, Budnick LD, Kirson I, et al: Hemolytic-uremic syndrome—An outbreak in Sacramento, California. West J Med 144:169–173, 1986.
5. Ceh S, Aisaka K, Mori H, et al: Effects of sitting position on uterine activity during labor. Obstet Gynecol 69:67–73, 1987.
6. Grizzle JE: Continuity correction in the χ^2 test for 2 × 2 tables. Am Statistician 21:28–32, 1967.
7. Remington RD, Schork MA: Statistics with Applications to the Biological and Health Sciences. 2nd ed. Englewood Cliffs: Prentice-Hall, 1985.
8. Upton GJG: A comparison of alternative tests for the 2 × 2 comparative trial. J Royal Statist Soc 145A:86–105, 1982.
9. Guderian RH, Mackenzie CD, Williams JF: High voltage shock treatment for snake bite (correspondence). Lancet 2:229, 1986.
10. Germain T: A clinical evaluation of the effect of tip integrity of I.V. catheters on phlebitis rates. J Nat Intraven Ther Assoc 9:115–117, 1986.
11. Schiffman SS, Buckley CE, Sampson HA, et al: Aspartame and susceptibility to headache. N Engl J Med 317:1181–1185, 1987.
12. Conover WJ: Practical Nonparametric Statistics. 2nd ed. New York: Wiley, 1980.
13. Tasota FJ, Hoffman LA, Zullo TG, et al: Evaluation of two methods used to stabilize oral endotracheal tubes. Heart Lung 16:140–146, 1987.
14. Salomon ME, Halperin R, Yee J: Evaluation of the two-needle strategy for reducing reactions to DPT vaccination. Am J Dis Child 141:796–798, 1987.
15. Woody AF, Ferguson S, Robertson LH, et al: Do patients learn what nurses say they teach? Nurs Manag 15:26–29, 1984.
16. Phelps RL, Sakol P, Metzger BE, et al: Changes in diabetic retinopathy during pregnancy. Correlations with regulation of hyperglycemia. Arch Ophthalmol 104:1806–1810, 1986.
17. Krane EJ, Jacobson LE, Lynn AM, et al: Caudal morphine for postoperative analgesia in children: A comparison with caudal bupivacaine and intravenous morphine. Anesth Analg 66:647–653, 1987.
18. Barker SB, Matthews PN, Philip PF, et al: Prospective study of intravesical dimethyl sulphoxide in the treatment of chronic inflammatory bladder disease. Br J Urol 59:142–144, 1987.
19. Domask ME, Childs S: Patient and nurse perceptions of analgesic administration times. J Nurs Qual Assur 2:64–69, 1988.
20. Elpern EH, Jacobs ER, Bone RC: Incidence of aspiration in tracheally intubated adults. Heart Lung 16:527–531, 1987.
21. Chantelau E, Lange G, Sonnenberg GE, et al: Acute cutaneous complications and catheter needle colonization during insulin-pump treatment. Diabetes Care 10:478–482, 1987.
22. Truman BI, Madore HP, Menegus MA, et al: Snow Mountain agent gastroenteritis from clams. Am J Epidemiol 126:516–525, 1987.
23. Glaser B, Sheinfeld M, Benmair J, et al: Magnetic resonance imaging of the pituitary gland. Clin Radiol 37:9–14, 1986.
24. Magnarelli LA, Anderson JF, Schreier AB, et al: Clinical and serologic studies of canine borreliosis. J Am Vet Med Assoc 191:1089–1094, 1987.
25. Bailit HL, Braun R: Is periodontal disease the primary cause of tooth extraction in adults? J Am Dent Assoc 114:40–45, 1987.
26. Niehaus CS, Meiller TF, Peterson DE, et al: Oral complications in children during cancer therapy. Canc Nurs 10:15–20, 1987.
27. Gross TL, Kwochka KW, Kunkle GA: Correlation of histologic and immunologic findings in cats with miliary dermatitis. J Am Vet Med Assoc 189:1322–1325, 1986.
28. Abel EL: Childhood homicide in Erie County, New York. Pediatrics 77:709–713, 1986.
29. Uhl JE, Wilkinson WE, Wilkinson CS: Aching backs? A glimpse into the hazards of nursing. AAOHN J 35:13–17, 1987.
30. Falahee MH, Matthews LS, Kauffer H: Resection arthroplasty as a salvage procedure for a knee with infection after a total arthroplasty. J Bone Joint Surg 69A:1013–1021, 1987.
31. Lough ME, Lindsey AM, Shinn JA, et al: Impact of symptom frequency and symptom distress on self-reported quality of life in heart transplant recipients. Heart Lung 16:193–200, 1987.

32. Haughey BP, Marshall JR, Mettlin C, et al: Nurses' ability to detect nodules in silicone breast models. Oncol Nurs Forum *11*:37–42, 1984.

33. Cordonnier C, Escudier E, Nicolas J, et al: Evaluation of three assays on alveolar lavage fluid in the diagnosis of cytomegalovirus pneumonitis after bone marrow transplantation. J Infect Dis *155*:495–500, 1987.

34. Whitney WO, Mehlhaff CJ: High-rise syndrome in cats. J Am Vet Med Assoc *191*:1399–1403, 1987.

35. Calvert PT, Packer NP, Stoker DJ, et al: Arthrography of the shoulder after operative repair of the torn rotator cuff. J Bone Joint Surg *68B*:147–150, 1986.

36. Gillmore D, McSwain NE, Browder IW: Hepatic trauma: To drain or not to drain? J Trauma *27*:898–902, 1987.

37. Eisenberg ES, Ambalu M, Szylagi G, et al: Colonization of skin and development of peritonitis due to coagulase-negative staphylococci in patients undergoing peritoneal dialysis. J Infect Dis *156*:478–482, 1987.

38. Foxall MJ, Ekberg JY, Griffith N: Comparative study of adjustment patterns of chronic obstructive pulmonary disease patients and peripheral vascular disease patients. Heart Lung *16*:354–363, 1987.

39. Chun Y, Berkelhamer JE, Herold TE: Dog bites in children less than 4 years old. Pediatrics *69*:119–120, 1982.

40. Frazee RC, Mucha P, Farnell MB, et al: Objective evaluation of blunt cardiac trauma. J Trauma *26*:510–520, 1986.

41. McDonald WS, Deitch EA. Hypertrophic skin grafts in burned patients: A prospective analysis of variables. J Trauma *27*:147–150, 1987.

11

NONPARAMETRIC STATISTICS

CHAPTER OBJECTIVES

*After studying this chapter and working the problems,
you should be able to:*

1. Carry out and interpret nonparametric hypothesis tests concerning population medians, population median differences, differences between two independent populations, differences among three or more independent populations, differences among three or more populations of repeated measurements, and correlation between two variables

2. Recognize data that violate assumptions required for nonparametric tests

3. Interpret SPSS and SAS output for nonparametric tests

4. Determine whether nonparametric tests reported in the medical and health care literature are appropriate

Many statistical procedures are based on fairly specific assumptions about the distribution of the population (e.g., normality or approximate normality). Statistical methods that require specific distributional assumptions are called *parametric statistics*. The t tests described in Chapter 7 are parametric statistics, as are analysis of variance (Chapters 8, 9, and 13) and correlation and regression (Chapter 12). When data do not satisfy the distributional assumptions required by parametric procedures, other statistical methods are needed. *Nonparametric statistical procedures* can sometimes be used to analyze such data. The distributional assumptions required for nonparametric procedures are usually less specific than those required for parametric procedures.

Nonparametric statistics are not the solution to every data analysis problem. Some distributional assumptions are required for nonparametric procedures, and data that fail to meet parametric assumptions may also fail to meet nonparametric assumptions. Many nonparametric tests have less power than the corresponding parametric tests. Because power should never be given up unless absolutely necessary, nonparametric methods should not be used when parametric methods are appropriate.

Like many parametric procedures, many nonparametric procedures cannot be used to test hypotheses about populations that consist of nominal data. As you may recall from Chapter 2, nominal data consist of arbitrary numerical labels for nonnumerical categories. The variable nursing specialty, with the values 1 = surgical, 2 = obstetric, 3 = oncology, and 4 = home care, produces nominal data. The numbers used to represent specialty are completely arbitrary. Most of the nonparametric procedures we will discuss are based on ranks. Because nominal data have no true numerical meaning, it does not make sense to rank them. Nonparametric procedures based on ranks can be used to test hypotheses about populations that consist of ordinal, interval, or ratio data.

We will describe some of the more commonly used nonparametric procedures. Many other nonparametric methods are available. A comprehensive discussion of nonparametric procedures is provided by Conover.[1] We will consider nonparametric methods for testing hypotheses about the following.

1. Population medians
2. Population median differences
3. Differences between two independent populations
4. Differences among three or more independent populations
5. Differences among three or more populations of repeated measurements
6. Association between two variables

11.1 HYPOTHESES ABOUT POPULATION MEDIANS

When the one-sample t test cannot be used to test hypotheses about population means, we can sometimes use nonparametric procedures to test hypotheses about population medians. Recall that the median is a middle number with half of the observations below it and half of the observations above it. Further discussion of the median can be found in Chapter 2.

Two nonparametric tests, the *Wilcoxon signed rank test* and the *sign test*, are used to test hypotheses about population medians. Because it has more power than the sign test, the Wilcoxon signed rank test is preferred when its assumptions are satisfied. When the assumptions required for the Wilcoxon signed rank test do not hold, the sign test can often be used instead. We will consider the Wilcoxon signed rank test first.

Suppose we have one sample of size n and we want to test the null hypothesis that the population median is equal to some number m_0:

$$H_0: \text{Population median} = m_0 \qquad (11.1)$$

The number m_0 (pronounced "m nought") is specified by the researcher and is not determined by any statistical procedure. The two-sided alternative hypothesis is

$$H_A: \text{Population median} \neq m_0 \qquad (11.2)$$

The Wilcoxon signed rank test can be used to test the null hypothesis (11.1) if the following assumptions hold.

1. Random Sampling. If the sample is not biased, random sampling is not essential.

2. Independence. The Wilcoxon signed rank test cannot be done if the observations are not independent.

3. Symmetry of the Population About the Median. Ideally, a vertical line drawn through the

population median should separate a graph of the population distribution into identical halves. If the population is approximately symmetric, the Wilcoxon signed rank test can still be done. If the population is extremely nonsymmetric, this test should not be done. The symmetry of the population is evaluated by examining a sample histogram, which should be symmetric or approximately symmetric.

Although the assumption of symmetry or approximate symmetry is less restrictive than the assumption of normality or approximate normality, it often fails to hold for medical and health care data. As we have seen, such data are often quite skewed. If the one-sample t test is ruled out because of extreme skewness, the Wilcoxon signed rank test is ruled out as well.

The test statistic used for the Wilcoxon signed rank test is based on the *ranks* of the data. This test statistic, called W, is calculated as follows:

STEP 1.   Subtract m_0 from each observation to get n new observations.

STEP 2.   Throw out all new observations that are equal to 0.

STEP 3.   Arrange the nonzero new observations in order of *increasing absolute value*. For example, -8 is placed after 3, since the absolute value of -8 (8) is larger than 3.

STEP 4.   Write the ranks of the absolute values of the new observations, starting with a rank of 1 for the new observation with the smallest absolute value. If two or more new observations are equal, they will be tied for the same rank. When this occurs, assign to each of the tied new observations the average of the ranks they would have if they were not tied.

STEP 5.   Assign to each rank the sign of the new observation to which it corresponds.

STEP 6.   Add all of the *positive* ranks. The resulting sum is W. If there are no positive ranks, $W = 0$.*

The calculation of W is best understood by working through an example. We will use data from a study of preoperative concerns of patients undergoing craniotomy.[2] Table 11.1 shows the number of concerns about loss of function expressed by 10 patients interviewed before craniotomy. A surgical nurse believes that the population median number of concerns about loss of function is 6. Do the data provide evidence that the population median is not 6? Here m_0 is 6, and we want to test the null hypothesis

$$H_0: \text{Population median} = 6 \qquad (11.3)$$

---

*If the number of ties is very large, an adjusted Wilcoxon signed rank test statistic is often used instead of W. A description of this adjusted statistic can be found in other texts.[1]

TABLE 11.1   NUMBER OF CONCERNS ABOUT LOSS OF FUNCTION

Patient No.	Number of Concerns
1	4
2	1
3	2
4	1
5	0
6	5
7	4
8	7
9	6
10	3

The alternative hypothesis is

$$H_A: \text{Population median} \neq 6 \qquad (11.4)$$

Before calculating W, let us consider whether the one-sample t test can be used to test the hypothesis that the population *mean* number of concerns about loss of function is 6. Because the one-sample t test has more power than the Wilcoxon signed rank test, the t test should be used if its assumptions are satisfied. But the number of possible values seems too small to justify the assumption of normality or approximate normality. The t test is not appropriate, and use of the Wilcoxon signed rank test is warranted.

To calculate W for the craniotomy data, we first need to subtract 6 from each observation in Table 11.1. The following 10 new observations are the result.

$$4 - 6 = -2 \qquad 1 - 6 = -5 \qquad 2 - 6 = -4$$
$$1 - 6 = -5 \qquad 0 - 6 = -6 \qquad 5 - 6 = -1$$
$$4 - 6 = -2 \qquad 7 - 6 = 1 \qquad 6 - 6 = 0$$
$$3 - 6 = -3$$

Arranging the nine *nonzero* new observations in order of increasing absolute value, we get

$$-1 \quad 1 \quad -2 \quad -2 \quad -3 \quad -4 \quad -5 \quad -5 \quad -6$$

Assigning ranks to the new observations according to absolute value, we have

new observations:
$$-1 \quad 1 \quad -2 \quad -2 \quad -3 \quad -4 \quad -5 \quad -5 \quad -6$$
ranks:
$$1.5 \quad 1.5 \quad 3.5 \quad 3.5 \quad 5 \quad 6 \quad 7.5 \quad 7.5 \quad 9$$

The ranks 1.5 are given to the new observations -1 and 1 because these values are tied for ranks 1 and 2. The average rank for ranks 1 and 2 is $(1 + 2)/2 = 1.5$. The other tied ranks are dealt with in a

similar way. Giving signs to the ranks, we obtain

signed ranks:
$$-1.5 \quad 1.5 \quad -3.5 \quad -3.5 \quad -5 \quad -6 \quad -7.5 \quad -7.5 \quad -9$$

There is only one positive rank, so the sum of the positive ranks is $W = 1.5$.

Why does W make sense as a test of the null hypothesis (11.1)? Suppose that the population median is m_0. Then we expect about half of the sample observations to be below m_0 and about half of them to be above m_0. Thus, we expect about half of the nonzero new observations to be negative and about half of them to be positive. Because the distribution is symmetric, we do *not* expect most of the positive new observations to be large and most of the negative new observations to be small, or vice versa.

When W is large, many of the new observations are positive, with large ranks. When W is small, few of the new observations are positive, and most of the positive new observations have small ranks. Thus, it makes sense to reject the null hypothesis (11.1) when W is very large or very small.

The p-value associated with the W statistic is used to determine whether W is large enough or small enough to warrant rejection of the null hypothesis (11.1). When W is extremely large or extremely small, its p-value is small. If the p-value for the W statistic is less than the significance level α, the null hypothesis (11.1) is rejected. If the p-value for the W statistic is greater than or equal to α, the null hypothesis (11.1) cannot be rejected. The p-value is interpreted in the usual way: it is the probability of getting a W statistic at least as extreme as the calculated W statistic if the null hypothesis (11.1) is true.

Approximate p-values for the W statistic can be obtained from Table E.9 in Appendix E. Let n_D be the number of *nonzero* new observations and let W_{calc} be the calculated value of the W statistic. To use Table E.9, we first determine n_D. We then proceed as follows to obtain approximate two-tailed p-values for W when the two-sided alternative hypothesis (11.2) is used.

STEP 1.   Check to see whether W_{calc} is one of the numbers listed in the column headed by the probability 0.10 and in the row for your n_D value. If so, the p-value is less than 0.10. If not, the p-value is greater than 0.10.

STEP 2.   If the p-value is greater than 0.10, no further information can be obtained from the table. If the p-value is less than 0.10, check to see whether W_{calc} is one of the numbers listed in the 0.05 column and in the row for your n_D value. If so, the p-value is less than 0.05. If not, the p-value is between 0.05 and 0.10.

STEP 3.   If the p-value is between 0.05 and 0.10, no further information can be obtained from the table. If the p-value is less than 0.05, check to see whether W_{calc} is one of the numbers listed in the 0.02 column and in the row for your n_D value. If so, the p-value is less than 0.02. If not, the p-value is between 0.02 and 0.05.

STEP 4. If the p-value is between 0.02 and 0.05, no further information can be obtained from the table. If the p-value is less than 0.02, check to see whether W_{calc} is one of the numbers listed in the 0.01 column and in the row for your n_D value. If so, the p-value is less than 0.01. If not, the p-value is between 0.01 and 0.02.

When "none" is listed in a row and column of Table E.9, no W_{calc} has a p-value greater than the probability for that column. Whatever the value of the W statistic, its p-value is greater than the probability for the column.

The use of Table E.9 is illustrated in the following example.

Example 11.1

What are the approximate p-values for the following calculated W statistics?

1. $W_{calc} = 36$, $n_D = 14$. In the row for $n_D = 14$ and in the 0.10 column, we find "≤ 25 or ≥ 80." Since 36 is *not* less than or equal to 25 or greater than or equal to 80, the approximate p-value is

$$p\text{-value} > 0.10$$

2. $W_{calc} = 1$, $n_D = 9$. In the row for $n_D = 9$ and in the 0.10 column, we find "≤ 8 or ≥ 37." Since 1 is less than 8, the p-value is less than 0.10. In the 0.05 column, we find "≤ 5 or ≥ 40." Since 1 is less than 5, the p-value is less than 0.05. In the 0.02 column, we find "≤ 3 or ≥ 42." Since 1 is less than 3, the p-value is less than 0.02. In the 0.01 column, we find "≤ 1 or ≥ 44." Since 1 is equal to 1, the approximate p-value is

$$p\text{-value} < 0.01$$

3. $W_{calc} = 170$, $n_D = 20$. In the row for $n_D = 20$ and in the 0.10 column, we find "≤ 60 or ≥ 150." Since 170 is greater than 150, the p-value is less than 0.10. In the 0.05 column, we find "≤ 52 or ≥ 158." Since 170 is greater than 158, the p-value is less than 0.05. In the 0.02 column, we find "≤ 43 or ≥ 167." Since 170 is greater than 167, the p-value is less than 0.02. In the 0.01 column, we find "≤ 37 or ≥ 173." Since 170 is *not* less than or equal to 37 or greater than or equal to 173, the p-value is greater than 0.01. The approximate p-value is

$$0.01 < p\text{-value} < 0.02$$

4. $W_{calc} = 0$, $n_D = 6$. In the row for $n_D = 6$ and in the 0.10 column, we find "≤ 2 or ≥ 19." Since 0 is less than 2, the p-value is less than 0.10. In the 0.05 column, we find "0 or 21." Since 0 is equal to 0, the p-value is less than 0.05. In the 0.02 column, we find "none." No W_{calc} has a p-value less than 0.02

when $n_D = 6$, so the p-value is greater than 0.02. The approximate p-value is

$$0.02 < p\text{-value} < 0.05$$

5. $W_{calc} = 10$, $n_D = 4$. In the row for $n_D = 4$ and in the 0.10 column, we find "none." No W_{calc} has a p-value less than 0.10 when $n_D = 4$, so the approximate p-value is

$$p\text{-value} > 0.10$$

One-sided Wilcoxon signed rank tests have the alternative hypotheses H_A: Population median $< m_0$ or H_A: Population median $> m_0$. In general, one-sided tests are not recommended, for the same reasons discussed in Chapter 7. The use of Table E.9 to obtain one-tailed p-values is more complicated than the use of this table to obtain two-tailed p-values. Consult a statistician if you need one-tailed p-values for the Wilcoxon signed rank test.

Before obtaining an approximate p-value for the W statistic from the craniotomy data, we need to check the assumptions required for the Wilcoxon signed rank test. Random sampling was not done, but this is not crucial. The independence assumption is reasonable if the patients did not have contact with one another, since the number of concerns for one patient tells us nothing about the number of concerns for another patient. Figure 11.1 shows a histogram of the number of concerns. Although the histogram is not perfectly symmetric, it does not suggest an extremely nonsymmetric population. The Wilcoxon signed rank test is appropriate. We will obtain an approximate p-value to test the null hypothesis (11.3), using a 0.05 significance level.

There are nine nonzero differences, and W is 1.5. In the row for $n_D = 9$ and in the 0.10 column in Table E.9, we find "≤ 8 or ≥ 37." Since 1.5 is less than 8, the p-value is less than 0.10. In the 0.05 column, we find "≤ 5 or ≥ 40." Since 1.5 is less than 5, the p-value is less than 0.05. In the 0.02 column, we find "≤ 3 or ≥ 42." Since 1.5 is less than 3, the p-value is less than 0.02. In the 0.01 column, we find "≤ 1 or ≥ 44." Since 1.5 is not less than or equal to 1 or greater than or equal to 44, the p-value is greater than 0.01. The approximate p-value is

$$0.01 < p\text{-value} < 0.02$$

Using a 0.05 significance level, we reject the hypoth-

```
0 – 1 | XXX
2 – 3 | XX
4 – 5 | XXX
6 – 7 | XX
```

Figure 11.1 Quick histogram of number of concerns

TABLE 11.2 AGE AT WHICH AUTISTIC SIBLINGS FIRST SAT UP

Family No.	Sibling No.	Age (mo)
1	1	8
1	2	6
1	3	5
2	4	6
2	5	6
2	6	6
3	7	5
3	8	7
3	9	6
4	10	5
4	11	7
4	12	6
5	13	8
5	14	7
5	15	8
5	16	7

esis that the population median number of concerns about loss of function is 6. We could not reject this hypothesis at the 0.01 significance level.

Example 11.2

In a study of autistic siblings, clinical data were obtained for five families with autistic siblings.[3] Table 11.2 shows the age at which these siblings first sat up. Can the Wilcoxon signed rank test be used to test the hypothesis that the population median age at which autistic children first sit up is equal to 7 months?

Because autistic children were obtained from the same families, the independence assumption is questionable. Knowing the age at which one sibling sat up may provide some idea of the ages at which other siblings from the family sat up. The Wilcoxon signed rank test cannot be used to analyze all 16 observations. We could select the oldest autistic sibling from each family to obtain five independent ages. If the histogram of the ages appeared symmetric or approximately symmetric, we could obtain a Wilcoxon signed rank test based on these five ages. No W value based on five observations can have a p-value less than 0.05, however, although a p-value less than 0.10 is possible.

When a histogram suggests an extremely nonsymmetric population, the Wilcoxon signed rank test cannot be used to test hypotheses about the population median. The sign test can often be used instead to test the null hypothesis (11.1). The sign test requires only one assumption: independence of the observations. If the independence assumption does not hold, the sign test cannot be done. Because the sign test assumes so little, it has even less power than the Wilcoxon signed rank test. The sign test should be used only when more powerful methods are not appropriate.

Suppose we have a sample of independent observations and we want to use the sign test to test the null hypothesis (11.1). The test statistic for the sign test is called S and is easily calculated as follows.

STEP 1. Subtract m_0 from each observation to get new observations.

STEP 2. Throw out any new observations that are equal to 0.

STEP 3. Record the signs $(+, -)$ of the nonzero new observations.

STEP 4. Count the number of *positive* $(+)$ signs. The resulting number is S. If there are no positive signs, S is 0.

Why does S make sense as a test statistic for testing the null hypothesis (11.1)? If the population median is m_0, half of the population values are less than m_0 and half of the population values are greater than m_0. We expect a sample from such a population to have about half of its observations below m_0 and about half of its observations above m_0. If most of the sample observations are larger than m_0, S will be large. If most of the sample observations are smaller than m_0, S will be small. Thus, it makes sense to reject the null hypothesis (11.1) when S is very large or very small.

S values that are very large or very small have small p-values. If the p-value for the S statistic is less than the significance level α, the null hypothesis (11.1) is rejected. If the p-value for the S statistic is greater than or equal to α, the null hypothesis (11.1) cannot be rejected. The p-value is interpreted in the usual way: it is the probability of getting an S statistic at least as extreme as the calculated S statistic if the null hypothesis (11.1) is true.

Approximate p-values for the S statistic can be obtained from Table E.8 in Appendix E. Let n_D be the number of *nonzero* new observations and let S_{calc} be the calculated value of the S statistic. To use Table E.8, we first determine n_D. We then proceed as follows to obtain approximate two-tailed p-values for S when the two-sided alternative hypothesis (11.2) is used.

STEP 1. Check to see whether S_{calc} is one of the numbers listed in the column headed by the probability 0.10 and in the row for your n_D value. If so, the p-value is less than 0.10. If not, the p-value is greater than 0.10.

STEP 2. If the p-value is greater than 0.10, no further information can be obtained from the table. If the p-value is less than 0.10, check to see whether S_{calc} is one of the numbers listed in the 0.05 column and in the row for your n_D value. If so, the p-value is less than 0.05. If not, the p-value is between 0.05 and 0.10.

STEP 3. If the p-value is between 0.05 and 0.10, no further information can be obtained from the table. If the p-value is less than 0.05, check to see whether S_{calc} is one of the numbers listed in the

0.02 column and in the row for your n_D value. If so, the p-value is less than 0.02. If not, the p-value is between 0.02 and 0.05.

STEP 4. If the p-value is between 0.02 and 0.05, no further information can be obtained from the table. If the p-value is less than 0.02, check to see whether S_{calc} is one of the numbers listed in the 0.01 column and in the row for your n_D value. If so, the p-value is less than 0.01. If not, the p-value is between 0.01 and 0.02.

When "none" is listed in a row and column of Table E.8, no S_{calc} has a p-value greater than the probability for that column. Whatever the value of the S statistic, its p-value is greater than the probability for the column.

The use of Table E.8 is illustrated in the following example.

Example 11.3 _____

What are the approximate p-values for the following calculated S statistics?

1. $S_{calc} = 17$, $n_D = 25$. In the row for $n_D = 25$ and in the 0.10 column, we find " ≤ 7 or ≥ 18." Since 17 is *not* less than or equal to 7 or greater than or equal to 18, the approximate p-value is

$$p\text{-value} > 0.10$$

2. $S_{calc} = 27$, $n_D = 33$. In the row for $n_D = 33$ and in the 0.10 column, we find " ≤ 11 or ≥ 22." Since 27 is greater than 22, the p-value is less than 0.10. In the 0.05 column, we find " ≤ 10 or ≥ 23." Since 27 is greater than 23, the p-value is less than 0.05. In the 0.02 column, we find " ≤ 9 or ≥ 24." Since 27 is greater than 24, the p-value is less than 0.02. In the 0.01 column, we find " ≤ 8 or ≥ 25." Since 27 is greater than 25, the approximate p-value is

$$p\text{-value} < 0.01$$

3. $S_{calc} = 12$, $n_D = 41$. In the row for $n_D = 41$ and in the 0.10 column, we find " ≤ 14 or ≥ 27." Since 12 is less than 14, the p-value is less than 0.10. In the 0.05 column, we find " ≤ 13 or ≥ 28." Since 12 is less than 13, the p-value is less than 0.05. In the 0.02 column, we find " ≤ 12 or ≥ 29." Since 12 is equal to 12, the p-value is less than 0.02. In the 0.01 column, we find " ≤ 11 or ≥ 30." Since 12 is *not* less than or equal to 11 or greater than or equal to 30, the p-value is greater than 0.01. The approximate p-value is

$$0.01 < p\text{-value} < 0.02$$

4. $S_{calc} = 6$, $n_D = 6$. In the row for $n_D = 6$ and in the 0.10 column, we find "0 or 6." Since 6 is equal to 6, the p-value is less than 0.10. In the 0.05 column, we find "0 or 6" again. Since 6 is equal to 6, the p-value is less than 0.05. In the 0.02 column,

we find "none." No S_{calc} has a p-value less than 0.02 when $n_D = 6$, so the p-value is greater than 0.02. The approximate p-value is

$$0.02 < p\text{-value} < 0.05$$

5. $S_{calc} = 4$, $n_D = 4$. In the row for $n_D = 4$ and in the 0.10 column, we find "none." No S_{calc} has a p-value less than 0.10 when $n_D = 4$, so the approximate p-value is

$$p\text{-value} > 0.10$$

One-sided sign tests have the alternative hypotheses H_A: Population median $< m_0$ or H_A: Population median $> m_0$. As usual, one-sided tests are generally not recommended. If you want to carry out one-sided sign tests, consult a statistician to obtain one-tailed p-values.

Example 11.4 _____

A study evaluated intrathecal morphine infusion via implanted pumps for intractable cancer pain.[4] Table 11.3 shows the highest daily morphine dose for 16 cancer patients with implanted pumps. An oncologist believes that the population median highest dose is 50 mg/day. She would like to use the sign test to test the hypothesis

$$H_0: \text{Population median} = 50$$

against the alternative hypothesis

$$H_A: \text{Population median} \neq 50$$

Is the sign test appropriate? The independence assumption is reasonable, since the highest dose for one patient tells us nothing about the highest dose

TABLE 11.3 HIGHEST DAILY MORPHINE DOSE FOR PATIENTS WITH IMPLANTED PUMPS

Patient No.	Highest Dose (mg/day)
1	1.5
2	7.5
3	14.0
4	8.0
5	22.5
6	8.0
7	30.0
8	48.0
9	80.0
10	7.5
11	50.0
12	4.0
13	20.0
14	22.5
15	100.0
16	15.0

```
0.0 – 14.9 | XXXXXXX
15.0 – 29.9 | XXXX
30.0 – 44.9 | X
45.0 – 59.9 | XX
60.0 – 74.9 |
75.0 – 89.9 | X
90.0 – 104.9 | X
```

Figure 11.2 Quick histogram of highest dose

for another patient. We will use the sign test with a 0.01 significance level.

Before carrying out the sign test, let us consider whether more powerful statistical methods could be used instead. The highest dose values are extremely skewed, with most values less than 30 and one value equal to 100. This skewness is evident in the histogram in Figure 11.2. Extreme nonnormality rules out the one-sample t test for testing the hypothesis that the population mean is 50. Marked skewness also rules out the Wilcoxon signed rank test for testing the hypothesis that the population median is 50. More powerful methods cannot be used, so the sign test is appropriate.

Subtracting 50 from each dose in Table 11.3 produces the following new observations.

−48.5	−42.5	−36.0	−42.0	−27.5	−42.0
−20.0	−2.0	30.0	−42.5	0.0	−46.0
−30.0	−27.5	50.0	−35.0		

Counting the number of positive *nonzero* new observations, we get $S = 2$. Since the number of nonzero new observations is 15, $n_D = 15$. In the row for $n_D = 15$ and in the 0.10 column in Table E.8, we find "≤ 3 or ≥ 12." Since 2 is less than 3, the p-value is less than 0.10. In the 0.05 column, we find "≤ 3 or ≥ 12" again. Since 2 is less than 3, the p-value is less than 0.05. In the 0.02 column, we find "≤ 2 or ≥ 13." Since 2 is equal to 2, the p-value is less than 0.02. In the 0.01 column, we find "≤ 2 or ≥ 13" again. Since 2 is equal to 2, the p-value is less than 0.01. We reject the hypothesis that the population median highest dose is 50 mg/day at the 0.01 significance level.

11.2 HYPOTHESES ABOUT POPULATION MEDIAN DIFFERENCES

If a sample of differences obtained from paired samples suggests an extremely nonnormal population of differences, the paired t test cannot be used to test hypotheses about the population mean difference. The Wilcoxon signed rank test or the sign test can often be used instead to test hypotheses about the population median difference. As before, the Wilcoxon signed rank test has more power than

the sign test and is preferred if its assumptions are satisfied. We will describe the use of the Wilcoxon signed rank test first.

Suppose we have two paired samples which we convert into one sample of differences. For each pair of observations, we subtract one observation from the other to obtain the difference between the two observations. If the observations for the first sample are denoted by x_{1i} and the observations for the second sample by x_{2i}, we calculate the difference

$$d_i = x_{1i} - x_{2i}$$

for each pair.

We want to test the null hypothesis that the population median difference is equal to some hypothesized value:

$$H_0: \text{Population median difference} = m_0 \quad (11.5)$$

The two-sided alternative hypothesis is

$$H_A: \text{Population median difference} \neq m_0 \quad (11.6)$$

Again, m_0 is a number specified by the researcher. In most cases, m_0 is 0.

The Wilcoxon signed rank test statistic for testing the null hypothesis (11.5) is again denoted by W. The test statistic W is calculated in the same way as the Wilcoxon signed rank test statistic described in Section 11.1, using the sample of differences. The assumptions given on p. 230 for the Wilcoxon signed rank test are required for the population of *differences*. Approximate two-tailed p-values for W are obtained from Table E.9 in the same way as before. Although one-sided tests are not usually recommended, Wilcoxon signed rank tests can be done with one-sided alternative hypotheses (H_A: Population median difference $< m_0$ or H_A: Population median difference $> m_0$).

Example 11.5 _____

A study evaluated the accuracy of children's blood pressure measurements obtained with the Dinamap monitor.[5] Table 11.4 shows the Dinamap systolic pressures, the direct radial artery systolic pressures, and the differences between the two pressures for 29 pediatric patients in an intensive care unit. A nurse believes that the population median difference between the two pressures is 0. In other words, he believes that positive differences and negative differences are equally likely. The null hypothesis is

$$H_0: \text{Population median difference} = 0 \quad (11.7)$$

and the alternative hypothesis is

$$H_A: \text{Population median difference} \neq 0 \quad (11.8)$$

Can we use the Wilcoxon signed rank test to test the null hypothesis (11.7)? Random sampling was

TABLE 11.4 DINAMAP SYSTOLIC PRESSURE, DIRECT RADIAL ARTERY SYSTOLIC PRESSURE, AND DIFFERENCE

Patient No.	Dinamap Systolic Pressure	Direct Systolic Pressure	Difference (Dinamap − Direct)
1	115	115	0
2	81	81	0
3	110	110	0
4	136	130	6
5	111	111	0
6	91	96	−5
7	118	118	0
8	97	102	−5
9	93	93	0
10	96	96	0
11	89	84	5
12	86	92	−6
13	99	99	0
14	99	97	2
15	113	113	0
16	127	131	−4
17	106	110	−4
18	111	111	0
19	91	91	0
20	96	97	−1
21	105	112	−7
22	93	94	−1
23	113	113	0
24	83	83	0
25	114	114	0
26	117	110	7
27	86	82	4
28	106	106	0
29	105	105	0

not done, but this is not essential. Since the difference for one patient tells us nothing about the difference for another patient, the assumption of independent differences is reasonable for these data. The histogram of the data shown in Figure 11.3 is nearly symmetric, so the assumption of symmetry appears to hold. The Wilcoxon signed rank test is appropriate. We will use a significance level of 0.10.

Before carrying out the Wilcoxon signed rank test, let us consider whether the paired t test could be used to test the hypothesis that the population mean difference is 0. Although the Dinamap and direct systolic pressures both have a large number of possible values, it is the distribution of the *dif-*

```
−7 – −5 | XXXX
−4 – −2 | XX
−1 – 1 | XXXXXXXXXXXXXXXXX
 2 – 4 | XX
 5 – 7 | XXX
```

Figure 11.3 Quick histogram of systolic pressure difference

ferences that matters. More than half of the differences in Table 11.4 are equal to 0, indicating an extremely nonnormal distribution. The paired t test cannot be used.

Since m_0 is 0, subtracting m_0 from the differences does not change them. The new differences are the same as the original differences. Arranging the 13 *nonzero* differences from Table 11.4 in increasing order of absolute value, we get

$$-1 \quad -1 \quad 2 \quad -4 \quad -4 \quad 4 \quad -5 \quad -5 \quad 5$$
$$6 \quad -6 \quad -7 \quad 7$$

Assigning ranks based on absolute values to the differences, we have

differences:	−1	−1	2	−4	−4	4	−5	−5
ranks:	1.5	1.5	3	5	5	5	8	8

differences:	5	6	−6	−7	7
ranks:	8	10.5	10.5	12.5	12.5

Giving the ranks the signs of the differences to which they correspond, we get

$$-1.5 \quad -1.5 \quad 3 \quad -5 \quad -5 \quad 5 \quad -8 \quad -8 \quad 8$$
$$10.5 \quad -10.5 \quad -12.5 \quad 12.5$$

Adding the positive ranks gives $W = 39$:

$$W = 3 + 5 + 8 + 10.5 + 12.5 = 39$$

Since there are 13 nonzero differences, $n_D = 13$. In the row for $n_D = 13$ and the 0.10 column in Table E.9, we find "≤ 21 or ≥ 70." Since 39 is *not* less than or equal to 21 or greater than or equal to 70, the p-value is greater than 0.10. We cannot reject the hypothesis that the population median difference is 0 at any reasonable significance level.

When a histogram of the differences is extremely nonsymmetric, the Wilcoxon signed rank test cannot be used to test hypotheses about the population median difference. The sign test should then be considered for testing the null hypothesis (11.5). As before, the sign test requires only one assumption: independence of the *differences*. If any of the differences are not independent, the sign test cannot be done. Because the sign test has so little power, it should be used only when more powerful methods are not appropriate.

To carry out the sign test of the null hypothesis (11.5), we first convert our paired samples into one sample of differences, as we did for the Wilcoxon signed rank test of this hypothesis. The sign test statistic S is obtained in the same way as the sign test statistic described in Section 11.1, using the sample of differences. Approximate two-tailed p-

TABLE 11.5 PERFORMANCE STATUS BEFORE AND AFTER HEPATIC ARTERIAL INFUSION

Patient No.	Before Infusion	After Infusion	Difference (After − Before)
1	2	1	−1
2	0	0	0
3	0	0	0
4	1	0	−1
5	3	3	0
6	1	0	−1
7	1	3	2
8	0	0	0
9	0	0	0
10	0	0	0
11	1	0	−1
12	1	1	0
13	2	1	−1
14	3	1	−2
15	0	0	0
16	0	0	0
17	0	3	3
18	2	3	1
19	2	3	1
20	3	2	−1
21	0	4	4
22	0	3	3
23	1	2	1
24	0	3	3
25	0	2	2
26	1	1	0
27	3	3	0
28	1	2	1
29	0	2	2

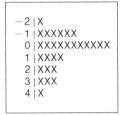

Figure 11.4 Quick histogram of performance status difference

Since the difference for one patient should not tell us anything about the difference for another patient, the independence assumption is reasonable. We will carry out the sign test with a 0.05 significance level.

Let us first consider whether more powerful statistical methods could be used to analyze the data. The paired t test is inappropriate for testing the hypothesis that the population mean difference is 0 because the differences have an extremely nonnormal distribution with only a few possible values. Figure 11.4 shows a histogram of the differences that suggests a fairly skewed population. The symmetry assumption does not seem reasonable for these data, so the Wilcoxon signed rank test is ruled out. More powerful methods cannot be used, and the sign test is appropriate.

Since m_0 is 0, subtracting m_0 from the differences in Table 11.5 does not change their values. Counting the number of positive *nonzero* differences in Table 11.5, we obtain $S = 11$. There are 18 nonzero differences, so $n_D = 18$. In the row for $n_D = 18$ and in the 0.10 column in Table E.8, we find "≤ 5 or ≥ 13." Since 11 is *not* less than or equal to 5 or greater than or equal to 13, the p-value is greater than 0.10. We cannot reject the hypothesis that the population median difference is 0 at any reasonable significance level.

Example 11.7

In a study of high-dose photoirradiation of esophageal cancer, dysphagia scores were obtained before and after 24 photodynamic therapy treatments of 14 patients with esophageal cancer.[7] These scores and their differences are shown in Table 11.6. The higher the score, the better the patient's ability to swallow. Can the sign test be used to test the hypothesis that the population median difference is −1?

Because 24 differences were obtained for 14 patients, some patients have more than one difference. Differences from the same patient cannot be considered independent, and the sign test cannot be done on all 24 differences. If we knew which differences belonged to each patient, we could select the differences for the first phototherapy session. A sign test then could be done on the resulting 14 independent differences.

values for S are obtained from Table E.8 in the same way as before.

The null hypothesis (11.5) is usually tested against the two-sided alternative hypothesis (11.6). In most cases, the number m_0 specified by the researcher is 0. One-sided sign tests can be done with the one-sided alternative hypotheses H_A: Population median difference $< m_0$ or H_A: Population median difference $> m_0$. Such tests usually are not recommended.

Example 11.6

A study evaluated hepatic arterial infusion of floxuridine and cisplatin for the treatment of liver metastases of colorectal cancer.[6] Table 11.5 shows the performance status scores before and after hepatic arterial infusion for 29 patients with colorectal cancer metastatic to the liver. Can we use the sign test to test the hypothesis that the population median population difference is 0? The null hypothesis is

$$H_0: \text{Population median difference} = 0$$

and the alternative hypothesis is

$$H_A: \text{Population median difference} \neq 0$$

TABLE 11.6 DYSPHAGIA SCORE BEFORE AND AFTER PHOTODYNAMIC THERAPY

Treatment No.	Before Therapy	After Therapy	Difference (Before − After)
1	1	3	−2
2	2	4	−2
3	2	4	−2
4	2	4	−2
5	1	3	−2
6	1	2	−1
7	1	2	−1
8	2	4	−2
9	2	4	−2
10	1	2	−1
11	2	3	−1
12	2	2	0
13	2	3	−1
14	2	2	0
15	2	2	0
16	2	2	0
17	4	2	2
18	3	3	0
19	3	3	0
20	3	3	0
21	3	4	−1
22	4	2	2
23	3	2	1
24	4	4	0

11.3 HYPOTHESES ABOUT DIFFERENCES BETWEEN TWO INDEPENDENT POPULATIONS

Extreme nonnormality often rules out the pooled-variance t test and the separate-variance t test for testing hypotheses about differences between the means of two independent populations. When this occurs, we can sometimes use the nonparametric *Mann-Whitney test* to test the null hypothesis that two independent populations are identical:

$$H_0: \text{The two populations are identical} \quad (11.9)$$

The two-sided alternative hypothesis is

$$H_A: \text{One population tends to produce larger observations than the other population} \quad (11.10)$$

The Mann-Whitney test does not require normality, or even approximate normality, but it does require the following assumptions.*

1. Random Samples. If the samples are not biased, random sampling is not necessary.

2. Independent Samples. The Mann-Whitney test cannot be done if the samples are not independent.

3. Independence Within Each Sample. If the observations within each sample are not independent, the Mann-Whitney test cannot be done.

The Mann-Whitney test statistic is based on the ranks of the data. This test statistic, called *MW*, is calculated as follows.

STEP 1. Combine the two samples into one sample. Underline the observations from the first sample in order to keep track of them.*

STEP 2. Arrange the observations in the combined sample in order of increasing size, keeping the lines under the observations from the first sample. Observations are ordered according to actual values, *not* absolute values.

STEP 3. Write the ranks of the observations, starting with a rank of 1 for the observation with the smallest value. Underline the ranks corresponding to observations from the first sample. If two or more observations are equal, they will be tied for the same rank. When this occurs, assign to each of the tied observations the average of the ranks they would have if they were not tied.

STEP 4. Add all of the ranks from the first sample. The resulting sum is *MW*.†

The calculation of *MW* is best understood by considering an example. We will use data from a study comparing transcutaneous nerve stimulation (TENS) and analgesic drugs for the relief of rib fracture pain.[8] Patients with multiple rib fractures were randomly assigned to receive either TENS or analgesic drugs. Table 11.7 shows the pain-relief scores for 23 of these patients. These scores measure the effectiveness and continuity of pain relief, with a high score indicating better pain relief. An anesthesiologist believes that the populations of pain relief scores are the same whether drugs or TENS treatments are used. Do the data provide evidence against her view? We would like to calculate *MW* to test the null hypothesis (11.9).

Before calculating *MW*, let us consider whether the pooled-variance t test or the separate-variance t test is appropriate for testing the hypothesis that the drug population relief score mean is equal to the TENS population relief score mean. Because

---

*The Mann-Whitney test is equivalent to another nonparametric test called the Wilcoxon rank sum test.[1]

*Either sample may be chosen as the first sample, as long as the same sample is consistently defined as the first sample throughout the calculation of *MW*. Although the value of *MW* depends on which sample is defined as the first sample, the *p*-value for *MW* does *not* depend on the first-sample designation.

†An alternative Mann-Whitney test statistic described in other texts is often used instead of *MW* if the number of ties is very large.[1]

TABLE 11.7 PAIN-RELIEF SCORE FOR PATIENTS WITH RIB FRACTURES

Drug Group		TENS Group	
PATIENT NO.	RELIEF SCORE	PATIENT NO.	RELIEF SCORE
1	7	13	15
2	6	14	14
3	4	15	17
4	11	16	16
5	16	17	16
6	4	18	16
7	10	19	14
8	6	20	12
9	9	21	14
10	3	22	17
11	13	23	16
12	5		

the pooled-variance t test and the separate-variance t test have slightly more power than the Mann-Whitney test, it does not make sense to use the Mann-Whitney test if the t test assumptions are satisfied. Approximate normality might be a reasonable assumption for the drug population, but it does not seem reasonable for the TENS population. The number of possible values for the TENS population seems quite small. The pooled-variance t test and the separate-variance t test are not appropriate, and use of the Mann-Whitney test is warranted.

To calculate MW, we first combine all of the relief scores and then sort the scores in order of increasing size. Let us arbitrarily designate the drug group as the first sample. The combined and sorted sample is shown in the following, with the observations from the drug group underlined.

3 4 4 5 6 6 7 9 10 11 12 13 14 14

14 15 16 16 16 16 16 17 17

Assigning ranks to the sorted scores, we get

scores: 3 4 4 5 6 6 7 9 10 11 12 13 14

ranks: 1 2.5 2.5 4 5.5 5.5 7 8 9 10 11 12 14

scores: 14 14 15 16 16 16 16 16 17 17

ranks: 14 14 16 19 19 19 19 19 22.5 22.5

Adding the ranks for the drug group observations (the underlined ranks), we get $MW = 86$:

$$MW = 1 + 2.5 + 2.5 + 4 + 5.5 + 5.5 + 7 + 8$$
$$+ 9 + 10 + 12 + 19$$
$$= 86$$

Why does MW make sense as a test of the null hypothesis (11.9)? If the two populations are identical, we expect the ranks to be evenly distributed between the two samples. We do *not* expect most of the ranks from the first sample to be large, nor do we expect most of the ranks from the first sample to be small. When MW is large, most of the ranks from the first sample are large. When MW is small, most of the ranks from the first sample are small. Thus, it makes sense to reject the hypothesis of identical populations when MW is very large or very small.

The p-value associated with the MW statistic is used to determine whether MW is large enough or small enough to warrant rejection of the null hypothesis (11.9). If MW is extremely large or extremely small, its p-value is small. If the p-value for the MW statistic is less than the significance level α, the null hypothesis (11.9) is rejected. If the p-value for the MW statistic is greater than or equal to α, the null hypothesis (11.9) cannot be rejected. The p-value is interpreted in the usual way: it is the probability of getting an MW statistic at least as extreme as the calculated MW statistic if the null hypothesis (11.9) is true.

Approximate p-values for the MW statistic can be obtained from Table E.10 in Appendix E. Let n_1 be the number of observations in the first sample and let n_2 be the number of observations in the second sample. The sample sizes n_1 and n_2 need not be equal. Let MW_{calc} be the calculated value of the MW statistic. To use Table E.10, we first locate the block of rows corresponding to n_1 and the column corresponding to n_2. We then proceed as follows to obtain approximate two-tailed p-values for MW when the two-sided alternative hypothesis (11.10) is used.

STEP 1. Check to see whether MW_{calc} is one of the numbers listed in the row beginning with the probability 0.10 and in the n_2 column, using the n_1 block. If so, the p-value is less than 0.10. If not, the p-value is greater than 0.10.

STEP 2. If the p-value is greater than 0.10, no further information can be obtained from the table. If the p-value is less than 0.10, check to see whether MW_{calc} is one of the numbers listed in the row beginning with the probability 0.05 and in the n_2 column, using the n_1 block. If so, the p-value is less than 0.05. If not, the p-value is greater than 0.05.

STEP 3. If the p-value is between 0.05 and 0.10, no further information can be obtained from the table. If the p-value is less than 0.05, check to see whether MW_{calc} is one of the numbers listed in the row beginning with the probability 0.02 and in the n_2 column, using the n_1 block. If so, the p-value is less than 0.02. If not, the p-value is greater than 0.02.

STEP 4. If the p-value is between 0.02 and 0.05, no further information can be obtained from the table. If the p-value is less than 0.02, check to see whether MW_{calc} is one of the numbers listed in the row beginning with the probability 0.01 and in the n_2 column, using the n_1 block. If so, the p-value is less than 0.01. If not, the p-value is greater than 0.01.

STEP 5. If the p-value is between 0.01 and 0.02, no further information can be obtained from the table. If the p-value is less than 0.01, check to see whether MW_{calc} is one of the numbers listed in the row beginning with the probability 0.002 and in the n_2 column, using the n_1 block. If so, the p-value is less than 0.002. If not, the p-value is greater than 0.002.

When "none" is listed in a row and column in Table E.10, no MW_{calc} has a p-value less than the probability for that column. Whatever the value of the MW statistic, its p-value is greater than the probability for the column.

The use of Table E.10 is illustrated in the following example.

Example 11.8

What are the approximate p-values for the following calculated MW statistics?

1. $MW_{calc} = 23$, $n_1 = 4$, $n_2 = 9$. In the column for $n_2 = 9$ and in the 0.10 row in the block for $n_1 = 4$, we find " ≤ 16 or ≥ 40." Since 23 is *not* less than or equal to 16 or greater than or equal to 40, the approximate p-value is

$$p\text{-value} > 0.10$$

2. $MW_{calc} = 168$, $n_1 = 10$, $n_2 = 13$. In the column for $n_2 = 13$ and in the 0.10 row in the block for $n_1 = 10$, we find " ≤ 92 or ≥ 148." Since 168 is greater than 148, the p-value is less than 0.10. In the column for $n_2 = 13$ and in the 0.05 row in the block for $n_1 = 10$, we find " ≤ 88 or ≥ 152." Since 168 is greater than 152, the p-value is less than 0.05. In the column for $n_2 = 13$ and in the 0.02 row in the block for $n_1 = 10$, we find " ≤ 82 or ≥ 158." Since 168 is greater than 158, the p-value is less than 0.02. In the column for $n_2 = 13$ and in the 0.01 row in the block for $n_1 = 10$, we find " ≤ 79 or ≥ 161." Since 168 is greater than 161, the p-value is less than 0.01. In the column for $n_2 = 13$ and in the 0.002 row in the block for $n_1 = 10$, we find " ≤ 72 or ≥ 168." Since 168 is equal to 168, the approximate p-value is

$$p\text{-value} < 0.002$$

3. $MW_{calc} = 141$, $n_1 = 15$, $n_2 = 8$. In the column for $n_2 = 8$ and in the 0.10 row in the block for $n_1 = 15$, we find " ≤ 153 or ≥ 207." Since 141 is less than 153, the p-value is less than 0.10. In the column for $n_2 = 8$ and in the 0.05 row in the block for $n_1 = 15$, we find " ≤ 149 or ≥ 211." Since 141 is less than 149, the p-value is less than 0.05. In the column for $n_2 = 8$ and in the 0.02 row in the block for $n_1 = 15$, we find " ≤ 144 or ≥ 216." Since 141 is less than 144, the p-value is less than 0.02. In the column for $n_2 = 8$ and in the 0.01 row in the block

for $n_1 = 15$, we find " ≤ 140 or ≥ 220." Since 141 is *not* less than or equal to 140 or greater than or equal to 220, the p-value is greater than 0.01. The approximate p-value is

$$0.01 < p\text{-value} < 0.02$$

4. $MW_{calc} = 202$, $n_1 = 10$, $n_2 = 20$. In the column for $n_2 = 20$ and in the 0.10 row in the block for $n_1 = 10$, we find " ≤ 117 or ≥ 193." Since 202 is greater than 193, the p-value is less than 0.10. In the column for $n_2 = 20$ and in the 0.05 row in the block for $n_1 = 10$, we find " ≤ 110 or ≥ 200." Since 202 is greater than 200, the p-value is less than 0.05. In the column for $n_2 = 20$ and in the 0.02 row in the block for $n_1 = 10$, we find " ≤ 102 or ≥ 208." Since 202 is *not* less than or equal to 102 or greater than or equal to 208, the p-value is greater than 0.02. The approximate p-value is

$$0.02 < p\text{-value} < 0.05$$

5. $MW_{calc} = 47$, $n_1 = 18$, $n_2 = 1$. In the column for $n_2 = 1$ and in the 0.10 row in the block for $n_1 = 18$, we find "none." No MW_{calc} has a p-value less than 0.10, so the approximate p-value is

$$p\text{-value} > 0.10$$

One-sided Mann-Whitney tests have the alternative hypotheses H_A: The first population tends to produce larger observations than the second population or H_A: The second population tends to produce larger observations than the first population. One-sided tests are not generally recommended, for the same reasons discussed in Chapter 7. Using Table E.10 to find one-tailed p-values is more complicated than using this table to find two-tailed p-values. Consult a statistician if you need one-tailed p-values for the Mann-Whitney test.

Before obtaining an approximate p-value from the pain-relief data, we need to check the assumptions required for the Mann-Whitney test. Random sampling was not done, but this is not crucial. If the patients had no contact with one another, both independence assumptions are reasonable. The pain-relief score for one patient tells us nothing about the pain-relief score for another patient. The Mann-Whitney test is appropriate. We will obtain an approximate p-value to test the null hypothesis (11.9), using a 0.05 significance level.

We have $n_1 = 12$, $n_2 = 11$, and $MW_{calc} = 86$. In the column for $n_2 = 11$ and in the 0.10 row in the block for $n_1 = 12$ in Table E.10, we find " ≤ 116 or ≥ 172." Since 86 is less than 116, the p-value is less than 0.10. In the column for $n_2 = 11$ and in the 0.05 row in the block for $n_1 = 12$, we find " ≤ 111 or ≥ 177." Since 86 is less than 111, the p-value is less than 0.05. In the column for $n_2 = 11$ and in the 0.02 row in the block for $n_1 = 12$, we find " ≤ 106 or ≥ 182." Since 86 is less than 106, the p-value is less than 0.02. In the column for $n_2 = 11$ and in the 0.01 row in the block for $n_1 = 12$, we find "≤ 102 or ≥ 186." Since 86 is less than 102, the p-value is less than 0.01. In the column for $n_2 = 11$ and in the 0.002 row in the block for $n_1 = 12$, we find "≤ 95 or ≥ 193." Since 86 is less than 95, the approximate p-value is

$$p\text{-value} < 0.002$$

Using a 0.05 significance level, we reject the hypothesis that the drug population of pain-relief scores is identical to the TENS population of pain relief scores.

Example 11.9

In a study of necrotizing enterocolitis (NEC) in infants of multiple gestation, 10 pairs of twins were investigated.[9] One or both twins in each pair had NEC. Table 11.8 shows the one-minute Apgar scores for 18 of these twins. Can we use the Mann-Whitney test to test the hypothesis that the population of Apgar scores for twins who develop NEC is identical to the population of Apgar scores for twins who do not develop NEC?

The independence assumption is questionable for Apgar scores from members of the same twin pair. Since the between-samples and within-samples independence assumptions may be violated, the Mann-Whitney test should not be used to analyze the data. If we knew which twins belonged together, we could select those twin pairs in which one twin developed NEC and the other twin did not develop NEC. This would produce two paired samples. We could then use the Wilcoxon signed rank test or the sign test to test the hypothesis that the population median difference between Apgar scores is 0.

TABLE 11.8 APGAR SCORE (1 MINUTE) FOR TWINS

NEC		No NEC	
PATIENT NO.	APGAR SCORE	PATIENT NO.	APGAR SCORE
1	7	13	8
2	9	14	1
3	6	15	3
4	8	16	8
5	8	17	7
6	9	18	4
7	6		
8	7		
9	8		
10	?		
11	7		
12	7		

11.4 HYPOTHESES ABOUT DIFFERENCES AMONG THREE OR MORE INDEPENDENT POPULATIONS

Suppose we have three or more independent samples and extreme nonnormality rules out one-way analysis of variance (Chapter 8) for testing the hypothesis of equal population means. We may be able to use a nonparametric test to test the hypothesis that all of the populations are identical. This test is a generalization of the Mann-Whitney test called the *Kruskal-Wallis test*.

If there are k samples, the null hypothesis tested by the Kruskal-Wallis test is

$$H_0: \text{All } k \text{ populations are identical} \qquad (11.11)$$

The alternative hypothesis is

$$H_A: \text{At least one population tends to produce larger observations than another population} \qquad (11.12)$$

If we reject the null hypothesis (11.11), we cannot conclude that all of the populations are different. We can conclude only that at least one of the populations is different.

We cannot carry out the Kruskal-Wallis test of (11.11) with any one-sided alternative hypothesis. This rules out alternative hypotheses like H_A: Population 1 tends to produce larger values than population 2 and population 2 tends to produce larger values than population 3.

The Kruskal-Wallis test does not require normality or approximate normality, but it does require other assumptions.

1. Random Samples. As usual, random sampling is not essential if the samples are not biased.

2. Independent Samples. If the samples are not independent, the Kruskal-Wallis test cannot be done.

3. Independence Within Each Sample. The Kruskal-Wallis test cannot be done if the observations within each sample are not independent.

Like the Mann-Whitney test, the Kruskal-Wallis test is based on the ranks of the data. To calculate the Kruskal-Wallis test, we proceed as follows.

STEP 1. Combine the k samples into one sample. Write the sample number above each observation in order to keep track of the sample from which each observation came.

STEP 2. Arrange the observations in the combined sample in order of increasing size, keeping the sample numbers above the observations. The observations are ordered by actual values, *not* by absolute values.

STEP 3. Write the ranks of the observations, with the observation having the smallest value re-

TABLE 11.9 IgE FOR HUMIDIFIER FEVER SUBJECTS

Symptomatic, HF Likely		Symptomatic, HF Unlikely		Asymptomatic	
SUBJECT NO.	IgE (mg/ml)	SUBJECT NO.	IgE (mg/ml)	SUBJECT NO.	IgE (mg/ml)
1	67	11	55	19	13
2	0	12	13	20	22
3	5	13	85	21	13
4	27	14	5	22	11
5	5	15	12	23	16
6	5	16	18	24	34
7	5	17	1000	25	38
8	0	18	19		
9	90				
10	78				

ceiving a rank of 1. If two or more observations are equal, they will be tied for the same rank. When this occurs, assign to each of the tied observations the average of the ranks they would have if they were not tied.

STEP 4. For each sample, calculate the sum of the ranks for the sample. This produces k sums of ranks, denoted by $R_1, R_2, \ldots, R_k$, where R_i is the sum of the ranks for the ith sample.

STEP 5. Let n_i be the sample size for the ith sample and let n_T be the size of the combined sample ($n_T = n_1 + n_2 + \cdots + n_k$). Calculate the Kruskal-Wallis test statistic according to the formula

$$\chi^2 = \left(\frac{12}{n_T(n_T + 1)} \times \sum_{i=1}^{k} \frac{R_i^2}{n_i} \right) \quad (11.13)$$
$$- [3(n_T + 1)]$$

We will refer to this statistic as the Kruskal-Wallis χ^2 statistic (pronounced "ki square statistic") or the KW χ^2 statistic.*

To illustrate the calculation of the Kruskal-Wallis χ^2 statistic, we will use data from a study of the serology of humidifier fever (HF).[10] Subjects were classified into three groups: symptomatic subjects considered likely to have HF, symptomatic subjects considered unlikely to have HF, and asymptomatic subjects. Table 11.9 shows the IgE values for 25 of these subjects. We would like to use the Kruskal-Wallis test to test the hypothesis that the symptomatic/HF likely population of IgE values, the symptomatic/HF unlikely population of IgE values, and the asymptomatic population of IgE values are identical.

Before calculating the KW χ^2 statistic, let us consider whether the more powerful one-way analy-

sis of variance procedure could be used to test the hypothesis that all three population IgE means are equal. One-way analysis of variance requires normal or approximately normal distributions for each population. Although the assumption of approximate normality might be reasonable for the asymptomatic population, it is not reasonable for the symptomatic/HF likely population or the symptomatic/HF unlikely population. In the symptomatic/HF likely sample, 60% of the IgE values are equal to 5 or 0. In the symptomatic/HF unlikely sample, the IgE values are extremely skewed, with most values less than 100 and one value equal to 1000. One-way analysis of variance is not appropriate, and use of the Kruskal-Wallis test is warranted.

To calculate the KW χ^2 statistic for the HF data, we first combine all 25 IgE values and arrange them in increasing order. We will treat the symptomatic/HF likely group as sample 1, the symptomatic/HF unlikely group as sample 2, and the asymptomatic group as sample 3. The assignment of sample numbers is arbitrary and does not affect the value of the KW χ^2 statistic. Assigning ranks to the sorted data, we get

sample:	1	1	1	1	1	1	2	3	2
observations:	0	0	5	5	5	5	5	11	12
ranks:	1.5	1.5	5	5	5	5	5	8	9

sample:	2	3	3	3	2	2	3	1	3
observations:	13	13	13	16	18	19	22	27	34
ranks:	11	11	11	13	14	15	16	17	18

sample:	3	2	1	1	2	1	2
observations:	38	55	67	78	85	90	1000
ranks:	19	20	21	22	23	24	25

Adding the ranks for each sample, we obtain the rank sums for the three samples:

$$R_1 = 1.5 + 1.5 + 5 + 5 + 5 + 5 + 17 + 21$$
$$+ 22 + 24 = 107$$
$$R_2 = 5 + 9 + 11 + 14 + 15 + 20 + 23 + 25 = 122$$
$$R_3 = 8 + 11 + 11 + 13 + 16 + 18 + 19 = 96$$

---

*If the number of ties is very large, an adjusted Kruskal-Wallis test statistic described in other texts is often used instead of the test statistic (11.13).[1]

Using the rank sums, the three sample sizes, and the total sample size of 25, we can apply formula (11.13) to calculate the KW χ^2 statistic:

$$\chi^2 = \left(\left(\frac{12}{(25)(25+1)} \right) \times \left(\frac{107^2}{10} + \frac{122^2}{8} + \frac{96^2}{7} \right) \right)$$
$$- [(3)(25+1)]$$
$$= \left(\frac{12}{650} \times (1144.90 + 1860.50 + 1316.57) \right) - 78$$
$$= 79.79 - 78 = 1.79$$

The rationale for the KW χ^2 statistic is not obvious. A description of the reasoning behind formula (11.13) requires a fairly technical discussion of probability. We will omit the rationale for the KW test and focus on the use of this test. Further information can be found in other texts.[1]

The hypothesis of identical populations is rejected when the KW χ^2 statistic is too large. The p-value associated with the KW χ^2 statistic is used to determine whether this statistic is large enough to warrant rejection of the null hypothesis (11.11). When the KW χ^2 statistic is extremely large, its p-value is small. If the p-value for the KW χ^2 statistic is less than the significance level α, the null hypothesis (11.11) is rejected. If the p-value for the KW χ^2 statistic is greater than or equal to α, the null hypothesis (11.11) cannot be rejected. The p-value is interpreted in the usual way: it is the probability of getting a KW χ^2 statistic at least as extreme as the calculated KW χ^2 statistic if the null hypothesis (11.11) is true.

It can be shown that the KW χ^2 statistic has an approximate chi-square distribution (pronounced "ki square distribution") with $k - 1$ degrees of freedom (df) if the Kruskal-Wallis test assumptions are satisfied and the sample sizes are large enough. Chi-square distributions, discussed in Chapter 10, are positively skewed distributions with frequency curves determined by their degrees of freedom. Random variables with chi-square distributions cannot have negative values. The frequency curves for several chi-square distributions are shown in Chapter 10 (p. 208).

The p-value for the KW χ^2 statistic is given by the probability

$$P\left(\chi^2 \text{ statistic} \geq \chi^2_{\text{calc}} \right)$$

where χ^2_{calc} is the calculated KW χ^2 statistic. Approximate p-values for KW χ^2 statistics can be obtained from Table E.7, which is based on upper percentage points of chi-square distributions. If χ^2_d is a random variable having a chi-square distribution with d degrees of freedom, the α upper percentage point of this distribution is the number $\chi^2_{\alpha, d}$ such that

$$P\left(\chi^2_d \geq \chi^2_{\alpha, d} \right) = \alpha$$

To obtain approximate p-values from Table E.7, we first locate the row for our degrees of freedom. We then find two adjacent numbers in this row such that χ^2_{calc} lies between these numbers, if possible. These numbers are upper percentage points, and the p-value lies between the probabilities to which they correspond. If χ^2_{calc} is very large, it will be larger than any of the appropriate upper percentage points given in the table. When this happens, we find the largest upper percentage point in the appropriate row. The p-value is *less* than the corresponding probability. If χ^2_{calc} is very small, it will be smaller than any of the appropriate upper percentage points listed. In this case, we find the smallest upper percentage point in the appropriate row. The p-value is *greater* than the corresponding probability. These possibilities are illustrated in Example 10.1 of Chapter 10. Refer to this example if you need practice using Table E.7.

Before obtaining an approximate p-value for the KW χ^2 statistic from the humidifier fever data, we need to check the assumptions required for the Kruskal-Wallis test. Random sampling was not done, but this is not essential. The independent-samples assumption and the within-samples independence assumption are reasonable, since the IgE for one subject tells us nothing about the IgE for another subject. The Kruskal-Wallis test is appropriate. We will obtain an approximate p-value to test the null hypothesis (11.11) with a 0.01 significance level.

Since there are three groups, the degrees of freedom are $3 - 1 = 2$. In the row for 2 df in Table E.7, the number 1.833 is very close to our χ^2 value of 1.79. This number is the 0.40 upper percentage point, so the approximate p-value is

$$p\text{-value} \cong 0.40$$

We cannot reject the null hypothesis (11.11) at any reasonable significance level.

If we cannot reject the hypothesis of identical populations, the analysis is finished. If we reject this hypothesis, we want to determine which populations are different. We cannot simply conclude that all of the populations differ. It is possible that only one population differs from the other populations, or that two populations differ from the other populations, and so on.

To determine which populations differ, we can carry out multiple Mann-Whitney tests to compare two populations at a time. When we obtain these tests, we need to adjust the significance level for each test to take the number of tests into account. The Bonferroni adjustment described in Chapter 7 is used to do this.

Suppose that the comparisons to be made are selected *before* examining the data, and define the number c by

$$c = \text{number of comparisons to be made}$$

If the comparisons are selected *after* examining the

data, we define c differently:

$$c = \text{total number of } possible \text{ comparisons}$$

In this case, c is the number of comparisons that *could* be made, whether we actually make these comparisons or not. If there are four populations and we select three comparisons after examining the data, c is not 3. There are six possible comparisons (population 1 versus population 2, population 1 versus population 3, population 1 versus population 4, population 2 versus population 3, population 2 versus population 4, and population 3 versus population 4), so c is 6. If we had selected three comparisons *before* examining the data, c would be 3.

If the desired overall significance level is α, the significance level used for each Mann-Whitney test is α/c. Extremely small overall significance levels (0.01 or less) are not recommended. The power of the Mann-Whitney test is greatly reduced when very small overall significance levels are used.

We cannot use the humidifier fever data to illustrate the use of Bonferroni-adjusted Mann-Whitney tests, since we cannot reject the hypothesis of identical populations. Instead, we will use data from a study of secretin provocation in patients with various disorders.[11] Table 11.10 shows the peak acid output (PAO) for 19 patients: seven hypochlorhydric patients, five patients with chronic renal failure, three postvagotomy patients, and four patients with gastrinoma. The KW χ^2 statistic for testing the hypothesis that the four populations of PAO values are identical is 13.36, with 3 df. Since the approximate p-value from Table E.7 is between 0.0005 and 0.005, we reject the null hypothesis (11.11) at the 0.01 significance level. We need to use Bonferroni-adjusted Mann-Whitney tests to determine which populations are different.

Let us use an overall significance level of 0.10. Suppose we knew, before examining the data, that we only wanted to compare the gastrinoma population with the other three populations. Since we selected these three comparisons before examining the data, $c = 3$. Dividing our overall significance level by 3, we get $0.10/3 = 0.033$. Since 0.033 is not one of the probabilities listed in Table E.10, we have to approximate with the closest probability in this table, which is 0.02. We will use a 0.02 significance level for each Mann-Whitney test to get an overall significance level of 0.10. The Mann-Whitney test statistics for comparing populations are obtained as follows.

Gastrinoma Versus Hypochlorhydric.

observations: 1   2   2   4   4   4   8   41   88   110   131
ranks: 1 2.5 2.5 5   5   5   7   8   9   10   11

$$MW = 8 + 9 + 10 + 11 = 38$$

$$n_1 = 4, \quad n_2 = 7, \quad 0.002 < p\text{-value} < 0.01$$

Gastrinoma Versus Renal Failure.

observations: 3   8   18   20   41   52   88   110   131
ranks: 1   2   3   4   5   6   7   8   9

$$MW = 5 + 7 + 8 + 9 = 29$$

$$n_1 = 4, \quad n_2 = 5, \quad 0.02 < p\text{-value} < 0.05$$

Gastrinoma Versus Postvagotomy.

observations: 11   22   41   41   88   110   131
ranks: 1   2   3.5 3.5   5   6   7

$$MW = 3.5 + 5 + 6 + 7 = 21.5$$

$$n_1 = 4, \quad n_2 = 3, \quad p\text{-value} > 0.10$$

Since the significance level for each Mann-Whitney test is 0.02, we reject the hypothesis that the gastrinoma and hypochlorhydric populations of PAO values are identical. We cannot reject the hypothesis that the gastrinoma and renal failure populations of PAO values are identical, nor can we reject the hypothesis that the gastrinoma and postvagotomy populations of PAO values are identical.

The Kruskal-Wallis test and the Bonferroni-adjusted Mann-Whitney tests can be inconsistent. It is possible to reject the hypothesis of k identical populations and then obtain Mann-Whitney tests that do not allow us to reject any of the hypotheses of two identical populations. Such inconsistencies are very annoying, since the Mann-Whitney tests fail to tell us which populations are different. This problem can sometimes be resolved by increasing the overall significance level until at least one of the Mann-Whitney tests leads to rejection of the hypothesis of identical populations.

TABLE 11.10   PEAK ACID OUTPUT FOR PATIENTS IN FOUR GROUPS

Patient No.	PAO	Patient No.	PAO
Hypochlorhydric patients		*Postvagotomy patients*	
1	1	13	41
2	4	14	22
3	8	15	11
4	4		
5	2	*Gastrinoma patients*	
6	4	16	88
7	2	17	41
		18	131
Renal failure patients		19	110
8	20		
9	3		
10	52		
11	18		
12	8		

TABLE 11.11 SYMPTOM SCORE BEFORE AND AFTER TREATMENT

Subject No.	0 Days	1 Day	10 Days	30 Days	150 Days
1	8	9	2	1	1
2	8	8	0	0	0
3	9	8	1	0	0
4	9	9	2	0	0
5	7	8	0	0	0
6	8	8	0	1	0
7	9	9	1	0	1
8	8	7	0	1	0
9	8	7	0	0	0
10	8	7	1	0	1
11	7	7	1	0	0
12	8	8	0	1	0
13	8	8	0	0	0
14	7	8	0	0	0
15	7	8	1	2	1

Example 11.10

In a study of eel-calcitonin for the treatment of headache, symptom scores were reported for 15 subjects with common migraine before treatment with eel-calcitonin and one, 10, 30, and 150 days after treatment.[12] These scores are shown in Table 11.11. The higher the score, the worse the symptoms. Can the Kruskal-Wallis test be used to test the hypothesis that the before-treatment population of scores and the four after-treatment populations of scores are identical?

Although the within-samples independence assumption is reasonable for these data, the between-samples independence assumption is not. The samples consist of repeated measurements on a group of subjects, and repeated measurements cannot be considered independent. The Kruskal-Wallis test cannot be used to analyze these data. The Friedman test described in the next section could be used instead.

11.5 HYPOTHESES ABOUT DIFFERENCES AMONG THREE OR MORE POPULATIONS OF REPEATED MEASUREMENTS

When data consist of three or more samples of repeated measurements, the Kruskal-Wallis test cannot be used to test the hypothesis of identical populations. If the data are extremely nonnormal, one-factor repeated-measures analysis of variance (Chapter 9) cannot be used to test the hypothesis of equal population means. The *Friedman test* can sometimes be used to compare extremely nonnormal populations of repeated measurements. Like the Kruskal-Wallis test, the Friedman test is based on ranks, although the Friedman ranks are calculated differently.

The null hypothesis tested by the Friedman test states that all possible rankings of the observations for any subject are equally likely:

$$H_0: \text{All possible rankings of the observations for any subject are equally likely} \quad (11.14)$$

This hypothesis implies that none of the populations tends to produce larger values than any of the other populations. The alternative hypothesis is

$$H_A: \text{At least one population tends to produce larger observations than another population} \quad (11.15)$$

If we reject the null hypothesis (11.14), we cannot conclude that all of the populations are different. We can conclude only that at least one of the populations is different.

One-sided alternative hypotheses cannot be used for the Friedman test. This rules out alternative hypotheses like H_A: Population 3 tends to produce larger values than population 2 and population 2 tends to produce larger values than population 1.

The Friedman test is based on the following assumptions.

1. Random Sample of Subjects. As long as the sample is not biased, random sampling is not crucial.

2. Repeated Measurements on a Group of Subjects. The Friedman test cannot be done if repeated measurements are not obtained.

3. Independence Within Each Sample of Repeated Measurements. All of the observations within the first sample must be independent, all of the observations within the second sample must be independent, and so on. Observations from *different* samples are not necessarily independent, since repeated measurements were obtained. If this assumption is violated, the Friedman test cannot be done.

A χ^2 statistic or F statistic based on ranks is used for the Friedman test. Ranks are not obtained for the combined sample but are obtained separately for each subject. It can be shown that better approximate p-values can be obtained for the Friedman F statistic than for the Friedman χ^2 statistic. For this reason, the Friedman F statistic is preferred to the Friedman χ^2 statistic.[1,13] Calculation of either statistic by hand is extremely tedious, especially when some of the observations are tied. We will omit the formulas for the Friedman test statistics and focus on the use of the Friedman test. These formulas can be found in other texts.[1]

It can be shown that the Friedman χ^2 statistic has an approximate chi-square distribution with $k - 1$ degrees of freedom, where k is the number of samples of repeated measurements. The Friedman

F statistic has an approximate F distribution with $k - 1$ numerator degrees of freedom and $(n - 1)(k - 1)$ denominator degrees of freedom, where n is the number of subjects. F distributions are positively skewed distributions with frequency curves determined by two sets of degrees of freedom: the numerator degrees of freedom and the denominator degrees of freedom. Random variables with F distributions cannot have negative values. The frequency curve for an F distribution is shown in Chapter 8 (p. 148).

The p-value for the Friedman χ^2 statistic is given by the probability

$$P\left(\chi^2 \text{ statistic} \geq \chi^2_{\text{calc}}\right)$$

where χ^2_{calc} is the calculated Friedman χ^2 statistic. The p-value for the Friedman F statistic is given by the probability

$$P\left(F \text{ statistic} \geq F_{\text{calc}}\right)$$

where F_{calc} is the calculated Friedman F statistic.

Approximate p-values for Friedman χ^2 statistics can be obtained from Table E.7. Approximate p-values for Friedman F statistics can be obtained from Table E.5, which is based on upper percentage points of F distributions. If F_{d_1, d_2} is a random variable having an F distribution with d_1 numerator degrees of freedom and d_2 denominator degrees of freedom, the α upper percentage point of this distribution is the number F_{α, d_1, d_2} such that

$$P\left(F_{d_1, d_2} \geq F_{\alpha, d_1, d_2}\right) = \alpha$$

To obtain approximate p-values from Table E.5, we first locate the column for our numerator degrees of freedom and the rows for our denominator degrees of freedom. We then find two adjacent numbers in this column and these rows such that F_{calc} lies between these numbers, if possible. These numbers are upper percentage points, and the p-value lies between the probabilities to which they correspond. If F_{calc} is very large, it will be larger than any of the appropriate upper percentage points given in the table. When this happens, we find the largest upper percentage point in the appropriate column and rows. The p-value is *less* than the corresponding probability. If F_{calc} is very small, it will be smaller than any of the appropriate upper percentage points listed. In this case, we find the smallest upper percentage point in the appropriate column and rows. The p-value is *greater* than the corresponding probability. These possibilities are illustrated in Example 8.1 of Chapter 8. Refer to this example if you need practice using Table E.5.

If the p-value for the Friedman test statistic is less than the significance level α, the null hypothesis (11.14) is rejected. If the p-value for the Friedman test statistic is greater than or equal to α, the null hypothesis (11.14) cannot be rejected. The

TABLE 11.12 INTRAPERICARDIAL PRESSURE (mm Hg) FOR PATIENTS WITH PERICARDIAL DISEASE

Patient No.	Tamponade	Intermediate Pericardio-centesis	Complete Pericardio-centesis
1	17	7	0
2	18	8	0
3	16	5	3
4	10	5	0
5	13	0	0
6	14	8	5
7	10	5	0
8	18	8	0
9	12	6	−1

p-value is interpreted in the usual way: it is the probability of getting a Friedman test statistic at least as extreme as the calculated Friedman test statistic if the null hypothesis (11.14) is true.

Let us consider data from a study of cardiac tamponade.[14] Table 11.12 shows the intrapericardial pressure during tamponade, intermediate pericardiocentesis, and complete pericardiocentesis for nine patients with pericardial disease. We would like to use the Friedman test to test the hypothesis that all possible rankings of the tamponade, intermediate, and complete pressures for any patient are equally likely.

Before using the Friedman test, we need to consider whether the more powerful one-factor· repeated-measures analysis of variance procedure (Chapter 9) could be used to test the hypothesis that all three population pressure means are equal. One-factor repeated-measures analysis of variance requires normal or approximately normal distributions for each population. Although the assumption of approximate normality might be reasonable for the tamponade population, it is not reasonable for the intermediate or complete pericardiocentesis populations. In the intermediate pericardiocentesis sample, 67% of the pressures are equal to 5 or 8. In the complete pericardiocentesis sample, 67% of the pressures are equal to 0. One-factor repeated-measures analysis of variance is not appropriate, and use of the Friedman test is warranted.

We also need to check the assumptions required for the Friedman test. Random sampling was not done, but this is not essential. Repeated measurements were obtained, and the within-samples independence assumption is reasonable. The pressures for one patient tell us nothing about the pressures for another patient. We will carry out the Friedman test with a 0.001 significance level.

The Friedman F statistic for the pericardial disease data is 307.00 with 2 and $(3 - 1)(9 - 1) = 16$ df. To find the approximate p-value in Table E.5, we have to use the rows for 15 denominator degrees of freedom, since 16 is not listed. In these rows and in the column for 2 numerator degrees of freedom, the largest number is 11.3. Since 11.3 is the 0.001

upper percentage point and 307.00 is greater than 11.3, the *p*-value for the Friedman *F* statistic is less than 0.001.

The Friedman χ^2 statistic for the pericardial disease data is 17.06, with 2 df. From Table E.7, we find that the approximate *p*-value for the Friedman χ^2 statistic is less than 0.0005. For these data, the Friedman *F* statistic and the Friedman χ^2 statistic both lead to rejection of the null hypothesis (11.14) at any reasonable significance level. In some cases, one Friedman test statistic may lead to rejection of the null hypothesis (11.14) while the other Friedman test statistic does not allow rejection of this hypothesis. If this occurs, the results of the Friedman *F* statistic should be used.

When the null hypothesis (11.14) is rejected, we often want to determine which populations are different. To do this, we can carry out multiple Wilcoxon signed rank tests or sign tests to compare populations. A Bonferroni adjustment of the significance level for each test must be used to take the number of tests into account.

Suppose that the comparisons to be made are selected *before* examining the data, and define the number *c* by

$$c = \text{number of comparisons to be made}$$

We define *c* differently if the comparisons are selected *after* examining the data:

$$c = \text{total number of } possible \text{ comparisons}$$

If the desired overall significance level is α, the significance level used for each Wilcoxon signed rank test or sign test is α/c. Extremely small overall significance levels (0.01 or less) greatly reduce power and should not be used.

Let us obtain multiple comparisons for the pericardial disease data. We rejected the hypothesis of equally likely rankings, so we would like to determine which of the populations of pressures differ. We will use an overall significance level of 0.10. There are three possible comparisons: tamponade versus intermediate, tamponade versus complete, and intermediate versus complete. All three comparisons are of interest, so $c = 3$. The significance level for each Wilcoxon signed rank test or sign test is $0.10/3 = 0.033$. But 0.033 is not listed in Table E.8 or Table E.9. Instead, we will use 0.02, the closest probability in these tables, as our significance level for each test.

We first calculate the differences among the three samples, which are shown in Table 11.13. Histograms of the differences are shown in Figures 11.5 through 11.7. The histogram of the difference between the tamponade pressures and the intermediate pressures suggests a symmetric or approximately symmetric U-shaped population. Since the symmetry assumption seems to hold for these differences, the more powerful Wilcoxon signed rank test can be used instead of the sign test to compare the tam-

TABLE 11.13 INTRAPERICARDIAL PRESSURE DIFFERENCES FOR PATIENTS WITH PERICARDIAL DISEASE

Patient No.	Tamponade − Intermediate	Tamponade − Complete	Intermediate − Complete
1	10	17	7
2	10	18	8
3	11	13	2
4	5	10	5
5	13	13	0
6	6	9	3
7	5	10	5
8	10	18	8
9	6	13	7

```
 4 – 6 | XXXX
 7 – 9 |
10 – 12 | XXXX
13 – 15 | X
```

Figure 11.5 Quick histogram of tamponade − intermediate difference

```
 9 – 11 | XXX
12 – 14 | XXX
15 – 17 | X
18 – 20 | XX
```

Figure 11.6 Quick histogram of tamponade − complete difference

```
0 – 3 | XXX
4 – 7 | XXXX
8 – 11 | XX
```

Figure 11.7 Quick histogram of intermediate − complete difference

ponade population and the intermediate population. We want to test the hypothesis that the population median difference between the tamponade and intermediate pressures is equal to 0.

When we carry out the calculations for the Wilcoxon signed rank test statistic, we obtain $W = 45$ and $n_D = 9$. From Table E.9, we get a *p*-value less than 0.01. We reject the hypothesis that the population median difference between the tamponade and intermediate pressures is equal to 0 at the 0.02 significance level.

The histogram of the difference between the tamponade and complete pressures suggests a skewed population. Since the symmetry assumption does not seem to hold, we will use the sign test to compare the tamponade and complete populations. Our null hypothesis states that the population median difference between the tamponade and complete pressures is 0. Our S value is 9, with $n_D = 9$. From Table E.8, we get a p-value less than 0.01, so we reject the hypothesis that the population median difference between the tamponade and complete pressures is equal to 0 at the 0.02 significance level.

Since the histogram of the difference between the intermediate and complete pressures suggests an approximately symmetric population, we will use the Wilcoxon signed rank test to compare the intermediate and complete populations of pressures. The null hypothesis states that the population median difference between the intermediate and complete pressures is 0. Our W value is 36, with $n_D = 8$. From Table E.9, the p-value is less than 0.01. We reject the null hypothesis at the 0.02 significance level. Based on our three comparisons, we conclude that all three populations are different.

The Friedman test and the Bonferroni-adjusted Wilcoxon signed rank tests or sign tests are sometimes inconsistent. In some cases, the Wilcoxon signed rank tests or sign tests do not allow us to say that any of the populations differ, even though the Friedman test allows us to reject the hypothesis of equally likely rankings. This problem can sometimes be resolved by increasing the overall significance level until at least one of the Wilcoxon signed rank tests or sign tests allows us to reject the hypothesis that the population median difference is 0.

Example 11.11

In a study of a female dispermic chimera, the levels of activity of H-, A-, and B-transferases in serum were reported for the chimera and her family members.[15] These activity levels are shown in Table 11.14. Can we use the Friedman test to test the hypothesis of equally likely rankings for any subject?

Although repeated measurements were obtained, the within-samples independence assumption may not hold. Since data were obtained for family members, the activity level for one family member may provide information about the activity levels for

other family members. The Friedman test cannot be used to analyze these data. No statistical method will allow us to use these data to test hypotheses about the population of all chimeras and family members of chimeras.

11.6 HYPOTHESES ABOUT ASSOCIATION BETWEEN TWO VARIABLES

In a study of corpus callosum section for the treatment of seizures, the numbers of partial complex seizures per month before and after callosotomy were reported for 21 patients.[16] These data are shown in Table 11.15. An obvious question of interest concerns whether the number of partial complex seizures changes after callosotomy. This question can be answered by using the sign test to test the hypothesis that the population median difference between the before-surgery number of seizures and the after-surgery number of seizures is equal to 0.

We might also want to investigate an entirely different question: Is the number of seizures before surgery related to the number of seizures after surgery? For example, do patients with more seizures than other patients before surgery also tend to have more seizures than other patients after surgery?

None of the procedures described in Sections 11.1 through 11.5 can be used to answer this question. Instead, we need a statistical procedure for determining the extent to which two variables are associated or *correlated*. Random variables are correlated if the values of one variable tend to be

TABLE 11.14 LEVELS OF ACTIVITY OF H-, A-, AND B-TRANSFERASES IN SERUM

Family Member	Incorporation of ^{14}C (%)		
	H	A	B
1	10.2	36.4	0
2	7.5	0	35.2
3	6.2	0	39.5
4	6.0	0	28.0
5	7.2	0	26.5
6	4.7	1.4	3.9
7	13.4	21.8	0

TABLE 11.15 NUMBER OF PARTIAL COMPLEX SEIZURES PER MONTH BEFORE AND AFTER CALLOSOTOMY

Patient No.	Preoperative	Postoperative
1	21	6
2	34	50
3	40	0
4	40	0
5	50	0
6	80	120
7	12	12
8	20	30
9	40	16
10	450	50
11	20	0
12	30	0
13	900	120
14	10	60
15	30	6
16	90	30
17	4	8
18	60	10
19	60	0
20	0	2
21	30	30

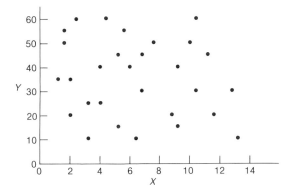

Figure 11.8 Scatterplot showing no relationship between variables X and Y

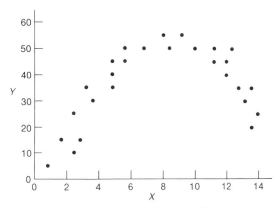

Figure 11.10 Scatterplot showing a nonlinear relationship between variables X and Y

associated in a linear way with the values of the other variable. When we say that variables are associated in a linear way, we mean that the relationship between the variables can be described by a straight line. If increasing values of one variable are associated in a linear way with increasing values of the other variable, the variables are *positively correlated*. If increasing values of one variable are associated in a linear way with decreasing values of the other variable, the variables are *negatively correlated*.

Consider the hypothetical data sets plotted in Figures 11.8 through 11.10. These plots are *scatterplots*, plots that allow us to see graphically how the values of one variable are related to the values of another variable. In Figure 11.8, no relationship is evident. The points in the plot appear to be randomly scattered with no pattern. In Figure 11.9, a linear relationship is present. A straight line could be drawn on the plot to represent the relationship between the values of the variable Y and the values of the variable X. In Figure 11.10, a *nonlinear* relationship is evident. Although the values of the variable Y are closely related to the values of the variable X, the relationship could not be described

with a straight line. A curve would have to be drawn on the plot to describe the relationship between these variables.

If one or both of two variables have normal or approximately normal distributions, the Pearson correlation coefficient described in Chapter 12 can be used to determine whether the variables are correlated. If both variables have extremely nonnormal distributions, the Pearson correlation coefficient is not appropriate. The *Spearman rank correlation coefficient* can often be used instead to measure the degree of linear association between the *ranks* of two variables.

The Spearman rank correlation coefficient can take any value between -1 and 1. If the population Spearman rank correlation coefficient is equal to 1, there is a perfect positive linear relationship between the ranks of one variable and the ranks of the other variable. If the population Spearman rank correlation coefficient is equal to -1, there is a perfect negative linear relationship between the ranks of one variable and the ranks of the other variable. In either case, the ranks of one variable can be perfectly predicted by knowing the ranks of the other variable. The closer the population Spearman rank correlation coefficient is to -1 or 1, the stronger the linear component of the relationship between the ranks of the two variables.

If the population Spearman rank correlation coefficient is 0, there is no *linear* relationship between the ranks of the two variables. A population Spearman rank correlation coefficient of 0 does *not* imply that there is no relationship at all between the ranks of the two variables. The ranks of the two variables could be closely related in a nonlinear fashion and have a population Spearman rank correlation coefficient of 0.

We will use the Greek letter ρ (rho, pronounced "rō") to denote the population Spearman rank correlation coefficient. The symbol r_s (pronounced "r sub s") will be used to denote the sample Spearman rank correlation coefficient. Although r_s can be calculated by hand, the computations are extremely

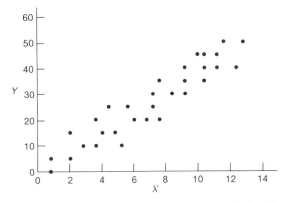

Figure 11.9 Scatterplot showing a linear relationship between variables X and Y

tedious. We will omit the formula for r_s and focus on the use of this coefficient. The formula for r_s can be found in other texts.[1]

When the sample Spearman rank correlation coefficient is obtained, the researcher is usually interested in making inferences about a population. She generally wants to test the hypothesis that there is no linear association between the ranks of the two variables. This is the null hypothesis that the population Spearman rank correlation coefficient is equal to 0:

$$H_0: \text{Spearman's } \rho = 0 \qquad (11.16)$$

The two-sided alternative hypothesis is

$$H_A: \text{Spearman's } \rho \neq 0 \qquad (11.17)$$

When a statistical software package is used to obtain r_s, the p-value for the test of the null hypothesis (11.16) is usually included in the output. If the p-value is less than the significance level α, the null hypothesis (11.16) is rejected. If the p-value is greater than or equal to α, the null hypothesis (11.16) cannot be rejected. The p-value is interpreted in the usual way: it is the probability of getting an r_s statistic at least as extreme as the calculated r_s statistic if the null hypothesis (11.16) is true.

One-sided tests of the null hypothesis (11.16) can be done, using the alternative hypotheses H_A: Spearman's $\rho < 0$ or H_A: Spearman's $\rho > 0$. Such tests are usually not recommended. Consult a statistician if you need a one-sided test of the null hypothesis (11.16).

The test of the null hypothesis (11.16) requires the following assumptions.

1. Random Sample of Subjects. If the sample is not biased, a random sample is not necessary.

2. Paired Samples. The Spearman rank correlation coefficient cannot be computed if the samples are not paired.

3. Independent Observations Within Each Sample. All of the observations within the first sample must be independent and all of the observations within the second sample must be independent. Observations from *different* samples are not necessarily independent, since paired samples were obtained. If this assumption is violated, the test of the null hypothesis (11.16) cannot be done.

Let us evaluate these assumptions for the seizure data. The patients are not a random sample, but this is not essential. The samples are obviously paired, and the within-samples independence assumption seems reasonable. Knowing the number of seizures for one patient should not tell us anything about the number of seizures for another patient. A test of the null hypothesis (11.16) is appropriate. We will use a 0.01 significance level.

For the seizure data, the Spearman rank correlation coefficient is 0.2299, with a two-tailed p-value

TABLE 11.16   RANKS FOR THE NUMBERS OF PARTIAL COMPLEX SEIZURES PER MONTH BEFORE AND AFTER CALLOSOTOMY

Patient No.	Preoperative	Postoperative
1	7	8.5
2	11	17.5
3	13	3.5
4	13	3.5
5	15	3.5
6	18	20.5
7	4	12
8	5.5	15
9	13	13
10	20	17.5
11	5.5	3.5
12	9	3.5
13	21	20.5
14	3	19
15	9	8.5
16	19	15
17	2	10
18	16.5	11
19	16.5	3.5
20	1	7
21	9	15

of 0.316. We cannot reject the hypothesis that the population Spearman rank correlation coefficient is 0 at any reasonable significance level. We conclude that the data provide no evidence of a *linear* relationship between the ranks of the presurgery numbers of seizures and the ranks of the postsurgery numbers of seizures.

We *cannot* conclude from this hypothesis test that the ranks are not related. It is possible that the ranks are related in a nonlinear way. To check this, we obtain a scatterplot of the presurgery ranks and the postsurgery ranks. These ranks are shown in Table 11.16, and an SPSS/PC scatterplot of the ranks is shown in Figure 11.11.* The ranks in Table 11.16 were calculated separately for each sample. No relationship of any kind is evident in the scatterplot. On the basis of the hypothesis test *and the scatterplot*, we conclude that the data provide no evidence that the ranks of the presurgery number of seizures are related to the ranks of the postsurgery number of seizures.

Can the Pearson correlation coefficient be used instead of the Spearman rank correlation coefficient to test the hypothesis of no correlation for the seizure data? The test of the hypothesis that the population Pearson correlation coefficient is 0 requires normal or approximately normal distributions for at least one of the two paired populations. The presurgery observations are extremely skewed, with

---

*In SPSS/PC scatterplots, points are represented by numbers. A "1" indicates one point, a "2" indicates two points, and so on.

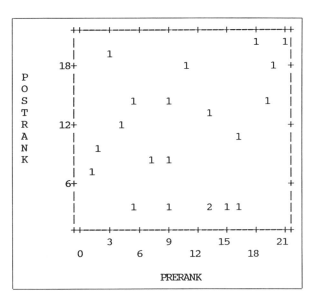

Figure 11.11 SPSS/PC scatterplot of presurgery and postsurgery ranks

90% of the values less than 100 and two extremely large values of 450 and 900. The postsurgery observations are less skewed, but more than one-fourth of these observations are equal to 0. Since both samples suggest extremely nonnormal populations, we cannot test the hypothesis that the population Pearson correlation coefficient is 0.

If we reject the hypothesis that the Spearman rank correlation coefficient is 0, we may be tempted to infer that a causal relationship exists. This would be a serious mistake, since *correlation never implies causation*. Although association of some kind must be demonstrated to show causation, the presence of association is not sufficient to show causation. Even a population Spearman rank correlation coefficient of 1 or −1 does not imply a causal relationship. Such a coefficient only means that the ranks of one variable can be predicted perfectly from the ranks of the other variable. There may be no causal relationship at all between the variables.

Example 11.12 _____

A study investigated the effect of corrective lenses on ocular refraction.[17] Table 11.17 shows the spherical equivalent refractive errors for 26 eyes from 13 subjects at their first and fifth refractions. Can we test the hypothesis that the population Spearman rank correlation coefficient for the first refraction error and the fifth refraction error is 0?

Because 26 eyes from 13 subjects were used, repeated measurements were obtained for each sample. The within-samples independence assumption is not reasonable for these data, and we cannot test the null hypothesis (11.16). If we knew which eyes belonged to each subject, we could analyze the right eye values and the left eye values separately. We could test the null hypothesis (11.16) for the population of right-eye observations and then test this hypothesis for the population of left-eye observations.

TABLE 11.17 SPHERICAL EQUIVALENT REFRACTIVE ERRORS FOR 26 EYES

Eye No.	First Refraction	Fifth Refraction
1	−1.25	−4.75
2	−0.75	−4.75
3	0.50	2.25
4	1.50	2.50
5	−0.75	−3.25
6	−0.50	−3.00
7	0.00	−3.50
8	0.00	−3.50
9	5.00	5.00
10	4.75	5.00
11	−1.25	−4.75
12	−1.25	−4.75
13	−2.25	−4.25
14	−2.25	−4.25
15	−1.00	−2.00
16	−1.00	−1.75
17	−4.00	−6.50
18	−3.25	−7.00
19	−1.25	−4.00
20	−1.00	−4.75
21	1.25	2.50
22	1.25	2.50
23	−4.25	−5.25
24	−7.50	−8.50
25	−0.25	−1.25
26	−0.25	−1.25

11.7 COMPUTER OUTPUT FOR NONPARAMETRIC TESTS

If a large data set is to be analyzed with nonparametric statistics based on ranks, a computer should be used. Sorting a large number of observations by hand is so tedious that errors are almost inevitable. Not only do computer programs perform time-consuming ranking procedures, they also provide *p*-values. Computer packages can be used to carry out all

```
Mean Rank     Cases

      6.50         8   - Ranks  (DINAMAP Lt DIRECT)
      7.80         5   + Ranks  (DINAMAP Gt DIRECT)
               16   Ties   (DINAMAP Eq DIRECT)
               --
               29   Total


      Z =   -.4543            2-tailed P =  .6496
```

Figure 11.12 SPSS/PC Wilcoxon signed rank test output for blood pressure data

```
Cases

      7   - Diffs (AFTER Lt BEFORE)
     11   + Diffs (AFTER Gt BEFORE)          (Binomial)
     11   Ties                              2-tailed P =     .4807
     --
     29   Total
```

Figure 11.13 SPSS/PC sign test output for hepatic infusion data

of the nonparametric tests discusssed in this chapter. The usual warnings about the computer's inability to check assumptions still apply.

In SPSS, the NPAR TESTS procedure is used to obtain the Wilcoxon signed rank test, the sign test, the Mann-Whitney test, the Kruskal-Wallis test, and the Friedman test. The Spearman rank correlation coefficient is obtained with the SPSS NONPAR CORR program. In SAS, the NPAR1WAY program is used to obtain the Mann-Whitney test and the Kruskal-Wallis test.

Figure 11.12 shows the SPSS/PC output for the Wilcoxon signed rank test for the blood pressure data. The Z statistic shown in the output is used to obtain an approximate p-value, listed after "2-tailed P = ." If the sample is large enough, this Z statistic has an approximately normal distribution. The use of the normal approximation to carry out the Wilcoxon signed rank test is described in other texts.[1] Figure 11.13 shows the SPSS/PC sign test output for the hepatic infusion data. The exact p-value is listed after "(Binomial) 2-tailed P = ."

The SPSS/PC Mann-Whitney test output for the pain-relief data is shown in Figure 11.14. In this output, the statistic listed under "W" is the MW test statistic when the TENS group is treated as the

first sample. We treated the drug group as the first sample, so our MW test statistic of 86 is not the same as the SPSS/PC MW test statistic of 190. The p-value is not affected by the choice of the first sample, and the p-value of 0.0001 given under "EXACT 2-tailed P" is consistent with our approximate p-value. A Z statistic that corrects for ties is listed under "Corrected for Ties." This statistic is based on a normal approximation described in other texts.[18] The statistic given under "U" is a test statistic that has the same p-value as the Mann-Whitney MW test statistic. The mean ranks listed under "Mean Rank" are the average ranks for the two samples.

In the SAS Mann-Whitney test output for the pain-relief data (Figure 11.15), the rank sums for the two samples are listed under "SUM OF SCORES" and the average ranks are listed under "MEAN SCORE." The number after "S = " is the MW test statistic when the TENS group is treated as the first sample. The p-value is based on a normal approximation and is given after "PROB > |Z| = ."

Figures 11.16 and 11.17 show the SPSS/PC and SAS Kruskal-Wallis test output for the humidifier fever data. In the SPSS/PC output, the Kruskal-

```
Mean Rank     Cases

      7.17        12   ANALGES = 1.00
     17.27        11   ANALGES = 2.00
               --
               23   Total

                               EXACT                    Corrected for Ties
      U              W        2-tailed P              Z          2-tailed P
      8.0          190.0       .0001             -3.5937          .0003
```

Figure 11.14 SPSS/PC Mann-Whitney test output for pain-relief data

```
                 WILCOXON SCORES (RANK SUMS)
                          SUM OF    EXPECTED    STD DEV      MEAN
  LEVEL            N      SCORES    UNDER H0    UNDER H0     SCORE

                1  12     86.00     144.00      16.14        7.17
                2  11    190.00     132.00      16.14       17.27
            WILCOXON 2-SAMPLE TEST (NORMAL APPROXIMATION)
            (WITH CONTINUITY CORRECTION OF .5)
            S=  190.00     Z= 3.5627     PROB >|Z|=0.0004
```

Figure 11.15 SAS Mann-Whitney test output for pain-relief data

```
  Mean Rank    Cases

      10.70       10   GROUP =     1
      15.25        8   GROUP =     2
      13.71        7   GROUP =     3
                   --
                   25   Total

                                          Corrected for Ties
     CASES     Chi-Square  Significance   Chi-Square  Significance
       25         1.7902       .4086        1.8076       .4050
```

Figure 11.16 SPSS/PC Kruskal-Wallis test output for humdifier fever data

Wallis χ^2 statistic is given under "Chi-Square" and its p-value is given under "Significance." A Kruskal-Wallis test statistic and p-value that have been corrected for ties are listed under "Corrected for Ties." The formula for this corrected statistic is described in other texts.[18] Average ranks for the three groups are given under "Mean Rank." In the SAS output, the corrected Kruskal-Wallis test statistic is listed after "CHISQ =." The p-value for this corrected statistic is given after "PROB >

CHISQ =." The values under "SUM OF SCORES" are the rank sums for the three groups and the values under "MEAN SCORE" are the average ranks for the three groups.

The SPSS/PC Friedman test output for the pericardial disease data is shown in Figure 11.18. Like most computer packages, SPSS calculates the Friedman χ^2 statistic instead of the Friedman F statistic. The χ^2 statistic is listed under "Chi-Square" and the p-value is listed under "Signifi-

```
                 WILCOXON SCORES (RANK SUMS)
                          SUM OF    EXPECTED    STD DEV      MEAN
  LEVEL            N      SCORES    UNDER H0    UNDER H0     SCORE

                1  10    107.00     130.00      17.94       10.70
                2   8    122.00     104.00      17.08       15.25
                3   7     96.00      91.00      16.44       13.71
            KRUSKAL-WALLIS TEST (CHI-SQUARE APPROXIMATION)
            CHISQ=   1.81     DF=  2    PROB > CHISQ=0.4050
```

Figure 11.17 SAS Kruskal-Wallis test output for humdifier fever data

Figure 11.18 SPSS/PC Friedman test output for pericardial disease data

```
  Mean Rank    Variable

      3.00     TMPONADE
      1.94     INTERMED
      1.06     COMPLETE

      Cases         Chi-Square      D.F.   Significance
        9            17.0556          2        .0002
```

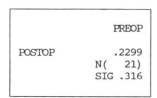

```
                    PREOP

POSTOP              .2299
            N(   21)
            SIG .316
```

Figure 11.19 SPSS Spearman rank correlation output for seizure data

cance." The average ranks for the three samples of repeated measurements are given under "Mean Rank."

Figure 11.19 shows the SPSS output for the Spearman rank correlation coefficient for the seizure data. The first number listed is r_s. The sample size is given in parentheses after N, and the p-value for testing the hypothesis of no correlation is given after "SIG."

SUMMARY

Parametric hypothesis tests require specific distributional assumptions, whereas nonparametric hypothesis tests usually require less specific distributional assumptions. Because nonparametric methods usually have less power than parametric methods, nonparametric methods should be used only when parametric methods are clearly inappropriate.

The Wilcoxon signed rank test and the sign test are used to test hypotheses about population medians and population median differences. The Mann-Whitney test is used to test the hypothesis that two populations are identical and the Kruskal-Wallis test is used to test the hypothesis that three or more populations are identical. When samples of repeated measurements are obtained, the Friedman test can be used to test the hypothesis that all possible rankings of the observations for any subject are equally likely. If the Kruskal-Wallis test leads to rejection of the hypothesis of identical populations, Bonferroni-adjusted Mann-Whitney tests can be used to determine which populations are different. If the Friedman test leads to rejection of the hy-

pothesis of equally likely rankings, Bonferroni-adjusted Wilcoxon signed rank tests or sign tests can be used to determine which populations are different.

The Spearman rank correlation coefficient is used to measure the degree of linear association between the ranks of two variables. The closer the population Spearman rank correlation coefficient is to −1 or 1, the stronger the linear component of the relationship between the ranks of the variables. If the population Spearman rank correlation coefficient is 0, the ranks of the variables can still be strongly related in a nonlinear way.

PROBLEMS

The following instructions apply to problems 3 through 29.

1. In each problem, data are presented and a question is asked about the data. Determine whether any of the tests described in this chapter are appropriate for answering this question. If no test is appropriate, state which assumptions are violated. Computer output that may or may not be appropriate is provided for some of the problems. Even though the Friedman F statistic is preferred to the Friedman χ^2 statistic, only computer output showing the Friedman χ^2 statistic is provided. Most computer packages do not calculate the Friedman F statistic.

2. If a statistical test is appropriate, carry out the test. Specify the null and alternative hypotheses. If appropriate computer output is given, use the test statistic or p-value from the output. If appropriate computer output is not given, calculate the test statistic and find the most exact p-value that can be obtained from the tables in this text. Interpret the p-value and use the test results to answer the question in the problem.

1. Construct a flowchart that will help you determine which of the nonparametric tests discussed in this chapter might be appropriate for particular data sets. The flowchart should begin as follows:

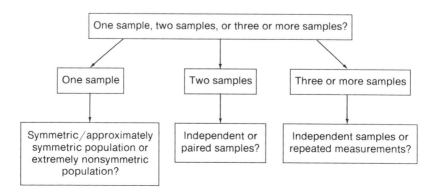

TABLE 11.18 NORTON SCORE FOR ELDERLY ORTHOPEDIC PATIENTS

Patients Who Did Not Develop Pressure Sores			Patients Who Developed Erythema	Patients Who Developed Pressure Sores
12	20	20	9	13
18	20	10	13	12
16	18	13	16	12
16	13	15	15	14
17	16	17	11	8
17	10	19	16	15
15	14	13	14	12
13	16	13	14	12
12	17	12	14	16
18	13	13	13	
19	14	11	13	
8	16	16	15	
16	16			

TABLE 11.19 AMOUNT OF PUS, DURATION OF DRAINAGE, AMOUNT RANKS, AND DURATION RANKS FOR PATIENTS WITH PYOGENIC LIVER ABCESSES

Patient No.	Amount of Pus (ml)	Amount Rank	Duration of Drainage (days)	Duration Rank
1	1000	11	14	8
2	40	4	8	6
3	30	3	3	1.5
4	5	1	12	7
5	110	8	25	10.5
6	15	2	6	3.5
7	335	10	16	9
8	120	9	25	10.5
9	60	6.5	7	5
10	50	5	3	1.5
11	60	6.5	6	3.5

```
                            AMOUNT

            DURATION        .6032
                        N(    11)
                        SIG .049
```

Figure 11.21 SPSS Spearman rank correlation output for amount of pus and duration of drainage

2. Indicate which parametric tests correspond to the nonparametric tests described in this chapter.

3. In a study of pressure sores in elderly orthopedic patients, Norton scores measuring physical and mental condition, activity, mobility, and incontinence were reported for elderly orthopedic patients.[19] Patients were classified into three groups: patients who did not develop pressure sores, patients who developed noticeable erythema, and patients who developed pressure sores. Table 11.18 shows the Norton scores for 59 of these patients. Do the data provide evidence that the three populations of Norton scores are not identical? Use a 0.01 significance level. If the hypothesis of identical populations is rejected, use a 0.05 overall significance level for multiple comparisons.

```
Mean Rank      Cases

    34.03          38     OUTCOME =    1
    25.58          12     OUTCOME =    2
    18.89           9     OUTCOME =    3
                   --
                   59     Total


    CASES       Chi-Square
      59          6.6482
```

Figure 11.20 SPSS/PC Kruskal-Wallis test output for Norton score

Figure 11.22 SPSS/PC scatterplot of duration ranks and amount ranks

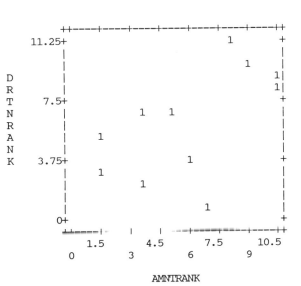

TABLE 11.20 DAYS SINCE LAST TRANSFUSION FOR CANCER PATIENTS WITH DELAYED HEMOLYTIC TRANSFUSION REACTIONS

Patient No.	Days
1	2
2	20
3	7
4	10
5	2
6	14
7	11
8	10
9	10
10	7
11	15
12	10
13	5

TABLE 11.22 MATERNAL ATTACHMENT SCORE BEFORE AND AFTER NURSING INTERVENTION

Patient No.	Before Intervention	After Intervention	Difference (After − Before)
1	23	25	2
2	10	23	13
3	9	19	10
4	6	17	11
5	13	23	10
6	12	23	11
7	12	23	11
8	7	17	10
9	8	19	11
10	10	12	2

4. A study evaluated the treatment of pyogenic liver abcesses by percutaneous aspiration and drainage.[20] Table 11.19 shows the amount of pus aspirated, the duration of drainage, and the ranks for these variables for 11 patients with pyogenic liver abcesses. Do the data provide evidence that the amount of pus and the duration of drainage are correlated? Use a 0.05 significance level.

5. In a study of transfusion reactions in cancer patients, the number of days since the last transfusion was reported for 13 cancer patients with delayed hemolytic transfusion reactions.[21] The data are shown in Table 11.20. An oncology nurse believes that the population median number of days is 10. Do the data provide evidence that the population median is not 10? Use a 0.01 significance level.

6. A study of the insulin autoimmune syndrome reported the immunoreactive insulin (IRI) levels for six patients with the insulin autoimmune syndrome and four patients with insulin-treated diabetes.[22] These values are shown in Table 11.21. Do the data provide evidence that the two populations of IRI values are not identical? Use a 0.05 significance level.

7. A study investigated the effect of nursing intervention on maternal attachment in mothers separated from their newborn infants for at least 24

hours after birth.[23] Table 11.22 shows the maternal attachment scores before and after nursing intervention for 10 mothers separated after delivery from their newborn infants. A nurse-midwife believes that the population median difference between the after-intervention scores and the before-intervention scores is 12. Do the data provide evidence that the population median difference is not 12? Use a 0.05 significance level.

8. A study evaluated the effectiveness of a live *Pasteurella haemolytica* vaccine in cattle.[24] Table

TABLE 11.23 IgG FOR FOUR GROUPS OF CALVES

Calf No.	IgG	Calf No.	IgG
Group 1		*Group* 3	
1	117	12	10
2	62	13	15
3	12	14	7
4	14	15	11
5	108	16	17
6	18	17	11
Group 2		*Group* 4	
7	23	18	2
8	64	19	1
9	8	20	3
10	39	21	1
11	19	22	3
		23	4

TABLE 11.21 IMMUNOREACTIVE INSULIN FOR TWO GROUPS OF PATIENTS

Insulin Autoimmune Syndrome		Insulin-Treated Diabetes	
PATIENT NO.	IRI (pmol/l)	PATIENT NO.	IRI (pmol/l)
1	53,813	7	1,873
2	16,503	8	1,815
3	6,307	9	223
4	5,094	10	1,421
5	790,613		
6	3,501		

```
Mean Rank     Cases

   17.67          6     GROUP =    1
   16.60          5     GROUP =    2
   11.00          6     GROUP =    3
    3.50          6     GROUP =    4
                 --
                 23     Total


   CASES      Chi-Square
    23         16.0428
```

Figure 11.23 SPSS/PC Kruskal-Wallis test output for IgG

11.23 shows the IgG antibody titer for four groups of calves 35 days after vaccination with the vaccine or a saline solution. The six calves in Group 1 were vaccinated twice with the vaccine, then stressed by being transported. The five calves in Group 2 were vaccinated once with the vaccine and once with saline, then stressed by being transported. The six calves in Group 3 were vaccinated twice with saline, then stressed by being transported. The six calves in Group 4 were vaccinated twice with saline, but were not stressed by being transported. Do the data provide evidence that the four populations of IgG titers are not identical? Use a 0.005 significance level. If the hypothesis of identical populations is rejected, assume that the only comparisons of interest are those between the population corresponding to Group 4 and the other three populations. Assume that these comparisons were selected before examining the data, and use a 0.05 overall significance level for multiple comparisons.

9. A study investigated clinicopathologic features of 30 patients who died within two years after

acute myocardial infarction (AMI) treated with selective intracoronary thrombolysis (SICT).[25] Table 11.24 shows the time from AMI onset to SICT. A cardiologist believes that the population median time from AMI onset to SICT is 6 hours. Do the

TABLE 11.24   TIME FROM AMI ONSET TO SICT FOR PATIENTS WHO DIED

Patient No.	Time (hours)
1	3
2	4
3	4
4	6
5	3
6	6
7	9
8	6
9	3
10	4
11	3
12	6
13	5
14	6
15	2
16	3
17	5
18	4
19	5
20	2
21	2
22	5
23	4
24	3
25	7
26	4
27	5
28	5
29	3
30	3

TABLE 11.25   TISSUE AND BODY FLUID CONCENTRATION OF α-TOCOPHEROL AND α-TOCOPHEROL ACETATE (μg/ml OR μg/g WET TISSUE) AND α-TOCOPHEROL AND α-TOCOPHEROL ACETATE RANKS FOR INFANTS

Infant No.	Specimen	α-Tocopherol	α-Tocopherol Rank	α-Tocopherol Acetate	Acetate Rank
1	Ascites	17	4	7	5
	Liver	4135	15	500	15
2	Serum	67	8	12	8
3	Ascites	18	5	2	3
	Liver	2054	14	82	14
	Lung	162	12	27	11
	Serum	87	10	13	9
	Spleen	223	13	46	13
4	Ascites	30	7	7	5
5	Ascites	16	3	7	5
	Serum	81	9	26	10
	Urine	0	1.5	0	1.5
6	Ascites	29	6	0	7
	Serum	134	11	41	12
	Urine	0	1.5	0	1.5

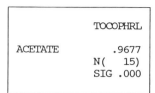

```
                    TOCOPHRL

    ACETATE           .9677
                    N(   15)
                    SIG .000
```

Figure 11.24 SPSS Spearman rank correlation output for α-tocopherol and α-tocopherol acetate

data provide evidence that the population median is not 6? Use a 0.05 significance level.

10. A study examined the association between illness and use of an intravenous vitamin E preparation in premature infants.[26] Table 11.25 shows the α-tocopherol and α-tocopherol acetate concentrations and their ranks for specimens from six infants who became ill after receiving this preparation. Do the data provide evidence that the α-tocopherol and α-tocopherol acetate concentrations are correlated? Use a 0.01 significance level.

11. In a study of tissue typing in human allografts of frozen bone, bone biopsies were performed after bone transplantation.[27] The specimens obtained were graded according to new bone formation in the periosteal, cortical, and trabecular areas of the transplant. Table 11.26 shows the new bone formation ratings for 13 specimens obtained from 10 patients. Do the data provide evidence that not all possible rankings of the periosteal, cortical, and trabecular ratings for a specimen are equally likely? Use a 0.01 significance level. If the hypothesis of equally likely rankings is rejected, use a 0.10 overall significance level for multiple comparisons.

12. A study investigated the effect of indomethacin on gastric mucosal prostaglandins.[28] Prostaglandin concentrations were measured for gastric mucosal biopsy specimens from 20 healthy

TABLE 11.26 NEW BONE FORMATION IN BIOPSY SPECIMENS*

Specimen No.	Transplant Area		
	PERIOSTEAL	CORTICAL	TRABECULAR
1	1	3	3
2	1	3	3
3	2	1	0
4	3	3	3
5	1	1	0
6	3	3	0
7	2	2	1
8	3	2	1
9	3	3	2
10	0	0	0
11	3	2	1
12	3	2	0
13	3	2	0

*0 = none, 1 = small number of surfaces with new bone formation, 2 = moderate number of surfaces with new bone formation, 3 = large number of surfaces with new bone formation

```
Mean Rank   Variable

   2.38     PERIOST
   2.23     CORTICAL
   1.38     TRABEC

   Cases           Chi-Square
    13               7.5385
```

Figure 11.26 SPSS/PC Friedman test output for new bone formation

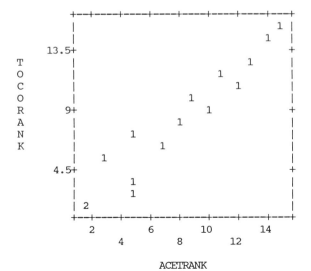

Figure 11.25 SPSS/PC scatterplot of α-tocopherol rank and α-tocopherol acetate rank

TABLE 11.27 6-KETO PROSTAGLANDIN $F_{1\alpha}$ AFTER ADMINISTRATION OF PLACEBO OR INDOMETHACIN

Placebo		Indomethacin	
Subject No.	6-Keto $PGF_{1\alpha}$	Subject No.	6-Keto $PGF_{1\alpha}$
1	14.4	11	42.2
2	23.3	12	25.0
3	38.6	13	20.6
4	10.1	14	0
5	50.6	15	0
6	0	16	41.4
7	67.8	17	0
8	2.8	18	0
9	12.2	19	22.7
10	6.6	20	28.4

TABLE 11.28 FETAL MOVEMENTS (% OF TIME) BEFORE AND AFTER CHORIONIC VILLUS SAMPLING

Patient No.	Before Sampling	After Sampling	Difference (Before − After)
1	25	18	7
2	24	27	−3
3	28	25	3
4	15	20	−5
5	20	17	3
6	23	24	−1
7	21	24	−3
8	20	22	−2
9	20	19	1
10	27	19	8

```
Mean Rank    Variable

  2.40       MYELO
  2.50       GRANULO
  1.10       MONO

  Cases           Chi-Square
    5               6.1000
```

Figure 11.27 SPSS/PC Friedman test output for monoclonal antibody percentages

subjects who received indomethacin or a placebo. Table 11.27 shows the 6-keto prostaglandin $F_{1\alpha}$ (6-keto $PGF_{1\alpha}$) concentrations in the antrum for these subjects. Do the data provide evidence that the two populations of antrum 6-keto $PGF_{1\alpha}$ concentrations are not identical? Use a 0.05 significance level.

13. In a study of the effect of chorionic villus sampling on fetal movements, ultrasound was used to record fetal movements before and after chorionic villus sampling.[29] Table 11.28 shows the percentage of time the fetus spent moving before and after sampling for 10 pregnant women. Do the data provide evidence that the population median difference between the movement percentage before

sampling and the movement percentage after sampling is not 0? Use a 0.10 significance level.

14. A study investigated discrepancies between the cytochemical cell pattern and the immunologic cell phenotype for patients with acute myeloblastic leukemia (AML).[30] Table 11.29 shows the monoclonal antibody percentages for five AML patients with discrepant cytochemical and immunologic results. Do the data provide evidence that not all possible rankings of the myelomonocytic, granulocytic, and monocytic percentages for a patient are equally likely? Use a 0.05 significance level. If the hypothesis of equally likely rankings is rejected, use a 0.10 overall significance level for multiple comparisons.

15. In a study of intrathyroidal dendritic cells, thyroid glands from nine patients without thyroid disease, 10 patients with sporadic nontoxic goiter,

TABLE 11.29 MONOCLONAL ANTIBODIES (PERCENTAGE OF POSITIVE BLAST CELLS) FOR PATIENTS WITH DISCORDANT AML

Patient No.	Myelomonocytic	Granulocytic	Monocytic
1	76	0	0
2	10	16	0
3	20	25	0
4	22	12	0
5	15	40	0

**TABLE 11.30 NUMBER OF ANTIGEN-PRESENTING
DENDRITIC CELLS / 10 MICROSCOPIC FIELDS**

No Thyroid Disease		Sporadic Nontoxic Goiter		Graves' Disease	
PATIENT NO.	NUMBER OF DENDRITIC CELLS	PATIENT NO.	NUMBER OF DENDRITIC CELLS	PATIENT NO.	NUMBER OF DENDRITIC CELLS
1	2	10	40	20	90
2	0	11	45	21	177
3	0	12	28	22	79
4	0	13	53	23	97
5	1	14	9	24	73
6	1	15	47	25	27
7	0	16	25	26	16
8	2	17	12	27	42
9	1	18	16	28	75
		19	23	29	135
				30	66
				31	70

```
Mean Rank     Cases

     5.00         9    DISEASE =     1
    16.05        10    DISEASE =     2
    24.21        12    DISEASE =     3
                 --
                 31    Total


  CASES      Chi-Square
    31         22.9542
```

Figure 11.28 SPSS/PC Kruskal-Wallis test output for number of antigen-presenting dendritic cells

and 12 patients with Graves' disease were examined for antigen-presenting dendritic cells.[31] Table 11.30 shows the number of antigen-presenting dendritic cells for these patients. Do the data provide evidence that the three populations of numbers of cells are not identical? Use a 0.01 significance level. If the hypothesis of identical populations is rejected, use a 0.10 overall significance level for multiple comparisons.

16. A study evaluated the use of lidocaine to reduce the pain caused by potassium chloride (KCl)

infusion.[32] Six subjects received intravenous infusions of a KCl solution with lidocaine and a KCl solution with a placebo. After each infusion, subjects were asked to rate the degree of pain felt. The higher the rating, the more severe the pain. Table 11.31 shows the pain ratings during the lidocaine KCl infusion and the placebo KCl infusion. Do the data provide evidence that the population median difference between the lidocaine rating and the placebo rating is not 0? Use a 0.10 significance level.

17. In a study of toxoplasmosis in sheep, ewes were innoculated orally with *Toxoplasma gondii* oocysts.[33] Table 11.32 shows the *T gondii* antibody titers for the ewes obtained by three methods: the modified agglutination test (MAT), the dye test (DT), and the latex agglutination test (LAT). Do the data provide evidence that not all possible rankings of the MAT, DT, and LAT titers for a ewe are equally likely? Use a 0.01 significance level. If the hypothesis of equally likely rankings is rejected, use a 0.10 overall significance level for multiple comparisons.

18. In a study of fibrin deposits in carotid artery plaques, 40 carotid endarterectomy specimens from 36 patients were evaluated for the presence of fibrin.[34] Table 11.33 shows the ratings that resulted

**TABLE 11.31 PAIN RATING DURING LIDOCAINE KCl
INFUSION AND PLACEBO KCl INFUSION**

Patient No.	Lidocaine KCl Infusion	Placebo KCl Infusion	Difference (Lidocaine − Placebo)
1	2	6	−4
2	6	6	0
3	3	7	−4
4	3	4	−1
5	2	7	−5
6	3	7	−4

TABLE 11.32 ANTIBODY TITERS AFTER INNOCULATION WITH *T GONDII* OOCYSTS

Ewe No.	Serotest		
	MAT	DT	LAT
1	4,096	1,296	64
2	4,096	1,296	256
3	4,096	1,296	256
4	16,384	1,296	64
5	4,096	1,296	256
6	16,384	1,296	256
7	16,384	1,296	1,024
8	16,384	1,296	256
9	16,384	3,888	4,096
10	4,096	1,296	256
11	16,384	1,296	4,096
12	16,384	1,296	16
13	16,384	3,888	256
14	65,536	1,296	4,096
15	65,536	3,888	4,096
16	65,536	1,296	4,096
17	65,536	1,296	256
18	65,536	1,296	4,096
19	65,536	3,888	4,096
20	65,536	1,296	1,024
21	65,536	3,888	1,024
22	65,536	1,296	4,096
23	65,536	1,296	1,024

TABLE 11.33 FIBRIN AND FIBRINOGEN DEPOSITS FOR CAROTID ENDARTERECTOMY SPECIMENS

Specimen No.	Deposits*	Specimen No.	Deposits
1	3	21	2
2	1	22	3
3	2	23	2
4	2	24	2
5	2	25	0
6	2	26	4
7	3	27	2
8	0	28	2
9	2	29	3
10	3	30	3
11	0	31	1
12	3	32	3
13	2	33	1
14	4	34	2
15	1	35	3
16	4	36	4
17	2	37	1
18	3	38	4
19	2	39	2
20	2	40	4

*0 = negative, 1 = rare discrete areas of staining, 2 = occasional discrete areas of staining, 3 = frequent discrete areas of staining, 4 = frequent, large, discrete areas of staining

```
Mean Rank    Variable

   3.00      MAT
   1.65      DT
   1.35      LAT

   Cases            Chi-Square
    23               35.5652
```

Figure 11.29 SPSS/PC Friedman test output for antibody titers

TABLE 11.34 TEST SCORE FOR NURSING STUDENTS TAUGHT BY DIFFERENT METHODS

Team Nursing		Primary Nursing		Control
93.0	85.0	98.5	85.0	92.5
91.0	85.0	92.5	85.0	88.0
91.0	85.0	91.0	85.0	88.0
91.0	85.0	89.5	83.5	85.0
91.0	85.0	89.5	83.5	85.0
91.0	83.5	89.5	82.0	83.5
89.5	79.0	88.0	81.75	79.0
89.5	77.5	86.5	80.5	73.0
89.5	77.5	86.5	77.5	
88.0	76.0	85.0	77.5	
88.0	74.5	85.0		

after staining the specimens for fibrin and fibrinogen deposits. A pathologist believes that the population median rating is 2. Do the data provide evidence that the population median is not 2? Use a 0.05 significance level.

19. A study compared the effectiveness of team nursing and primary nursing for teaching neurological nursing to associate-degree nursing students.[35] Fifty-one students were divided into three groups that used different methods of instruction: a team nursing group, a primary nursing group, and a control group that received clinical instruction through traditional case assignment. Table 11.34 shows the final test scores for these students. Do the data provide evidence that the three populations of test scores are not identical? Use a 0.05 significance level. If the hypothesis of identical populations is rejected, use a 0.05 overall significance level for multiple comparisons.

```
Mean Rank    Cases

   27.52       22      METHOD =    1
   25.57       21      METHOD =    2
   22.94        8      METHOD =    3
               --
               51      Total


   CASES        Chi-Square
    51             .5878
```

Figure 11.30 SPSS/PC Kruskal-Wallis test output for test score

TABLE 11.35 PLATELET COUNT (PLATELETS/μl OF BLOOD) AND COUNT RANKS BEFORE AND AFTER SPLENECTOMY

Dog No.	Before Count	Before Rank	After Count	After Rank
1	202,000	6	260,000	4
2	157,000	5	220,000	3
3	302,000	7	310,000	5.5
4	11,400	4	74,000	2
5	2,751	1	6,000	1
6	4,400	2	310,000	5.5
7	11,240	3	380,000	7

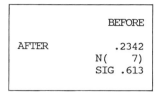

Figure 11.31 SPSS Spearman rank correlation output for platelet counts

20. A study evaluated splenectomy as adjunctive therapy for dogs with immune-mediated hematologic disorders.[36] Table 11.35 shows the platelet counts before and after splenectomy and the ranks for these counts for seven dogs with hematologic disorders. Do the data provide evidence that the presplenectomy platelet count and the postsplenectomy platelet count are correlated? Use a 0.01 significance level.

21. In a study of heart transplantation in children, the time between transplantation and rejection was reported for 27 rejection episodes in 14 children.[37] Table 11.36 shows these times for children taking 0.1 to 0.3 mg/kg/d of prednisone and children taking 0.4 to 1.0 mg/kg/d of prednisone. Do the data provide evidence that the two populations of times are not identical? Use a 0.05 significance level.

22. A study investigated the response of patients with bronchial asthma to the immunogen Helix pomatia Haemocyanin (HPH).[38] Table 11.37 shows the diameters of delayed skin reactions in 11 asthmatic patients 24 hours and 48 hours after intradermal challenge with 10.0 μg of HPH. Do the data provide evidence that the population median difference between the 24-hour diameter and the 48-hour diameter is not 0? Use a 0.10 significance level.

23. In a study of eating disorders and pregnancy, the duration of gestation for 23 pregnancies in 15 women with eating disorders was reported.[39] These values are shown in Table 11.38. Three groups of women were studied: women treated for anorexia nervosa and in remission, women with anorexia nervosa, and women with bulimia nervosa. Do the data provide evidence that the three populations of gestation durations are not identical? Use a 0.01 significance level. If the hypothesis of identical populations is rejected, use a 0.10 overall significance level for multiple comparisons.

24. In a study of gonadal dysgenesis, basal luteinizing hormone (LH) values were reported for children with bilateral anorchism.[40] Table 11.39 shows the LH values for 16 samples from eight children. An endocrinologist believes that the population median LH is 0.5. Do the data provide evidence that the population median is not 0.5? Use a 0.05 significance level.

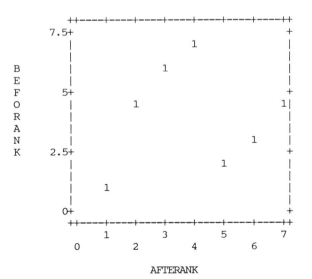

AFTERANK

Figure 11.32 SPSS/PC scatterplot of presplenectomy rank and postsplenectomy rank

TABLE 11.36 TIME BETWEEN TRANSPLANTATION AND REJECTION

0.1–0.3 mg/kg/d Prednisone		0.4–1.0 mg/kg/d Prednisone	
REJECTION NO.	TIME (months)	REJECTION NO.	TIME (months)
1	0.4	13	2.0
2	3.0	14	0.2
3	24.0	15	2.0
4	0.5	16	3.0
5	0.2	17	5.0
6	2.0	18	6.0
7	4.0	19	1.0
8	0.5	20	0.5
9	9.0	21	2.0
10	0.4	22	3.0
11	1.2	23	5.0
12	3.0	24	1.0
		25	2.0
		26	4.0
		27	0.5

TABLE 11.37 DIAMETER OF DELAYED SKIN REACTIONS (mm) AFTER INTRADERMAL CHALLENGE WITH HPH

Subject No.	24 Hours	48 Hours	Difference (24 hours − 48 hours)
1	0	0	0
2	7	8	−1
3	0	0	0
4	6	0	6
5	5	7	−2
6	10	10	0
7	6	5	1
8	30	24	6
9	14	22	−8
10	8	21	−13
11	5	8	−3

TABLE 11.38 DURATION OF GESTATION (WEEKS) FOR PREGNANCIES OF WOMEN WITH EATING DISORDERS

Pregnancy No.	Duration of Gestation	Pregnancy No.	Duration of Gestation
Remission		*Anorexia nervosa*	
1	37	14	15
2	38	15	39
3	38	16	39
4	39	17	40
5	39	18	36
6	39	19	38
7	40	20	12
8	40		
9	40		
10	39	*Bulimia nervosa*	
11	10	21	37
12	40	22	36
13	40	23	38

```
Mean Rank      Cases

    14.38          13     GROUP  =    1
     9.79           7     GROUP  =    2
     6.83           3     GROUP  =    3
                    --
                    23     Total



    CASES       Chi-Square
     23            4.0941
```

Figure 11.33 SPSS/PC Kruskal-Wallis test output for pregnancy duration

TABLE 11.39   BASAL LUTEINIZING HORMONE FOR PLASMA SAMPLES FROM CHILDREN WITH BILATERAL ANORCHISM

Sample No.	Basal LH (ng/ml)
1	5.9
2	0.7
3	0.5
4	0.5
5	0.5
6	0.3
7	0.4
8	0.8
9	1.5
10	0.6
11	0.5
12	0.4
13	1.9
14	2.0
15	3.3
16	2.2

TABLE 11.40   CHRONICITY INDEX FOR PATIENTS TREATED WITH CYCLOSPORINE

Patient No.	Chronicity Index
1	2
2	6
3	5
4	3
5	5
6	4
7	2
8	5
9	4
10	4
11	7
12	3
13	2
14	4
15	4
16	3
17	3

TABLE 11.41   DAILY INTAKE OF n-3 FATTY ACIDS IN GASTRIC-TUBE-FED PATIENTS

Patient No.	n-3 Fatty Acids (mg/24 hr)
1	34
2	10
3	19
4	24
5	1500
6	116
7	135

TABLE 11.42   DURATION OF INFERTILITY FOR WOMEN WHO DID NOT BECOME PREGNANT

Patient No.	Years Infertile
1	4
2	2
3	7
4	1
5	6
6	5
7	2
8	3

TABLE 11.43   GLASGOW COMA SCORE, RECOVERY SCORE, GLASGOW RANKS, AND RECOVERY RANKS FOR CHILDREN WITH INTRACEREBRAL HEMATOMA

Patient No.	Glasgow Coma Score	Glasgow Rank	Recovery Score	Recovery Rank
1	11	6	16	8
2	13	8	13	3
3	15	10	16	8
4	6	2	12	2
5	3	1	4	1
6	9	5	14	4
7	13	8	15	5
8	7	3.5	16	8
9	7	3.5	16	8
10	13	8	16	8

25. A study investigated renal abnormalities associated with long-term cyclosporine therapy.[41] Renal biopsy specimens from 17 patients treated with cyclosporine were evaluated and graded according to the severity of histopathologic alterations. The resulting chronicity index values are shown in Table 11.40. The higher the chronicity index, the more severe the renal abnormalities. A nephrology nurse believes that the population median chronicity index is 6. Do the data provide evidence that the population median is not 6? Use a 0.01 significance level.

26. In a study of alpha-linolenic acid deficiency in patients on long-term gastric-tube feeding, the

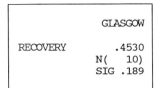

Figure 11.34 SPSS Spearman rank correlation output for coma score and recovery score

daily intake of fatty acids was reported for seven gastric-tube-fed patients.[42] Table 11.41 shows the daily intake of certain n-3 fatty acids for these patients. A nurse believes that the population median intake of these acids is 150. Do the data provide evidence that the population median is not 150? Use a 0.05 significance level.

27. A study investigated the results of laparoscopic treatment of ovarian endometriomas.[43] Table 11.42 shows the duration of infertility for eight infertile women who did not become pregnant after laparoscopy for ovarian endometriomas. A gynecologist believes that the population median duration of infertility is 2 years. Do the data provide evidence that the population median is not 2? Use a 0.01 significance level.

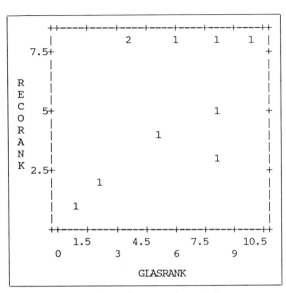

Figure 11.35 SPSS/PC scatterplot of Glasgow coma score rank and recovery score rank

28. In a study of recovery from intracerebral hematoma, Glasgow coma scores and recovery

TABLE 11.44 NUMBER OF REPORTED CHANGES FOR RADIATION THERAPY OUTPATIENTS

Patient No.	Food and Water	Solitude and Social Interaction	Protection From Hazards	Normality
1	5	1	6	3
2	3	3	4	6
3	3	0	2	2
4	3	0	3	2
5	4	1	5	6
6	8	1	6	5
7	1	0	2	2
8	7	1	4	4
9	2	0	2	3
10	3	0	4	3
11	3	0	4	3
12	8	1	1	2
13	3	1	1	1
14	4	1	6	3
15	1	1	4	3
16	5	3	9	6
17	3	1	6	1
18	3	1	3	2
19	5	2	2	2
20	3	1	2	2
21	3	1	4	3
22	2	2	5	3
23	3	1	1	1
24	3	1	3	2
25	3	0	3	2
26	4	1	2	2
27	4	1	2	3
28	2	1	3	3
29	2	1	3	5
30	6	3	11	9

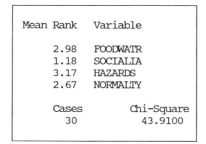

Mean Rank	Variable
2.98	FOODWATR
1.18	SOCIALIA
3.17	HAZARDS
2.67	NORMALTY

Cases	Chi-Square
30	43.9100

Figure 11.36 SPSS/PC Friedman test output for reported changes

scores were reported for 10 children with intracerebral hematoma.[44] These scores and their ranks are shown in Table 11.43. Do the data provide evidence that the coma score and the recovery score are correlated? Use a 0.05 significance level.

29. A study investigated changes in the lives of outpatients receiving external radiation therapy.[45] Thirty radiation therapy outpatients were asked to describe changes that took place in their lives after the initiation of radiation therapy. Table 11.44 shows the number of reported changes related to food and water, solitude and social interaction, protection from hazards, and normality. Do the data provide evidence that not all possible rankings of the numbers of reported changes for each patient are equally likely? Use a 0.05 significance level. If the hypothesis of equally likely rankings is rejected, assume that the only comparisons of interest are those between the population corresponding to the social interaction category and the other three populations. Assume that these comparisons were selected before examining the data, and use a 0.05 overall significance level for multiple comparisons.

30. Find an article in a medical or health care journal in which a nonparametric procedure was incorrectly used to analyze nonindependent data. Photocopy the article and write a letter to the journal editor that clearly describes the statistical error.

REFERENCES

1. Conover WJ: Practical Nonparametric Statistics. 2nd ed. New York: Wiley, 1980.
2. Markin DA: Preoperative concerns of the patient undergoing craniotomy. J Neurosci Nurs 18:275–278, 1986.
3. Ritvo ER, Mason-Brothers A, Jenson WP, et al: A report of one family with four autistic siblings and four families with three autistic siblings. J Am Acad Child Adol Psychiatr 26:339–341, 1987.
4. Paice JA: Intrathecal morphine infusion for intractable cancer pain: A new use for implanted pumps. Oncol Nurs Forum 13:41–47, 1986.
5. Park MK, Menard SM: Accuracy of blood pressure measurement by the Dinamap monitor in infants and children. Pediatrics 79:907–914, 1987.
6. Patt YZ, Boddie AW, Charnsangavej C, et al: Hepatic arterial infusion with floxuridine and cisplatin: Overriding importance of antitumor effect versus degree of tumor burden as determinants of survival among patients with colorectal cancer. J Clin Oncol 4:1356–1364, 1986.
7. Thomas RJ, Abbott M, Bhathal PS, et al: High-dose photoirradiation of esophageal cancer. Ann Surg 206:193–199, 1987.
8. Sloan JP, Muwanga CL, Waters EA, et al: Multiple rib fractures: Transcutaneous nerve stimulation versus conventional analgesia. J Trauma 26:1120–1122, 1986.
9. Samm M, Curtis-Cohen M, Keller M, et al: Necrotizing enterocolitis in infants of multiple gestation. Am J Dis Child 140:937–939, 1986.
10. McSharry C, Anderson K, Boyd G: Serological and clinical investigation of humidifier fever. Clin Allergy 17:15–22, 1987.
11. Brady CE, Utts SJ, Hyatt JR, et al: Secretin provocation: Gastrin results in various clinical situations. Am J Gastroenterol 83:130–135, 1988.
12. Patti F, Scapagnini U, Nicoletti F, et al: A short-term trial of an analogue of eel-calcitonin in headache. Headache 27:334–339, 1987.
13. Iman RL, Davenport JM: Approximations of the critical region of the Friedman statistic. Commun Statist A9:571–595, 1980.
14. Boltwood CM: Ventricular performance related to transmural filling pressure in clinical cardiac tamponade. Circulation 75:941–955, 1987.
15. Moores PP, Watkins WM, Greenwell P, et al: Zulu XX/XX dispermic chimaera from natal with two populations of red blood cells and patchy skin pigmentation. Vox Sang 54:52–56, 1988.
16. Gates JR, Rosenfeld WE, Maxwell RE, et al: Response of multiple seizure types to corpus callosum section. Epilepsia 28:28–34, 1987.
17. Medina A: A model for emmetropization. The effect of corrective lenses. Acta Ophthalmol 65:565–571, 1987.
18. SPSS, Inc. SPSS Statistical Algorithms. Chicago: SPSS, 1985.
19. Goldstone LA, Roberts BV: A preliminary discriminant function analysis of elderly orthopedic patients who will or will not contract a pressure sore. Int J Nurs Stud 17:17–23, 1980.
20. Attar B, Levendoglu H, Cuasay NS: CT-guided percutaneous aspiration and catheter drainage of pyogenic liver abcesses. Am J Gastroenterol 81:550–555, 1986.
21. Huh YO, Lichtiger B: Transfusion reactions in patients with cancer. Am J Clin Pathol 87:253–257, 1987.
22. Wasada T, Eguchi Y, Takayama S, et al: Reverse phase high performance liquid chromatographic analysis of circulating insulin in the insulin autoimmune syndrome. J Clin Endocrinol Metab 66:153–158, 1988.
23. Boudreaux M: Maternal attachment of high-risk mothers with well newborns. A pilot study. JOGN Nurs 10:366–369, 1981.
24. Blanchard-Channell MT, Ashfaq MK, Kadel WL: Efficacy of a streptomycin-dependent, live *Pasteurella*

haemolytica vaccine against challenge exposure to *Pasteurella haemolytica* in cattle. Am J Vet Res *48*:637–642, 1987.

25. Fujiwara H, Onodera T, Tanaka M, et al: A clinico-pathologic study of patients with hemorrhagic my-ocardial infarction treated with selective coronary thrombolysis with urokinase. Circulation *73*:749–757, 1986.

26. Martone WJ, Williams WW, Mortensen ML, et al: Illness with fatalities in premature infants: Associa-tion with an intravenous vitamin E preparation, E-Ferol. Pediatrics *78*:591–600, 1986.

27. Muscolo DL, Caletti E, Schajowicz F, et al: Tissue-typing in human massive allografts of frozen bone. J Bone Joint Surg *69A*:583–595, 1987.

28. Redfern JS, Lee E, Feldman M: Effect of in-domethacin on gastric mucosal prostaglandins in hu-mans. Correlation with mucosal damage. Gastroen-terology *92*:969–977, 1987.

29. Boogert A, Mantingh A, Visser GHA: The immedi-ate effects of chorionic villus sampling on fetal move-ments. Am J Obstet Gynecol *157*:137–139, 1987.

30. del Canizo MC, San Miguel JF, Gonzalez M, et al: Discrepancies between morphologic, cytochemical, and immunologic characteristics in acute myeloblastic leukemia. Am J Clin Pathol *88*:38–42, 1987.

31. Kabel PJ, Voorbij HAM, De Haan M, et al: Intrathy-roidal dendritic cells. J Clin Endocrinol Metab *66*:199–207, 1988.

32. Morrill GB, Katz MD: The use of lidocaine to reduce the pain induced by potassium chloride infusion. J Intrav Nurs *11*:105–108, 1988.

33. Dubey JP, Emond JP, Desmonts G, et al: Serodiag-nosis of postnatally and prenatally induced toxoplas-mosis in sheep. Am J Vet Res *48*:1239–1243, 1987.

34. Fisher M, Sacoolidge JC, Taylor CR: Patterns of fibrin deposits in carotid artery plaques. Angiology *38*:393–399, 1987.

35. Williams A: Student learning: Team vs primary nurs-ing. Nurs Manag *12*:48–51, 1981.

36. Feldman BF, Handagama P, Lubberink AAME: Splenectomy as adjunctive therapy for immune-medi-ated thrombocytopenia and hemolytic anemia in the dog. J Am Vet Med Assoc *187*:617–619, 1985.

37. Fricker FJ, Griffith BP, Hardesty RL, et al: Experi-ence with heart transplantation in children. Pedi-atrics *79*:138–146, 1987.

38. Weller FR, Kallenberg CGM, Orie NGM, et al: Primary cell-mediated immune response in bronchial asthma. Relationship between primary *in vitro* and *in vivo* cell-mediated and antibody responses in pa-tients with asthma and healthy controls. Clin Allergy *16*:241–250, 1986.

39. Stewart DE, Raskin J, Garfinkel PE, et al: Anorexia nervosa, bulimia, and pregnancy. Am J Obstet Gy-necol *157*:1194–1198, 1987.

40. Lustig RH, Conte FA, Kogan BA, et al: Ontogeny of gonadotropin secretion in congenital anorchism: Sex-ual dimorphism versus syndrome of gonadal dysgene-sis and diagnostic considerations. J Urol *138*:587–591, 1987.

41. Palestine AG, Austin HA, Balow JE, et al: Renal histopathologic alterations in patients treated with cyclosporine for uveitis. N Engl J Med *314*:1293–1298, 1986.

42. Bjerve KS, Mostad IL, Thoresen L: Alpha-linolenic acid deficiency in patients on long-term gastric-tube feeding: Estimation of linolenic acid and long-chain unsaturated n-3 fatty acid requirement in man. Am J Clin Nutr *45*:66–77, 1987.

43. Reich H, McGlynn F: Treatment of ovarian en-dometriomas using laparoscopic surgical techniques. J Reprod Med *31*:577–584, 1986.

44. Eggleston C, Cruvant D: Review of recovery from intracerebral hematoma in children and adults. J Neurosurg Nurs *15*:128–135, 1983.

45. Kubricht DW: Therapeutic self-care demands ex-pressed by outpatients receiving external radiation therapy. Canc Nurs *7*:43–52, 1984.

12

CORRELATION AND REGRESSION

CHAPTER OBJECTIVES

After studying this chapter and working the problems, you should be able to:

1. Explain the concept of linear association

2. Carry out and interpret hypothesis tests concerning population Pearson correlation coefficients and population regression coefficients

3. Calculate and interpret confidence intervals for population regression coefficients

4. Recognize data that violate assumptions required for correlation and regression hypothesis tests and regression confidence intervals

5. Explain the rationale for data transformation

6. Interpret SPSS correlation and regression output and SAS regression output

7. Determine whether correlation and regression analyses reported in the medical and health care literature are appropriate

Many medical and health care studies focus on the issue of *association*: Are the values of one variable related to the values of another variable? Can the values of one variable be used to predict the values of another variable? We might investigate whether an illness score is related to the length of hospital stay. Or we might consider whether clotting time is related to the serum level of a new drug. Or we might evaluate whether the number of pack-years of smoking can be used to predict the severity of emphysema.

We cannot determine whether the values of two variables are related by comparing means. Thus, we cannot use *t* tests (Chapter 7), analysis of variance

(Chapters 8 and 13), or repeated-measures analysis of variance (Chapter 9) to investigate association between the values of two variables. If two variables have only a few possible values, the chi-square test of association described in Chapter 10 can often be used to determine whether the variables are associated. If one or both variables have a large number of possible values, correlation or regression analysis can often be done to determine whether the variables are associated.

We will focus on the use and interpretation of correlation and regression results rather than the calculation of these results. Because the calculations for correlation and regression coefficients are extremely tedious, they are almost always done by a computer. The formulas used for correlation and regression analyses can be found in other texts.[1]

12.1 CORRELATION

In a study of carbon dioxide sensitivity in panic anxiety, scores for the Hamilton Anxiety Scale (HAS) and the Patient-Rated Anxiety Scale (PRAS) were reported for 14 subjects with panic anxiety.[2] These scores are shown in Table 12.1. We would like to determine whether the HAS scores and the PRAS scores are related. To do this, we need a statistical procedure for determining the extent to which two variables are *correlated*.

Random variables are correlated if the values of one variable tend to be associated *in a linear way* with the values of the other variable. Variables are related in a linear way when the relationship between them can be described by a straight line. If increasing values of one variable are associated in a linear way with increasing values of the other variable, the variables are *positively correlated*. If increasing values of one variable are associated in a linear way with decreasing values of the other variable, the variables are *negatively correlated*.

Consider the hypothetical data plotted in Figures 12.1 through 12.4. These plots are *scatterplots*, plots that show how the values of one variable are related to the values of another variable. In Figure 12.1, there is no relationship between the variables X and Y. The points in the plot appear to be randomly scattered.

In Figures 12.2 and 12.3, each scatterplot shows a linear relationship. A straight line could be drawn on each plot to represent the relationship between the values of the variable X and those of the variable Y. Figure 12.2 shows variables that are positively correlated and Figure 12.3 shows variables that are negatively correlated.

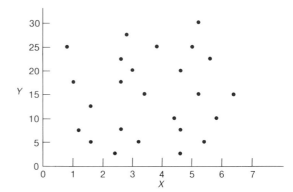

Figure 12.1 Scatterplot showing no relationship between variables X and Y

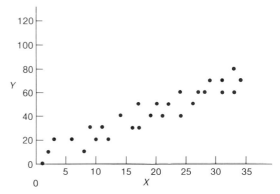

Figure 12.2 Scatterplot showing a positive linear relationship between variables X and Y

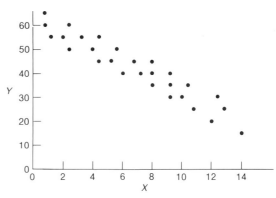

Figure 12.3 Scatterplot showing a negative linear relationship between variables X and Y

A *nonlinear* relationship is evident in Figure 12.4. Although the values of X are closely related to the values of Y, the relationship could not be described accurately with a straight line. A curve would have to be drawn to describe the relationship.

The *Pearson correlation coefficient* is used to measure the degree to which two variables are linearly

TABLE 12.1 HAS AND PRAS SCORES FOR PATIENTS WITH PANIC ANXIETY

Subject No.	HAS Score	PRAS Score
1	8	11
2	20	40
3	23	46
4	9	14
5	20	52
6	10	14
7	23	46
8	22	45
9	18	30
10	23	54
11	21	43
12	16	35
13	20	59
14	10	20

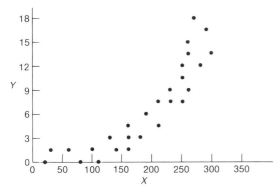

Figure 12.4 Scatterplot showing a nonlinear relationship between variables X and Y

related. This coefficient can take any value between -1 and 1. If the population Pearson correlation coefficient is equal to 1, there is a perfect positive linear relationship between the values of one variable and those of the other variable. If the population Pearson correlation coefficient is equal to -1, there is a perfect negative linear relationship between the values of one variable and those of the other variable. In either case, the values of one variable can be perfectly predicted by knowing the values of the other variable. The closer the Pearson correlation coefficient is to -1 or 1, the stronger the linear component of the relationship between the variables.

If the population Pearson correlation coefficient is equal to 0, there is no *linear* relationship between the two variables. This does *not* imply that there is no relationship at all between the two variables. Uncorrelated variables can be perfectly related in a nonlinear way.

We will use the letter r to denote the sample Pearson correlation coefficient. Although Pearson's r can be calculated by hand, the calculations are extremely tedious. We will omit the formula for Pearson's r and focus on the use of this coefficient. The formula can be found in other texts.[1]

When the sample Pearson correlation coefficient is obtained, inferences about a population are usually of interest. Researchers often use the sample coefficient to test the hypothesis that there is no linear association between two variables in the population. This is the null hypothesis that the population Pearson correlation coefficient is equal to 0:

$$H_0: \text{ Population Pearson correlation} \atop \text{coefficient} = 0 \qquad (12.1)$$

The two-sided alternative hypothesis is

$$H_A: \text{ Population Pearson correlation} \atop \text{coefficient} \neq 0 \qquad (12.2)$$

If a statistical software package is used to obtain the sample Pearson correlation coefficient, the

p-value for a test of the null hypothesis (12.1) is usually given in the output. If this p-value is not given, a t statistic based on r can be used to obtain it. This t statistic is given by the formula

$$t = \frac{r \times \sqrt{n-2}}{\sqrt{1-r^2}} \qquad (12.3)$$

where n is the number of subjects. The rationale for the t statistic (12.3) is not obvious and we will not discuss it. Our primary concern is the use and interpretation of this statistic.

If the null hypothesis (12.1) is true and certain assumptions are satisfied, the t statistic (12.3) has a t distribution with $n-2$ (*not* $n-1$) degrees of freedom (df). The two-tailed p-value for this t statistic is

$$P(t \text{ statistic} \leq -|t_{\text{calc}}| \quad \text{or} \quad t \text{ statistic} \geq |t_{\text{calc}}|)$$

where t_{calc} is the calculated value of the t statistic.

Table E.4 is used to obtain two-tailed p-values for the t statistic (12.3) in essentially the same way as described in Chapter 7. Only the degrees of freedom are different. If the p-value is less than the significance level α, the null hypothesis (12.1) is rejected. If the p-value is greater than or equal to α, the null hypothesis (12.1) cannot be rejected. The p-value is interpreted in the usual way: it is the probability of getting a t statistic at least as extreme as the calculated t statistic if the null hypothesis (12.1) is true.

One-sided tests of the null hypothesis (12.1) have the alternative hypotheses H_A: Population Pearson correlation coefficient < 0 or H_A: Population Pearson correlation coefficient > 0. In general, such tests are not recommended, for the same reasons discussed in Chapter 7. A statistician can be consulted to obtain one-tailed p-values for the t statistic (12.3).

The t test of the null hypothesis (12.1) requires the following assumptions.

1. Random Sample of Subjects. Random sampling is not required if the sample is not biased.

2. Paired Samples. If the samples are not paired, the Pearson correlation coefficient cannot be obtained.

3. Independent Observations for at Least One Variable. All of the sample values for at least one of the variables must be independent. Observations for *different* variables are not necessarily independent, since paired data were obtained. If the observations for the first variable are not independent *and* the observations for the second variable are not independent, the t test of the null hypothesis (12.1) cannot be done.

Suppose we want to test the hypothesis that the population Pearson correlation coefficient for the variables drug dose and duration of response is equal to 0. Then the drug dose observations must be independent or the duration observations must be independent. The drug doses might have been systematically assigned to subjects in a way that makes them nonindependent. As long as the duration observations are independent, the independence assumption is satisfied.

4. Normality. At least one of the variables with independent observations must have a normal or approximately normal distribution. If the sample values of both variables satisfy the independence assumption, normality is required for only one of the variables. The null hypothesis (12.1) cannot be tested if both variables have extremely nonnormal distributions (e.g., if both variables have only a few possible values).

5. Constant Variance. Let Y be the variable that satisfies the independence and normality assumptions. The variability of the Y values should not change as the values of the other variable change. To check this assumption, we examine a scatterplot of the variables with Y on the vertical axis. The amount of vertical scatter in different parts of the plot should not differ greatly. In other words, points should be evenly spread out vertically throughout the plot. If points in one part of the plot are very close together vertically and those in another part are very far apart vertically, the constant variance assumption is questionable. If both variables satisfy the independence and normality assumptions, constant variance is required for only one of the variables.

6. Linearity. If a relationship exists between the two variables, it must be linear. The Pearson correlation coefficient is not appropriate when two variables are related in a nonlinear way. This assumption is evaluated by checking a scatterplot of the two variables for evidence of a curve.

Let us evaluate these assumptions for the anxiety data. The subjects are not a random sample, but this is not essential. The samples are obviously paired, and the independence assumption seems reasonable for both variables. Knowing the HAS or PRAS score for one subject should not tell us anything about the HAS or PRAS score for another subject. Histograms of the HAS and PRAS scores are shown in Figures 12.5 and 12.6. Although these histograms do not look exactly normal, they are not so extremely nonnormal that a t test of the null hypothesis (12.1) is ruled out.

An SPSS/PC scatterplot of the HAS and PRAS scores is shown in Figure 12.7.* Although the points in the upper-right-hand corner of the plot are slightly more scattered than the points in the rest of the plot, the plot does not suggest extreme violations of the constant variance assumption. No curve

---

*Points are represented as numbers in SPSS/PC scatterplots. A "1" indicates one point, a "2" indicates two points, and so on.

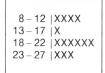

Figure 12.5   Quick histogram of HAS score

```
10 – 23 |XXXX
24 – 37 |XX
38 – 51 |XXXXX
52 – 65 |XXX
```

Figure 12.6   Quick histogram of PRAS score

is evident, so the linearity assumption seems to hold. A straight line could be drawn on the plot to represent the relationship between the HAS scores and the PRAS scores. We will use a 0.05 significance level to test the null hypothesis (12.1).

The sample Pearson correlation coefficient for the HAS and PRAS scores is 0.9214. Applying formula (12.3), we obtain the t statistic for testing the null hypothesis (12.1).

$$t = \frac{0.9214 \times \sqrt{14 - 2}}{\sqrt{1 - 0.9214^2}}$$

$$= \frac{3.192}{0.389} = 8.21$$

The degrees of freedom are $14 - 2 = 12$. In the row for 12 df in Table E.4, the largest number is 4.318. Since this number is the 0.0005 upper percentage point and 8.21 is greater than 4.318, the two-tailed p-value is less than $2 \times 0.0005 = 0.001$:

$$p\text{-value} < 0.001$$

We reject the hypothesis that the population Pearson correlation coefficient is equal to 0 at any reasonable significance level.*

Can we conclude from this t test that the HAS and PRAS scores are linearly related? The answer is *no*. The relationship between two variables can be nonlinear even if the population Pearson correlation coefficient does not equal zero. Only a population Pearson correlation coefficient of 1 or -1 rules out a nonlinear relationship. If the population

---

*The hypothesis that the population Pearson correlation coefficient is equal to some nonzero number can also be tested, and confidence intervals for the population Pearson correlation coefficient can be obtained. These tests and confidence intervals require the assumption of bivariate normality, which implies that *both* variables have normal distributions. Further information can be found in other texts.[3]

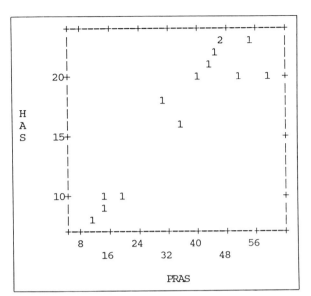

Figure 12.7 SPSS/PC scatterplot of HAS and PRAS scores

Pearson correlation coefficient does not equal 1 or −1, the variables may be related in a nonlinear way. A scatterplot must always be obtained to check linearity when a correlation coefficient is computed.

As we saw earlier, the SPSS/PC scatterplot of the HAS and PRAS scores (Figure 12.7) is consistent with a linear relationship. *Together*, the scatterplot *and* the *t* test indicate that the HAS and PRAS scores are linearly related. We cannot use the *t* test alone to reach this conclusion.

How strong is the linear relationship between the HAS and PRAS scores? Our *t* test of the null hypothesis (12.1) only allows us to decide that the population Pearson correlation coefficient is not 0. To evaluate the strength of a linear relationship, we examine the *square* of the sample Pearson correla-

TABLE 12.2   AGE AND THEOPHYLLINE CLEARANCE FOR 51 ADMISSIONS

Admission No.	Age (mo)	Theophylline Clearance (ml/kg/h)	Admission No.	Age (mo)	Theophylline Clearance (ml/kg/h)
1	7	63	27	37	106
2	13	105	28	29	98
3	14	125	29	31	85
4	16	115	30	33	103
5	17	141	31	67	70
6	24	126	32	35	55
7	29	103	33	37	65
8	39	75	34	41	86
9	16	148	35	48	74
10	19	139	36	35	84
11	24	136	37	44	72
12	16	124	38	46	80
13	22	134	39	51	84
14	29	100	40	52	74
15	35	130	41	58	80
16	24	55	42	35	82
17	30	64	43	37	121
18	33	66	44	39	127
19	35	42	45	43	105
20	26	62	46	36	41
21	34	71	47	38	58
22	53	110	48	43	53
23	66	70	49	36	88
24	26	78	50	38	110
25	27	90	51	41	116
26	34	76			

tion coefficient, r^2. If r^2 is equal to 1, the sample observations have a perfect linear relationship. The closer r^2 is to 1, the stronger the linear component of the relationship.

For the anxiety data, $r^2 = 0.9214^2 = 0.8490$. This value suggests a fairly strong linear relationship between the HAS and PRAS scores. The population squared Pearson correlation coefficient may be smaller, since r^2 is just a sample estimate of the population squared coefficient.

Example 12.1

In a study of theophylline clearance in pediatric asthmatics, age and theophylline clearance were reported for pediatric patients with multiple admissions for status asthmaticus.[4] Table 12.2 shows the age and theophylline clearance for 51 admissions for 12 patients. Can we test the hypothesis that the population Pearson correlation coefficient for age and theophylline clearance is 0?

Because there are far more admissions than patients, repeated measurements were obtained for some patients. The independence assumption is not reasonable for age or theophylline clearance, and we cannot test the null hypothesis (12.1). If we knew which admissions belonged to each patient, we could select the data for the first admissions. This would produce 12 independent age values and 12 independent theophylline clearance values. We could then use these data to test the null hypothesis (12.1) if the other correlation assumptions were satisfied.

Example 12.2

A study evaluated the effect of programmed ventricular stimulation in patients without structural heart disease, patients with idiopathic dilated cardiomyopathy, and patients with coronary artery disease.[5] Table 12.3 shows the percentage of coronary artery

stenosis in the left anterior descending coronary artery (LAD) and the right coronary artery (RCA) for these 17 patients. Can we test the hypothesis that the population Pearson correlation coefficient for LAD stenosis and RCA stenosis is 0?

Although the independence assumption seems reasonable, both the LAD stenosis percentages and the RCA stenosis percentages have extremely nonnormal distributions. We cannot test the hypothesis that the population Pearson correlation coefficient is equal to 0. The Spearman rank correlation coefficient described in Chapter 11 could be used instead to test the hypothesis that the population Spearman rank correlation coefficient is 0.

12.2 BIVARIATE REGRESSION

In a study of fibrin glue use during cardiac operations, the chest tube output 24 hours and 48 hours after cardiac surgery was reported for 20 patients who were treated with glue and 20 patients who were not treated with glue.[6] Table 12.4 shows the output values for the 20 untreated patients. An SPSS/PC scatterplot of the 48-hour and 24-hour output values is shown in Figure 12.8.

The scatterplot suggests a linear relationship between the 24-hour output and the 48-hour output. We would like to describe this relationship by drawing a straight line on the scatterplot. Such a line should fit the data well by being close to as many data points as possible.

How can we draw such a line through the data? We could fit it by eye, trying to sketch a line that comes close to most of the data points. If we were

TABLE 12.3 CORONARY ARTERY STENOSIS (PERCENT OF DIAMETER)

Patient No.	LAD	RCA
1	0	0
2	0	0
3	0	0
4	0	0
5	0	0
6	0	0
7	0	0
8	0	0
9	100	50
10	95	95
11	80	100
12	80	100
13	60	100
14	90	90
15	90	100
16	100	0
17	80	100

TABLE 12.4 CHEST-TUBE OUTPUT (ml) 24 AND 48 HOURS AFTER CARDIAC SURGERY

Patient No.	24 Hrs	48 Hrs
1	520	610
2	340	625
3	530	640
4	1393	1543
5	1093	1253
6	156	261
7	2211	3006
8	1654	1864
9	555	555
10	610	720
11	995	1225
12	1365	1505
13	1220	1300
14	1240	1560
15	1075	1280
16	1330	1615
17	690	690
18	1035	1035
19	1280	1425
20	1035	1035

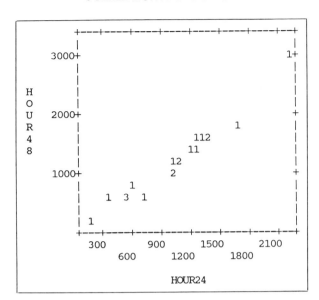

Figure 12.8 SPSS/PC scatterplot of 48-hour output and 24-hour output

to ask two different researchers to do this, they most likely would produce two different lines. How do we decide which line is better? To avoid disagreements, we need a standard method for obtaining a line that fits the data as well as possible.

The most commonly used method for obtaining a straight line to describe a linear relationship between two variables is *bivariate regression*. (The term "bivariate" means "two-variable.") Formulas described in other texts can be used to obtain a *regression equation* for a straight line that fits the data as well as possible.[1] If X and Y are random variables, the regression equation describing the line for *sample* values of X and Y has the general form

$$\text{estimated } Y = b_0 + b_1 X \qquad (12.4)$$

The term "estimated Y" in equation (12.4) refers to the estimated values of the variable Y given by the sample regression equation. We will describe the use of sample regression equations to obtain estimated values in a later section. Estimated values are also called *fitted values* and are often denoted by $\hat{Y}$ (pronounced "Y hat"). The numbers b_0 (pronounced "b nought") and b_1 (pronounced "b sub one") are calculated from the data according to regression formulas described in other texts.[1] These numbers are called the *sample regression coefficients*. Equation (12.4) can be used to draw a line called the *sample regression line* on the scatterplot of the data.* This line fits the data as well as possible.

In equation (12.4), the variable Y is the *dependent variable* and the variable X is the *independent vari-*

able. This terminology is used because equation (12.4) expresses the estimated values of Y in terms of the values of X. For some data, the choice of independent and dependent variables is arbitrary. For other data, one of the variables makes more sense as the independent variable. If one variable is used to predict the values of the other variable, the variable used for prediction is the independent variable and the predicted variable is the dependent variable. With the chest-tube data, it makes sense to try to use the 24-hour output to predict the 48-hour output. If this is done, the 24-hour output is the independent variable and the 48-hour output is the dependent variable. By convention, dependent variables are plotted on the vertical axis and independent variables on the horizontal axis of a scatterplot.

The regression equation (12.4) is the equation for the *sample* regression line. This equation is used to estimate the unknown *population* regression line, which is described by the population regression equation

$$\text{estimated } Y = \beta_0 + \beta_1 X \qquad (12.5)$$

Here estimated Y refers to the estimated values of the variable Y given by the population regression line. The unknown numbers β_0 (pronounced "beta nought") and β_1 (pronounced "beta sub one") are called the *population regression coefficients*. The number β_0 is the population *intercept* of the regression line.* The number β_1 is the population *slope* of the regression line.

The intercept of a line is the point on the vertical axis of a scatterplot where the line crosses (intercepts) this axis. The slope of a line is a number that

---

*We will not describe the procedure for drawing sample regression lines. Information about drawing lines from linear equations can be found in most elementary algebra texts.

---

*The regression intercept is also called the regression *constant term*.

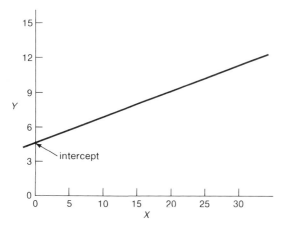

Figure 12.9 Line with positive slope

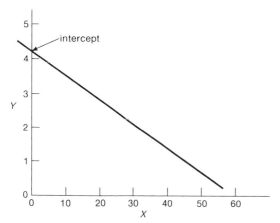

Figure 12.10 Line with negative slope

indicates whether the line rises or falls and how steeply the line rises or falls. If the slope is positive, the line has an upward slant. If the slope is negative, the line has a downward slant. Figure 12.9 shows a line with a positive slope and Figure 12.10 shows one with a negative slope.

If the population regression slope is positive, the independent and dependent variables are positively correlated. If the population regression slope is negative, the independent and dependent variables are negatively correlated. The b_0 coefficient in equation (12.4) is the sample regression intercept and is used to estimate the population regression intercept. The b_1 coefficient is the sample regression slope and is used to estimate the population regression slope. As we shall see in the next sections, the sample regression coefficients can be used to obtain confidence intervals and tests concerning the population regression coefficients.

For the chest-tube data, b_0 is equal to -52.78 and b_1 is equal to 1.22. (These values were obtained from the SPSS/PC REGRESSION program.) The positive b_1 value suggests a positive relationship between the 24-hour output and the 48-hour output, as we would expect. The sample regression equation for the chest-tube data is

estimated 48-hour output

$$= -52.78 + 1.22(\text{24-hour output})$$

In this equation, the estimated 48-hour output is expressed in terms of the 24-hour output. The sample regression line given by this equation is shown in Figure 12.11. Most of the data values are quite close to the regression line, indicating that the regression line fits the data fairly well.

In most regression analyses, the primary concern is not the sample regression equation itself but the

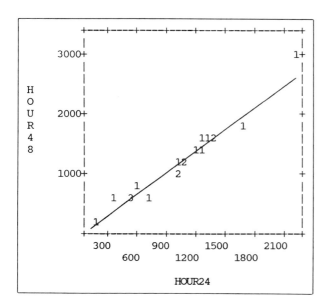

Figure 12.11 SPSS/PC scatterplot of 48-hour output and 24-hour output with sample regression line

use of this equation to make inferences about the population regression equation. Such inferences are made by obtaining confidence intervals to estimate population regression coefficients or by testing hypotheses about population regression coefficients.

12.3 CONFIDENCE INTERVALS FOR REGRESSION COEFFICIENTS

Just as we often want to use confidence intervals to estimate population means or proportions, we often want to use confidence intervals to estimate population regression coefficients. Confidence intervals for the population regression slope and intercept are easy to calculate if the sample regression coefficients and their standard errors have been obtained from a computer.

Let $se(b_1)$ denote the estimated standard error (standard deviation) of the sample regression slope and let $se(b_0)$ denote the estimated standard error of the sample regression intercept. These standard errors need not be calculated by hand, since they are usually included in computer regression output. The formulas can be found in other texts.[1]

Let $t_{\alpha/2, n-2}$ be the $\alpha/2$ upper percentage point of the t distribution with $n - 2$ degrees of freedom. As before, n is the number of subjects. A $100(1 - \alpha)\%$ confidence interval for the population regression slope is given by the formula

$$
\begin{aligned}
\big(b_1 - (t_{\alpha/2, n-2})(se(b_1)), \\
b_1 + (t_{\alpha/2, n-2})(se(b_1))\big)
\end{aligned}
\tag{12.6}
$$

A $100(1 - \alpha)\%$ confidence interval for the population regression intercept is given by the formula

$$
\begin{aligned}
\big(b_0 - (t_{\alpha/2, n-2})(se(b_0)), \\
b_0 + (t_{\alpha/2, n-2})(se(b_0))\big)
\end{aligned}
\tag{12.7}
$$

If formula (12.6) is used to obtain a 95% confidence interval for the population regression slope, 95% of all possible samples will produce confidence intervals that contain the population slope. Five percent of all possible samples will produce confidence intervals that do not contain the population slope. We interpret a 95% confidence interval for the population regression slope by saying that we are 95% sure that the confidence interval contains the population slope.

If formula (12.7) is used to obtain a 99% confidence interval for the population regression intercept, 99% of all possible samples will produce confidence intervals that contain the population intercept. One percent of all possible samples will produce confidence intervals that do not contain the population intercept. We interpret a 99% confidence interval for the population regression intercept by saying that we are 99% sure that the confidence interval contains the population intercept.

Confidence intervals for regression coefficients require the following assumptions.

1. Random Sample of Subjects. As long as the sample is not biased, random sampling is not crucial.

2. Paired Samples. Regression coefficients cannot be obtained if the samples are not paired.

3. Independent Observations for the Dependent Variable. All of the observations for the dependent variable must be independent. If this assumption is violated, confidence intervals cannot be obtained for population regression coefficients. The observations for the independent variable need not be independent.

4. Normality of the Dependent Variable. The dependent variable must have a normal or approximately normal distribution. Confidence intervals cannot be obtained for population regression coefficients if the dependent variable has an extremely nonnormal distribution (e.g., if the dependent variable has only a few possible values). If the independent variable has a nonnormal distribution but the dependent variable has a normal or approximately normal distribution, confidence intervals can still be obtained for population regression coefficients.

5. Constant Variance. The variability of the values of the dependent variable should not change as the values of the independent variable change. To check this assumption, we examine a scatterplot of the dependent and independent variables. The amount of vertical scatter in different parts of the plot should not differ greatly. In other words, points should be evenly spread out vertically throughout the plot. If points in one part of the plot are very close together vertically and those in another part are very far apart vertically, the constant variance assumption is questionable.

6. Linearity. Any relationship between the independent and dependent variables must be linear. Bivariate regression is not appropriate when two variables are related in a nonlinear way. To evaluate this assumption, we examine a scatterplot of the dependent and independent variables for evidence of a curve.

In addition, confidence intervals for the population regression intercept are obtained only when the independent variable can equal 0 and some of the sample values for the independent variable are equal to or close to 0. It can be shown that the regression intercept is the estimated value of the dependent variable when the independent variable is equal to 0. If the independent variable cannot equal 0, there is no point in making inferences about the intercept. If all of the sample values for the independent variable are far from 0, we do not have enough information about the intercept to obtain a confidence interval for the population intercept.

```
   0 –  499 |X
 500 –  999 |XXXXX
1000 – 1499 |XXXXXX
1500 – 1999 |XXXX
2000 – 2499 |
2500 – 2999 |
3000 – 3499 |X
```

Figure 12.12 Quick histogram of 48-hour output

Let us evaluate these assumptions for the chest-tube data. Although the subjects are not a random sample, this is not essential. The samples are obviously paired, and the independence assumption seems reasonable. Knowing the 48-hour output for one patient should not tell us anything about the 48-hour output for another patient. A histogram of the 48-hour output values is shown in Figure 12.12. The large value in the last interval may indicate a skewed population, or it may be an unusually large observation from an approximately normal population. The histogram does not suggest the sort of extreme nonnormality that would rule out confidence intervals for population regression coefficients.

The scatterplot of the 48-hour and 24-hour output (Figure 12.8) does not show marked differences in the degree to which points are vertically scattered. The constant variance assumption is reasonable for these data. Since no evidence of a curve is apparent in the scatterplot, the linearity assumption seems to hold as well. A confidence interval for the population regression slope is appropriate.

Although the distributional assumptions needed for confidence intervals are reasonable for the chest-tube data, the smallest 24-hour output is 156, which is quite far from 0. A chest-tube output of 0 is extremely unlikely 24 hours after cardiac surgery. For this reason, a confidence interval for the population intercept has little practical value. We will calculate this confidence interval just to illustrate the use of formula (12.7).

Let us use a 95% level of confidence for each confidence interval. The degrees of freedom are $20 - 2 = 18$. In Table E.4, we find the 0.025 upper percentage point of the t distribution with 18 df: $t_{.025, 18} = 2.101$. We can get the sample regression coefficients and their estimated standard errors from a computer package:

$$b_1 = 1.22 \qquad se(b_1) = 0.07$$

$$b_0 = -52.78 \qquad se(b_0) = 75.57$$

Using these sample coefficients and standard errors, we apply formulas (12.6) and (12.7) to obtain our 95% confidence intervals for the population regression slope and intercept:

TABLE 12.5 PERFUSION (ml/100 ml/min)

Limb No.	Occasion 1	Occasion 2
1	13.3	13.5
2	20.0	19.1
3	19.6	19.5
4	15.3	13.4
5	15.1	13.6
6	4.6	4.4
7	6.5	6.7
8	13.3	14.1
9	11.1	11.1

Confidence Interval for β_1.

$(1.22 - (2.101)(0.07), \quad 1.22 + (2.101)(0.07))$

$(1.22 - 0.15, \quad 1.22 + 0.15)$

$(1.07, \quad 1.37)$

Confidence Interval for β_0.

$(-57.28 - (2.101)(75.57), \quad -57.28 + (2.101)(75.57))$

$(-57.28 - 158.77, \quad -57.28 + 158.77)$

$(-216.05, \quad 101.49)$

We are 95% sure that the population regression slope is between 1.07 and 1.37. If the confidence interval for b_0 had been appropriate, we would have been 95% sure that the population regression intercept is between -216.05 and 101.49.

Example 12.3 _____

A study evaluated the use of technetium-labeled red blood cells for the measurement of limb blood flow.[7] Table 12.5 shows the perfusion measurements on two occasions for nine limbs from five subjects. Can we obtain a confidence interval for the slope of the population regression equation with the second measurement as the dependent variable and the first measurement as the independent variable?

Nine limbs from five subjects were used, so repeated measurements were obtained for each variable. Not all of the observations for the dependent variable are independent, and a confidence interval cannot be obtained for the population slope. If we knew which limbs belonged to each subject, we could select the first pair of measurements from each subject. The resulting data should satisfy the independence assumption. If these data satisfied the other regression assumptions, they could be used to obtain a confidence interval for the regression slope.

12.4 TESTING REGRESSION HYPOTHESES

Hypotheses about regression coefficients are often of interest. Just as we might want to test the hypothesis that a population mean is equal to some hypothesized value, we might want to test the hypothesis that the population regression slope or intercept is equal to some hypothesized value.

Hypotheses about the population slope are of interest much more often than hypotheses about the population intercept. The general null hypothesis for the population slope is

$$H_0: \beta_1 = \beta_{10} \qquad (12.8)$$

The number β_{10} (pronounced "beta sub one nought") is some number specified by the researcher. It is not derived statistically. The two-sided alternative hypothesis is

$$H_A: \beta_1 \neq \beta_{10} \qquad (12.9)$$

In most cases, β_{10} is 0. When the population regression slope is equal to 0, there is no linear relationship between the independent and dependent variables. A line with a slope of 0 is a horizontal line, a line that is parallel to the horizontal axis of a scatterplot. Figure 12.13 shows a line with a slope of 0. If the relationship between two variables can be described by a line with a slope of 0, the estimated value of the dependent variable is the same no matter what the value of the independent variable is. The hypothesis that the population regression slope is equal to 0 is the most frequently tested hypothesis in regression analysis.

To test the null hypothesis (12.8), we use a t statistic given by the formula

$$t = \frac{b_1 - \beta_{10}}{\text{se}(b_1)} \qquad (12.10)$$

As before, $\text{se}(b_1)$ is the estimated standard error of the sample regression slope. If the null hypothesis (12.8) is true and certain assumptions are satisfied, this t statistic has a t distribution with $n - 2$ degrees of freedom, where n is the number of subjects. The t test of the null hypothesis (12.8) requires the same assumptions as the confidence interval for the population regression slope (p. 277).

The t statistic (12.10) has the usual test statistic format. The top part of this t statistic is the difference between our sample estimate of the population slope and its hypothesized value. In other words, the top part measures the discrepancy between what we got and what we expect to get if the null hypothesis is true. The bottom part of this t statistic is an estimate of the variability of the sample regression slope.

If the discrepancy between the sample slope and the hypothesized slope is large relative to the variability of the sample slope, the t statistic will be large in absolute value. If the discrepancy between the sample slope and the hypothesized slope is small relative to the variability of the sample slope, the t statistic will be small in absolute value. Thus, it makes sense to reject the null hypothesis (12.8) if the t statistic is large in absolute value.

The two-tailed p-value for the t statistic (12.10) is given by

$$P(t \text{ statistic} \leq -|t_{\text{calc}}| \quad \text{or} \quad t \text{ statistic} \geq |t_{\text{calc}}|)$$

where t_{calc} is the calculated value of the t statistic. Table E.4 is used to obtain p-values. If the p-value is less than the significance level α, the null hypothesis (12.8) is rejected. If the p-value is greater than or equal to α, the null hypothesis (12.8) cannot be rejected. The p-value is interpreted in the usual way: it is the probability of getting a t statistic at least as extreme as the calculated t statistic if the null hypothesis (12.8) is true.

One-sided tests of the null hypothesis (12.8) can be done with the alternative hypotheses $H_A: \beta_1 < \beta_{10}$ or $H_A: \beta_1 > \beta_{10}$, although such tests are not usually recommended. Consult a statistician if you need one-tailed p-values for testing the null hypothesis (12.8).

It can be shown that the hypothesis that β_1 is equal to 0 is the same as the hypothesis that the population Pearson correlation coefficient is equal to 0. A population regression slope of 0 implies a population Pearson correlation coefficient of 0, and a population Pearson correlation coefficient of 0

Figure 12.13 Line with slope of 0

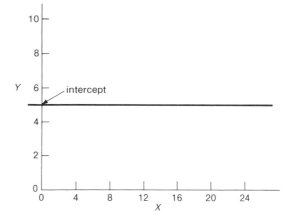

implies a population regression slope of 0. It can also be shown that the t statistic (12.10) for testing the hypothesis that the population slope is zero is identical to the t statistic (12.3) for testing the hypothesis that the population Pearson correlation coefficient is zero. Since the degrees of freedom for these t statistics are the same, the p-values for these statistics are always the same. The two t tests are equivalent.

Let us use the chest-tube data to test the null hypothesis that the population regression slope is equal to 0:

$$H_0: \beta_1 = 0 \qquad (12.11)$$

Our two-sided alternative hypothesis states that the population regression slope is not equal to 0:

$$H_A: \beta_1 \neq 0 \qquad (12.12)$$

From the previous section, we know that the assumptions required for this test are satisfied. We will use a 0.005 significance level.

The sample regression slope is 1.22 and the estimated standard error of the sample regression slope is 0.07. Applying formula (12.10), we can calculate our t statistic for testing the null hypothesis (12.11):

$$t = \frac{1.22 - 0}{0.07} = 17.43$$

The degrees of freedom are $20 - 2 = 18$. In the row for 18 df in Table E.4, the largest number is 3.922. Since this number is the 0.0005 upper percentage point and 17.43 is larger than 3.922, the two-tailed p-value is less than 2×0.0005:

$$p\text{-value} < 0.001$$

We reject the hypothesis that the population regression slope is equal to 0 at any reasonable significance level.

The interpretation of the t test of the null hypothesis (12.11) is a frequent source of confusion. If we cannot reject the hypothesis that the population regression slope is equal to 0, we conclude only that the data provide no evidence of a *linear* relationship between the independent variable and the dependent variable. We *cannot* conclude that there is no relationship at all between the variables. The population regression slope can equal 0 when the independent and dependent variables are perfectly related in a nonlinear way.

If we reject the hypothesis that the population regression slope is equal to 0, we cannot conclude that the relationship between the independent variable and the dependent variable is linear. Nonzero population regression slopes are quite common when variables have a nonlinear relationship. The t test of the null hypothesis (12.11) cannot be used by itself to determine whether the dependent variable is related to the independent variable. The t test

must always be interpreted in conjunction with a scatterplot. If the scatterplot indicates a nonlinear relationship, the t statistic (12.10) should not be used.

The scatterplot of the chest-tube data (Figure 12.8), together with the results of the t test, indicate that the 48-hour output is linearly related to the 24-hour output. Does this mean that the 24-hour output can be used to make accurate predictions of the 48-hour output? The answer is no. The amount of scatter in Figure 12.8 suggests that extremely accurate predictions of the 48-hour output cannot be made from the 24-hour output. The linear relationship is strong enough to allow approximate predictions, however. Whether these predictions are accurate enough to be of clinical value is a medical issue and not a statistical one. A regression equation can be used to obtain intervals for predicting values of the dependent variable from values of the independent variable. Formulas for such prediction intervals can be found in other texts.[1]

Hypotheses about the population regression intercept are sometimes of interest in medical and health care research. The general null hypothesis is

$$H_0: \beta_0 = \beta_{00} \qquad (12.13)$$

where β_{00} (pronounced "beta nought nought") is a number specified by the researcher. In many cases, β_{00} is equal to 0. The two-sided alternative hypothesis is

$$H_A: \beta_0 \neq \beta_{00} \qquad (12.14)$$

Hypotheses about the population intercept are tested much less frequently than hypotheses about the population slope.

As before, let $se(b_0)$ denote the estimated standard error of the sample regression intercept. To test the null hypothesis (12.13), we use a t statistic given by the formula

$$t = \frac{b_0 - \beta_{00}}{se(b_0)} \qquad (12.15)$$

If the null hypothesis (12.13) is true and certain assumptions are satisfied, this t statistic has a t distribution with $n - 2$ degrees of freedom. The t test of the null hypothesis (12.13) requires the same assumptions as the confidence interval for the population regression intercept (p. 277). In addition, this t test should be done only if the independent variable can equal 0 and some of the sample values of the independent variable are equal to 0 or close to 0.

The two-tailed p-value for the t statistic (12.15) is given by

$$P(t \text{ statistic} \leq -|t_{calc}| \quad \text{or} \quad t \text{ statistic} \geq |t_{calc}|)$$

where t_{calc} is the calculated value of the t statistic. Table E.4 is used to obtain p-values. If the p-value is less than the significance level α, the null hypothesis (12.13) is rejected. If the p-value is greater than or equal to α, the null hypothesis (12.13) cannot be rejected. The p-value is interpreted in the usual way: it is the probability of getting a t statistic at least as extreme as the calculated t statistic if the null hypothesis (12.13) is true.

One-sided tests of the null hypothesis (12.13) can be done but usually are not recommended. Such tests have the alternative hypotheses H_A: $\beta_0 < \beta_{00}$ or H_A: $\beta_0 > \beta_{00}$. A statistician can be consulted to obtain one-tailed p-values for the t statistic (12.15).

A test of the null hypothesis (12.13) is not appropriate for the chest-tube data. None of the 24-hour chest-tube output values is close to 0, and a 24-hour chest-tube output value of 0 after cardiac surgery is nearly impossible. We will carry out this test anyway in order to illustrate the use of formula (12.15). Let us arbitrarily select a β_{00} value of 5 and a significance level of 0.01. Our null hypothesis states that the population regression intercept is equal to 5:

$$H_0: \beta_0 = 5$$

$$H_A: \beta_0 \neq 5$$

The sample regression intercept is -52.78, and the estimated standard error of the sample regression intercept is 75.57. Using these values and our β_{00} value of 5, we apply formula (12.15) to calculate our t statistic:

$$t = \frac{-52.78 - 5}{75.57} = -0.76$$

The degrees of freedom are $20 - 2 = 18$. In the row for 18 df in Table E.4, 0.76 lies between the numbers 0.534 and 0.862. Since these numbers are the 0.30 and 0.20 upper percentage points, the approximate p-value is

$$0.40 < p\text{-value} < 0.60$$

We cannot reject the hypothesis that the population regression intercept is equal to 5 at any reasonable significance level.

Tests concerning the population regression intercept tell us nothing about the linearity of the relationship between the independent variable and the dependent variable. Remember that the regression intercept is simply the point at which the regression line crosses the vertical axis.

Confidence intervals for population regression coefficients are always consistent with hypothesis tests concerning population regression coefficients. Suppose the hypothesis that a population regression coefficient is equal to some specified value is rejected at the significance level α. Then the $100(1 - \alpha)\%$ confidence interval for the population regression coefficient will not include the hypothesized value. If the hypothesis that a population regression coefficient is equal to some specified

value is not rejected at the significance level α, the $100(1 - \alpha)\%$ confidence interval for the population regression coefficient will include the hypothesized value.

Example 12.4

A study evaluated indirect calorimetry and the Fick method for determining resting energy expenditure (REE).[8] Table 12.6 shows the REE obtained by each method for 19 patients. Figure 12.14 shows a scatterplot of the Fick REE and the indirect REE, and Figure 12.15 shows a histogram of the Fick REE. The scatterplot suggests a linear relationship between the Fick REE and the indirect REE. The histogram is consistent with approximate normality of the population of Fick REE values. Although there is a slight increase in vertical scatter at the center of the scatterplot, it is not large enough to suggest that the constant variance assumption is violated. Paired samples were obviously obtained, and the Fick REE observations appear to be independent. The assumptions required for regression analysis with the Fick REE as the dependent variable are reasonable for these data.

SPSS/PC output gives us the sample regression coefficients for the REE data: $b_0 = 239.13$ and $b_1 = 0.80$. The sample regression equation is

estimated Fick REE = 239.13 + 0.80(indirect REE)

Hypotheses about the population regression intercept are not of interest, since REE does not take values anywhere near 0 in living subjects. We do want to test the hypothesis that the population regression slope is 0. If the population regression slope is equal to 0, there is no linear relationship between the indirect REE and the Fick REE. A

TABLE 12.6   INDIRECT REE AND FICK REE

Patient No.	Indirect REE	Fick REE
1	1969	1722
2	1325	1213
3	1464	1188
4	874	823
5	950	1100
6	916	1028
7	1134	1333
8	1181	1028
9	1410	1457
10	1530	1417
11	819	982
12	1396	1265
13	1365	1299
14	1924	2019
15	1700	1706
16	1450	1332
17	1479	1375
18	1526	1427
19	1372	1480

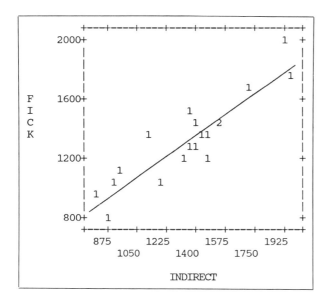

Figure 12.14 SPSS/PC scatterplot of Fick REE and indirect REE with sample regression line

```
700 – 999  |XX
1000 – 1299 |XXXXXXX
1300 – 1599 |XXXXXXX
1600 – 1899 |XX
1900 – 2199 |X
```

Figure 12.15 Quick histogram of Fick REE

zero population regression slope would mean that the Fick results are not equivalent to the indirect results.

We will use a 0.01 significance level to test the hypothesis that the population regression slope is equal to 0. From SPSS/PC output, the estimated standard error of b_1 is 0.09. Using this standard error and the value of b_1 (0.80) in formula (12.10), we obtain our t statistic for testing the null hypothesis that the population slope is equal to 0:

$$t = \frac{0.80 - 0}{0.09} = 8.89$$

The degrees of freedom are $19 - 2 = 17$. From Table E.4, the approximate p-value is

$$p\text{-value} < 0.001$$

We reject the hypothesis that the population regression slope is equal to 0 at any reasonable significance level.

For these data, another hypothesis about the population regression slope is also of interest. If the Fick method and the indirect method are equivalent, they will produce identical REE values, on average. In this case, the relationship between these variables can be described by the population regression equation

$$\text{estimated Fick REE} = \text{indirect REE}$$

Writing this equation with the population regression intercept and slope, we have

$$\text{estimated Fick REE} = 0 + 1(\text{indirect REE})$$

If the Fick method and the indirect method are equivalent, the population regression slope is equal to 1. If the population regression slope is not equal to 1, the Fick method and the indirect method are not equivalent.

To determine further whether the data provide evidence that the two methods are not equivalent, we also test the null hypothesis

$$H_0: \beta_1 = 1 \qquad (12.16)$$

The alternative hypothesis is

$$H_A: \beta_1 \neq 1 \qquad (12.17)$$

We will use a 0.01 significance level. Applying formula (12.10), we obtain the t statistic

$$t = \frac{0.80 - 1}{0.09} = -2.22$$

The degrees of freedom are still $19 - 2 = 17$. From Table E.4, we get the approximate p-value:

$$p\text{-value} \cong 0.04$$

We cannot reject the null hypothesis (12.16) at the 0.01 significance level.

If we had rejected the hypothesis that the population regression slope is equal to 1, we would have concluded that the Fick method and the indirect method are not equivalent. Can we conclude that the two methods are equivalent because we did not reject this hypothesis? The answer is no. Although the data do not provide evidence that the two methods are not equivalent, they do not demon-

TABLE 12.7   COMPLAINT SCORES FOR PATIENTS WITH SPASMODIC TORTICOLLIS

Patient No.	Deflexion of Head	Neck and Head Pain
1	4	0
2	3	2
3	3	2
4	5	3
5	3	2
6	3	4
7	2	1
8	2	2
9	3	0
10	4	2
11	2	1
12	1	1
13	3	3
14	3	2
15	5	4
16	4	2
17	1	1

strate that the methods are equivalent. Even if the population regression slope is equal to 1, many of the Fick REE values and the indirect REE values could be quite different. In fact, the values shown in Table 12.6 are fairly discrepant for many patients. The clinical importance of these discrepancies is a medical issue and not a statistical one.

Example 12.5

In a study of spasmodic torticollis (ST), the subjective symptom complaint scores shown in Table 12.7 were reported for 17 patients with idiopathic ST.[9] High scores indicate greater severity of the symptom. Can we test the hypothesis that the slope is equal to 0 for the population regression equation with neck and head pain as the dependent variable and deflexion of the head as the independent variable?

Although the paired-samples assumption holds and the pain score observations appear to be independent, the pain scores have an extremely nonnormal distribution, with only five different values. We cannot test the hypothesis that the population regression slope is equal to 0. If we wanted to determine whether the pain and deflexion scores are correlated, we could obtain the Spearman rank correlation coefficient described in Chapter 11. We could then test the hypothesis that the population Spearman rank correlation coefficient is 0.

12.5   RESIDUAL ANALYSIS

Some of the assumptions required for regression analysis can be evaluated by examining the *residuals* from the sample regression equation. The residuals,

denoted by e_i, are the differences between the actual values of the dependent variable and the estimated values of the dependent variable:

e_i = residual for ith subject

  = dependent variable value for ith subject

    − estimated dependent variable value

    for ith subject

How do we calculate the estimated values of the dependent variable? We first obtain the sample regression equation, and then use the values of the independent variable in this equation to obtain the estimated values. For the chest-tube data, the sample regression equation is

estimated 48-hour output

  $= -52.78 + 1.22(\text{24-hour output})$

From Table 12.4, we find that the 24-hour output for the first patient is 520 ml. Using this value in the sample regression equation, we get an estimated 48-hour output of 581.62 ml for the first patient:

estimated 48-hour output for first patient

  $= -52.78 + 1.22(520)$

  $= -52.78 + 634.40$

  $= 581.62$

The actual 48-hour output for the first patient is 610 ml, from Table 12.4. Subtracting the estimated output from the actual output, we get the residual for the first patient:

$$e_1 = 610 - 581.62 = 28.38$$

Table 12.8 shows the estimated 48-hour output values and the residuals for all 20 patients.

It can be shown that the independence, normality, linearity, and constant variance assumptions required for regression hypothesis tests and confidence intervals can be stated in terms of the residuals. Specifically, we require independent residuals with a normal or approximately normal distribution and constant variance. By examining plots of the residuals, we can check some of these assumptions.

The normality assumption can be checked by obtaining a histogram of the residuals. Ideally, the residual histogram should be consistent with a normal or approximately normal population. A large sample size can compensate for skewness, however. Figure 12.16 shows a histogram of the chest-tube regression residuals in Table 12.8. Although the histogram suggests a skewed population, the sample size is large enough to compensate for the degree of skewness indicated.

A scatterplot of the residuals and the estimated values can be used to check the linearity and constant variance assumptions. In this plot, the residuals are plotted on the vertical axis and the estimated

TABLE 12.8   ESTIMATED 48-HOUR OUTPUT VALUES AND RESIDUALS

Patient No.	Estimated 48-Hour Output	Residual
1	$-52.78 + 1.22(520) = 581.62$	$610 - 581.62 = 28.38$
2	$-52.78 + 1.22(340) = 362.02$	$625 - 362.02 = 262.98$
3	$-52.78 + 1.22(530) = 593.82$	$640 - 593.82 = 46.18$
4	$-52.78 + 1.22(1393) = 1646.68$	$1543 - 1646.68 = -103.68$
5	$-52.78 + 1.22(1093) = 1280.68$	$1253 - 1280.68 = -27.68$
6	$-52.78 + 1.22(156) = 137.54$	$261 - 137.54 = 123.46$
7	$-52.78 + 1.22(2211) = 2644.64$	$3006 - 2644.64 = 361.36$
8	$-52.78 + 1.22(1654) = 1965.10$	$1864 - 1965.10 = -101.10$
9	$-52.78 + 1.22(555) = 624.32$	$555 - 624.32 = -69.32$
10	$-52.78 + 1.22(610) = 691.42$	$720 - 691.42 = 28.58$
11	$-52.78 + 1.22(995) = 1161.12$	$1225 - 1161.12 = 63.88$
12	$-52.78 + 1.22(1365) = 1612.52$	$1505 - 1612.52 = -107.52$
13	$-52.78 + 1.22(1220) = 1435.62$	$1300 - 1435.62 = -135.62$
14	$-52.78 + 1.22(1240) = 1460.02$	$1560 - 1460.02 = 99.98$
15	$-52.78 + 1.22(1075) = 1258.72$	$1280 - 1258.72 = 21.28$
16	$-52.78 + 1.22(1330) = 1569.82$	$1615 - 1569.82 = 45.18$
17	$-52.78 + 1.22(690) = 789.02$	$690 - 789.02 = -99.02$
18	$-52.78 + 1.22(1035) = 1209.92$	$1035 - 1209.92 = -174.92$
19	$-52.78 + 1.22(1280) = 1508.82$	$1425 - 1508.82 = -83.82$
20	$-52.78 + 1.22(1035) = 1209.92$	$1035 - 1209.92 = -174.92$

```
 -200.00 - -100.01 |XXXXX
 -100.00 - -0.01   |XXXX
    0.00 -  99.99  |XXXXXXX
  100.00 - 199.99  |X
  200.00 - 299.99  |X
  300.00 - 399.99  |X
```

Figure 12.16 Quick histogram of chest-tube regression residuals

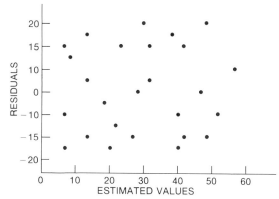

Figure 12.17 Hypothetical ideal scatterplot of residuals and estimated values

values on the horizontal axis. The ideal scatterplot shows a randomly scattered blob of points, such as the hypothetical plot in Figure 12.17. If the scatterplot shows points that form a curve, a linear relationship may not hold. When a straight line is used to describe a nonlinear relationship, the residual scatterplot often shows a curve. A hypothetical example of this sort of plot is shown in Figure 12.18.

If the residual scatterplot shows points in the shape of a horizontal funnel, the constant variance assumption may be violated. Figure 12.19 shows a hypothetical example of such a plot. In this plot, the residuals become more scattered as the estimated values increase. This suggests that residuals corresponding to large estimated values have a larger variance than residuals corresponding to small estimated values. If the residuals have constant variance, the amount of vertical scatter is usually about the same in all parts of the scatterplot.

An SPSS/PC scatterplot of the residuals and the estimated values from the chest-tube regression is shown in Figure 12.20. In this plot, the points appear to be randomly scattered with no curve or

funnel pattern.* The plot suggests that the constant variance and linearity assumptions are both reasonable for these data.

The circled point in Figure 12.20 is an *outlier*, a point far outside the range of the rest of the data. This plot illustrates yet another use for residuals: the detection of outliers. In some cases, outliers result from errors. Data values corresponding to residual outliers should always be checked. An out-

---

*The residuals in this plot have been *standardized*: each residual has been divided by the sample standard deviation of the residuals. The interpretation of the residual scatterplot is the same whether or not the residuals have been standardized.

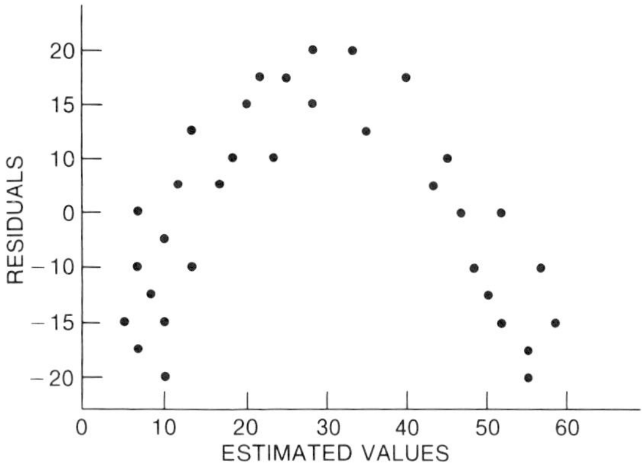

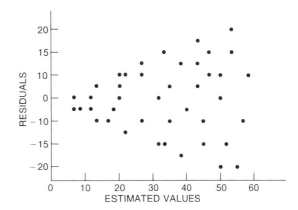

Figure 12.18 Hypothetical scatterplot of residuals and estimated values with curve pattern

Figure 12.19 Hypothetical scatterplot of residuals and estimated values with funnel pattern

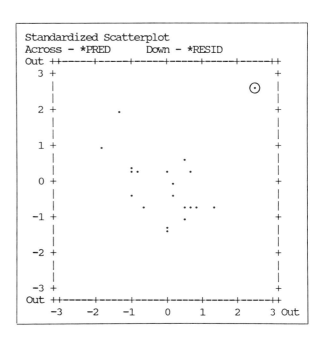

Figure 12.20 SPSS/PC scatterplot of chest-tube output regression residuals and estimated values

TABLE 12.9 PULMONARY ARTERY PRESSURE AND RELATIVE FLOW VELOCITY CHANGE FOR 30 PATIENTS

Patient No.	PAP (mm Hg)	ΔPV%
1	28	12
2	69	−27
3	41	−14
4	37	−10
5	34	−19
6	48	−25
7	42	−18
8	57	−21
9	81	−19
10	85	−25
11	63	−30
12	46	−21
13	38	−12
14	46	−21
15	47	−27
16	11	26
17	8	6
18	11	42
19	16	22
20	20	7
21	17	15
22	10	68
23	13	27
24	13	36
25	20	16
26	13	26
27	11	9
28	18	19
29	15	24
30	20	15

lier that is not the result of an error cannot be arbitrarily excluded from the regression analysis, even if it causes the regression line to fit the data poorly. If an outlier corresponds to a subject who should not have been included in the study (such as a hemophiliac in a study of cancer surgery), the subject can be excluded from the analysis. Whenever data are excluded, the researcher must report and justify the exclusions. Outliers sometimes indicate unusual responses that are of considerable clinical interest.

12.6 DATA TRANSFORMATION

Correlation coefficients or regression analyses are often desired when the data suggest nonlinear relationships, extremely skewed distributions, or nonconstant variance. These problems can sometimes be resolved by *transforming* one or both of the variables. Instead of analyzing a variable in milligrams, we might analyze it in square-root milligrams. Or we might analyze a variable in logarithm minutes instead of minutes. Although data transformations make us work with unfamiliar units of measurement, they often allow us to apply correlation or regression methods that otherwise would be inappropriate.

We will discuss the use of data transformations to deal with nonlinear relationships. The use of data transformations to correct violations of other regression assumptions is described in other texts.[1]

Let us consider data from a study of echocardiography for noninvasive evaluation of pulmonary hypertension.[10] Table 12.9 shows the average pulmonary artery pressure (PAP) and relative flow velocity change (ΔPV%) for 30 patients admitted for diagnostic cardiac catheterization. Figure 12.21 shows a scatterplot of the PAP and ΔPV% values, with the sample regression line drawn in. This regression line is given by the sample regression equation

$$\text{estimated PAP} = 34.55 + -0.72(\Delta PV\%)$$

The PAP and ΔPV% values seem to be related, but the regression line does not accurately describe

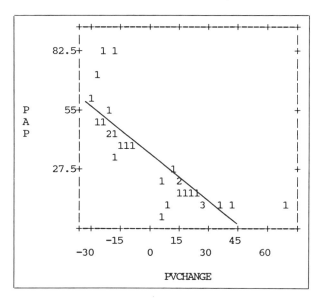

Figure 12.21 SPSS/PC scatterplot of PAP and ΔPV% with sample regression line

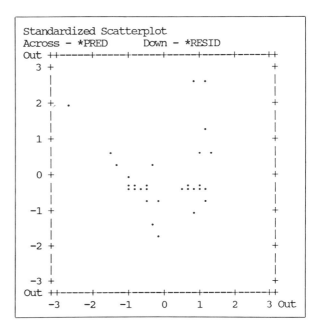

Figure 12.22 SPSS/PC scatterplot of PAP and ΔPV% regression residuals and estimated values

the relationship between these variables. In Figure 12.22, the SPSS/PC scatterplot of the residuals and the estimated values shows a curve, providing further evidence that the regression equation is not appropriate. To describe the nonlinear relationship

TABLE 12.10   LOG PULMONARY ARTERY PRESSURE

Patient No.	Log PAP (log mm Hg)
1	3.33
2	4.23
3	3.71
4	3.61
5	3.53
6	3.87
7	3.74
8	4.04
9	4.39
10	4.44
11	4.14
12	3.83
13	3.64
14	3.83
15	3.85
16	2.40
17	2.08
18	2.40
19	2.77
20	3.00
21	2.83
22	2.30
23	2.56
24	2.56
25	3.00
26	2.56
27	2.40
28	2.89
29	2.71
30	3.00

between PAP and ΔPV%, we need a curve instead of a straight line.

Suppose we transform PAP by taking logarithms to obtain log PAP values. Table 12.10 shows the log PAP values, and Figure 12.23 shows a scatterplot of the log PAP values and the ΔPV% values. The sample regression equation for log PAP and ΔPV% is

$$\text{estimated log PAP} = 3.32 + -0.02(\Delta PV\%)$$

The regression line given by this equation is shown in Figure 12.23. This line appears to accurately summarize the relationship between log PAP and ΔPV%. In Figure 12.24, the residual scatterplot for this regression equation shows fairly random scatter. An outlier is present, but no curve is evident. By transforming the data, we obtain new units of measurement (log mm Hg instead of mm Hg) and a linear relationship.

How would we know in advance that taking the logarithm of PAP would produce a linear relationship? A person familiar with mathematical functions can see that the curve in the scatterplot of the original data (Figure 12.21) resembles an exponential curve. If you are not familiar with mathematical functions, you will not be able to see this. If you want to learn how to recognize mathematical functions that describe commonly encountered curves, you should consult a more advanced text.[1] The logarithmic function, the square-root function, and the reciprocal function are some of the more frequently encountered functions in regression analysis. If you are not interested in mathematical functions, you will need to consult a statistician to analyze data with nonlinear relationships.

Data transformation often strikes students as cheating. Transforming a nonlinear relationship to

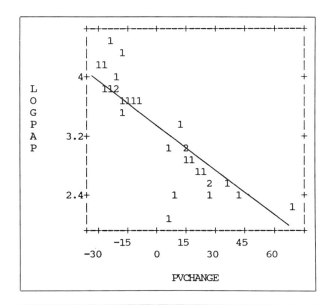

Figure 12.23 SPSS/PC scatterplot of log PAP and ΔPV% with sample regression line

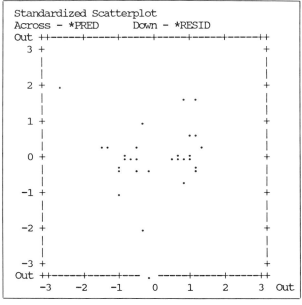

Figure 12.24 SPSS/PC scatterplot of log PAP and ΔPV% regression residuals and estimated values

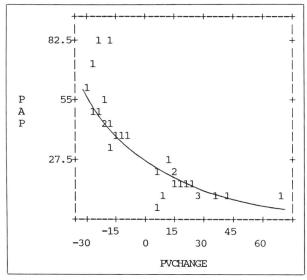

Figure 12.25 SPSS/PC scatterplot of PAP and ΔPV% with curve from log PAP and ΔPV% regression

get a linear relationship may seem like a sleazy statistical trick. But data transformation is an honest method of data analysis. We are simply changing the *units* in which the data are measured. Just as it is reasonable to measure weight in kilograms instead of pounds, it is reasonable to measure blood pressure in log mm Hg instead of mm Hg. The fact that a unit of measurement is unfamiliar does not make it illegitimate.

In addition, regression analyses based on transformed variables can be used to estimate curves that describe the relationships between the untransformed variables. It can be shown that the sample regression equation for the log PAP and ΔPV% regression can be used to obtain the curve shown in Figure 12.25. This scatterplot shows the untransformed PAP and ΔPV% values. By obtaining regression equations for transformed variables, we can obtain curves that describe nonlinear relationships between the untransformed variables.

12.7 MULTIPLE REGRESSION

More than one independent variable can be used to estimate or predict the values of a dependent variable. When two or more independent variables are used, the data are analyzed with *multiple regression* methods. Multiple regression allows us to obtain regression equations that relate two or more independent variables to a single dependent variable. If k independent variables $X_1, X_2, \ldots, X_k$ are used to estimate the dependent variable Y, the sample multiple regression equation has the form

$$\text{estimated } Y = b_0 + b_1 X_1 + b_2 X_2 + \cdots + b_k X_k \quad (12.18)$$

Estimated Y refers to the estimated values of Y given by the sample regression equation. The population multiple regression equation is

$$\text{estimated } Y = \beta_0 + \beta_1 X_1 + \beta_2 X_2 + \cdots + \beta_k X_k \quad (12.19)$$

In this formula, estimated Y refers to the estimated values of Y given by the population regression equation.

A regression equation with two or more independent variables does not describe a line, and the regression coefficients β_0 and β_1 are not the intercept and slope of a line. The interpretation of multiple regression coefficients is more complicated than the interpretation of bivariate regression coefficients. Further information about multiple regression coefficients can be found in other texts.[1]

When sample multiple regression equations are obtained, hypotheses about the population regression coefficients β_i are usually tested. Confidence intervals for population regression coefficients can also be calculated. A computer is required to obtain multiple regression coefficients, and most computer regression output includes the information needed to obtain hypothesis tests and confidence intervals.

We will not describe multiple regression confidence intervals and hypothesis tests. A complete discussion of multiple regression would require an entire book. The interested reader should consult a more advanced text.[1]

12.8 COMPUTER OUTPUT FOR CORRELATION AND BIVARIATE REGRESSION

In SPSS, Pearson correlation coefficients are obtained with the CORRELATION and PLOT programs. The PLOT program is also used to obtain scatterplots. Bivariate regression results are calculated with the SPSS REGRESSION and PLOT programs. In SAS, the REG procedure is used to obtain regression results. The usual warnings about the computer's inability to check assumptions still apply.

Figure 12.26 shows SPSS/PC correlation output for the anxiety data. Three-fourths of this output consists of useless or redundant information. The value 1.0000 is the sample Pearson correlation coefficient for HAS and itself and the sample Pearson correlation coefficient for PRAS and itself. Any variable is always perfectly correlated with itself, producing a Pearson correlation coefficient of 1. The sample Pearson correlation coefficient for HAS and PRAS (0.9214) is given twice. The value in parentheses under this coefficient is the sample size. Under the sample size, the p-value for the two-sided t test of the hypothesis that the population Pearson correlation coefficient is 0 appears after "P=."

SPSS/PC regression output for the chest-tube output data is shown in Figure 12.27. The sample regression coefficients are given in the column labeled "B." The sample regression slope is given in this column and in the row beginning with "HOUR24." The sample regression intercept appears under the slope in the row beginning with "(Constant)." Estimated standard errors of the sample regression coefficients are given in the "SE B" column. The column labeled "Beta" contains the standardized sample regression slope, which we will not discuss. The "T" column contains t statistics for

```
Correlations:  HAS          PRAS

     HAS       1.0000       .9214
               (   14)      (   14)
               P= .         P= .000


     PRAS      .9214        1.0000
               (   14)      (   14)
               P= .000      P= .
```

Figure 12.26 SPSS/PC correlation output for anxiety data

```
------------------- Variables in the Equation -------------------

Variable              B          SE B       Beta          T   Sig T

HOUR24           1.22018       .06733      .97367     18.122   .0000
(Constant)     -52.77564     75.56590                   -.698   .4938
```

Figure 12.27 SPSS/PC regression output for chest-tube output data

```
Correlation  .97367 R Squared  .94804  S.E. of Est  143.33856 Sig.  .0000
Intercept(S.E.)  -52.77564( 75.56590)  Slope(S.E.)      1.22018(  .06733)
```

Figure 12.28 SPSS/PC PLOT correlation and regression output for chest-tube output data

		PARAMETER	STANDARD	T FOR H0:	
VARIABLE	DF	ESTIMATE	ERROR	PARAMETER=0	PROB > |T|
INTERCEP	1	-52.775643	75.565896	-0.698	0.4938
HOUR24	1	1.220176	0.067331	18.122	0.0001

Figure 12.29 SAS regression output for chest-tube output data

testing hypotheses about population regression coefficients. The first t statistic, 18.122, is the t statistic for testing the hypothesis that the population regression slope is equal to 0. This t statistic differs from our calculated t statistic on p. 280 because of rounding error. The second t statistic, -0.698, is the t statistic for testing the hypothesis that the population regression intercept is equal to 0. P-values for these t statistics are given in the "Sig T" column. The first p-value listed is 0.0000, which means that the p-value is less than or equal to 0.00005. It does not mean that the p-value is 0.

In Figure 12.28, SPSS/PC PLOT correlation and regression output for the chest-tube data is shown. The sample Pearson correlation coefficient is listed after "Correlation" and the squared sample Pearson correlation coefficient is given after "R Squared." The p-value for testing the hypothesis that the population Pearson correlation coefficient is 0 appears after "Sig." The output after "S.E. of Est" is of no use to us and will not be discussed here. The sample regression intercept is given after "Intercept(S.E.)," followed by its estimated standard error in parentheses. The sample regression slope and its estimated standard error appear after "Slope(S.E.)."

Figure 12.29 shows SAS regression output for the chest-tube output data. The column labeled "DF" is of no use to us. The sample regression intercept is given in the "PARAMETER ESTIMATE" column

and in the row beginning with "INTERCEP." The sample regression slope is listed in this column and in the row beginning with "HOUR24." The estimated standard errors of these coefficients appear in the "STANDARD ERROR" column. The t statistics for testing the hypothesis that the population regression intercept is equal to 0 and the hypothesis that the population regression slope is equal to 0 are given in the column labeled "T FOR H0: PARAMETER = 0." The p-values for these tests are listed in the column labeled "PROB > |T|."

12.9 CORRELATION AND REGRESSION PITFALLS

Correlation and regression analyses are frequently misused in the medical and health care literature. Some of the more common sources of trouble are worth discussing here.

1. Nominal Data. Correlation and regression should not be done if either variable produces nominal data. As you may recall from Chapter 2, nominal data consist of arbitrary numerical labels for categories. The variable "type of surgery" (with the values 1 = orthopedic, 2 = cardiac, 3 = gastrointestinal, and 4 = gynecologic) produces nominal data. The numbers used to represent type of surgery are completely arbitrary. Because nominal data have no real numerical meaning, correlation and regression

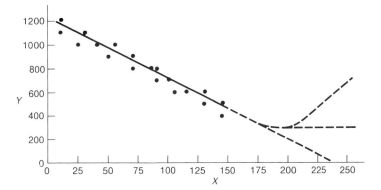

Figure 12.30 Hypothetical scatterplot

coefficients do not make sense for nominal data. If association between two variables that produce nominal data is of interest, the chi-square test of association (Chapter 10) should be considered.*

2. Association Versus Linear Association. Correlation and regression methods are used to measure the degree of *linear* association between variables. If the hypothesis of no correlation is not rejected, we cannot conclude that there is no association between the variables. If the hypothesis of no correlation is rejected, we cannot conclude that the association is linear. Nonlinear association can be ruled out only if the population Pearson correlation coefficient is equal to 1 or −1. When correlation or regression coefficients are calculated, scatterplots should always be obtained to evaluate linearity.

3. Correlation and Causality. If two variables are correlated, we cannot assume that the variables are causally related. Conversely, a lack of correlation does not indicate that variables are not causally related. Even a correlation coefficient of 1 or −1 does not imply a causal relationship, and a correlation coefficient of 0 does not rule out a causal relationship. In the same way, the presence or absence of a regression relationship has nothing to do with causality.

4. Correlation and Independence. The assumption that uncorrelated variables are independent is a common error. We cannot determine whether variables are independent by testing the hypothesis that the population Pearson correlation coefficient is 0. If two variables are correlated, they are not independent. But if two variables are not correlated, they may or may not be independent. Two

variables can be completely nonindependent and still have a population correlation coefficient of 0.

5. Statistical Significance Versus Clinical Significance. When statistically significant correlation or regression coefficients are obtained, it does not follow that the results are clinically significant. When we reject the hypothesis that the population Pearson correlation coefficient is 0, we cannot conclude that the independent variable can be used to obtain clinically useful predictions of the values of the dependent variable. Very small *p*-values are often obtained for correlation coefficients and regression equations with no practical value whatsoever.

6. Extrapolation. When a regression equation is used for prediction, predictions should be based on values of the independent variable that are within or close to the range of values for which data were obtained. Attempting predictions based on values far outside the range of the data is called *extrapolation*. Serious mistakes often result when extrapolation is done, since the regression relationship that holds for a particular range of data may not hold outside this range.

Consider the hypothetical scatterplot in Figure 12.30. A linear relationship seems to hold within the range of the data, but we have no information about what happens outside this range. Several possibilities are illustrated in the plot. The line describing the relationship might continue unchanged, or it might flatten out, or it might curve back up. Since we have no information about what happens outside the range of the data, we cannot rule out any of these possibilities.

---

*Special regression methods can be used to analyze nominal data produced by *indicator variables*, variables that take only the values 0 and 1. *Dummy variable regression* is used when any of the independent variables are indicator (dummy) variables. *Logistic regression* is used when the dependent variable is an indicator variable. A discussion of these methods can be found in other texts.[1]

SUMMARY

Correlation and bivariate regression analyses are used to evaluate linear association between two variables when at least one of the variables has a normal or approximately normal distribution. The Pearson correlation coefficient measures the degree of linear association. A positive population Pearson correlation coefficient indicates that increasing values of one variable are linearly related to increasing values of the other variable. A negative population Pearson correlation coefficient indicates that increasing values of one variable are linearly related to decreasing values of the other variable. A t test is used to test the hypothesis that the population Pearson correlation coefficient is 0. Two variables can be associated in a nonlinear way even when the population Pearson correlation coefficient is 0.

In bivariate regression, the values of an independent variable are used to estimate or predict the values of a dependent variable. A straight line that fits the data as well as possible is obtained. The sample regression intercept and slope for this line are used to estimate the regression intercept and slope for the population regression line. Confidence intervals and hypothesis tests based on t distributions can be obtained for the regression intercept and slope, although inferences about the population regression intercept usually are not made. The most commonly tested hypothesis about the population regression slope is the hypothesis that the slope is equal to 0. If the equivalence of two measurements is studied, the hypothesis that the population regression slope is equal to 1 is also tested. Data must sometimes be transformed before using bivariate regression in order to correct violations of the normality, constant variance, or linearity assumptions. These assumptions can be evaluated by examining scatterplots of the data and residual plots.

Common regression pitfalls include the use of variables that produce nominal data, the belief that linear association is equivalent to association, the misuse of correlation coefficients to evaluate causality or independence, the confusion of statistical significance with clinical significance, and extrapolation.

FORMULAS FOR CONFIDENCE INTERVALS FOR POPULATION REGRESSION COEFFICIENTS

Population Regression Coefficient	$100(1 - \alpha)\%$ Confidence Interval
β_1	$(b_1 - (t_{\alpha/2, n-2})(\text{se}(b_1)), \quad b_1 + (t_{\alpha/2, n-2})(\text{se}(b_1)))$
β_0	$(b_0 - (t_{\alpha/2, n-2})(\text{se}(b_0)), \quad b_0 + (t_{\alpha/2, n-2})(\text{se}(b_0)))$

FORMULAS FOR CORRELATION AND REGRESSION TEST STATISTICS

Null Hypothesis	Test Statistic	Distribution of Test Statistic
H_0: Population Pearson correlation coefficient $= 0$	$t = \dfrac{r \times \sqrt{n-2}}{\sqrt{1 - r^2}}$	t distribution with $n - 2$ df
H_0: $\beta_1 = \beta_{10}$	$t = \dfrac{b_1 - \beta_{10}}{\text{se}(b_1)}$	t distribution with $n - 2$ df
H_0: $\beta_0 = \beta_{00}$	$t = \dfrac{b_0 - \beta_{00}}{\text{se}(b_0)}$	t distribution with $n - 2$ df

PROBLEMS

The following instructions apply to problems 1 through 19.

1. In each problem, data are presented and a question is asked about the data. Computer output that may or may not be helpful is provided. Determine whether the tests and confidence intervals suggested in the problems are appropriate. If they are not appropriate, state which assumptions are violated.

2. If the suggested tests and confidence intervals are appropriate, carry out the tests and calculate the confidence intervals. Specify the null and alternative hypotheses and find the most exact p-value that can be obtained from the tables in this text. Interpret the p-value and use the test results and confidence intervals to answer the question in the problem.

1. A study investigated the effect of prognostic expectations of myocardial infarction (MI) patients on their health status after discharge.[11] Table 12.11 shows the McMaster Health Status Index scores for 19 MI patients two days before discharge and eight

TABLE 12.11 MCMASTER HEALTH STATUS INDEX SCORE FOR MI PATIENTS BEFORE AND AFTER DISCHARGE

Patient No.	Before Discharge	8 Weeks Post-MI
1	24	22
2	29	30
3	22	32
4	26	27
5	21	23
6	26	21
7	25	28
8	23	29
9	25	23
10	23	25
11	23	22
12	25	28
13	28	27
14	22	24
15	28	26
16	30	26
17	28	24
18	34	31
19	23	22

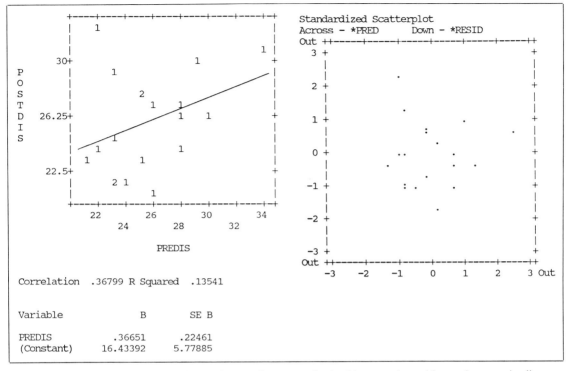

```
              +----+----+----+----+----+----+----+                    Standardized Scatterplot
          |    1                                   |                   Across - *PRED      Down - *RESID
          |                                        |                   Out ++----+----+----+----+----+----++
          |                                   1 |              3 +                                      +
       30+             1                       +                  |
  P       |        1                           |              2 +              .                         +
  O       |                                    |                  |
  S       |             2                       |              1 +                   .                    +
  T       |           1   1                     |                  |                     :           .    +
  D    26.25+            1   1                  +              1 +                  :               .    +
  I       |                                    |                  |                      .                +
  S       |      1                              |              0 +            . .           .             +
          |    1            1                   |                  |         .                             +
          |  1          1                       |             -1 +            : .        .                +
     22.5+                                       +                  |
          |       2 1                            |             -2 +                    .                   +
          |            1                         |                  |
          +----+----+----+----+----+----+----+              -3 +                                          +
              22        26        30        34               Out ++----+----+----+----+----+----++
                 24        28        32                              -3   -2   -1    0    1    2    3 Out
                          PREDIS

  Correlation  .36799  R Squared  .13541

  Variable              B          SE B

  PREDIS             .36651      .22461
  (Constant)       16.43392     5.77885
```

Figure 12.31 SPSS/PC correlation and regression output for health status data with sample regression line

weeks post-MI. Do the data provide evidence that the eight-week post-MI McMaster score is linearly related to the before-discharge McMaster score?

a. Test the hypothesis that the population regression slope is equal to 0, using a 0.05 significance level.
b. Obtain a 95% confidence interval for the population regression slope.
c. Test the hypothesis that the population regression intercept is equal to 0, using a 0.05 significance level.
d. Obtain a 95% confidence interval for the population regression intercept.

2. A study compared coagulation studies obtained for arterial and venous blood specimens.[12] Table 12.12 shows the activated partial thromboplastin time (APTT) for arterial and venous blood specimens from 50 patients. Do the data provide

```
    -6.00 - -4.01 | X
    -4.00 - -2.01 | XXXXX
    -2.00 - -0.01 | XXXX
     0.00 - 1.99 | XXX
     2.00 - 3.99 | XXXX
     4.00 - 5.99 | X
     6.00 - 7.99 | X
```

Figure 12.32 Quick histogram of health status regression residuals

evidence that the arterial APTT and the venous APTT are not equivalent?

a. Test the hypothesis that the population regression slope is equal to 0, using a 0.01 significance level.
b. Test the hypothesis that the population regression slope is equal to 1, using a 0.01 significance level.
c. Test the hypothesis that the population regression intercept is equal to 0, using a 0.05 significance level.
d. Obtain a 95% confidence interval for the population regression intercept.

3. In a study of ethambutol kinetics in patients with decreased renal function, the serum creatinine and creatinine clearance were reported for 13 patients with impaired renal function.[13] These data are shown in Table 12.13. Do the data provide evidence that creatinine clearance is linearly related to serum creatinine?

a. Test the hypothesis that the population regression slope is equal to 0, using a 0.01 significance level.
b. Obtain a 99% confidence interval for the population regression slope.
c. Test the hypothesis that the population regression intercept is equal to 50, using a 0.01 significance level.
d. Obtain a 99% confidence interval for the population regression intercept.

TABLE 12.12 APTT FOR ARTERIAL AND VENOUS BLOOD SPECIMENS

Patient No.	Arterial Specimen	Venous Specimen	Patient No.	Arterial Specimen	Venous Specimen
1	38.6	38.5	26	32.1	30.4
2	26.2	26.9	27	19.3	19.3
3	38.2	36.5	28	22.5	22.8
4	22.5	21.7	29	19.3	20.0
5	32.7	32.1	30	19.6	19.3
6	22.0	24.2	31	16.4	16.0
7	30.5	30.9	32	33.4	31.3
8	28.4	28.2	33	24.9	27.2
9	24.8	25.4	34	77.7	78.4
10	22.8	22.9	35	90.0	80.2
11	27.8	24.5	36	21.3	21.6
12	27.5	26.7	37	42.3	40.5
13	24.8	24.5	38	30.9	30.3
14	33.4	30.9	39	24.7	24.9
15	47.3	44.3	40	21.4	21.0
16	27.7	29.3	41	23.6	23.5
17	21.5	21.7	42	24.2	22.8
18	25.5	26.8	43	21.1	21.1
19	50.1	70.5	44	35.0	34.3
20	26.4	26.0	45	24.1	23.4
21	23.5	23.5	46	25.6	24.8
22	28.0	28.2	47	42.2	44.4
23	20.8	20.3	48	23.2	23.3
24	31.0	30.4	49	24.8	24.2
25	25.1	24.2	50	23.6	23.6

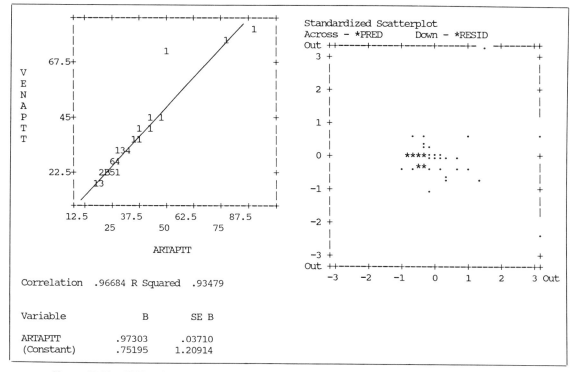

Figure 12.33 SPSS/PC correlation and regression output for APTT data with sample regression line

```
 - 10.00 - - 7.51 | X
  - 7.50 - - 5.01 |
  - 5.00 - - 2.51 | X
  - 2.50 - - 0.01 | XXXXXXXXXXXXXXXXXXXXXXXXXXXXXXX
    0.00 - 2.49 | XXXXXXXXXXXXXX
    5.00 - 7.49 | X
    7.50 - 9.99 |
   10.00 - 12.49 |
   12.50 - 14.99 |
   15.00 - 17.49 |
   17.50 - 19.99 |
   20.00 - 22.49 | X
```

Figure 12.34 Quick histogram of APTT regression residuals

TABLE 12.13   SERUM CREATININE AND CREATININE CLEARANCE FOR PATIENTS WITH IMPAIRED RENAL FUNCTION

Patient No.	Serum Creatinine (mg / dl)	Creatinine Clearance (ml / min)
1	2.8	27
2	3.9	36
3	1.6	81
4	9.3	12
5	1.4	54
6	5.6	23
7	1.8	54
8	4.2	13
9	2.4	29
10	5.0	26
11	10.6	13
12	1.9	40
13	6.1	5

4. A study evaluated several methods for measuring cardiac output.[14] Table 12.14 shows the thermodilution cardiac output (CO) determined with room-temperature (RT) injectate and with iced-temperature (IT) injectate for 29 patients who underwent cardiac catheterization. Do the data provide evidence that the IT method and the RT method are not equivalent?

   a. Test the hypothesis that the population regression slope is equal to 0, using a 0.05 significance level.
   b. Test the hypothesis that the population regression slope is equal to 1, using a 0.05 significance level.
   c. Test the hypothesis that the population regression intercept is equal to 0, using a 0.05 significance level.
   d. Obtain a 95% confidence interval for the population regression intercept.

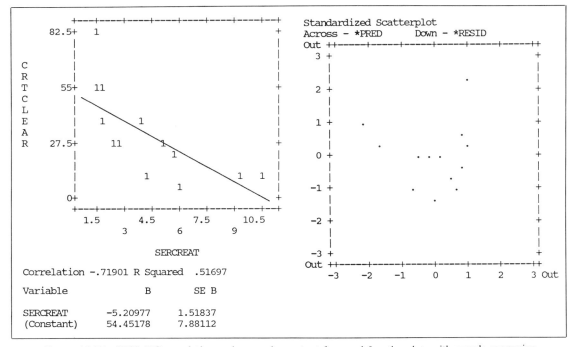

Figure 12.35 SPSS/PC correlation and regression output for renal function data with sample regression line

```
 -20.00 - -10.01 |XXXX
 -10.00 - -0.01 |XXX
   0.00 - 9.99 |XXXX
  10.00 - 19.99 |X
  20.00 - 29.99 |
  30.00 - 39.99 |X
```

Figure 12.36 Quick histogram of renal function regression residuals

TABLE 12.14 ROOM-TEMPERATURE AND ICED-TEMPERATURE THERMODILUTION CARDIAC OUTPUT

Patient No.	RT CO	IT CO
1	2.60	3.02
2	5.16	5.47
3	6.18	5.72
4	3.22	4.22
5	4.99	4.89
6	3.62	3.50
7	3.31	3.08
8	4.11	4.11
9	5.24	4.86
10	4.27	4.73
11	3.42	3.78
12	4.70	4.26
13	5.42	4.97
14	5.36	5.47
15	2.63	2.62
16	3.70	3.87
17	5.39	5.30
18	5.44	4.79
19	3.86	3.75
20	6.68	6.38
21	5.35	5.30
22	3.26	3.86
23	4.06	4.28
24	2.64	2.88
25	5.40	5.63
26	5.93	6.08
27	5.90	6.15
28	4.11	4.51
29	4.44	3.26

5. A study investigated the hemodynamic effects of hydralazine in infants with idiopathic dilated cardiomyopathy.[15] Table 12.15 shows the cardiac index (CI) and systemic arteriolar resistance (Rs) after hydralazine administration for 12 infants with dilated cardiomyopathy. Do the data provide evidence that the cardiac index after hydralazine is linearly related to the systemic arteriolar resistance after hydralazine?

    a. Test the hypothesis that the population Pearson correlation coefficient is equal to 0, using a 0.10 significance level.

    b. Obtain a 90% confidence interval for the population regression slope.

    c. Test the hypothesis that the population regression intercept is equal to 0, using a 0.10 significance level.

    d. Obtain a 90% confidence interval for the population regression intercept.

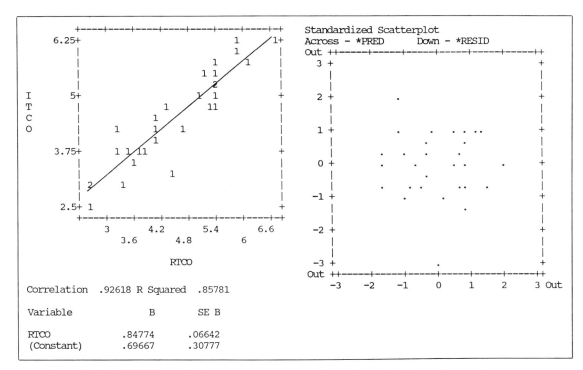

Figure 12.37 SPSS/PC correlation and regression output for cardiac output data with sample regression line

```
−1.20 − −0.91 | X
−0.90 − −0.61 |
−0.60 − −0.31 | XXXXX
−0.30 − −0.01 | XXXXXXX
 0.00 − −0.29 | XXXXXXXX
 0.30 − 0.59 | XXXXXX
 0.60 − 0.89 | X
```

Figure 12.38 Quick histogram of cardiac output regression residuals

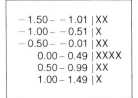

```
−1.50 − −1.01 | XX
−1.00 − −0.51 | X
−0.50 − −0.01 | XX
 0.00 − 0.49 | XXXX
 0.50 − 0.99 | XX
 1.00 − 1.49 | X
```

Figure 12.40 Quick histogram of hemodynamic regression residuals

TABLE 12.15 CI AND Rs VALUES AFTER HYDRALAZINE FOR INFANTS WITH DILATED CARDIOMYOPATHY

Patient No.	CI (L/min/m^2)	Rs (U/m^2)
1	4.93	9.5
2	5.88	10.2
3	4.54	13.9
4	5.66	12.9
5	5.34	10.9
6	5.40	9.8
7	4.37	16.9
8	3.28	15.5
9	3.20	14.1
10	6.30	7.6
11	3.90	10.3
12	4.62	12.3

6. In a study of mycoplasmal pneumonia, the IgM rheumatoid factor (IgM-RF) concentrations in Table 12.16 were reported for 20 patients with mycoplasmal pneumonia.[16] Do the data provide evidence that the peak IgM-RF concentration is linearly related to the acute-phase IgM-RF concentration?

a. Test the hypothesis that the population regression slope is equal to 0, using a 0.001 significance level.

b. Obtain a 99.9% confidence interval for the population regression slope.

c. Test the hypothesis that the population regression intercept is equal to 0, using a 0.001 significance level.

d. Obtain a 99.9% confidence interval for the population regression intercept.

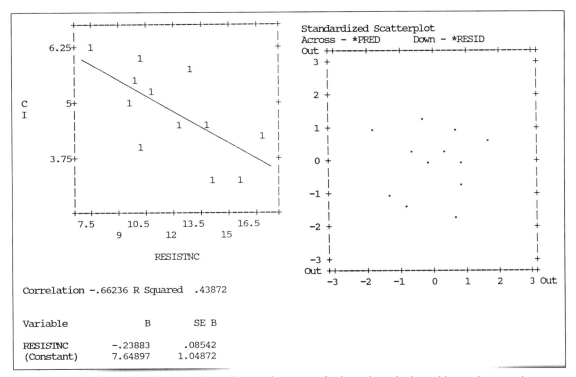

Figure 12.39 SPSS/PC correlation and regression output for hemodynamic data with sample regression line

TABLE 12.16 IgM-RF CONCENTRATION (EXPRESSED IN E_{405} IN ELISA)

Patient No.	In Acute Phase	Peak
1	0.548	0.708
2	0.420	0.431
3	0.550	0.762
4	0.370	0.487
5	0.596	0.664
6	0.660	0.693
7	0.361	0.451
8	0.520	0.750
9	0.383	0.404
10	0.353	0.592
11	0.374	0.824
12	0.311	0.546
13	0.162	0.485
14	0.252	0.340
15	0.226	0.352
16	0.135	0.237
17	0.163	0.218
18	0.139	0.166
19	0.156	0.164
20	0.161	0.160

```
 - 0.200 - - 0.101 | XXXXX
 - 0.100 - - 0.001 | XXXXXXX
   0.000 - 0.099 | XXXX
   0.100 - 0.199 | XX
   0.200 - 0.299 | X
   0.300 - 0.399 | X
```

Figure 12.42 Quick histogram of IgM-RF regression residuals

TABLE 12.17 CARDIAC OUTPUT (l/min) WHILE LYING FLAT AND IN 20-DEGREE BACK-REST POSITION

Patient No.	Flat	20 Degrees
1	6.43	7.04
2	8.73	8.68
3	1.90	1.96
4	6.87	6.15
5	6.15	5.74
6	7.16	6.71
7	4.35	3.94
8	6.01	6.25
9	8.15	7.02
10	8.30	7.87
11	9.36	9.31
12	4.74	4.50
13	5.94	5.08
14	8.80	9.19
15	3.40	3.10

7. A study evaluated the effect of the back-rest position on measurements of cardiac output obtained by the thermodilution method.[17] Table 12.17 shows the cardiac output for 15 acutely ill patients while lying flat and in a 20-degree back-rest position. Do the data provide evidence that flat cardiac

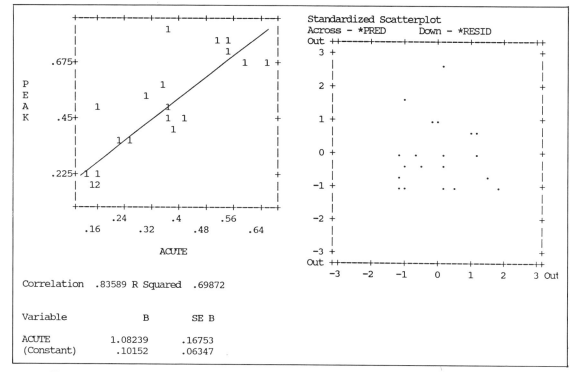

Correlation .83589 R Squared .69872

Variable	B	SE B
ACUTE	1.08239	.16753
(Constant)	.10152	.06347

Figure 12.41 SPSS/PC correlation and regression output for IgM-RF data with sample regression line

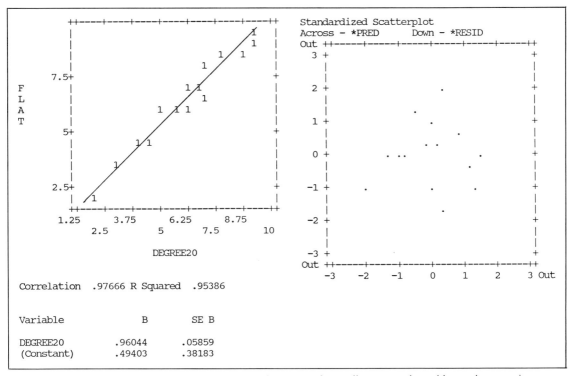

Figure 12.43 SPSS/PC correlation and regression output for cardiac output data with sample regression line

```
-1.00 - -0.61 | X
-0.60 - -0.21 | XXX
-0.20 - 0.19 | XXXXXX
 0.20 - 0.59 | XXXX
 0.60 - 0.99 | X
```

Figure 12.44 Quick histogram of cardiac output regression residuals

output and 20-degree cardiac output are not equivalent?

    a. Test the hypothesis that the population regression slope is equal to 0, using a 0.01 significance level.

    b. Test the hypothesis that the population regression slope is equal to 1, using a 0.01 significance level.

    c. Test the hypothesis that the population regression intercept is equal to 0, using a 0.05 significance level.

    d. Obtain a 95% confidence interval for the population regression intercept.

    8. A study of oak toxicosis in cattle reported the creatinine and BUN values for 16 calves with oak toxicosis.[10] These data are shown in Table 12.18. Do the data provide evidence that creatinine is linearly related to BUN?

TABLE 12.18 CREATININE AND BUN FOR CALVES WITH OAK TOXICOSIS

Calf No.	Creatinine (mg/dl)	BUN (mg/dl)
1	16.4	100
2	22.0	133
3	16.3	141
4	3.4	75
5	10.9	156
6	6.4	71
7	3.7	29
8	12.2	104
9	15.0	132
10	5.8	54
11	16.5	164
12	7.2	67
13	17.3	232
14	1.8	25
15	0.9	23
16	3.0	33

    a. Test the hypothesis that the population regression slope is equal to 0, using a 0.05 significance level.

    b. Obtain a 95% confidence interval for the population regression slope.

    c. Test the hypothesis that the population regression intercept is equal to 0.5, using a 0.05 significance level.

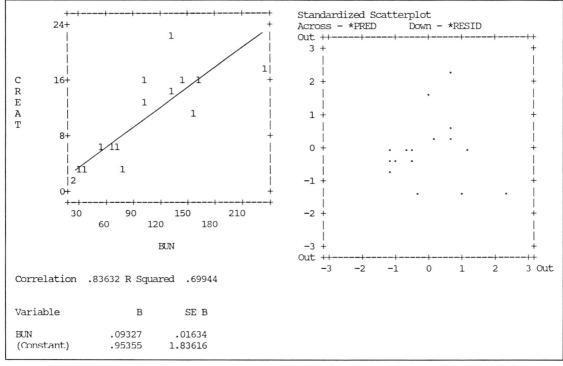

Correlation .83632 R Squared .69944

Variable	B	SE B
BUN	.09327	.01634
(Constant.)	.95355	1.83616

Figure 12.45 SPSS/PC correlation and regression output for renal function data with sample regression line

```
− 6.00 − − 3.01 | XXX
− 3.00 − − 0.01 | XXXXXX
  0.00 −  2.99 | XXXXX
  3.00 −  5.99 |
  6.00 −  8.99 | XX
```

Figure 12.46 Quick histogram of renal function regression residuals

d. Obtain a 95% confidence interval for the population regression intercept.

9. A study evaluated two-dimensional echocardiography (2D ECHO) for the assessment of left ventricular diastolic filling.[19] Table 12.19 shows the half-filling fraction (1/2FF) obtained by 2D ECHO and angiography for 27 patients who underwent diagnostic cardiac catheterization. Do the data provide evidence that the angiography 1/2FF and the 2D ECHO 1/2FF are not equivalent?

a. Test the hypothesis that the population regression slope is equal to 0, using a 0.01 significance level.
b. Test the hypothesis that the population regression slope is equal to 1, using a 0.01 significance level.
c. Test the hypothesis that the population regression intercept is equal to 0, using a 0.01 significance level.

TABLE 12.19   2D ECHO 1/2FF AND ANGIOGRAPHY 1/2FF

Patient No.	2D ECHO 1/2FF	Angiography 1/2FF
1	0.61	0.55
2	0.67	0.75
3	0.50	0.55
4	0.36	0.26
5	0.54	0.43
6	0.73	0.74
7	0.69	0.73
8	0.75	0.71
9	0.38	0.44
10	0.61	0.63
11	0.57	0.43
12	0.58	0.52
13	0.52	0.73
14	0.69	0.74
15	0.44	0.51
16	0.54	0.58
17	0.59	0.68
18	0.78	0.73
19	0.42	0.40
20	0.45	0.38
21	0.90	0.70
22	0.36	0.35
23	0.57	0.52
24	0.70	0.74
25	0.64	0.67
26	0.85	0.77
27	0.35	0.39

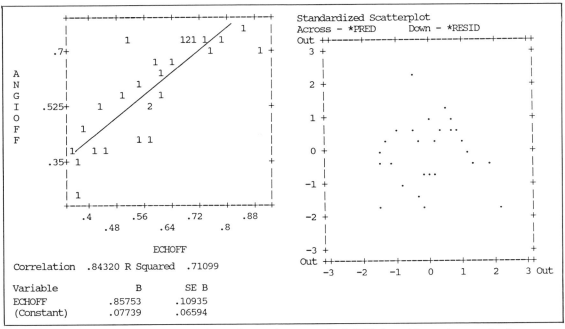

Figure 12.47 SPSS/PC correlation and regression output for 1/2 FF data with sample regression line

```
-0.15 - -0.11 |XXXX
-0.10 - -0.06 |X
-0.05 - -0.01 |XXXXXXXX
 0.00 - 0.04 |XXXXXXX
 0.05 - 0.09 |XXXX
 0.10 - 0.14 |XX
 0.15 - 0.19 |
 0.20 - 0.24 |X
```

Figure 12.48 Quick histogram of 1/2FF regression residuals

d. Obtain a 99% confidence interval for the population regression intercept.

10. In a study of pulmonary embolism diagnosis, age and the FEV_1/FVC ratio were reported for patients suspected of having pulmonary embolism.[20] Table 12.20 shows these data for 69 patients found not to have pulmonary embolism or believed to have a low probability of pulmonary embolism. Do the data provide evidence that the FEV_1/FVC ratio is linearly related to age?

a. Test the hypothesis that the population regression slope is equal to 0, using a 0.05 significance level.

b. Obtain a 95% confidence interval for the population regression slope.

c. Test the hypothesis that the population regression intercept is equal to 80, using a 0.05 significance level.

d. Obtain a 95% confidence interval for the population regression intercept.

11. In a study of hemorrhagic cerebral infarction, neurological symptom scores before and after

TABLE 12.20   AGE AND FEV₁/FVC

Patient No.	Age	$\dfrac{FEV_1}{FVC}$ (%)	Patient No.	Age	$\dfrac{FEV_1}{FVC}$ (%)
1	26	78	36	42	66
2	32	89	37	54	68
3	25	87	38	60	76
4	45	69	39	46	81
5	53	73	40	60	81
6	21	74	41	54	62
7	40	81	42	58	58
8	65	66	43	42	100
9	38	72	44	43	70
10	57	64	45	47	76
11	60	85	46	58	78
12	43	84	47	47	71
13	30	66	48	52	82
14	47	78	49	82	82
15	60	72	50	61	78
16	65	81	51	63	74
17	48	73	52	42	54
18	67	57	53	56	88
19	44	65	54	61	72
20	47	53	55	45	47
21	39	80	56	41	83
22	70	52	57	39	80
23	40	28	58	81	69
24	27	74	59	47	73
25	52	67	60	60	82
26	67	71	61	47	76
27	63	63	62	51	83
28	20	87	63	58	71
29	62	59	64	56	77
30	71	60	65	62	80
31	62	74	66	17	100
32	73	63	67	56	71
33	63	67	68	34	76
34	75	65	69	26	81
35	63	69			

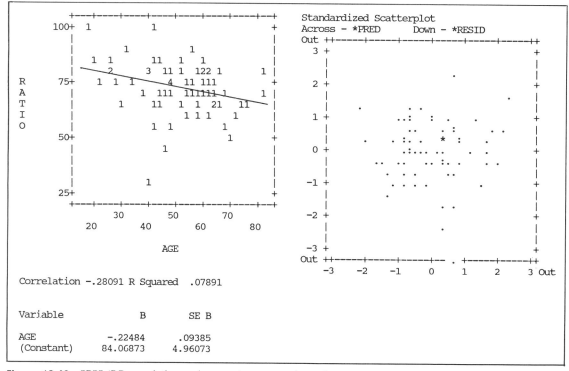

Figure 12.49 SPSS/PC correlation and regression output for pulmonary embolism data with sample regression line

```
−50.00 − −45.01 |X
−45.00 − −40.01 |
−40.00 − −35.01 |
−35.00 − −30.01 |
−30.00 − −25.01 |X
−25.00 − −20.01 |XX
−20.00 − −15.01 |X
−15.00 − −10.01 |XXXX
−10.00 − −5.01 |XXXXXXXX
 −5.00 − −0.01 |XXXXXXXXXXXXXXXXX
  0.00 − 4.99 |XXXXXXXXXXXX
  5.00 − 9.99 |XXXXXXXXXXX
 10.00 − 14.99 |XXXXXX
 15.00 − 19.99 |XXX
 20.00 − 24.99 |
 25.00 − 29.99 |X
```

Figure 12.50 Quick histogram of pulmonary embolism regression residuals

hemorrhage were reported for 28 patients with ischemic cerebral infarction.[21] These scores measure the severity of neurological symptoms and can range from 1 to 29. The higher the score, the greater the neurological deficit. Table 12.21 shows the reported scores. Do the data provide evidence that the post-hemorrhage score is linearly related to the prehemorrhage score?

TABLE 12.21 NEUROLOGICAL SYMPTOM SCORE BEFORE AND AFTER HEMORRHAGE

Patient No.	Before Hemorrhage	After Hemorrhage
1	20	18
2	18	21
3	14	21
4	15	13
5	10	9
6	14	11
7	18	21
8	19	18
9	9	6
10	21	18
11	20	17
12	13	12
13	7	4
14	7	5
15	16	16
16	19	19
17	16	15
18	17	16
19	18	17
20	9	9
21	8	8
22	6	5
23	12	12
24	8	8
25	12	2
26	15	14
27	15	14
28	14	13

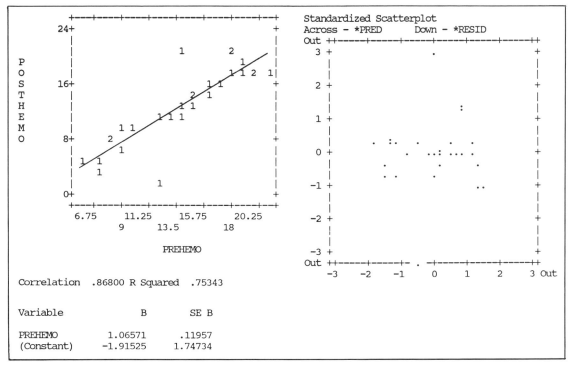

Figure 12.51 SPSS/PC correlation and regression output for cerebral infarction data with sample regression line

```
− 9.00 − − 6.01 | X
− 6.00 − − 3.01 |
− 3.00 − − 0.01 | XXXXXXXXXXXXXX
  0.00 − 2.99 | XXXXXXXXX
  3.00 − 5.99 | XX
  6.00 − 8.99 | X
```

Figure 12.52 Quick histogram of cerebral infarction regression residuals

a. Test the hypothesis that the population Pearson correlation coefficient is equal to 0, using a 0.01 significance level.
b. Obtain a 99% confidence interval for the population regression slope.
c. Test the hypothesis that the population regression intercept is equal to 0, using a 0.01 significance level.
d. Obtain a 99% confidence interval for the population regression intercept.

12. A study investigated the exposure of nurses to radiation from patients receiving diagnostic radionuclides.[22] Table 12.22 shows the maximum weekly radiation exposure and the cumulative quarterly radiation exposure for 13 nurses involved in the care of patients who received diagnostic radionuclides. Do the data provide evidence that the maximum exposure is linearly related to the cumulative exposure?

a. Test the hypothesis that the population regression slope is equal to 0, using a 0.05 significance level.
b. Obtain a 95% confidence interval for the population regression slope.
c. Test the hypothesis that the population regression intercept is equal to 0, using a 0.05 significance level.
d. Obtain a 95% confidence interval for the population regression intercept.

TABLE 12.22   MAXIMUM WEEKLY RADIATION EXPOSURE AND CUMULATIVE QUARTERLY RADIATION EXPOSURE FOR 13 NURSES

Subject No.	Maximum 5-day Week Dose Equivalent per Person (mrem)	Cumulative Quarterly Dose Equivalent per Person (mrem)
1	8.4	32.5
2	3.1	5.5
3	1.6	2.3
4	3.8	5.6
5	1.6	1.6
6	10.4	17.2
7	6.2	6.3
8	7.8	7.8
9	3.7	13.3
10	5.1	17.8
11	6.3	25.8
12	6.0	9.9
13	0.0	0.0

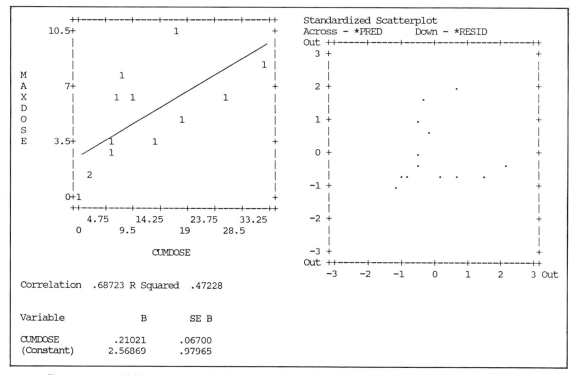

Figure 12.53 SPSS/PC correlation and regression output for radiation exposure data with sample regression line

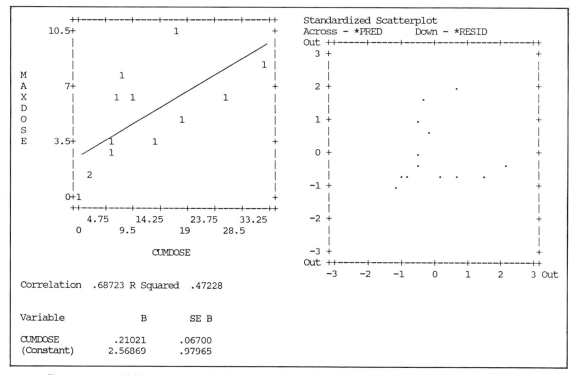

Figure 12.54 Quick histogram of radiation exposure regression residuals

13. A study of white clot syndrome reported the platelet count before heparin and the lowest platelet count after heparin for 20 patients with white clot syndrome.[23] The logarithms of these counts are shown in Table 12.23. Do the data provide evidence that the lowest log platelet count after heparin is linearly related to the log platelet count before heparin?

a. Test the hypothesis that the population regression slope is equal to 0, using a 0.01 significance level.

b. Obtain a 99% confidence interval for the population regression slope.

c. Test the hypothesis that the population regression intercept is equal to 30, using a 0.01 significance level.

d. Obtain a 99% confidence interval for the population regression intercept.

TABLE 12.23 LOG PLATELET COUNT (LOG(PLATELETS / μl)) BEFORE HEPARIN AND LOWEST LOG PLATELET COUNT (LOG(PLATELETS / μl)) AFTER HEPARIN FOR PATIENTS WITH HEPARIN-INDUCED THROMBOCYTOPENIA

Patient No.	Before Heparin	Lowest
1	12.31	10.24
2	12.03	9.21
3	11.70	10.17
4	12.68	9.21
5	11.90	11.11
6	12.38	9.62
7	12.48	9.47
8	12.92	9.85
9	12.41	9.85
10	12.51	9.21
11	12.53	9.85
12	12.00	10.95
13	12.30	10.49
14	13.03	10.93
15	12.75	8.70
16	12.40	10.62
17	12.38	11.49
18	12.69	9.85
19	12.36	10.88
20	12.23	10.78

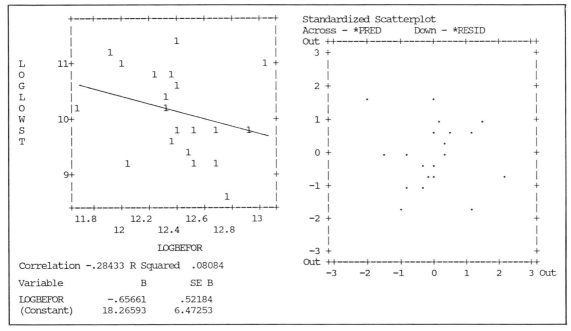

Figure 12.55 SPSS/PC correlation and regression output for platelet data with sample regression line

```
- 1.20 - - 0.81 | XXX
- 0.80 - - 0.41 | XXXX
- 0.40 - - 0.01 | XXX
  0.00 - 0.39 | XXX
  0.40 - 0.79 | XXXXX
  0.80 - 1.19 |
  1.20 - 1.59 | XX
```

Figure 12.56 Quick histogram of platelet regression residuals

14. In a study of acute pancreatitis, initial and final serum amylase values were reported for 32 episodes of acute pancreatitis in 21 patients with end-stage renal disease.[24] These data are shown in Table 12.24. Do the data provide evidence that the final serum amylase is linearly related to the initial serum amylase?

  a. Test the hypothesis that the population Pearson correlation coefficient is equal to 0, using a 0.01 significance level.
  b. Obtain a 99% confidence interval for the population regression slope.
  c. Test the hypothesis that the population regression intercept is equal to 110, using a 0.01 significance level.
  d. Obtain a 99% confidence interval for the population regression intercept.

15 In a study of tetralogy of Fallot in the dog, the hematocrit (Hct) and plasma protein were reported for 13 dogs with tetralogy of Fallot.[25] These data are shown in Table 12.25. Do the data provide

TABLE 12.24 INITIAL AND FINAL SERUM AMYLASE (U/I) FOR EPISODES OF ACUTE PANCREATITIS IN PATIENTS WITH END-STAGE RENAL DISEASE

Episode No.	Initial	Final
1	756	47
2	334	125
3	360	274
4	392	300
5	367	196
6	533	112
7	564	177
8	754	110
9	748	30
10	668	63
11	235	62
12	313	115
13	481	371
14	1940	4
15	1565	124
16	1870	151
17	520	59
18	113	120
19	236	185
20	741	788
21	1014	200
22	1320	134
23	204	167
24	176	170
25	162	136
26	398	283
27	203	196
28	1254	130
29	178	108
30	424	217
31	542	327
32	1360	206

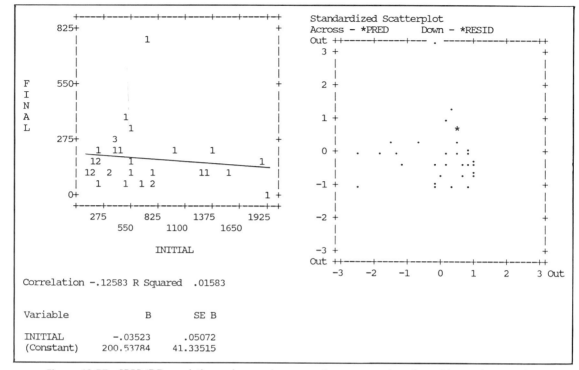

Figure 12.57 SPSS/PC correlation and regression output for serum amylase data with sample regression line

```
 −200.00 − −100.01 | XXXXXX
  −100.00 − −0.01  | XXXXXXXXXXXXX
     0.00 − 99.99  | XXXXXXX
   100.00 − 199.99 | XXX
   200.00 − 299.99 |
   300.00 − 399.99 |
   400.00 − 499.99 |
   500.00 − 599.99 |
   600.00 − 699.99 | X
```

Figure 12.58 Quick histogram of serum amylase regression residuals

TABLE 12.25 HEMATOCRIT AND PLASMA PROTEIN FOR DOGS WITH TETRALOGY OF FALLOT

Dog No.	Hct (%)	Plasma Protein (g/dl)
1	44	7.4
2	53	7.5
3	65	6.1
4	44	6.8
5	48	6.5
6	76	5.5
7	62	6.7
8	51	6.5
9	50	7.0
10	43	6.7
11	40	7.5
12	43	5.8
13	40	6.5

evidence that plasma protein is linearly related to Hct?

   a. Test the hypothesis that the population Pearson correlation coefficient is equal to 0, using a 0.05 significance level.
   b. Obtain a 95% confidence interval for the population regression slope.
   c. Test the hypothesis that the population regression intercept is equal to 0, using a 0.05 significance level.
   d. Obtain a 95% confidence interval for the population regression intercept.

16. A study investigated the effect of increased fluid intake on urinary stone formation in patients with Foley catheters.[26] Table 12.26 shows the patient–average daily fluid intake and the urine pH for 17 patients with indwelling Foley catheters. Do the data provide evidence that daily fluid intake is linearly related to urine pH?

   a. Test the hypothesis that the population Pearson correlation coefficient is equal to 0, using a 0.05 significance level.
   b. Obtain a 95% confidence interval for the population regression slope.
   c. Test the hypothesis that the population regression intercept is equal to 2500, using a 0.05 significance level.

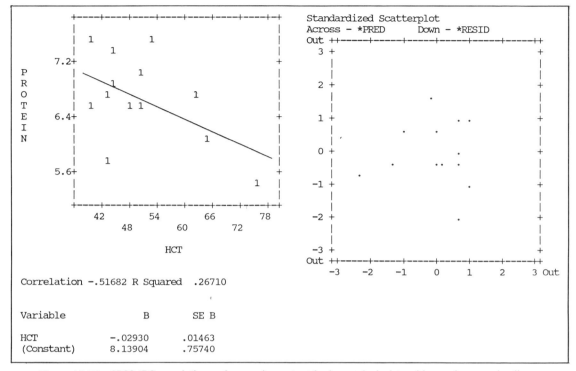

Figure 12.59 SPSS/PC correlation and regression output for hematologic data with sample regression line

```
- 1.50 - - 1.01 | X
- 1.00 - - 0.51 |
- 0.50 - - 0.01 | XXXXXXX
  0.00 - 0.49 | XX
  0.50 - 0.99 | XXX
```

Figure 12.60 Quick histogram of hematologic regression residuals

d. Obtain a 95% confidence interval for the population regression intercept.

17. A study evaluated the accuracy of preoperative two-dimensional echocardiography (2D ECHO) for measuring the mitral and aortic annulus diameter in children undergoing valve replacement.[27] Table 12.27 shows the 2D ECHO annulus diameter and the diameter of the prosthetic valve used for 14 patients. Do the data provide evidence that the measured annulus diameter and the prosthetic valve diameter are not equivalent?

a. Test the hypothesis that the population regression slope is equal to 0, using a 0.05 significance level.

b. Test the hypothesis that the population regression slope is equal to 1, using a 0.05 significance level.

c. Test the hypothesis that the population regression intercept is equal to 0, using a 0.05 significance level.

TABLE 12.26 PATIENT–AVERAGE DAILY FLUID INTAKE AND URINE pH FOR PATIENTS WITH INDWELLING FOLEY CATHETERS

Patient No.	Average Daily Fluid Intake (ml)	Urine pH
1	2715	6.0
2	767	7.5
3	1081	6.5
4	1726	9.0
5	1891	9.0
6	1070	5.0
7	3661	6.5
8	1049	9.0
9	1282	6.0
10	988	7.5
11	1470	9.0
12	1226	8.0
13	908	9.0
14	1293	8.0
15	1830	6.0
16	1792	7.5
17	2532	6.0

d. Obtain a 95% confidence interval for the population regression intercept.

18. In a study of serological testing for antibody to *Borrelia burgdorferi*, IFA titers of antibody to *B. burgdorferi* were obtained from several laboratories.[28] Table 12.28 shows the titers from two labora-

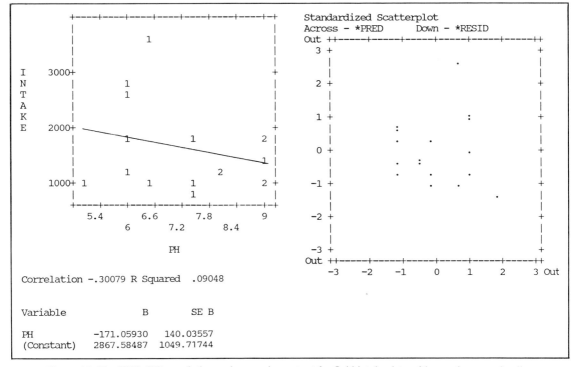

Figure 12.61 SPSS/PC correlation and regression output for fluid intake data with sample regression line

```
−1000 − −501 | XXXXX
 −500 − −1 | XXXXX
    0 − 499 | XXX
  500 − 999 | XXX
 1000 − 1499 |
 1500 − 1999 | X
```

Figure 12.62 Quick histogram of fluid intake regression residuals

tories for nine national forest employees at risk for Lyme disease. Do the data provide evidence that titers from the two laboratories are not equivalent?

    a. Test the hypothesis that the population Pearson correlation coefficient is equal to 0, using a 0.10 significance level.

    b. Test the hypothesis that the population regression slope is equal to 1, using a 0.10 significance level.

    c. Test the hypothesis that the population regression intercept is equal to 75, using a 0.10 significance level.

    d. Obtain a 90% confidence interval for the population regression intercept.

19. A study investigated fluctuations in pulmonary artery systolic (PAS) pressures in acutely ill patients.[29] Table 12.29 shows the initial PAS pressure and the PAS pressure taken 30 minutes later for 22 acutely ill patients in intensive care units. Do the data provide evidence that the 30-minute PAS

TABLE 12.27 MEASURED ANNULUS DIAMETER AND PROSTHETIC VALVE DIAMETER

Patient No.	ECHO Annulus Diameter (mm)	Prosthetic Diameter (mm)
1	14	15
2	26	25
3	16	15
4	24	23
5	36	35
6	28	27
7	31	30
8	24	23
9	18	17
10	28	28
11	18	19
12	22	21
13	31	29
14	29	29

TABLE 12.28 TITERS OF ANTIBODY TO B. BURGDORFERI

Employee No.	Laboratory 1	Laboratory 2
1	1024	64
2	1024	64
3	512	128
4	256	64
5	256	32
6	128	128
7	128	64
8	64	64
9	64	16

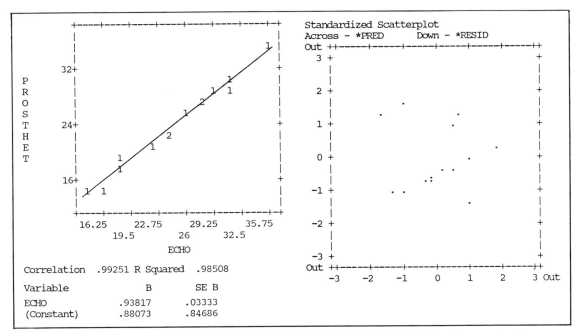

Figure 12.63 SPSS/PC correlation and regression output for diameter data with sample regression line

```
−1.00 − −0.51 | XXXX
−0.50 − −0.01 | XXXX
 0.00 −  0.49 | XX
 0.50 −  0.99 | XXX
 1.00 −  1.49 | X
```

Figure 12.64 Quick histogram of diameter regression residuals

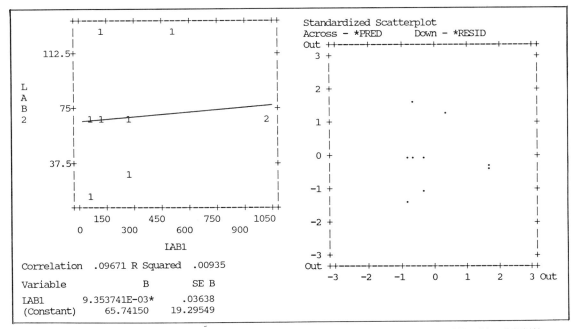

Correlation .09671 R Squared .00935

Variable	B	SE B
IAB1	9.353741E-03*	.03638
(Constant)	65.74150	19.29549

*SPSS/PC uses the symbols "E−" and "E+" to indicate scientific notation. Thus, 9.353741E−03 = 9.353741 × 10⁻³ = 0.009353741.

Figure 12.65 SPSS/PC correlation and regression output for antibody titer data with sample regression line

```
-60.00 - -30.01 | XX
-30.00 - -0.01  | XXXXX
  0.00 - 29.99  |
 30.00 - 59.99  | X
 60.00 - 89.99  | X
```

Figure 12.66 Quick histogram of antibody titer regression residuals

TABLE 12.29 INITIAL AND 30-MINUTE PAS PRESSURES FOR ACUTELY ILL PATIENTS

Patient No.	Initial PAS	30-Minute PAS
1	34	36
2	24	26
3	35	32
4	37	42
5	24	26
6	30	34
7	35	36
8	35	37
9	55	53
10	25	22
11	26	22
12	21	22
13	26	27
14	45	48
15	31	31
16	22	20
17	56	59
18	31	32
19	45	44
20	19	21
21	30	28
22	19	16

```
-6.00 - -4.01 | X
-4.00 - -2.01 | XXXXX
-2.00 - -0.01 | XXX
 0.00 - 1.99  | XXXXXXXXX
 2.00 - 3.99  | XXX
 4.00 - 5.99  | X
```

Figure 12.68 Quick histogram of PAS pressure regression residuals

pressure and the initial PAS pressure are linearly related?

a. Test the hypothesis that the population Pearson correlation coefficient is equal to 0, using a 0.01 significance level.

b. Obtain a 99% confidence interval for the population regression slope.

c. Test the hypothesis that the population regression intercept is equal to 0, using a 0.01 significance level.

d. Obtain a 99% confidence interval for the population regression intercept.

20. Find an article in a medical or health care journal in which hypothesis tests or confidence intervals concerning correlation or regression coefficients were incorrectly used to analyze nonindependent or extremely nonnormal data. Photocopy the article and write a letter to the journal editor that clearly describes the statistical error.

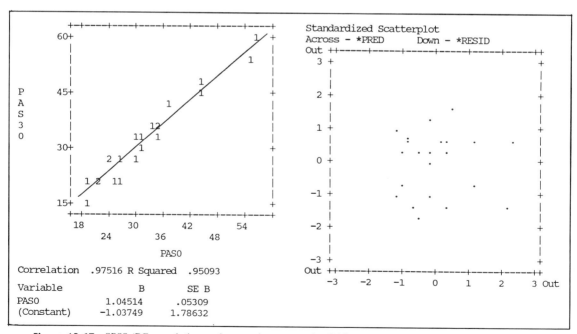

Figure 12.67 SPSS/PC correlation and regression output for PAS pressure data with sample regression line

REFERENCES

1. Neter J, Wasserman W, Kutner MH: Applied Linear Statistical Models. Regression, Analysis of Variance, and Experimental Designs. 2nd ed. Homewood: Irwin, 1985.
2. Woods SW, Charney DS, Loke J, et al: Carbon dioxide sensitivity in panic anxiety. Ventilatory and anxiogenic response to carbon dioxide in healthy subjects and patients with panic anxiety before and after alprazolam treatment. Arch Gen Psychiatry *43*:900–909, 1986.
3. Kleinbaum DG, Kupper LL, Muller KE: Applied Regression Analysis and Other Multivariable Methods. 2nd ed. Boston: PWS-Kent, 1988.
4. Kolski GB, Levy J, Anolik R: The use of theophylline clearance in pediatric status asthmaticus. I. Interpatient and intrapatient theophylline clearance variability. Am J Dis Child *141*:282–287, 1987.
5. Morady F, DiCarlo LA, Krol RB, et al: Effect of programmed ventricular stimulation on myocardial lactate extraction in patients with and without coronary artery disease. Am Heart J *111*:252–257, 1986.
6. Spotnitz WD, Dalton MS, Baker JW, et al: Reduction of perioperative hemorrhage by anterior mediastinal spray application of fibrin glue during cardiac operations. Ann Thorac Surg *44*: 529–531, 1987.
7. Parkin A, Robinson PJ, Wiggins PA, et al: The measurement of limb blood flow using technetium-labelled red blood cells. Br J Radiol *59*:493–497, 1986.
8. Liggett SB, St. John RE, Lefrak SS: Determination of resting energy expenditure utilizing the thermodilution pulmonary artery catheter. Chest *91*:562–566, 1987.
9. van Hoof JJM, Horstink MWI, Berger HJC, et al: Spasmodic torticollis: The problem of pathophysiology and assessment. J Neurol *234*:322–327, 1987.
10. Zeiher AM, Bonzel T, Wollschlager H, et al: Noninvasive evaluation of pulmonary hypertension by quantitative contrast M-mode echocardiography. Am Heart J *111*:297–306, 1986.
11. Meagher DM: MI patient expectations and health status. Rehabil Nurs *12*:128–131, 1987.
12. Pryor AC: The intra-arterial line: A site for obtaining coagulation studies. Heart Lung *12*:586–590, 1983.
13. Varughese A, Brater DC, Benet LZ, et al: Ethambutol kinetics in patients with impaired renal function. Am Rev Respir Dis *134*:34–38, 1986.
14. Daily EK, Mersch J: Thermodilution cardiac outputs using room and ice temperature injectate: Comparison with the Fick method. Heart Lung *16*:294–300, 1987.
15. Artman M, Parrish MD, Appleton S, et al: Hemodynamic effects of hydralazine in infants with idiopathic dilated cardiomyopathy and congestive heart failure. Am Heart J *113*:144–150, 1987.
16. Mizutani H, Mizutani H: Immunoglobulin M rheumatoid factor in patients with mycoplasmal pneumonia. Am Rev Respir Dis *134*:1237–1240, 1986.
17. Grose BL, Woods SL, Laurent DJ: Effect of backrest position on cardiac output measured by the thermodilution method in acutely ill patients. Heart Lung *10*:661–665, 1981.
18. Spier SJ, Smith BP, Seawright AA, et al: Oak toxicosis in cattle in northern California: Clinical and pathologic findings. J Am Vet Med Assoc *191*:958–964, 1987.
19. Zoghbi WA, Rokey R, Linmacher MC, et al: Assessment of left ventricular diastolic filling by two-dimensional echocardiography. Am Heart J *113*:1108–1113, 1987.
20. Burki NK: The dead space to tidal volume ratio in the diagnosis of pulmonary embolism. Am Rev Respir Dis *133*:679–685, 1986.
21. Hornig CR, Dorndorf W, Agnoli AL: Hemorrhagic cerebral infarction—A prospective study. Stroke *17*:179–185, 1986.
22. Burks J, Griffith P, McCormick K, et al: Radiation exposure to nursing personnel from patients receiving diagnostic radionuclides. Heart Lung *11*:217–220, 1982.
23. Chang JC: White clot syndrome associated with heparin-induced thrombocytopenia: A review of 23 cases. Heart Lung *16*:403–407, 1987.
24. Rutsky EA, Robards M, Van Dyke JA, et al: Acute pancreatitis in patients with end-stage renal disease without transplantation. Arch Intern Med *146*:1741–1745, 1986.
25. Ringwald RJ, Bonagura JD: Tetralogy of Fallot in the dog: Clinical findings in 13 cases. J Am Anim Hosp Assoc *24*:33–43, 1988.
26. Hart M, Adamek C: Do increased fluids decrease urinary stone formation? Geriatr Nurs *5*:245–248, 1984.
27. Caldwell RL, Girod DA, Hurwitz RA, et al: Preoperative two-dimensional echocardiographic prediction of prosthetic aortic and mitral valve size in children. Am Heart J *113*:873–878, 1987.
28. Hedburg CW, Osterholm MT, MacDonald KL, et al: An interlaboratory study of antibody to *Borrelia burgdorferi*. J Infect Dis *155*:1325–1327, 1987.
29. Nemens EJ, Woods SL: Normal fluctuations in pulmonary artery and pulmonary capillary wedge pressures in acutely ill patients. Heart Lung *11*:393–398, 1982.

TWO-WAY ANALYSIS
OF VARIANCE

CHAPTER OBJECTIVES

*After studying this chapter and working the problems,
you should be able to:*

1. Interpret two-way analysis of variance results

2. Explain the concept of interaction

3. Recognize data that violate assumptions required for two-way analysis of variance

4. Interpret SPSS and SAS two-way analysis of variance output

5. Calculate and interpret Tukey and Bonferroni confidence intervals for two-way analysis of variance

6. Determine whether two-way analyses of variance reported in the medical and health care literature are appropriate

When one-way analysis of variance (ANOVA) is done, we compare population means in order to determine the effect of one *factor*, a characteristic used to classify subjects into different groups. For the burn data in Chapter 8, the factor is the survival outcome, since survival outcome is used to classify patients into three different groups. Other examples of factors are race, drug, dose, disease, and treatment. The *levels* of a factor are the possible categories of the factor. The survival outcome factor in Chapter 8 has three levels: (1) death within three days, (2) death within five to 48 days, and (3) survival.

We sometimes want to compare population means in order to evaluate the effects of two factors. When the data are independent observations, comparison of means involving two factors often can be done with two-way analysis of variance.

13.1 HYPOTHESIS TESTS

A study investigated the physical and mental health of elderly women engaged in long-term or short-term care of their husbands.[1] Three groups of women were studied: (1) long-term caregivers, whose husbands were permanently impaired; (2) short-term caregivers, whose husbands were temporarily impaired; and (3) non-caregivers, whose husbands were not impaired. Table 13.1 shows a quality-of-life score for these subjects. This score measures the subject's evaluation of her health, her frequency of social contact outside the home, and her feelings of control over events in her life. The higher the score, the better the subject's perceived quality of life. We will examine the effects of two factors on the population mean quality-of-life score: *education* (college or no

**TABLE 13.1   QUALITY-OF-LIFE SCORE FOR ELDERLY WOMEN
WITH MEANS AND STANDARD DEVIATIONS**

	Caregiving status		
Education	LONG-TERM CAREGIVER	SHORT-TERM CAREGIVER	NON-CAREGIVER
College	33 31 40 38	41 39	38 28
	46 36 37 36	46 43	39
	32 31 36 40	48 44	40
	35 43 34 32	47 38	42
	45 39 24 37	37 39	33
	36 36 46 41	42 43	36
	41 35 36 41	40	41
	42 46 47 39	41	37
	38 26 41	44	45
	37.6 ± 5.4	42.1 ± 3.3	37.9 ± 4.8
No college	26 27 28 42	31 43	32 39
	27 21 38 29	28	39 37
	41 29 27 44	37	36 40
	32 31 38 28	38	33 41
	36 35 34 38	39	41 38
	32 22 35 37	36	42 43
	26 43 31 38	40	43
	29 36 31 27	25	42
	27 29 34	31	33
	34 29 32	44	39
	32.2 ± 5.6	35.6 ± 6.1	38.6 ± 3.6

college) and *caregiving status* (long-term caregiver, short-term caregiver, or non-caregiver).

In general, we want to determine the effects of two factors by comparing the population means for different factor levels. Each combination of levels for two factors is called a *cell*. The mean and standard deviation of the observations in a cell are called the *cell mean* and *cell standard deviation*. The number of observations in a cell is called the *cell size*. Let us refer to the factors as Factor A and Factor B. We will denote the levels of Factor A by $1, 2, \ldots, a$ and the levels of Factor B by $1, 2, \ldots, b$. The number of Factor A levels is denoted by a and the number of Factor B levels is denoted by b. The sample cell mean, sample cell standard deviation, and cell size for level i of Factor A and level j of Factor B are denoted by $\bar{x}_{AiBj}$, s_{AiBj}, and n_{AiBj}. Each sample cell mean $\bar{x}_{AiBj}$ has a corresponding population cell mean μ_{AiBj}.

The caregiver data in Table 13.1 have six cells. We will treat education as Factor A (level 1 = college, level 2 = no college), and caregiving status as Factor B (level 1 = long-term caregiver, level 2 = short-term caregiver, level 3 = non-caregiver).* The sample cell means, sample cell standard deviations, and cell sizes for these data can be obtained

---

*The assignment of the labels "Factor A" and "Factor B" is arbitrary. To avoid confusion, the same labels should be used throughout the analysis.

from Table 13.1:

$\bar{x}_{A1B1} = 37.6$	$s_{A1B1} = 5.4$	$n_{A1B1} = 35$
$\bar{x}_{A1B2} = 42.1$	$s_{A1B2} = 3.3$	$n_{A1B2} = 15$
$\bar{x}_{A1B3} = 37.9$	$s_{A1B3} = 4.8$	$n_{A1B3} = 10$
$\bar{x}_{A2B1} = 32.2$	$s_{A2B1} = 5.6$	$n_{A2B1} = 38$
$\bar{x}_{A2B2} = 35.6$	$s_{A2B2} = 6.1$	$n_{A2B2} = 11$
$\bar{x}_{A2B3} = 38.6$	$s_{A2B3} = 3.6$	$n_{A2B3} = 16$

A *factor mean* for a particular factor level is the average of all of the cell means for that level. The sample Factor A mean for level i is denoted by $\bar{x}_{Ai}$, and the sample Factor B mean for level j is denoted by $\bar{x}_{Bj}$. Each sample Factor A mean $\bar{x}_{Ai}$ has a corresponding population Factor A mean μ_{Ai}, and each sample Factor B mean $\bar{x}_{Bj}$ has a corresponding population Factor B mean μ_{Bj}. A population factor mean for a particular factor level is the average of all of the population cell means for that level. The sample factor means for the caregiver data are calculated as follows, using the sample cell means in Table 13.1.

Sample Education Factor Means.

$$\bar{x}_{A1} = \frac{(37.6 + 42.1 + 37.9)}{3} = 39.2$$

$$\bar{x}_{A2} = \frac{(32.2 + 35.6 + 38.6)}{3} = 35.5$$

**TABLE 13.2 HYPOTHETICAL CELL MEANS
FOR SEVERITY OF DIARRHEA**

Sex	Dose		
	5 mg/kg	10 mg/kg	15 mg/kg
Female	30.0	44.2	60.9
Male	20.5	28.1	20.6

Sample Caregiving Factor Means.

$$\bar{x}_{B1} = \frac{(37.6 + 32.2)}{2} = 34.9$$

$$\bar{x}_{B2} = \frac{(42.1 + 35.6)}{2} = 38.8$$

$$\bar{x}_{B3} = \frac{(37.9 + 38.6)}{2} = 38.2$$

Whenever two factors are examined, the possibility of *interaction* exists. Interaction occurs when the effect of one factor depends on the level of the other factor. Suppose a new chemotherapy drug for lymphosarcoma is evaluated in women and men. Two factors are examined, sex and dose (5 mg/kg, 10 mg/kg, and 15 mg/kg). A very common side effect of the drug is severe diarrhea, which is measured by the number of loose stools per week. Suppose the population cell means for severity of diarrhea are those shown in Table 13.2. If we plot these cell means as in Figure 13.1, it becomes clear that the effect of drug dose depends on sex. In women, increasing the dose greatly increases the severity of diarrhea. In men, increasing the dose has little effect on the severity of diarrhea. There is an interaction between dose and sex.

Figures 13.2 through 13.4 show plots of other hypothetical population cell means. In Figure 13.2, there is no interaction and no dose effect, but there is a sex effect. For all doses, the mean severity is higher for women. In Figure 13.3, sex and dose effects are both evident, but interaction is not present. Women and men have the same magnitude of increase in mean severity when the dose is in-

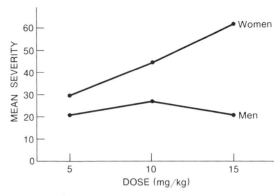

Figure 13.1 Plot of hypothetical cell means for severity of diarrhea showing interaction

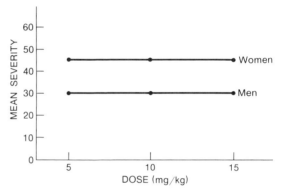

Figure 13.2 Plot of hypothetical cell means for severity of diarrhea showing sex effect

creased. The mean severity for women is higher at each dose than the mean severity for men, but the effect of changing the dose does not depend on sex.

Figure 13.4 suggests interaction between dose and sex. For women, a sharp increase in mean severity occurs when the dose changes from 5 mg/kg to 10 mg/kg. A slight increase in mean severity occurs when the dose changes from 10 mg/kg to 15 mg/kg. For men, a slight increase in mean severity

Figure 13.3 Plot of hypothetical cell means for severity of diarrhea showing sex and dose effects but no interaction

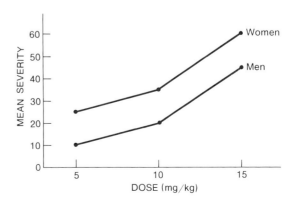

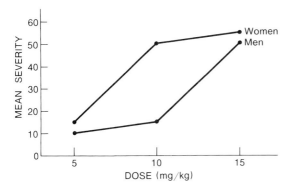

Figure 13.4 Plot of hypothetical cell means for severity of diarrhea showing interaction

is evident when the dose changes from 5 mg/kg to 10 mg/kg. A sharp increase in mean severity is evident when the dose changes from 10 mg/kg to 15 mg/kg. In other words, the effect of dose depends on sex.

It is important to determine whether factors interact because interaction affects our interpretation of the results. The first hypothesis tested in two-way ANOVA is the null hypothesis that there is no interaction:

$$H_0: \text{No interaction} \qquad (13.1)$$

The alternative hypothesis states that interaction is present:

$$H_A: \text{Interaction present} \qquad (13.2)$$

If we cannot reject the hypothesis of no interaction, we go on to test two other null hypotheses. One of these hypotheses states that all of the Factor A population means are equal:

$$H_0: \mu_{A1} = \mu_{A2} = \mu_{A3} = \cdots = \mu_{Aa} \qquad (13.3)$$

The alternative hypothesis is

H_A: At least one Factor A population mean does not equal another Factor A   (13.4) population mean

We also test the null hypothesis that all of the Factor B population means are equal:

$$H_0: \mu_{B1} = \mu_{B2} = \mu_{B3} = \cdots = \mu_{Bb} \qquad (13.5)$$

The alternative hypothesis is

H_A: At least one Factor B population mean does not equal another Factor B   (13.6) population mean

If we reject the hypothesis of no interaction, there is no point in testing the null hypotheses (13.3) or (13.5). We already know that Factor A and Factor B have effects, which are interactive. Interaction can occur in such a way that the null hypothe-

ses (13.3) and (13.5) cannot be rejected. The presence of interaction still implies that Factor A and Factor B both have effects.*

When we conclude that interaction is present, the next step is the comparison of population *cell* means in order to determine the nature of the interaction. Plots of the sample cell means, like those in Figures 13.1 through 13.4, are often useful. Multiple comparison confidence intervals for differences between population cell means are usually obtained.

If we cannot reject the hypothesis of no interaction, but we conclude that at least one of the population factor means is different, we obtain multiple comparison confidence intervals for differences between population *factor* means. Multiple comparison procedures for two-way ANOVA are described in Sections 13.4 and 13.5.

If we cannot reject the hypothesis of no interaction or the hypothesis of equal population Factor A means, the data do not provide evidence for a Factor A effect. If we cannot reject the hypothesis of no interaction or the hypothesis of equal population Factor B means, the data do not provide evidence for a Factor B effect.

To test the null hypotheses (13.1), (13.3), and (13.5), we use F statistics based on mean squares. These mean squares are described by simple formulas only when all of the cell sizes are equal. Even then, calculating mean squares by hand is extremely tedious. When the cell sizes are not equal, a method called the regression approach is often used by a computer to obtain mean squares. We will not describe the details of this method or the formulas for two-way ANOVA mean squares. Further information can be found in other texts.[2]

We will concentrate on the interpretation of two-way ANOVA results. When two-way ANOVA is done with a statistical software package, the output usually includes a two-way analysis of variance table.

---

*The term "factor effect" is a statistical term that is not meant to imply causality. When we say that a factor has an effect, we mean that some of the population factor means or cell means differ. In other words, the population means are related to the factor.

Source	Degrees of Freedom	Sum of Squares	Mean Square
Factor A	$a - 1$	SSA	MSA
Factor B	$b - 1$	SSB	MSB
Interaction	$(a - 1)(b - 1)$	SSAB	MSAB
Error	$n_T - ab$	SSE	MSE
Total	$n_T - 1$	SST	

Figure 13.5 Two-way analysis of variance table format

This table has the format shown in Figure 13.5. In this figure, a is the number of Factor A levels, b is the number of Factor B levels, and n_T is the total number of observations.

The mean squares in the two-way ANOVA table are used to obtain F statistics for testing the null hypotheses (13.1), (13.3), and (13.5). To test the hypothesis of no interaction, we use the F statistic obtained by dividing the interaction mean square by the error mean square:

$$F = \frac{\text{MSAB}}{\text{MSE}} \qquad (13.7)$$

If the null hypothesis (13.1) is true and the data satisfy certain assumptions, this statistic has an F distribution with $(a - 1)(b - 1)$ numerator degrees of freedom and $n_T - ab$ denominator degrees of freedom. These degrees of freedom are the interaction degrees of freedom and the error degrees of freedom in the two-way ANOVA table.

To test the hypothesis that all of the Factor A population means are equal, we use another F statistic. The Factor A F statistic is obtained by dividing the Factor A mean square by the error mean square:

$$F = \frac{\text{MSA}}{\text{MSE}} \qquad (13.8)$$

If the null hypothesis (13.3) is true and the data meet certain assumptions, this F statistic has an F distribution with $a - 1$ numerator degrees of freedom and $n_T - ab$ denominator degrees of freedom. These degrees of freedom are the Factor A degrees of freedom and the error degrees of freedom in the two-way ANOVA table.

Another F statistic is used to test the hypothesis that all of the Factor B population means are equal. The Factor B F statistic is calculated by dividing the Factor B mean square by the error mean square:

$$F = \frac{\text{MSB}}{\text{MSE}} \qquad (13.9)$$

If the null hypothesis (13.5) is true and the required

assumptions hold, this F statistic has an F distribution with $b - 1$ numerator degrees of freedom and $n_T - ab$ denominator degrees of freedom. These degrees of freedom are the Factor B degrees of freedom and the error degrees of freedom in the two-way ANOVA table.

For each hypothesis test, a large F statistic provides evidence against the null hypothesis and a small F statistic does not provide evidence against the null hypothesis. The p-value for the F statistic and the previously selected significance level α determine whether the F statistic is large enough to warrant rejection of the null hypothesis. If the p-value is less than α, the null hypothesis is rejected. If the p-value is greater than or equal to α, the null hypothesis cannot be rejected at this significance level. The p-value is interpreted in the usual way: it is the probability of getting an F statistic at least as extreme as the calculated F statistic if the null hypothesis is true.

For all three F statistics, the p-value is given by

$$p\text{-value} = P(F \text{ statistic} \geq F_{\text{calc}})$$

where F_{calc} is the calculated value of the F statistic. The approximate p-value can be obtained from Table E.5 in essentially the same way as described in Chapter 8. Only the degrees of freedom are different.

Two-way ANOVA requires the following assumptions.

1. Random Samples. As usual, random sampling is not essential if the samples are not biased.

2. Independent Observations. If any of the observations are not independent, two-way ANOVA cannot be done. This rules out the use of two-way ANOVA to analyze repeated measurements.

3. Normal Populations. The observations in each cell should come from a normal or approximately normal population. If the cell sizes are large enough, the populations need not be exactly normal, but two-way ANOVA cannot be done when any of the populations are extremely nonnormal (e.g., when the data have only a few possible values).

4. Equal Variances. The populations from which the cell observations are taken should have equal or similar variances. Examination of the sample cell variances provides some idea of whether this assumption is reasonable, but there is no simple rule for determining whether the population cell variances are equal. When in doubt, consult a statistician.*

---

*Neter, Wasserman, and Kutner describe the use of ANOVA *residual plots* to evaluate the independence, normality, and equal-variance assumptions.[2] The use of residual plots in regression analysis is discussed in Chapter 12.

```
24 – 27 | XX
28 – 31 | XX
32 – 35 | XXXXX
36 – 39 | XXXXXXXXXXX
40 – 43 | XXXXXXX
44 – 47 | XXXXX
```

Figure 13.6 Quick histogram of quality-of-life score for long-term caregivers with college education

```
35 – 38 | XX
39 – 42 | XXXXXX
43 – 46 | XXXXX
47 – 50 | XX
```

Figure 13.7 Quick histogram of quality-of-life score for short-term caregivers with college education

```
28 – 32 | X
33 – 37 | XXX
38 – 42 | XXXXX
43 – 47 | X
```

Figure 13.8 Quick histogram of quality-of-life score for non-caregivers with college education

```
20 – 23 | XX
24 – 27 | XXXXXX
28 – 31 | XXXXXXXXX
32 – 35 | XXXXXXX
36 – 39 | XXXXXX
40 – 43 | XXX
44 – 47 | X
```

Figure 13.9 Quick histogram of quality-of-life score for long-term caregivers with no college education

```
25 – 29 | XX
30 – 34 | XX
35 – 39 | XXXX
40 – 44 | XXX
```

Figure 13.10 Quick histogram of quality-of-life score for short-term caregivers with no college education

```
30 – 32 | X
33 – 35 | XX
36 – 38 | XXX
39 – 41 | XXXXXX
42 – 44 | XXXX
```

Figure 13.11 Quick histogram of quality-of-life score for non-caregivers with no college education

TABLE 13.3   TWO-WAY ANOVA TABLE FOR CAREGIVER DATA

Source	Degrees of Freedom	Sum of Squares	Mean Square
Education	1	333.8	333.8
Caregiver status	2	407.8	203.9
Interaction	2	208.3	104.2
Error	119	3101.0	26.1
Total	124	4427.2	

Let us evaluate how well the caregiver data satisfy these assumptions. The data are not a random sample, but this is not crucial. Since the quality-of-life score for one subject tells us nothing about the quality-of-life score for another subject, the observations are independent. Histograms of the data for each cell (Figures 13.6 through 13.11) are consistent with sampling from approximately normal or moderately skewed populations. From Table 13.1, the ratio of the largest cell variance to the smallest cell variance is $(6.1)^2/(3.3)^2 = 3.4$. Given six cells, a ratio of this size is not extremely unlikely if the population cell variances are equal or similar. Two-way ANOVA seems appropriate for these data.

The two-way ANOVA table for the caregiver data is shown in Table 13.3. We will use a 0.01

significance level for all hypothesis tests. We first need to test the hypothesis of no interaction. From Table 13.3, we obtain the mean squares needed to calculate the interaction F statistic (13.7):

$$F = \frac{104.2}{26.1} = 3.99$$

The degrees of freedom for this F statistic can also be obtained from Table 13.3: 2 numerator degrees of freedom and 119 denominator degrees of freedom. From Table E.5, we get the approximate p-value

$$0.01 < p\text{-value} < 0.025$$

We cannot reject the hypothesis of no interaction at the 0.01 significance level, although we would reject this hypothesis at the 0.05 significance level.

Since we cannot reject the hypothesis of no interaction at the 0.01 significance level, we need to test the hypothesis that all of the population education factor means are equal and the hypothesis that all of the population caregiving factor means are equal. Using the appropriate mean squares in Table 13.3, we calculate the F statistic for testing the hypothesis of equal population education factor means:

$$F = \frac{333.8}{26.1} = 12.79$$

From Table 13.3, we also get 1 and 119 degrees of freedom. Table E.5 gives the approximate p-value:

$$p\text{-value} < 0.001$$

We reject the hypothesis that the two population education factor means are equal at any reasonable significance level.

To test the hypothesis of equal population caregiving factor means, we calculate an F statistic based on the appropriate mean squares in Table 13.3.

$$F = \frac{203.9}{26.1} = 7.81$$

The degrees of freedom are 2 and 119, from Table 13.3. Using Table E.5, we get the approximate p-value

$$p\text{-value} < 0.001$$

We reject the hypothesis that all of the population caregiving factor means are equal at any reasonable significance level.

Because we rejected the hypothesis that all of the population caregiving factor means are equal, further analysis is needed to determine which population means are different. We will carry out this analysis in Sections 13.4 and 13.5. We do not need further analysis to determine which population education factor means are different because there are only two of these means.

Example 13.1

In a study of carbon dioxide (CO_2) vulnerability in patients with panic disorders, 12 subjects with panic disorders and 11 control subjects were asked to record the degree of distress felt after inhalation of a 35% CO_2/65% oxygen mixture.[3] Distress was measured by the Subjective Units of Disturbance Scale (SUDS), which measures distress on a continuum ranging from 0 ("no anxiety at all") to 100 ("the most terrifying experience one can imagine"). The SUDS scores before and after inhalation are shown in Table 13.4. Can two-way ANOVA be used to determine whether the data provide evidence that the population SUDS score means are related to CO_2 inhalation and panic disorder?

Although scores for different subjects are independent, the preinhalation and postinhalation scores for the same subjects are not independent. In addition, the preinhalation scores for the control subjects seem to have an extremely nonnormal distribution, with more than half of the scores equal to 0. Two-way ANOVA cannot be used to analyze these

TABLE 13.4 SUDS SCORE BEFORE AND AFTER INHALATION

Patients		Controls	
PRE	POST	PRE	POST
50	100	0	5
30	80	5	25
22.5	90	20	25
50	75	8	12
70	100	5	80
85	100	0	0
0	60	0	15
10	60	0	15
30	65	40	30
30	80	0	5
60	75	0	20
40	75		

data. Instead, we could use the sign test described in Chapter 11 to test the hypothesis that the panic disorder population median difference between the preinhalation and postinhalation scores is 0. We could then use the sign test again to test the hypothesis that the control population median difference between the pre and post scores is 0.

Example 13.2

A study investigated the effect of tumor size and intraoperative monitoring of facial nerve function on the facial function remaining after acoustic neuroma removal.[4] Table 13.5 shows the immediate postoperative facial function ratings for 96 patients. Can two-way ANOVA be used to determine whether the data provide evidence that the population func-

TABLE 13.5 IMMEDIATE POSTOPERATIVE FACIAL FUNCTION*

Tumor Size	Intraoperative Monitoring					
	MONITORED			NOT MONITORED		
Small	1	2	1	3	1	2
	2	2	1	1	1	1
	1	2	1	2	2	2
	1	1	2	2	2	2
	2	1		2	1	
Medium	2	3	3	3	3	2
	1	2	2	1	2	2
	2	2	2	2	2	2
	2	2	2	2	2	3
	3	2	2	2	3	2
	2	3	3	2	3	2
	2	2		3	2	
	3	2		3	2	
Large	2	3	2	3	3	3
	3	3	3	3	3	2
	3	3	3	2	2	3
	2	2	3	3	2	3

*1 = normal, 2 = weak, 3 = paralyzed

tion rating means are related to monitoring and tumor size?

The independence assumption should hold, since the rating for one patient gives no information about the rating for another patient. But the ratings have an extremely nonnormal distribution, with only three possible values. Two-way ANOVA cannot be used to analyze these data. Instead, we could use the Mann-Whitney test described in Chapter 11 to test the hypothesis that the monitored population of ratings is identical to the nonmonitored population of ratings for patients with small tumors. We could then use the Mann-Whitney test two more times to test the hypothesis of identical monitored and non-monitored populations for patients with medium tumors and for patients with large tumors.

13.2 COMPUTER OUTPUT

In SPSS, two-way ANOVA calculations are done by the ANOVA and MANOVA programs. In SAS,

they are done by the ANOVA and GLM programs. The usual warnings about the computer's inability to check assumptions still apply.

SPSS/PC and SAS two-way ANOVA output for the caregiver data is shown in Figures 13.12 and 13.13. Both SPSS and SAS output include two-way ANOVA tables with formats similar to the format in Figure 13.5. In the SPSS/PC output, the error sum of squares is called the residual sum of squares. We will not use the SPSS/PC main effects sum of squares or the SPSS/PC explained sum of squares. Exact p-values are given under "Signif of F."

In SAS two-way ANOVA output, the factor and interaction sums of squares are listed under "TYPE III SS." The interaction sum of squares is called the $A*B$ sum of squares (EDUCATN*CAREGVNG for the caregiver output). We will not use the SAS model sum of squares, which is the same as the SPSS/PC explained sum of squares. Exact p-values are listed under "PR > F." All of the SPSS/PC and SAS p-values are consistent with the approximate p-values we obtained from Table E.5.

Source of Variation	Sum of Squares	DF	Mean Square	F	Signif of F
Main Effects	754.356	3	251.452	9.649	.000
EDUCATN	333.809	1	333.809	12.810	.001
CAREGVNG	407.821	2	203.910	7.825	.001
2-way Interactions	208.337	2	104.169	3.997	.021
EDUCATN CAREGVNG	208.337	2	104.169	3.997	.021
Explained	1326.161	5	265.232	10.178	.000
Residual	3101.039	119	26.059		
Total	4427.200	124	35.703		

Figure 13.12 SPSS/PC two-way ANOVA output for caregiver data

SOURCE	DF	SUM OF SQUARES	MEAN SQUARE	
MODEL	5	1326.16068581	265.23213716	
ERROR	119	3101.03931419	26.05915390	
CORRECTED TOTAL	124	4427.20000000		

SOURCE	DF	TYPE III SS	F VALUE	PR > F
EDUCATN	1	333.80883820	12.81	0.0005
CAREGVNG	2	407.82061535	7.82	0.0006
EDUCATN*CAREGVNG	2	208.33702442	4.00	0.0209

Figure 13.13 SAS two-way ANOVA output for caregiver data

13.3 MULTIPLE COMPARISONS

Multiple-comparison procedures are appropriate when two-way ANOVA F tests indicate that factor effects are present. If we decide that one or both factors have an effect, we want to determine which population cell means differ or which population factor means differ. Multiple-comparison procedures for comparing population means are used to do this.

When interaction is NOT present, population factor means are compared. When interaction IS present, population cell means are compared. Because cell means depend on the levels of *both* factors, comparison of cell means allows us to determine the nature of the interaction. Factor means depend only on the levels of one factor. They are compared only when interaction is not present. If interaction is not present and we cannot reject the hypothesis of equal population Factor A means or the hypothesis of equal population Factor B means, further analysis is not required. There is no point in trying to find differences between population means when we cannot reject the hypothesis that all of the population means are equal.

For the caregiver data, we did not reject the hypothesis of no interaction. We did reject the hypothesis of equal population education factor means and the hypothesis of equal population caregiving factor means. Comparison of the population caregiving factor means will allow us to describe the effect of caregiving status on the population mean quality-of-life score.

We will describe the Tukey and Bonferroni procedures for multiple comparisons in two-way ANOVA.* Both procedures require independent observations. If this assumption is violated, neither method can be used.

13.4 THE TUKEY METHOD FOR MULTIPLE COMPARISONS

Multiple-comparison procedures require estimated variances of sample cell means or sample factor means. It can be shown that the estimated variance of a sample cell mean is given by the formula

$$\text{var}(\bar{x}_{AiBj}) = \frac{\text{MSE}}{n_{AiBj}} \quad (13.10)$$

The cell size in this formula is the sample size for

the cell from which the mean $\bar{x}_{AiBj}$ was obtained. The estimated variance of a sample Factor A mean is given by the formula

$$\text{var}(\bar{x}_{Ai}) = \quad (13.11)$$

$$\frac{\text{MSE}}{b^2}\left(\frac{1}{n_{AiB1}} + \frac{1}{n_{AiB2}} + \cdots + \frac{1}{n_{AiBb}}\right)$$

The estimated variance of a sample Factor B mean is given by the formula

$$\text{var}(\bar{x}_{Bj}) = \quad (13.12)$$

$$\frac{\text{MSE}}{a^2}\left(\frac{1}{n_{A1Bj}} + \frac{1}{n_{A2Bj}} + \cdots + \frac{1}{n_{AaBj}}\right)$$

The MSE value is obtained from the two-way ANOVA table. In formulas (13.11) and (13.12), the MSE is divided by the square of the number of levels of the *other* factor. The cell sizes in formulas (13.11) and (13.12) are the sample sizes for the cells whose means were averaged to obtain the factor mean.

Using the caregiver data cell sizes on p. 314 and the MSE from Table 13.3, we can apply formula (13.12) to obtain the estimated variances for the sample caregiving factor means:

$$\text{var}(\bar{x}_{B1}) = \frac{26.1}{2^2}\left(\frac{1}{35} + \frac{1}{38}\right) = 0.36$$

$$\text{var}(\bar{x}_{B2}) = \frac{26.1}{2^2}\left(\frac{1}{15} + \frac{1}{11}\right) = 1.03$$

$$\text{var}(\bar{x}_{B3}) = \frac{26.1}{2^2}\left(\frac{1}{10} + \frac{1}{16}\right) = 1.06$$

Although we will not compare the education factor means, the estimated variances of the sample education factor means are shown in the following to illustrate the use of formula (13.11).

$$\text{var}(\bar{x}_{A1}) = \frac{26.1}{3^2}\left(\frac{1}{35} + \frac{1}{15} + \frac{1}{10}\right) = 0.57$$

$$\text{var}(\bar{x}_{A2}) = \frac{26.1}{3^2}\left(\frac{1}{38} + \frac{1}{11} + \frac{1}{16}\right) = 0.52$$

Formula (13.10) will be used later in Example 13.3.

Like the Tukey method for one-way ANOVA, the Tukey method for two-way ANOVA is based on studentized range distributions. Let $q_{\alpha, ab, n_T - ab}$ be the α upper percentage point of the studentized range distribution with ab numerator degrees of freedom and $n_T - ab$ denominator degrees of freedom. The $100(1 - \alpha)\%$ Tukey confidence intervals for differences between population *cell* means are

---

*Another multiple-comparison procedure for two-way ANOVA, the Scheffé method, is described in other texts.[2]

given by the formula

$$(13.13)$$

$$\left((\bar{x}_{AiBj} - \bar{x}_{AkBl}) - \frac{q_{\alpha, ab, n_T - ab}}{\sqrt{2}} \sqrt{\mathrm{var}(\bar{x}_{AiBj}) + \mathrm{var}(\bar{x}_{AkBl})} , \right.$$

$$\left. (\bar{x}_{AiBj} - \bar{x}_{AkBl}) + \frac{q_{\alpha, ab, n_T - ab}}{\sqrt{2}} \sqrt{\mathrm{var}(\bar{x}_{AiBj}) + \mathrm{var}(\bar{x}_{AkBl})} \right)$$

The variance formula (13.10) is used to obtain the estimated variances in formula (13.13).

Let $q_{\alpha, a, n_T - ab}$ be the α upper percentage point of the studentized range distribution with a numerator degrees of freedom and $n_T - ab$ denominator degrees of freedom. The $100(1 - \alpha)\%$ Tukey confidence intervals for differences between population *Factor A* means are given by the formula

$$(13.14)$$

$$\left((\bar{x}_{Ai} - \bar{x}_{Ak}) - \frac{q_{\alpha, a, n_T - ab}}{\sqrt{2}} \sqrt{\mathrm{var}(\bar{x}_{Ai}) + \mathrm{var}(\bar{x}_{Ak})} , \right.$$

$$\left. (\bar{x}_{Ai} - \bar{x}_{Ak}) + \frac{q_{\alpha, a, n_T - ab}}{\sqrt{2}} \sqrt{\mathrm{var}(\bar{x}_{Ai}) + \mathrm{var}(\bar{x}_{Ak})} \right)$$

The variance formula (13.11) is used to obtain the estimated variances in formula (13.14).

Let $q_{\alpha, b, n_T - ab}$ be the α upper percentage point of the studentized range distribution with b numerator degrees of freedom and $n_T - ab$ denominator degrees of freedom. The $100(1 - \alpha)\%$ Tukey confidence intervals for differences between population *Factor B* means are given by the formula

$$(13.15)$$

$$\left((\bar{x}_{Bj} - \bar{x}_{Bl}) - \frac{q_{\alpha, b, n_T - ab}}{\sqrt{2}} \sqrt{\mathrm{var}(\bar{x}_{Bj}) + \mathrm{var}(\bar{x}_{Bl})} , \right.$$

$$\left. (\bar{x}_{Bj} - \bar{x}_{Bl}) + \frac{q_{\alpha, b, n_T - ab}}{\sqrt{2}} \sqrt{\mathrm{var}(\bar{x}_{Bj}) + \mathrm{var}(\bar{x}_{Bl})} \right)$$

The variances in formula (13.15) are obtained from the variance formula (13.12).

Let us use the caregiver data to obtain 95% Tukey confidence intervals for differences between the population caregiving factor means. We want to determine which population caregiving factor means are different. Our studentized range upper percentage point is $q_{.05, 3, 119}$, since the caregiving factor has three levels and $n_T - ab = 125 - (2 \times 3) = 119$. The error degrees of freedom $n_T - ab$ can also be obtained from the two-way ANOVA table (Table 13.3). Since 119 df are not listed in Table E.6, we have to approximate. Looking up 3 in the top row and 120 in the first column of the $\alpha = 0.05$ section of Table E.6, we obtain $q_{.05, 3, 119} \cong q_{.05, 3, 120} = 3.36$. Using the sample caregiving factor means on p. 315 and the estimated variances on p. 321, we can apply formula (13.15) to get the following Tukey confidence intervals.

Confidence Interval for $\mu_{B1} - \mu_{B2}$ (Long-Term Caregivers Versus Short-Term Caregivers).

$$\left((34.9 - 38.8) - \frac{3.36}{\sqrt{2}} \sqrt{0.36 + 1.03} , \right.$$

$$\left. (34.9 - 38.8) + \frac{3.36}{\sqrt{2}} \sqrt{0.36 + 1.03} \right)$$

$$(-3.9 - 2.8, \quad -3.9 + 2.8)$$

$$(-6.7, -1.1)$$

Confidence Interval for $\mu_{B1} - \mu_{B3}$ (Long-Term Caregivers Versus Non-Caregivers).

$$\left((34.9 - 38.2) - \frac{3.36}{\sqrt{2}} \sqrt{0.36 + 1.06} , \right.$$

$$\left. (34.9 - 38.2) + \frac{3.36}{\sqrt{2}} \sqrt{0.36 + 1.06} \right)$$

$$(-3.3 - 2.8, \quad -3.3 + 2.8)$$

$$(-6.1, -0.5)$$

Confidence Interval for $\mu_{B2} - \mu_{B3}$ (Short-Term Caregivers Versus Non Caregivers).

$$\left((38.8 - 38.2) - \frac{3.36}{\sqrt{2}} \sqrt{1.03 + 1.06} , \right.$$

$$\left. (38.8 - 38.2) + \frac{3.36}{\sqrt{2}} \sqrt{1.03 + 1.06} \right)$$

$$(0.6 - 3.4, \quad 0.6 + 3.4)$$

$$(-2.8, 4.0)$$

We are 95% sure that the following is true.

1. The population mean quality-of-life score for long-term caregivers is smaller than the population mean quality-of-life score for short-term caregivers. The difference appears to be small (between 1.1 and 6.7).

2. The population mean quality-of-life score for long-term caregivers is smaller than the population mean quality-of-life score for non-caregivers. The difference appears to be small (between 0.5 and 6.1).

3. We cannot say that the population mean quality-of-life score for short-term caregivers differs from the population mean quality-of-life score for non-caregivers.

Because the *overall* confidence level is 95%, we are 95% sure that all of these conclusions are correct. We can summarize the results of our F tests and confidence intervals as follows:

1. The data do not provide evidence for interaction between education and caregiving status.

2. The data provide evidence that the population mean quality-of-life score for women with college education differs from the population mean quality-of-life score for women without college education.

3. The data provide evidence that the population mean quality-of-life score for long-term caregivers is slightly smaller than the population mean quality-of-life score for short-term caregivers and the population mean quality of life score for non-caregivers. The data do not provide evidence that the population mean quality-of-life score for short-term caregivers differs from the population mean quality-of-life score for non-caregivers.

Example 13.3

A study reported the serum levels of a glycoprotein antigen, CA125, in ovarian cancer patients receiving platinum therapy.[5] Table 13.6 shows the square root of the serum CA125 level before platinum therapy for 21 of these patients, grouped by tumor size and clinical response to platinum therapy. (The data were transformed by taking square roots in order to reduce skewness and make the variances more similar.) Sample cell means and sample cell standard deviations are also shown in this table.

We want to determine whether the population mean square-root CA125 level is related to two factors: clinical response and tumor size. The clinical response factor has two levels (1 = no response, 2 = complete response or no evaluable disease), and the tumor size factor has two levels (1 = less than 10 cm, 2 = at least 10 cm). We can assume that the observations are independent, since the square-root CA125 level for one patient should not tell us anything about the square-root CA125 level for another patient. Histograms of the observations in the two cells with at least five observations suggest slightly skewed populations, as you can verify. (Histograms for cells of size less than 5 are not helpful.) The ratio of the largest cell variance to the smallest cell variance is 5.5. Given four cells with small sample sizes, this ratio is consistent with similar population variances. Two-way ANOVA seems appropriate for analyzing these data.

The SPSS/PC two-way ANOVA table for the cancer data is shown in Figure 13.14. Let us use a significance level of 0.01 to test the hypothesis of no interaction. Since the p-value for the interaction F statistic is 0.002, we reject the hypothesis of no interaction. Because we have decided that interaction is present, we need to compare cell means rather than factor means.

A graph of the sample cell means, shown in Figure 13.15, can be used to help us select cell mean comparisons. This graph suggests that the population mean square-root CA125 levels for different tumor sizes differ when patients with no response are considered. When patients who respond are considered, the mean square-root CA125 levels for different tumor sizes do not seem to differ.

TABLE 13.6 SQUARE-ROOT SERUM CA125 LEVEL BEFORE PLATINUM THERAPY FOR OVARIAN CANCER PATIENTS WITH CELL MEANS AND STANDARD DEVIATIONS

Response	Tumor Size			
	< 10 CM		≥ 10 CM	
None	9.9		20.6	
	3.7		28.2	
	6.5		25.1	
	6.7 ± 3.1		23.7	
			24.4 ± 3.2	
Complete response	3.2	7.7	10.6	15.5
or no evaluable	22.4	20.5	21.2	14.2
disease	10.3	22.4	11.6	
	13.2	19.5	11.8	
	14.9 ± 7.3		14.2 ± 3.9	

Source of Variation	Sum of Squares	DF	Mean Square	F	Signif of F
Main Effects	351.492	2	175.746	5.963	.011
RESPONSE	4.839	1	4.839	.164	.690
SIZE	328.095	1	328.095	11.132	.004
2-way Interactions	387.222	1	387.222	13.138	.002
RESPONSE SIZE	387.222	1	387.222	13.138	.002
Explained	560.802	3	186.934	6.343	.004
Residual	501.043	17	29.473		
Total	1061.846	20	53.092		

Figure 13.14 SPSS/PC two-way ANOVA output for cancer data

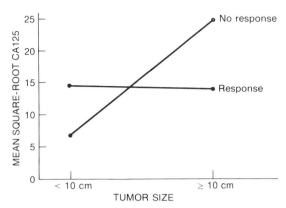

Figure 13.15 Plot of sample cell means for cancer data

We will use formula (13.13) to obtain a 90% Tukey confidence interval comparing the population mean square-root CA125 levels for different tumor sizes for patients who fail to respond. Just to confirm our impression from the graph, we will also obtain a 90% Tukey confidence interval comparing the population mean square-root CA125 levels for different tumor sizes for patients who respond. Let us arbitrarily consider clinical response to be Factor A and tumor size to be Factor B. Using formula (13.10) and the MSE in Figure 13.14, we get the estimated variances for the sample cell means:

$$\text{var}(\bar{x}_{A1B1}) = \frac{29.473}{3} = 9.82$$

$$\text{var}(\bar{x}_{A1B2}) = \frac{29.473}{4} = 7.37$$

$$\text{var}(\bar{x}_{A2B1}) = \frac{29.473}{8} = 3.68$$

$$\text{var}(\bar{x}_{A2B2}) = \frac{29.473}{6} = 4.91$$

Our studentized range upper percentage point is $q_{.10, 4, 17} = 3.50$, since $ab = 2 \times 2 = 4$ and $n_T - ab = 21 - 4 = 17$. The error (residual) degrees of freedom $n_T - ab$ can also be obtained from the two-way ANOVA table in Figure 13.14. Using the cell means in Table 13.6 and our estimated variances, we calculate the following 90% Tukey confidence intervals.

Confidence Interval for $\mu_{A1B1} - \mu_{A1B2}$ (Nonresponders with Small Tumors Versus Nonresponders with Large Tumors).

$$\left((6.7 - 24.4) - \frac{3.50}{\sqrt{2}} \sqrt{9.82 + 7.37}, \right.$$

$$\left. (6.7 - 24.4) + \frac{3.50}{\sqrt{2}} \sqrt{9.82 + 7.37} \right)$$

$$(-17.7 - 10.3, \quad -17.7 + 10.3)$$

$$(-28.0, -7.4)$$

Confidence Interval for $\mu_{A2B1} - \mu_{A2B2}$ (Responders with Small Tumors Versus Responders with Large Tumors).

$$\left((14.9 - 14.2) - \frac{3.50}{\sqrt{2}} \sqrt{3.68 + 4.91}, \right.$$

$$\left. (14.9 - 14.2) + \frac{3.50}{\sqrt{2}} \sqrt{3.68 + 4.91} \right)$$

$$(0.7 - 7.3, \quad 0.7 + 7.3)$$

$$(-6.6, 8.0)$$

Since the overall confidence level is 90%, we are 90% sure that the following is true.

1. When patients who fail to respond to platinum therapy are considered, the population mean square-root CA125 for patients with small tumors is smaller than the population mean square-root CA125 for patients with large tumors. The difference might be large (no less than 7.4) or extremely large (as high as 28.0).
2. When patients who respond to platinum therapy are considered, we cannot say that the population mean square-root CA125 for patients with small tumors differs from the population mean square-root CA125 for patients with large tumors.

We cannot make statements about any other differences between population cell means unless we calculate appropriate confidence intervals. It can be shown that there are six possible cell mean comparisons, and we obtained only two of these comparisons. For example, we did not compare the population means for small-tumor nonresponders and small-tumor responders, nor did we compare the population means for large-tumor nonresponders and large-tumor responders.

13.5 THE BONFERRONI METHOD FOR MULTIPLE COMPARISONS

Like the Bonferroni procedure for one-way ANOVA described in Chapter 8, the Bonferroni procedure for two-way ANOVA is based on adjusted upper percentage points of t distributions. If the comparisons to be made are selected *before* examining the sample means, the number c is defined by

$$c = \text{number of comparisons to be made}$$

If the comparisons are selected *after* examining the sample means, c is defined by

$$c = \text{total number of } possible \text{ comparisons}$$

In both cases, c refers to the number of cell mean

comparisons, the number of Factor A mean comparisons, or the number of Factor B mean comparisons.

To obtain Bonferroni confidence intervals, $\alpha/2c$ upper percentage points of the t distribution with $n_T - ab$ degrees of freedom are used. The $100(1 - \alpha)\%$ Bonferroni confidence intervals for differences between population *cell* means are given by the formula

$$(13.16)$$

$$\left((\bar{x}_{AiBj} - \bar{x}_{AkBl}) - t_{\alpha/2c, n_T - ab} \sqrt{\text{var}(\bar{x}_{AiBj}) + \text{var}(\bar{x}_{AkBl})} \right. ,$$

$$\left. (\bar{x}_{AiBj} - \bar{x}_{AkBl}) + t_{\alpha/2c, n_T - ab} \sqrt{\text{var}(\bar{x}_{AiBj}) + \text{var}(\bar{x}_{AkBl})} \right)$$

The variance formula (13.10) is used to obtain the estimated variances in formula (13.16).

The $100(1 - \alpha)\%$ Bonferroni confidence intervals for differences between population *Factor A* means are given by the formula

$$(13.17)$$

$$\left((\bar{x}_{Ai} - \bar{x}_{Ak}) - t_{\alpha/2c, n_T - ab} \sqrt{\text{var}(\bar{x}_{Ai}) + \text{var}(\bar{x}_{Ak})} \right. ,$$

$$\left. (\bar{x}_{Ai} - \bar{x}_{Ak}) + t_{\alpha/2c, n_T - ab} \sqrt{\text{var}(\bar{x}_{Ai}) + \text{var}(\bar{x}_{Ak})} \right)$$

The estimated variances in formula (13.17) are obtained from the variance formula (13.11).

The $100(1 - \alpha)\%$ Bonferroni confidence intervals for differences between population *Factor B* means are given by the formula

$$(13.18)$$

$$\left((\bar{x}_{Bj} - \bar{x}_{Bl}) - t_{\alpha/2c, n_T - ab} \sqrt{\text{var}(\bar{x}_{Bj}) + \text{var}(\bar{x}_{Bl})} \right. ,$$

$$\left. (\bar{x}_{Bj} - \bar{x}_{Bl}) + t_{\alpha/2c, n_T - ab} \sqrt{\text{var}(\bar{x}_{Bj}) + \text{var}(\bar{x}_{Bl})} \right)$$

The variance formula (13.12) is used to obtain the estimated variances in formula (13.18).

Let us obtain 95% Bonferroni confidence intervals for the differences between the caregiving factor means, using the caregiver data. There are three possible caregiving factor comparisons, so $c = 3$, and $0.05/(2 \times 3) = 0.0083$. Our t upper percentage point is $t_{.0083, 119} \cong t_{.0075, 120} = 2.468$. Using the fac-

tor means on p. 315 and the estimated variances on p. 321 in formula (13.18), we get the following Bonferroni confidence intervals.

Confidence Interval for $\mu_{B1} - \mu_{B2}$ (Long-Term Caregivers Versus Short-Term Caregivers).

$$\left((34.9 - 38.8) - 2.468\sqrt{0.36 + 1.03} \right. ,$$

$$\left. (34.9 - 38.8) + 2.468\sqrt{0.36 + 1.03} \right)$$

$$(-3.9 - 2.9, \quad -3.9 + 2.9)$$

$$(-6.8, -1.0)$$

Confidence Interval for $\mu_{B1} - \mu_{B3}$ (Long-Term Caregivers Versus Non-Caregivers).

$$\left((34.9 - 38.2) - 2.468\sqrt{0.36 + 1.06} \right. ,$$

$$\left. (34.9 - 38.2) + 2.468\sqrt{0.36 + 1.06} \right)$$

$$(-3.3 - 2.9, \quad -3.3 + 2.9)$$

$$(-6.2, -0.4)$$

Confidence Interval for $\mu_{B2} - \mu_{B3}$ (Short-Term Caregivers Versus Non-Caregivers).

$$\left((38.8 - 38.2) - 2.468\sqrt{1.03 + 1.06} \right. ,$$

$$\left. (38.8 - 38.2) + 2.468\sqrt{1.03 + 1.06} \right)$$

$$(0.6 - 3.6, \quad 0.6 + 3.6)$$

$$(-3.0, 4.2)$$

These confidence intervals are interpreted in the same way as the 95% Tukey confidence intervals on p. 322. For these data, the Bonferroni confidence intervals are slightly wider than the Tukey confidence intervals. In this case, the Tukey confidence intervals are preferred because they are slightly more precise.

We can also obtain 90% Bonferroni confidence intervals for differences between population cell means for the cancer data. We will use the same two comparisons we used for the Tukey confidence intervals. There are six possible cell mean comparisons, and we selected our two comparisons *after* examining the sample means, so $c = 6$. Since $0.10/(2 \times 6) = 0.0083$, our t upper percentage point is $t_{.0083, 17} \cong t_{.0075, 17} = 2.706$. Using the cell means in Table 13.6 and the estimated variances on p. 324, we apply formula (13.16) to calculate the following Bonferroni confidence intervals:

Confidence Interval for $\mu_{A1B1} - \mu_{A1B2}$ *(Nonresponders with Small Tumors Versus Nonresponders with Large Tumors).*

$$((6.7 - 24.4) - 2.706\sqrt{9.82 + 7.37},$$

$$(6.7 - 24.4) + 2.706\sqrt{9.82 + 7.37})$$

$$(-17.7 - 11.2, \quad -17.7 + 11.2)$$

$$(-28.9, -6.5)$$

Confidence Interval for $\mu_{A2B1} - \mu_{A2B2}$ *(Responders with Small Tumors Versus Responders with Large Tumors).*

$$((14.9 - 14.2) - 2.706\sqrt{3.68 + 4.91},$$

$$(14.9 - 14.2) + 2.706\sqrt{3.68 + 4.91})$$

$$(0.7 - 7.9, \quad 0.7 + 7.9)$$

$$(-7.2, 8.6)$$

Again, the Bonferroni confidence intervals are wider (less precise) than the Tukey confidence intervals, so the Tukey confidence intervals are preferred in this case. The Bonferroni confidence intervals are interpreted in the same way as the Tukey confidence intervals on p. 324.

The Bonferroni procedure for two-way ANOVA tends to produce narrower confidence intervals than the Tukey procedure when there is a large number of possible comparisons and only a few of these are selected *before* looking at the sample means. The Tukey procedure tends to produce narrower confidence intervals than the Bonferroni procedure when all of the possible comparisons are of interest or when comparisons are selected *after* looking at the sample means.

To determine which procedure will produce the narrowest confidence intervals for a particular confidence level, we obtain both the Tukey studentized range upper percentage point and the Bonferroni t upper percentage point. If the studentized range value divided by $\sqrt{2}$ is less than the t value, the Tukey confidence intervals will be narrower. If the studentized range value divided by $\sqrt{2}$ is greater than the t value, the Bonferroni confidence intervals will be narrower. If the studentized range value divided by $\sqrt{2}$ is equal to the t value, the Tukey and Bonferroni confidence intervals will be the same. For the cancer data, $q_{.10, 4, 17}/\sqrt{2} = 2.47$ and $t_{.0083, 17} \cong 2.706$ when all possible comparisons are taken into account. Since 2.47 is less than 2.706, we would choose the Tukey procedure for these data.

Multiple-comparison confidence intervals can be inconsistent with two-way ANOVA F statistics. It is possible for all $100(1 - \alpha)\%$ multiple-comparison confidence intervals to include 0 even when the hypothesis of equal population means is rejected at the significance level α. This problem can usually be resolved by reducing the confidence level until at least one of the confidence intervals does not include 0.

When three or more factors are investigated, three-way or higher analysis of variance can often be done to compare population means in order to determine the effects of the factors. These ANOVAs are also based on sums of squares and F statistics, and their tables look familiar to anyone acquainted with two-way ANOVA. The possible interaction effects are more complicated when more than two factors are examined. In three-way ANOVA, all three factors may interact, or the first two factors may interact, or the second two factors may interact, or the first and third factors may interact. The reader interested in this type of ANOVA should consult a more advanced text.[2]

If two factors are of interest and one or both of them involve repeated measurements, two-way analysis of variance cannot be used to compare population means. Two-factor repeated-measures analysis of variance should be considered instead. This procedure is an extension of one-factor repeated-measures ANOVA. A discussion of two-factor repeated-measures ANOVA can be found in other texts.[6,7]

SUMMARY

Two-way analysis of variance is used to determine whether population means are related to two factors. Independent observations, normal or approximately normal populations, and equal or similar population cell variances are required for two-way ANOVA. Interaction between the factors exists if the effect of one factor depends on the level of the other factor. The hypothesis of no interaction is the first hypothesis tested. If this hypothesis is rejected, no further hypothesis tests are done. If the hypothesis of no interaction is not rejected, the hypothesis of equal population factor means is tested for each factor.

If any of the null hypotheses are rejected, multiple comparisons are done to determine which population means are different. Cell means are compared if the hypothesis of no interaction is rejected. Factor means are compared if the hypothesis of no interaction is not rejected but at least one hypothesis of equal population factor means is rejected. Two commonly used multiple-comparison procedures are the Tukey method and the Bonferroni method. The multiple-comparison procedure that produces the narrowest confidence intervals should be used.

FREQUENTLY USED TWO-WAY ANOVA FORMULAS

F statistic for testing H_0: No interaction

$$F = \frac{\text{MSAB}}{\text{MSE}}$$

F statistic for testing H_0: $\mu_{A1} = \mu_{A2} = \mu_{A3} = \cdots = \mu_{Aa}$

$$F = \frac{\text{MSA}}{\text{MSE}}$$

F statistic for testing H_0: $\mu_{B1} = \mu_{B2} = \mu_{B3} = \cdots = \mu_{Bb}$

$$F = \frac{\text{MSB}}{\text{MSE}}$$

Estimated variance of cell mean

$$\text{var}(\bar{x}_{AiBj}) = \frac{\text{MSE}}{n_{AiBj}}$$

Estimated variance of Factor A mean

$$\text{var}(\bar{x}_{Ai}) = \frac{\text{MSE}}{b^2}\left(\frac{1}{n_{AiB1}} + \frac{1}{n_{AiB2}} + \cdots + \frac{1}{n_{AiBb}}\right)$$

Estimated variance of Factor B mean

$$\text{var}(\bar{x}_{Bj}) = \frac{\text{MSE}}{a^2}\left(\frac{1}{n_{A1Bj}} + \frac{1}{n_{A2Bj}} + \cdots + \frac{1}{n_{AaBj}}\right)$$

$100(1 - \alpha)\%$ Tukey confidence interval for difference between population cell means

$$\left((\bar{x}_{AiBj} - \bar{x}_{AkBl}) - \frac{q_{\alpha,\,ab,\,n_T-ab}}{\sqrt{2}}\sqrt{\text{var}(\bar{x}_{AiBj}) + \text{var}(\bar{x}_{AkBl})},\right.$$

$$\left.(\bar{x}_{AiBj} - \bar{x}_{AkBl}) + \frac{q_{\alpha,\,ab,\,n_T-ab}}{\sqrt{2}}\sqrt{\text{var}(\bar{x}_{AiBj}) + \text{var}(\bar{x}_{AkBl})}\right)$$

$100(1 - \alpha)\%$ Tukey confidence interval for difference between population Factor A means

$$\left((\bar{x}_{Ai} - \bar{x}_{Ak}) - \frac{q_{\alpha,\,a,\,n_T-ab}}{\sqrt{2}}\sqrt{\text{var}(\bar{x}_{Ai}) + \text{var}(\bar{x}_{Ak})},\right.$$

$$\left.(\bar{x}_{Ai} - \bar{x}_{Ak}) + \frac{q_{\alpha,\,a,\,n_T-ab}}{\sqrt{2}}\sqrt{\text{var}(\bar{x}_{Ai}) + \text{var}(\bar{x}_{Ak})}\right)$$

$100(1 - \alpha)\%$ Tukey confidence interval for difference between population Factor B means

$$\left((\bar{x}_{Bj} - \bar{x}_{Bl}) - \frac{q_{\alpha,\,b,\,n_T-ab}}{\sqrt{2}}\sqrt{\text{var}(\bar{x}_{Bj}) + \text{var}(\bar{x}_{Bl})},\right.$$

$$\left.(\bar{x}_{Bj} - \bar{x}_{Bl}) + \frac{q_{\alpha,\,b,\,n_T-ab}}{\sqrt{2}}\sqrt{\text{var}(\bar{x}_{Bj}) + \text{var}(\bar{x}_{Bl})}\right)$$

$100(1 - \alpha)\%$ Bonferroni confidence interval for difference between population cell means

$$\left((\bar{x}_{AiBj} - \bar{x}_{AkBl}) - t_{\alpha/2c,\,n_T-ab}\sqrt{\text{var}(\bar{x}_{AiBj}) + \text{var}(\bar{x}_{AkBl})},\right.$$

$$\left.(\bar{x}_{AiBj} - \bar{x}_{AkBl}) + t_{\alpha/2c,\,n_T-ab}\sqrt{\text{var}(\bar{x}_{AiBj}) + \text{var}(\bar{x}_{AkBl})}\right)$$

$100(1 - \alpha)\%$ Bonferroni confidence interval for difference between population Factor A means

$$\left((\bar{x}_{Ai} - \bar{x}_{Ak}) - t_{\alpha/2c,\,n_T-ab}\sqrt{\text{var}(\bar{x}_{Ai}) + \text{var}(\bar{x}_{Ak})},\right.$$

$$\left.(\bar{x}_{Ai} - \bar{x}_{Ak}) + t_{\alpha/2c,\,n_T-ab}\sqrt{\text{var}(\bar{x}_{Ai}) + \text{var}(\bar{x}_{Ak})}\right)$$

$100(1 - \alpha)\%$ Bonferroni confidence interval for difference between population Factor B means

$$\left((\bar{x}_{Bj} - \bar{x}_{Bl}) - t_{\alpha/2c,\,n_T-ab}\sqrt{\text{var}(\bar{x}_{Bj}) + \text{var}(\bar{x}_{Bl})},\right.$$

$$\left.(\bar{x}_{Bj} - \bar{x}_{Bl}) + t_{\alpha/2c,\,n_T-ab}\sqrt{\text{var}(\bar{x}_{Bj}) + \text{var}(\bar{x}_{Bl})}\right)$$

PROBLEMS

The following instructions apply to problems 2 through 14.

1. In each problem, data are described, SPSS/PC two-way ANOVA output is presented, and a question is asked about the data. Determine whether two-way ANOVA is appropriate for analyzing the data. If it is not appropriate, state which assumptions are violated.

2. If the two-way ANOVA assumptions are satisfied, carry out all appropriate F tests. Specify the null and alternative hypotheses and find the most exact p-values that can be obtained from Table E.5. Interpret the p-values.

3. If any of the null hypotheses are rejected, carry out an appropriate multiple-comparison procedure. You must calculate sample factor means when population factor mean comparisons are appropriate, since only sample cell means are given. Use the confidence intervals and p-values to answer the question in the problem.

You may wish to obtain quick histograms for each cell. Histograms are not helpful when the cell size is less than 5. Do not worry about slightly or moderately nonnormal histograms if the data have a large number of possible values. Unless the data are extremely nonnormal and the sample is very small, you can assume that the central limit theorem applies to the data.

1. Construct a flowchart that will help you carry out two-way ANOVA tests in the correct order and select population cell means or factor means for comparison. The flowchart should begin as follows:

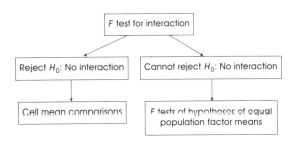

TABLE 13.7   PCV (%) WITH CELL MEANS AND STANDARD DEVIATIONS

Neutrophil Morphology	Age (yr)		
	≤ 1	$> 1 \& < 5$	≥ 5
Toxic vacuolation	22.5	25.0 20.0	26.0
	24.0	22.0 22.0	27.0
	23.5	27.5 16.0	15.5
	15.5	15.5 13.0	18.0
	35.0	21.5 32.0	31.0
	30.0	27.0 24.0	25.0
	17.0	15.0	28.0
		11.0	20.0
	23.9 ± 6.8	13.5	34.5
		20.3 ± 6.2	25.0 ± 6.2
Normal	27.0	27.0 15.0	34.0 28.0
	38.0	13.5 17.0	23.0 21.0
	36.0	21.0 27.0	34.0 4.5
	34.5	34.0 35.0	19.0
	38.0	19.5	27.0
	34.7 ± 4.6	23.2 ± 7.9	23.8 ± 9.6

2. In a study of methods for detecting antineutrophil antibody in cat serum, the packed cell volumes (PCVs) in Table 13.7 were reported for 53 clinically neutropenic cats.[8] Two factors are of interest: age (level 1 = one year or less, level 2 = greater than one year and less than five years, level 3 = at least five years) and neutrophil morphology (level 1 = toxic vacuolation, level 2 = normal). Do the data provide evidence that the population PCV means are related to these factors? Use a 0.10 significance level and a 90% overall confidence level for multiple comparisons. If interaction is present, assume that the only comparisons of interest are those between cats one year old or less with normal neutrophil morphology and the three age groups of cats with toxic vacuolation. Also assume that these comparisons were selected after examining the sample means. (There are 15 possible cell mean comparisons.)

TABLE 13.8   DAYS OF PREVIOUS VENTILATOR SUPPORT WITH CELL MEANS AND STANDARD DEVIATIONS

Outcome	COPD	
	PRESENT	ABSENT
Successful	2	2 3
	4	5 2
	3.0 ± 1.4	2 2
		2 2
		2.5 ± 1.1
Unsuccessful	58	77
	47	3
	82	9
	62.3 ± 17.9	19
		27.0 ± 34.0

3. In a study of weaning from mechanical ventilation, the number of days of previous ventilator support shown in Table 13.8 was reported for 17 patients.[9] Two factors are of interest: outcome of weaning attempt (level 1 = successful, level 2 = unsuccessful) and chronic obstructive pulmonary disease (COPD) (level 1 = present, level 2 = absent). Do the data provide evidence that the population mean numbers of days are related to these factors? Use a 0.01 significance level for hypothesis tests and a 95% overall confidence level for multiple comparisons.

4. In a study of attachment in children with developmental disorders, children with developmental disorders were videotaped after being left by their parents in a playroom.[10] Table 13.9 shows the score on the Behavior Checklist for Deviant Preschoolers (BCDP) for 33 of these children. The higher the BCDP score, the greater the severity of behavioral symptoms. Two factors are of interest: negative mood change after separation from parent (level 1 = present, level 2 = absent) and diagnosis

```
Source of Variation          Sum of      DF       Mean
                             Squares              Square

Main Effects                 631.371      3      210.457
    AGE                      436.416      2      218.208
    MORPH                    205.579      1      205.579

2-way Interactions           249.037      2      124.518
    AGE       MORPH          249.037      2      124.518

Explained                    788.836      5      157.767

Residual                    2343.372     47       49.859

Total                       3132.208     52       60.235
```

Figure 13.16   SPSS/PC two-way ANOVA results for PCV

Figure 13.17 SPSS/PC two-way ANOVA results for days of previous support

Source of Variation	Sum of Squares	DF	Mean Square
Main Effects	8578.970	2	4289.485
OUTCOME	5816.299	1	5816.299
COPD	1062.644	1	1062.644
2-way Interactions	1004.161	1	1004.161
OUTCOME COPD	1004.161	1	1004.161
Explained	8579.098	3	2859.699
Residual	4114.667	13	316.513
Total	12693.765	16	793.360

TABLE 13.9   BCDP SCORE WITH CELL MEANS AND STANDARD DEVIATIONS

Negative Mood Change	Diagnosis		
	DEVELOPMENTAL LANGUAGE DISORDER	ATYPICAL PERVASIVE DEVELOPMENTAL DISORDER	AUTISM
Present	7	13	31 32
	8	14	37 41
	18	17	44 51
		31	53 68
			54
	11.0 ± 6.1	18.8 ± 8.3	45.7 ± 12.0
Absent	8	13	39
	18	18	41
	28	27	42
	35	41	42
	55	15	46
		27	51
	28.8 ± 17.9	23.5 ± 10.4	43.5 ± 4.3

Figure 13.18 SPSS/PC two-way ANOVA results for BCDP score

Source of Variation	Sum of Squares	DF	Mean Square
Main Effects	4530.115	3	1510.038
MOODCHGE	338.400	1	338.400
DIAGNSIS	4507.347	2	2253.674
2-way Interactions	491.519	2	245.759
MOODCHGE DIAGNSIS	491.519	2	245.759
Explained	4981.995	5	996.399
Residual	3346.550	27	123.946
Total	8328.545	32	260.267

TABLE 13.10 BLOOD ARSENIC AND ICG HALF-LIFE (MINUTES) WITH CELL MEANS AND STANDARD DEVIATIONS

Sex	Chemical	
	ARSENIC	ICG
Female	58.2	7.1
	28.4	5.9
	83.4	11.6
	56.7 ± 27.5	8.2 ± 3.0
Male	33.7	6.6
	20.5	6.5
	33.9	6.7
	29.4 ± 7.7	6.6 ± 0.1

TABLE 13.11 LOG (GDS + 1) WITH CELL MEANS AND STANDARD DEVIATIONS

Sex	Thyroid Function			
	EUTHYROID		HYPOTHYROID	
Female	0.00	1.95	1.61	1.61
	1.61	2.40	2.30	1.61
	1.61	0.69	1.39	3.18
	0.69		1.10	
	1.28 ± 0.84		1.83 ± 0.70	
Male	1.61	1.95	2.56	2.71
	0.00	1.79	2.20	1.10
	1.39	1.39	0.00	1.39
	0.00	3.14	0.69	1.95
	2.08		1.39	
	1.48 ± 0.99		1.55 ± 0.89	

(level 1 = developmental language disorder, level 2 = atypical pervasive developmental disorder, level 3 = autism). Do the data provide evidence that the population BCDP means are related to these factors? Use a 0.01 significance level for hypothesis tests and a 90% overall confidence level for multiple comparisons. If only the hypothesis of equal population diagnosis factor means is rejected, assume that the only comparisons of interest are those between autistic children and the other two groups of children. Also assume that these comparisons were selected before examining the sample means.

5. A study of the disposition kinetics of thiacetarsamide in dogs presented the blood arsenic and indocyanine green (ICG) half-lives shown in Table 13.10.[11] Each of the six dogs studied was given both thiacetarsamide and ICG. Two factors are of interest: sex (level 1 = female, level 2 = male) and chemical (level 1 = arsenic, level 2 = ICG). Do the data provide evidence that the population half-life means are related to these factors? Use a 0.05 significance level for hypothesis tests and a 95% overall confidence level for multiple comparisons.

6. In a study of depression and hypothyroidism in nursing-home residents, Geriatric Depression Scale (GDS) scores were reported for 16 hypothyroid nursing-home residents and 16 euthyroid nursing-home residents.[12] Table 13.11 shows the logarithms of these GDS scores. (The number 1 was added to each score before taking logarithms, since some of the scores were equal to 0. The data were transformed in this way to reduce skewness and obtain more similar variances.) The higher the log(GDS + 1) score, the greater the depression. Two factors are of interest: sex (level 1 = female, level 2 = male) and thyroid function (level 1 = euthyroid, level 2 = hypothyroid). Do the data provide evidence that the population log(GDS + 1) means are related to these factors? Use a 0.01 significance level for hypothesis tests and a 99% overall confidence level for multiple comparisons.

7. A testicular hypothermia device was evaluated in 64 men with subfertile semen and elevated testicular temperature.[13] The logarithm of the motile oval index after treatment for these men is shown in Table 13.12. (The number 1 was added to the index values before taking logarithms, since some of the values were equal to 0. The data were transformed in this way to reduce skewness and obtain more similar variances.) Two factors are of interest: diagnosis (level 1 = no varicocele, level

Source of Variation	Sum of Squares	DF	Mean Square
Main Effects	4432.048	2	2216.024
SEX	626.407	1	626.407
CHEMICAL	3805.641	1	3805.641
2-way Interactions	495.368	1	495.368
SEX CHEMICAL	495.368	1	495.368
Explained	4927.416	3	1642.472
Residual	1652.053	8	206.507
Total	6579.469	11	598.134

Figure 13.19 SPSS/PC two-way ANOVA results for half-life

Source of Variation	Sum of Squares	DF	Mean Square
Main Effects	.769	2	.385
THYROID	.759	1	.759
SEX	.010	1	.010
2-way Interactions	.449	1	.449
THYROID SEX	.449	1	.449
Explained	1.089	3	.363
Residual	21.326	28	.762
Total	22.415	31	.723

Figure 13.20 SPSS/PC two-way ANOVA results for log(GDS + 1) score

TABLE 13.12 LOG(MOTILE OVAL INDEX + 1) AFTER TREATMENT WITH CELL MEANS AND STANDARD DEVIATIONS

Diagnosis	Initial Motile Oval Index		
	< 1 MILLION/ml	1–4.8 MILLION/ml	> 4.8 MILLION/ml
No varicocele	0.00 2.22 0.47 0.53 0.64 0.69 1.03 0.00 2.26 2.30	0.00 2.52 1.31 2.48 0.00	1.70 1.72 2.70 2.99 3.10 3.16 3.69
	1.01 ± 0.91	1.26 ± 1.25	2.72 ± 0.75
Failed varicocele operation	0.00 0.53 2.28 0.26 0.00 0.74 1.19 0.00 2.82 3.14	0.00 1.28 1.69 2.09 2.10	1.90 2.05 2.19 2.26 2.42 2.59 4.27
	1.10 ± 1.22	1.43 ± 0.87	2.53 ± 0.80
Varicocele	0.26 0.34 0.41 1.61 1.65 1.95 2.27 2.34 2.46 3.01	0.74 1.65 2.29 1.56 ± 0.78	1.59 2.56 2.76 2.80 3.38 3.91 4.45
	1.63 ± 0.98		3.06 ± 0.94

Source of Variation	Sum of Squares	DF	Mean Square
Main Effects	33.361	4	8.340
DIAGNSIS	1.888	2	.944
INDEX	30.743	2	15.371
2-way Interactions	.466	4	.116
DIAGNSIS INDEX	.466	4	.116
Explained	34.488	8	4.311
Residual	52.518	55	.955
Total	87.006	63	1.381

Figure 13.21 SPSS/PC two-way ANOVA results for log(index + 1)

TABLE 13.13 HAMILTON DEPRESSION SCORE WITH CELL MEANS AND STANDARD DEVIATIONS

Age	Duration of Pain	
	< 5 YEARS	≥ 5 YEARS
< 40 years	24.0 2.0	8.0
	5.0 23.0	27.0
	2.0 4.0	16.0
	18.0	18.0
	12.0	21.0
	11.2 ± 9.3	18.0 ± 7.0
≥ 40 years	21.0 22.0	18.0 5.0
	20.0	13.0 5.0
	18.0	18.0 11.0
	8.0	8.0 6.0
	18.0	12.0
	17.8 ± 5.1	10.7 ± 5.1

TABLE 13.14 PERCENTAGE OF VALID BREATHS WITH CELL MEANS AND CELL STANDARD DEVIATIONS

Calibration Volume	Subject	Validation Volume		
		LOW	NORMAL	HIGH
Low	1	92.3	84.6	92.3
	2	100.0	0.0	0.0
	3	100.0	100.0	0.0
	4	94.1	94.1	35.3
	5	94.1	88.2	17.6
	6	75.0	25.0	41.7
	7	100.0	100.0	0.0
	8	100.0	100.0	33.3
		94.4 ± 8.5	74.0 ± 39.0	27.5 ± 31.3
Normal	1	100.0	100.0	100.0
	2	13.3	93.3	93.3
	3	100.0	100.0	0.0
	4	100.0	100.0	6.2
	5	100.0	100.0	72.7
	6	42.1	89.5	89.5
	7	100.0	100.0	65.0
	8	81.8	100.0	45.5
		79.6 ± 33.6	97.8 ± 4.1	59.0 ± 38.7
High	1	88.2	94.1	100.0
	2	64.3	100.0	100.0
	3	0.0	0.0	100.0
	4	0.0	0.0	87.5
	5	100.0	100.0	100.0
	6	66.7	93.3	93.3
	7	7.7	23.1	100.0
	8	41.2	58.8	64.7
		46.0 ± 40.0	58.7 ± 44.8	93.2 ± 12.4

2 = failed varicocele operation, level 3 = varicocele) and initial (before-treatment) motile oval index (level 1 = less than 1 million/ml, level 2 = at least 1 million/ml but no more than 4.8 million/ml, level 3 = more than 4.8 million per ml). Do the data provide evidence that the population log(index + 1) means are related to these factors? Use a 0.01 significance level for hypothesis tests and a 90% overall confidence level for multiple comparisons.

8. In a study of chronic facial pain, Hamilton depression scores were reported for 28 patients with chronic oral-facial pain.[14] These data are shown in Table 13.13. Two factors are of interest: age (level 1 = less than 40 years, level 2 = at least 40 years) and duration of pain (level 1 = less than five years, level 2 = at least five years). Do the data provide evidence that the population Hamilton depression score means are related to these factors? Use a 0.10 significance level for hypothesis tests and an 80% overall confidence level for multiple comparisons. If the hypothesis of no interaction is rejected, assume that only the duration comparisons within the age groups are of interest. Also assume that these comparisons were selected before examining the sample means. Use the Bonferroni procedure to obtain multiple comparisons.

9. A study investigated whether the size of the breaths used for calibrating the respiratory induc-

Source of Variation	Sum of Squares	DF	Mean Square
Main Effects	1.517	2	.758
AGE	.933	1	.933
DURATION	.288	1	.288
2-way Interactions	321.302	1	321.302
AGE DURATION	321.302	1	321.302
Explained	325.774	3	108.591
Residual	1140.333	24	47.514
Total	1466.107	27	54.300

Figure 13.22 SPSS/PC two-way ANOVA results for Hamilton depression score

Source of Variation	Sum of Squares	DF	Mean Square
Main Effects	6629.571	4	1657.393
CALIBRTN	2795.268	2	1397.634
VALIDTN	3834.303	2	1917.152
2-way Interactions	30556.272	4	7639.068
CALIBRTN VALIDTN	30556.272	4	7639.068
Explained	37185.843	8	4648.230
Residual	62739.031	63	995.858
Total	99924.874	71	1407.393

Figure 13.23 SPSS/PC two-way ANOVA results for percentage of valid breaths

tive plethysmograph (RIP) affected the accuracy of the RIP.[15] Eight healthy, nonsmoking male subjects were asked to perform low-tidal-volume breathing, normal-tidal-volume breathing, and high-tidal-volume breathing. Table 13.14 shows the percentage of RIP breaths within 10% of actual spirometric volumes (percentage of valid breaths). Two factors are of interest: the tidal volume used to calibrate the RIP, or calibration volume (level 1 = low, level 2 = normal, level 3 = high), and the actual spirometer volume, or validation volume (level 1 = low, level 2 = normal, level 3 = high). Do the data provide evidence that the population mean percentages of valid breaths are related to these factors? Use a 0.01 significance level for hypothesis tests and a 90% overall confidence level for multiple comparisons.

10. In a study of neuroendocrine function and endogenous depression, Hamilton depression scores were reported for 40 patients with endogenous depression.[16] Table 13.15 shows the logarithm of the depression score for these patients. (The data were transformed by taking logarithms in order to reduce skewness and obtain more similar variances.) The larger the log depression score, the greater the depression. Two factors are of interest: dexametha-

TABLE 13.15 LOG HAMILTON DEPRESSION SCORE WITH CELL MEANS AND STANDARD DEVIATIONS

DST Result	Previous Episodes of Depression		
	NONE	AT LEAST ONE	
Suppressed	3.53	3.22	3.37
	2.94	3.00	3.50
	3.47	3.00	3.09
	3.33	2.83	3.58
	3.30	3.09	3.09
	3.00	3.40	3.18
		3.40	3.33
	3.26 ± 0.24	3.56	3.47
		2.94	3.40
		3.26	
		3.25 ± 0.22	
Not suppressed	3.18	3.74	
	3.00	3.00	
	3.18	3.14	
	3.40	3.09	
	3.74	3.37	
	3.58	2.89	
	3.26	3.30	
		3.40	
	3.33 ± 0.26		
		3.24 ± 0.27	

Source of Variation	Sum of Squares	DF	Mean Square
Main Effects	.039	2	.020
DST	.009	1	.009
EPISODES	.023	1	.023
2-way Interactions	.014	1	.014
DST EPISODES	.014	1	.014
Explained	.044	3	.015
Residual	2.075	36	.058
Total	2.118	39	.054

Figure 13.24 SPSS/PC two-way ANOVA results for log depression score

TABLE 13.16 SIGNED SQUARE-ROOT HEIGHT DEVIATE WITH CELL MEANS AND STANDARD DEVIATIONS

Height at Start of Treatment	Pubertal Rating at Start of Treatment		
	I	II–III	IV–V
Less than mean for girl's age	0.52	−1.00	−1.01
	−0.49	−0.26	−1.20
	−1.12	0.42	0.55
	−1.09		
		−0.28 ± 0.71	−0.56 ± 0.96
	−0.54 ± 0.77		
Greater than or equal to mean for girl's age	0.52 0.82	1.40	0.00 0.73
	0.92 1.50	1.62	1.41 0.00
	1.03 0.00	−0.73	0.00 0.82
	1.03 1.22	1.36	1.27
	1.32 1.44	1.15	1.33
	0.00 1.33	1.18	0.88
	1.06 0.00		−0.35
		1.00 ± 0.86	
	0.87 ± 0.54		0.61 ± 0.65

standardized height deviates for 40 girls with thyrotoxicosis. (The square root of the height deviate's absolute value was calculated and then given the same sign as the height deviate. The data were transformed in this way to reduce skewness and obtain more similar variances.) A negative square-root height deviate indicates that the girl's height is below the mean height for her age. A positive square-root height deviate indicates that the girl's height is above the mean height for her age. A square-root height deviate of 0 indicates that the girl's height is equal to the mean height for her age. Two factors are of interest: height at the start of treatment (level 1 = less than the mean height for child's age, level 2 = greater than or equal to the mean height for child's age) and Tanner pubertal rating at the start of treatment (level 1 = I, level

sone suppression test (DST) result (level 1 = suppressed, level 2 = not suppressed) and previous episodes of depression (level 1 = none, level 2 = at least one). Do the data provide evidence that the population log depression score means are related to these factors? Use a 0.10 significance level for hypothesis tests and a 90% overall confidence level for multiple comparisons.

11. In a study of the effect of thyrotoxicosis on growth, standardized height deviates at the end of follow-up were reported for children who developed thyrotoxicosis after infancy.[17] These standardized deviates were calculated as follows.

standardized height deviate

$$= \frac{\text{child's height} - \text{mean height for child's age}}{\text{standard deviation of heights for child's age}}$$

Table 13.16 shows the signed square roots of these

TABLE 13.17 SQUARE-ROOT KYPHOSIS (SQUARE-ROOT DEGREES) WITH CELL MEANS AND STANDARD DEVIATIONS

Treatment	No. of Vertebrae in Curve		
	3–7	8–13	14–16
None	7.00 5.83	7.28 5.83	5.92
	6.56 6.56	6.71 6.48	6.71
	6.86 5.39	5.10 5.57	6.40
	6.08 6.63	5.00 6.48	5.48
	6.93 5.66	5.66 5.92	6.13 ± 0.54
	6.71 6.63	6.56 5.66	
	7.00 6.78	3.46 6.63	
	6.32 6.48	6.40 5.29	
	6.48 6.71	5.66 5.57	
	6.71	5.00	
	6.49 ± 0.45	5.80 ± 0.86	
Brace	5.57	5.48	4.58
	6.56	6.16	4.69
	4.69	5.57	4.24
	6.32	8.25	4.50 ± 0.23
	5.10	6.36 ± 1.29	
	5.65 ± 0.79		

Source of Variation	Sum of Squares	DF	Mean Square
Main Effects	12.129	3	4.043
PUBERTY	.475	2	.238
STARTHT	11.881	1	11.881
2-way Interactions	.085	2	.043
PUBERTY STARTHT	.085	2	.043
Explained	13.081	5	2.616
Residual	15.863	34	.467
Total	28.943	39	.742

Figure 13.25 SPSS/PC two-way ANOVA results for square-root height deviate

Source of Variation	Sum of Squares	DF	Mean Square
Main Effects	7.083	3	2.361
TREATMNT	3.178	1	3.178
VERTEBRA	3.204	2	1.602
2-way Interactions	6.333	2	3.167
TREATMNT VERTEBRA	6.333	2	3.167
Explained	13.192	5	2.638
Residual	25.413	48	.529
Total	38.605	53	.728

Figure 13.26 SPSS/PC two-way ANOVA results for square-root kyphosis

TABLE 13.18 SQUARE-ROOT LVEF (SQUARE-ROOT %) WITH CELL MEANS AND STANDARD DEVIATIONS

Sex	Endomyocardial Biopsy Results		
	NORMAL	NONSPECIFIC CHANGE	MYOCARDITIS
Female	4.80	6.71	7.48
	3.46	5.48	6.00
	4.58		5.83
	4.13 ± 0.95	3.16	5.20
		4.90	4.47
		4.97 ± 1.30	6.08
			5.84 ± 1.01
Male	4.47	4.47 5.39	8.12
	6.63	4.24 4.58	7.94
	4.69	6.63 3.87	3.87
	6.00	4.12 5.39	
			6.64 ± 2.40
	5.45 ± 1.04	4.84 ± 0.91	

$2 = $ II–III, level $3 = $ IV–V). Do the data provide evidence that the population square-root height deviate means are related to these factors? Use a 0.01 significance level for hypothesis tests and a 95% overall confidence level for multiple comparisons.

12. A study examined methods for measuring the back in patients with scoliosis.[18] Table 13.17 shows the square root of the kyphosis for 54 patients with adolescent idiopathic scoliosis. (The data were transformed by taking square roots in order to obtain more similar variances.) The larger the square-root kyphosis, the larger the kyphosis. Two factors are of interest: treatment (level $1 = $ none, level $2 = $ brace) and number of vertebrae in the curve (level $1 = $ three to seven, level $2 = $ eight to 13, level $3 = $ 14 to 16). Do the data provide evidence that the population square-root kyphosis means are related to these factors? Use a 0.01 significance level for hypothesis tests and a 90% overall confidence level for multiple comparisons. If the hypothesis of no interaction is rejected, assume that the only comparisons of interest are those between untreated patients and patients treated

Source of Variation	Sum of Squares	DF	Mean Square
Main Effects	10.973	3	3.658
BIOPSY	10.481	2	5.241
SEX	2.516	1	2.516
2-way Interactions	2.282	2	1.141
BIOPSY SEX	2.282	2	1.141
Explained	12.300	5	2.460
Residual	33.254	22	1.512
Total	45.554	27	1.687

Figure 13.27 SPSS/PC two-way ANOVA results for square-root LVEF

with a brace. Also assume that these comparisons were selected after examining the sample means. (There are 15 possible cell mean comparisons.)

13. In a study of antimyosin antibody imaging for the diagnosis of acute myocarditis, the left ventricular ejection fraction (LVEF) was reported for 28 patients who presented with possible acute myocarditis.[19] Table 13.18 shows the square roots of these LVEF values. (The data were transformed by taking square roots in order to reduce skewness and obtain more similar variances.) Two factors are of interest: sex (level 1 = female, level 2 = male) and endomyocardial biopsy result (level 1 = normal, level 2 = nonspecific change, level 3 = myocarditis). Do the data provide evidence that the population

square-root LVEF means are related to these factors? Use a 0.05 significance level for hypothesis tests and a 95% overall confidence level for multiple comparisons.

14. A study evaluated the effectiveness of the Salter innominate osteotomy for the treatment of congenital hip dislocation.[20] Table 13.19 shows the logarithm of the age at surgery for 50 children with hip dislocations treated with the Salter osteotomy. (The data were transformed by taking logarithms in order to reduce skewness and obtain more similar variances.) The larger the log age, the older the child. Two factors are of interest: previous treatment (level 1 = closed reduction of the hip, level 2 = open reduction of the hip, level 3 = open reduction and innominate osteotomy) and clinical results of Salter osteotomy (level 1 = poor or fair, level 2 = good or excellent). Do the data provide evidence that the population log age means are related to these factors? Use a 0.01 significance level for hypothesis tests and a 90% overall confidence level for multiple comparisons.

15. Find an article in a medical or health care journal in which two-way ANOVA was incorrectly used to analyze nonindependent or extremely nonnormal data. Photocopy the article and write a letter to the journal editor that clearly describes the statistical error.

TABLE 13.19 LOGARITHM OF AGE (LOG MONTHS) AT TIME OF SALTER OSTEOTOMY WITH CELL MEANS AND STANDARD DEVIATIONS

Clinical Results	Previous Treatment		
	CLOSED REDUCTION	OPEN REDUCTION	OPEN REDUCTION + OSTEOTOMY
Poor or fair	4.19	3.87	3.74
	4.30	4.30	4.13
	4.34	4.76	4.38
	4.34		
	4.43	4.31 + 0.45	4.08 ± 0.32
	4.80		
	4.40 ± 0.21		
Good or excellent	2.89 3.33	2.89 3.91	2.89
	3.04 3.33	3.04 4.13	3.00
	3.04 3.50	3.53 4.23	3.04
	3.09 3.71	3.56 4.74	3.22
	3.14 3.87	3.58	3.22
	3.14 4.30	3.58	3.33
	3.22 4.52	3.64	3.50
	3.26 4.92	3.76	3.78
	3.33	3.85	
			3.25 ± 0.29
	3.51 ± 0.58	3.73 ± 0.48	

REFERENCES

1. Gaynor SE: The Effects of Home Care on Elderly Female Caregivers. (Unpublished doctoral dissertation.) Chicago: Rush University, 1988. (Data provided by Dr. Gaynor.)
2. Neter J, Wasserman W, Kutner MH: Applied Linear Statistical Models. 2nd ed. Homewood: Irwin, 1985.
3. Griez EJL, Lousberg H, van den Hout MA, et al: CO_2 vulnerability in panic disorder. Psychiatry Res 20:87–95, 1987.
4. Harner SG, Daube JR, Ebersold MJ, et al: Improved preservation of facial nerve function with use of

Source of Variation	Sum of Squares	DF	Mean Square
Main Effects	5.840	3	1.947
TREATMNT	.676	2	.338
RESULTS	4.899	1	4.899
2-way Interactions	.153	2	.077
TREATMNT RESULTS	.153	2	.077
Explained	6.788	5	1.358
Residual	9.524	44	.216
Total	16.312	49	.333

Figure 13.28 SPSS/PC two-way ANOVA results for log age

electrical monitoring during removal of acoustic neuromas. Mayo Clin Proc *62*:92–102, 1987.

5. Fish RG, Shelley MD, Maughan T, et al: The clinical value of serum CA125 levels in ovarian cancer patients receiving platinum therapy. Eur J Cancer Clin Oncol *23*:831–835, 1987.

6. Winer, BJ: Statistical Principles in Experimental Design. 2nd ed. New York: McGraw-Hill, 1971.

7. Norusis MJ, SPSS Inc: SPSS/PC+ Advanced Statistics V3.0 for the IBM PC/XT/AT and PS/2. Chicago: SPSS, 1989.

8. Chickering WR, Prasse KW, Dawe DL: Development and clinical application of methods for detection of antineutrophil antibody in serum of the cat. Am J Vet Res *46*:1809–1814, 1985.

9. Tobin MJ, Perez W, Guenther SM, et al: Unsuccessful trials of weaning from mechanical ventilation. Am Rev Respir Dis *134*:1111–1118, 1986.

10. Shapiro T, Sherman M, Calamari G, et al: Attachment in autism and other developmental disorders. J Amer Acad Child Adol Psychiatry *26*:480–484, 1987.

11. Holmes RA, Wilson RC, McCall JW: Thiacetarsamide in dogs: Disposition kinetics and correlations with selected indocyanine green kinetic values. Am J Vet Res *47*:1338–1340, 1986.

12. Drinka PJ, Voeks SK: Psychological depressive symptoms in Grade II hypothyroidism in a nursing home. Psychiatry Res *21*:199–204, 1987.

13. Zorgniotti AW, Cohen MS, Sealfon AI: Chronic scrotal hypothermia: Results in 90 infertile couples. J Urol *135*:944–947, 1986.

14. Sharav Y, Singer E, Schmidt E, et al: The analgesic effect of amitriptyline on chronic facial pain. Pain *31*:199–209, 1987.

15. Millman RP, Chung DC, Shore ET: Importance of breath size in calibrating the respiratory inductive plethysmograph. Chest *89*:840–845, 1986.

16. Rubin RT, Poland RE, Lesser IM, et al: Neuroendocrine aspects of primary endogenous depression. I. Cortisol secretory dynamics in patients and matched controls. Arch Gen Psychiatry *44*:328–336, 1987.

17. Buckler JMH, Willgerodt H, Keller E: Growth in thyrotoxicosis. Arch Dis Child *61*:464–471, 1986.

18. Stokes IAF, Moreland MS: Measurement of the shape of the surface of the back in patients with scoliosis. The standing and forward-bending positions. J Bone Joint Surg *69A*:203–211, 1987.

19. Yasuda T, Palacios IF, Dec GW, et al: Indium 111-monoclonal antimyosin antibody imaging in the diagnosis of acute myocarditis. Circulation *76*:306–311, 1987.

20. Barret WP, Staheli LT, Chew DE: The effectiveness of the Salter innominate osteotomy in the treatment of congenital dislocation of the hip. J Bone Joint Surg *68A*:79–87, 1986.

Glossary

Absolute value: The value of a number after any negative sign present is removed

Adjusted univariate approach: A method for repeated-measures analysis of variance that decreases the univariate degrees of freedom and requires fewer variance-covariance assumptions than the univariate approach to repeated-measures analysis of variance

Alternative hypothesis: The hypothesis that is accepted if the null hypothesis is rejected

Analysis of variance: A statistical method used to test the hypothesis that population means are related to one or more factors

Analysis-of-variance table: A table that presents the results of an analysis of variance

ANOVA: An abbreviation for analysis of variance

Bayes' rule: A formula used to calculate conditional probabilities from unconditional probabilities and other conditional probabilities

Between-groups mean square: In one-way analysis of variance, the between-groups sum of squares divided by the between-groups degrees of freedom

Between-groups sum of squares: In one-way analysis of variance, a quantity that measures the discrepancy between the sample means and the overall mean

Between-subjects mean square: In one-factor repeated-measures analysis of variance, the between-subjects sum of squares divided by the between-subjects degrees of freedom

Between-subjects sum of squares: In one-factor repeated-measures analysis of variance, a quantity that measures the discrepancy between the subject means and the overall mean

Bimodal: Having two modes

Binomial distribution: The distribution of a sum of independent random variables that take only the values 0 and 1 and have the same probability of taking the value 1

Bivariate: Involving two variables

Bivariate regression: A statistical method for obtaining a straight line that describes the relationship between two variables

Blind study: A double-blind or single-blind study

Bonferroni adjustment: Reduction of a significance level by dividing it by the number of statistical tests done; or increase of a confidence level by dividing 1 minus the confidence level by the number of confidence intervals obtained

Bonferroni procedure: A type of multiple-comparison procedure used with a variety of statistical methods

Carryover effect: A confounded effect that results when a new treatment is given while the effects of previous treatments are still present

Cell: In two-way analysis of variance, any combination of levels for two factors

Cell mean: The mean of all the observations in a cell

Cell size: The number of observations in a cell

Cell standard deviation: The standard deviation of all the observations in a cell

Censored data: Waiting times that result when patients are lost to follow-up or when the event of interest does not occur; or measurements that result when concentrations are below the detection limit of an instrument

Central limit theorem: A statistical theorem that states that the sample mean has an approximately normal distribution when based on sufficiently large random samples from any infinitely large population with a finite variance

Chi-square distribution: A positively skewed distribution with one degrees-of-freedom parameter

Chi-square statistic: A statistic that has a chi-square distribution

Chi-square test: A hypothesis test based on a statistic that has a chi-square distribution

Chi-square test of association: A statistical test of the hypothesis that two variables used to obtain a contingency table are not associated

Chi-square test of hypothesized proportions: A statistical test of the hypothesis that two or more population proportions are equal to hypothesized values

Column percentage: A sample percentage that uses a column total from a contingency table as the base

Column total: The sum of all the frequencies in a column of a contingency table

Column variable: The variable whose categories are listed in the columns of a contingency table

Complementary event: The event that happens when a given event does not occur

Conditional probability: A probability based on the knowledge that some event has occurred

Conditioning event: The event taken into account when calculating a conditional probability

Confidence interval: An interval estimate constructed in a way that ensures that the interval will include the population parameter it estimates a specified percentage of the time

Confidence level: The degree of certainty that a confidence interval includes the population parameter it estimates

Confounded effect: An effect that is mixed up with other effects and cannot be distinguished from them

Confounding: The presence of confounded effects

Constant term: In bivariate regression, the regression intercept

Constant variance: Unchanging variability of a variable when the values of another variable change

Contingency table: A table obtained by cross-classifying data according to two variables

Continuous: Having no gaps between possible values

Control group: A group of subjects in an experiment who are left untreated or are treated with standard methods

Correlation: Linear association between two variables

Covariance: A measure of the degree to which two variables are associated in a linear way

Cumulative frequency: The number of observations in a specified interval or any preceding interval; or the number of observations equal to a particular value or any preceding value

Cumulative frequency distribution: A listing of intervals that shows the number or percentage of observations in each interval or any preceding interval; or a listing of values that shows the number or percentage of observations equal to each value or any preceding value

Cumulative percentage: The percentage of observations in a specified interval or any preceding interval; or the percentage of observations equal to a particular value or any preceding value

Data transformation: The expression of data in units other than the original units of measurement

Degrees of freedom: A parameter of certain types of distributions

Denominator: The bottom part of a ratio

Denominator degrees of freedom: The degrees of freedom associated with the denominator of a statistic

Dependent variable: A variable whose values are estimated or predicted by a regression equation

Descriptive statistics: Numerical or graphical summaries of data

Discrete: Having gaps between all possible values

Disjoint events: Events that cannot occur at the same time

Distribution: A table, graph, or formula that gives the probabilities with which a random variable takes different values or ranges of values

Double-blind study: A study in which neither the researchers nor the subjects know which subjects are in the control group and which subjects are in the treatment groups

Dummy variable: A variable that takes only the values 0 and 1

Dummy variable regression: Regression analysis in which some or all of the independent variables are indicator variables

Error mean square: In analysis of variance, the error sum of squares divided by the error degrees of freedom

Error sum of squares: In one-way analysis of variance, the within-groups sum of squares; in one-factor repeated-measures analysis of variance, the total sum of squares minus the factor sum of squares and the between-subjects sum of squares

Estimated values: In regression analysis, the estimated values of the dependent variable given by the regression equation

Estimation: The use of sample statistics to estimate population parameters

Expected frequencies: The frequencies expected in a sample if the hypothesis specifying the values of population proportions is true; or the frequencies expected in a contingency table if the hypothesis of no association is true

Experimental design: The structure of an experiment; specifically, the experimental procedures, the selection of subjects, and the allocation of subjects to experimental groups

Experimental study: A study in which the researcher assigns subjects to the groups studied

Extrapolation: The use of predictions based on values far outside the range of the data

F distribution: A positively skewed distribution with two degrees-of-freedom parameters

F statistic: A statistic that has an F distribution

F test: A hypothesis test based on a statistic that has an F distribution

Factor: A characteristic used to classify observations into different groups

Factor A mean square: In two-way analysis of variance, the mean square that is the numerator of the F statistic used to test the hypothesis of equal population Factor A means

Factor B mean square: In two-way analysis of variance, the mean square that is the numerator of the F statistic used to test the hypothesis of equal population Factor B means

Factor effect: A difference between population factor means or between population cell means

Factor level: Any of the possible forms of a factor

Factor mean square: In one-factor repeated-measures analysis of variance, the factor sum of squares divided by the factor degrees of freedom

Factor sum of squares: In one-factor repeated-measures analysis of variance, a quantity that measures the discrepancy between the factor means and the overall mean

Fifty-fifty fallacy: The erroneous belief that events are equally likely when only two events are possible

Fisher's exact test: A statistical test of the hypothesis of no association between two variables used to obtain a contingency table with two rows and two columns

Fitted values: In regression analysis, the estimated values of the dependent variable given by the regression equation

Frequency: The number of observations in a specified interval; or the number of observations equal to a particular value

Frequency curve: A curve used to obtain probabilities by calculating areas under the curve

Frequency distribution: A listing that shows the numbers or percentages of observations in specified intervals; or a listing that shows the numbers or percentages of observations equal to particular values

Friedman test: A nonparametric test used to compare three or more populations of repeated measurements

Gambler's fallacy: The erroneous belief that the repeated occurrence of an event increases the probability that the opposite event will occur

Grand mean: The mean for the combined sample with all the observations

Greenhouse-Geisser adjusted univariate approach: An adjusted univariate procedure for repeated-measures analysis of variance that uses the Greenhouse-Geisser epsilon to reduce the univariate degrees of freedom

Greenhouse-Geisser epsilon: A number used to reduce the univariate degrees of freedom when the Greenhouse-Geisser adjusted univariate approach is used

Histogram: A graphical representation of a frequency distribution

Hotelling's trace: A test statistic used in the multivariate approach to repeated-measures analysis of variance

Huynh-Feldt adjusted univariate approach: An adjusted univariate procedure for repeated-measures analysis of variance that uses the Huynh-Feldt epsilon to reduce the univariate degrees of freedom

Huynh-Feldt epsilon: A number used to reduce the univariate degrees of freedom when the Huynh-Feldt adjusted univariate approach is used

Hypothesis: A statement about the world that can be tested

Hypothesis test: A formal test of a hypothesis in which a test statistic calculated from the data is used to determine whether or not the hypothesis should be rejected

Independent events: Events such that the conditional probability of one event, given the other event, is equal to the unconditional probability of the event

Independent observations: Observations such that the random variables representing the first, second, third, ..., and nth observations are all independent

Independent populations: Populations such that all the observations in any population are independent of all the observations in any of the other populations

Independent random variables: Random variables such that information about one random variable gives no information about any of the other random variables

Independent samples: Samples such that all the observations in any sample are independent of all the observations in any of the other samples

Independent variable: In a contingency table, a variable controlled by the researcher; in regression analysis, a variable used to estimate or predict the values of another variable

Indicator variable: A variable that takes only the values 0 and 1

Integer: Any of the numbers $0, 1, 2, 3, \ldots$ or the numbers $-1, -2, -3, \ldots$

Interaction: In two-way analysis of variance, the dependence of one factor's effects on the level of another factor

Interaction mean square: In two-way analysis of variance, the mean square that is the numerator of the F statistic used to test the hypothesis of no interaction

Intercept of a line: The point on the vertical axis of a scatterplot where the line crosses this axis

Interval data: Data that can be ordered and used to compute meaningful distances but lack a nonarbitrary zero point

Interval endpoints: The first and last numbers in an interval

Interval estimate: An estimate consisting of a range of numbers

Kruskal-Wallis test: A nonparametric test based on ranks that is used to test the hypothesis that three or more independent populations are identical

Latent effect: A confounded effect that results when the effects of previous treatments are reactivated by later treatments

Learning effect: A confounded effect that results when the mere repetition of a treatment or activity changes subjects' responses

Linear association: Association between two variables that can be described by a straight line

Logistic regression: A type of regression analysis in which the dependent variable is an indicator variable

Lower tail: The left tail of a distribution

Lower-tail probability: A probability calculated by computing an area in the lower tail of a distribution

Mann-Whitney test: A nonparametric test of the hypothesis that two independent populations are identical

Mauchly's test: A test used in repeated-measures analysis of variance to determine whether the variance-covariance assumptions of the univariate approach hold

McNemar test for paired proportions: A statistical test of the hypothesis that two paired population proportions are equal

Mean: The arithmetic average of the observations

Measure of central tendency: A number that represents a central value around which the data seem to be grouped

Measure of variability: A number that represents the degree to which the observations vary

Median: A middle number such that half of the observations are below this number and half of the observations are above it

Mode: The most frequently occurring data value

Multiple-comparison procedure: A method for determining which populations differ or which population parameters differ that reduces the risk of mistakenly concluding that identical populations are different or that identical population parameters are different

Multiple regression: A statistical method for obtaining an equation that describes the relationship between a dependent variable and two or more independent variables

Multiplicity problem: The tendency for a large number of tests to lead to rejection of some of the null hypotheses even when all of the null hypotheses are true

Multivariate approach: A procedure for repeated-measures analysis of variance that uses multivariate test statistics and requires fewer variance-covariance assumptions than the univariate approach to repeated-measures analysis of variance

Multivariate normality: A type of distribution for a group of random variables that implies that each random variable has a normal distribution

Mutually exclusive categories: Categories such that no observation can be classified into more than one category

Negative correlation: Linear association of increasing values of one variable with decreasing values of another variable

Negatively skewed: Skewed with the tail on the left

Nominal data: Data that consist of arbitrary numerical labels for categories

Nonparametric statistics: Statistical tests that require less restrictive distributional assumptions than parametric statistics

Nonstandard normal distribution: A normal distribution with a mean other than 0 or a standard deviation other than 1

Normal distribution: A continuous distribution with a bell-shaped frequency curve given by a mathematical formula for normal distributions

Null hypothesis: The hypothesis tested by a statistical test

Numerator: The top part of a ratio

Numerator degrees of freedom: The degrees of freedom associated with the numerator of a statistic

Observational study: A study in which the researcher cannot assign subjects to the groups studied

Observed frequencies: The frequencies obtained for a sample or contingency table

One-factor repeated-measures analysis of variance: A statistical method requiring repeated measurements that is used to test the hypothesis that three or more population means are equal

One-sample t test: A statistical test of the hypothesis that the population mean is equal to some hypothesized value

One-sided alternative hypothesis: An alternative hypothesis that states that a population parameter is less than a hypothesized value; or an alternative hypothesis that states that a population parameter is greater than a hypothesized value

One-sided test: A statistical test with a one-sided alternative hypothesis

One-tailed p-value: A p-value for a one-sided test

One-way analysis of variance: A statistical method requiring independent samples that is used to test the hypothesis that three or more population means are equal

Opposite event: The event that happens when a given event does not occur

Ordinal data: Data that consist of rankings according to some criterion

Outlier: A data value far outside the range of the rest of the data

Overall confidence level: The degree of certainty that a group of confidence intervals all include the population parameters they estimate

Overall mean: The mean for the combined sample with all the observations

Overall significance level: An upper bound for the probability of mistakenly rejecting any of a group of null hypotheses when all of the null hypotheses are true

Overall standard deviation: The standard deviation for the combined sample with all the observations

Overall variance: The variance for the combined sample with all the observations

Paired populations: Populations obtained by pairing subjects to obtain two populations of measurements or by measuring something twice for a single population of subjects

Paired proportions: Proportions obtained from paired populations or paired samples

Paired samples: Samples obtained by pairing subjects to obtain two samples or by measuring something twice for a single sample of subjects

Paired-samples confidence interval: A confidence interval for the difference between two population means that is based on paired samples

Paired t test: A statistical test of the hypothesis that two population means are equal that is based on paired samples

Pairwise disjoint events: Events such that no two events can happen at the same time

Parameter: A characteristic of a population or distribution

Parametric statistics: Statistical tests that require specific distributional assumptions

Pearson correlation coefficient: A measure of the degree to which two variables are associated in a linear way

Pillai's trace: A test statistic used in the multivariate approach to repeated-measures analysis of variance

Placebo: An inert substance administered in the same way as the treatment medication

Point estimate: An estimate consisting of a single number

Pooled-variance confidence interval: A confidence interval for the difference between two population means that is based on independent samples and assumes that the population variances are equal

Pooled-variance t test: A statistical test of the hypothesis that two population means are equal that is based on independent samples and assumes that the population variances are equal

Population: All possible observations of interest

Positive correlation: Linear association of increasing values of one variable with increasing values of another variable

Positively skewed: Skewed with the tail on the right

Power: The probability of rejecting the null hypothesis when it is false

Probability: The long-run proportion of times an event will occur

Probability sample: A sample obtained in a way that ensures that every member of the population has a known, nonzero probability of being included in the sample

P-value: The probability of getting a test statistic at least as extreme as the calculated test statistic if the null hypothesis is true

Random assignment: The assignment of subjects to treatment and control groups by using a chance-governed mechanism

Random number table: A table of numbers constructed in a way that ensures that (1) each of the numbers 0 through 9 has probability $1/10$ of occurring in any position in the table and (2) the occurrence of any number in one part of the table is independent of the occurrence of any number in any other part of the table

Random sample: A simple random sample

Random variable: A potential quantity whose values are determined by a chance-governed mechanism

Randomization: The assignment of subjects to treatment and control groups by using a chance-governed mechanism

Range: The difference between the largest data value and the smallest data value

Ratio data: Data that have a nonarbitrary 0 point and that can be ordered and used to compute meaningful distances

Regression: A statistical method for obtaining an equation that describes the linear relationship between a dependent variable and one or more independent variables

Regression coefficients: In bivariate regression, the regression intercept and slope; in multiple regression, the numbers that specify the multiple regression equation

Regression equation: An equation that describes the linear relationship between a dependent variable and one or more independent variables

Regression intercept: The intercept of a regression line

Regression line: A line obtained by regression methods to describe the linear relationship between two variables

Regression slope: The slope of a regression line

Repeated measurements: Measurements of some quantity obtained more than once for the same subjects

Repeated-measures analysis of variance: A statistical method based on repeated measurements that is used to test the hypothesis that population means are related to one or more factors

Residual mean square: In analysis of variance, the error mean square

Residual sum of squares: In analysis of variance, the error sum of squares

Residual plot: In regression analysis, any plot of the residuals used to check regression assumptions

Residuals: In regression analysis, the differences between the actual values of the dependent variable and the estimated values of the dependent variable given by the sample regression equation

Row percentage: A sample percentage that uses a row total from a contingency table as the base

Row total: The sum of all the frequencies in a row of a contingency table

Row variable: The variable whose categories are listed in the rows of a contingency table

Roy's largest root: A test statistic used in the multivariate approach to repeated-measures analysis of variance

Sample: The data collected by the researcher

Sampling distribution: The distribution of a statistic when all samples of a given size are considered

SAS: A statistical software package. SAS is a registered trademark of SAS Institute, Inc.

Scatterplot: A plot that shows how the values of one variable are related to the values of another variable

SD: An abbreviation for standard deviation

Selection bias: Bias in the assignment of subjects to control or treatment groups

Separate-variance confidence interval: A confidence interval for the difference between two population means that is based on independent samples and does not assume that the population variances are equal

Separate-variance *t* test: A statistical test of the hypothesis that two population means are equal that is based on independent samples and does not assume that the population variances are equal

Sham procedure: A procedure that closely resembles the treatment procedure but is not intended to provide effective treatment

Sign test: A nonparametric test based on signs that is used to test hypotheses about population medians or population median differences

Signed rank: A rank that has been given the sign of the observation to which it corresponds

Significance level: A cutoff value for evaluating *p*-values which is equal to the probability of rejecting the null hypothesis when it is true

Simple random sample: A sample obtained in a way that ensures that (1) every member of the population has the same probability of being included in the sample and (2) different members of the population are selected independently

Single-blind study: A study in which the researchers do not know which subjects are in the control group and which subjects are in the treatment groups but each subject knows which group she is in; or a study in which the researchers know which subjects are in the control group and which subjects are in the treatment groups but the subjects do not know which groups they are in

Skewed distribution: A distribution in which most of the observations are clumped toward one end, with observations at the other end forming a stretched-out tail

Skewed to the left: Skewed with the tail on the left

Skewed to the right: Skewed with the tail on the right

Slope of a line: A number that indicates whether a line rises or falls and how steeply the line rises or falls

Spearman rank correlation coefficient: A measure of the degree of linear association between the ranks of two variables

SPSS: A statistical software package. SPSS is a trademark of SPSS Inc.

SPSS/PC: A statistical software package for personal computers. SPSS/PC is a trademark of SPSS Inc.

Standard deviation: The square root of the variance, widely used as a measure of variability

Standard error: The standard deviation of a sample statistic

Standard normal distribution: The normal distribution with a mean equal to 0 and a standard deviation equal to 1

Standardized residuals: In regression analysis, residuals that have been divided by the sample standard deviation of the residuals

Statistic: A characteristic of a sample

Statistical inference: The use of sample statistics to reach conclusions about population parameters

Statistically significant test: A hypothesis test that leads to rejection of the null hypothesis

Statistics: The science of collecting, analyzing, and interpreting data

Stratified random sample: A sample obtained by combining simple random samples from different strata

Stratum: A subgroup of a population

Student's *t* distribution: A type of symmetric distribution that resembles the standard normal distribution

Student's *t* test: A hypothesis test based on a statistic that has a *t* distribution

Studentized range distribution: A distribution used to obtain confidence intervals with the Tukey multiple-comparison procedure

Subject mean: The mean of all the observations for a subject

Subject standard deviation: The standard deviation of all the observations for a subject

Subject variance: The variance of all the observations for a subject

Symmetric distribution: A distribution whose two halves are mirror images of each other

Systematic sample: A sample obtained by selecting every *k*th name in a list

***t* distribution:** A type of symmetric distribution that resembles the standard normal distribution

***t* statistic:** A statistic that has a *t* distribution

***t* test:** A hypothesis test based on a statistic that has a *t* distribution

Tail probability: A probability calculated from an area in the tail or tails of a distribution

Test statistic: A statistic used to carry out a hypothesis test

Total sum of squares: In one-way analysis of variance and repeated-measures analysis of variance, the overall variance times the total number of observations minus 1

Treatment group: A group of subjects in an experiment who are given the treatment being studied

Treatment mean square: In one-factor repeated-measures analysis of variance, the factor mean square

Treatment sum of squares: In one-factor repeated-measures analysis of variance, the factor sum of squares

Tukey procedure: A multiple-comparison procedure used in one-way and two-way analysis of variance

Two-factor repeated-measures analysis of variance: A statistical method based on samples of repeated measurements that is used to determine whether population means are related to two factors

Two-sided alternative hypothesis: An alternative hypothesis that states that a population parameter does not equal a hypothesized value

Two-sided test: A statistical test with a two-sided alternative hypothesis

Two-tailed probability: A probability calculated from areas in both tails of a distribution

Two-tailed *p*-value: A *p*-value for a two-sided test

Two-way analysis of variance: A statistical method requiring independent samples that is used to determine whether population means are related to two factors

Type I error: Rejection of the null hypothesis when it is true

Type II error: Failure to reject the null hypothesis when it is false

Unbiased statistic: A statistic whose mean is equal to the population parameter it estimates

Unimodal: Having one mode

Univariate approach: A procedure for repeated-measures analysis of variance that is based on sums of squares and requires more variance-covariance assumptions than the multivariate or adjusted univariate approaches to repeated-measures analysis of variance

Upper percentage point of a distribution: A number such that the probability that a random variable with the distribution is greater than or equal to that number is equal to some specified value

Upper tail: The right tail of a distribution

Upper-tail probability: A probability calculated by computing an area in the upper tail of a distribution

Variable: Random variable

Variance: A commonly used measure of variability

Variance-covariance assumptions: Assumptions about the variances and covariances of random variables that are required for repeated-measures analysis of variance

Waiting time: The time until the occurrence of some event

Welch's t test: The separate-variance t test

Wilcoxon signed rank test: A nonparametric test based on ranks that is used to test hypotheses about population medians or population median differences

Wilks' lambda: A test statistic used in the multivariate approach to repeated-measures analysis of variance

Within-groups mean square: In one-way analysis of variance, the within-groups sum of squares divided by the within-groups degrees of freedom

Within-groups sum of squares: In one-way analysis of variance, a weighted sum of the sample variances

Within-subjects mean square: In one-factor repeated-measures analysis of variance, the within-subjects sum of squares divided by the within-subjects degrees of freedom

Within-subjects sum of squares: In one-factor repeated-measures analysis of variance, a weighted sum of the subject variances

Yates-corrected χ^2 statistic: A modified chi-square statistic sometimes used for the chi-square test of association for two variables with only two categories

Z statistic: A statistic that has a standard normal distribution

Z test: A hypothesis test based on a statistic that has a standard normal distribution

Glossary of Symbols

α (alpha): the significance level

b_i (b sub i): the sample regression coefficient for the independent variable X_i

b_0 (b nought): the sample regression intercept

b_1 (b sub one): the sample regression slope

β_i (beta sub i): the population regression coefficient for the independent variable X_i

β_0 (beta nought): the population regression intercept or constant term

β_{00} (beta nought nought): the hypothesized value of the population regression intercept

β_1 (beta sub one): the population regression slope

β_{10} (beta sub one nought): the hypothesized value of the population regression slope

χ^2: (kī square): a random variable with a chi-square distribution

$\chi^2_{\alpha,d}$ (kī sub alpha d square): the α upper percentage point of the chi-square distribution with d degrees of freedom

χ^2_{calc} (kī square calc): the calculated value of a chi-square statistic

χ^2_d (kī sub d square): a random variable with a chi-square distribution having d degrees of freedom

column pct_{ij} (column per cent i j): the column percentage for category i of the row variable and category j of the column variable of a contingency table

d: degrees of freedom

$\bar{d}$ (d bar): the mean of a sample of differences

d_i (d sub i): the ith difference

d_1 (d sub one): the numerator degrees of freedom

d_2 (d sub two): the denominator degrees of freedom

Δ_0 (delta nought): the hypothesized value of the difference between two population means

df: degrees of freedom

e_i (e sub i): the sample regression residual for the ith subject

E_i (e sub i): the expected frequency for the ith category of a variable when the chi-square test of hypothesized proportions is done

E_{ij} (e sub i j): the expected frequency for the ith category of the row variable and the jth category of the column variable of a contingency table when the chi-square test of association is done

f: the degrees of freedom for the separate-variance confidence interval and the separate-variance t test

F: a random variable with an F distribution

F_{α,d_1,d_2} (F sub alpha d one d two): the α upper percentage point of the F distribution with d_1 numerator degrees of freedom and d_2 denominator degrees of freedom

F_{calc} (F calc): the calculated value of an F statistic

F_{d_1,d_2} (F sub d one d two): a random variable with an F distribution having d_1 numerator degrees of freedom and d_2 denominator degrees of freedom

H_A (h sub a): the alternative hypothesis

$\hat{}$ (hat): a symbol that denotes a sample estimate of a population parameter

H_0 (h nought): the null hypothesis

M: the McNemar test statistic

M_{calc} (M calc): the calculated value of the McNemar test statistic

m_0 (m nought): the hypothesized value of the population median or population median difference

MSA: the Factor A mean square in two-way analysis of variance

MSAB: the interaction mean square in two-way analysis of variance

MSB: the between-groups mean square in one-way analysis of variance; or the Factor B mean square in two-way analysis of variance

MSBS: the between-subjects mean square in one-factor repeated-measures analysis of variance

MSE: the error mean square in analysis of variance

MSF: the factor mean square in one-factor repeated-measures analysis of variance

MSW: the within-groups mean square in one-way analysis of variance

MSWS: the within-subjects mean square in one-factor repeated-measures analysis of variance

μ (mew): the population mean; or the mean of a random variable

μ_{Ai} (mew sub a i): the population factor mean for the ith level of Factor A

μ_{AiBj} (mew sub a i b j): the population cell mean for the ith level of Factor A and the jth level of Factor B

μ_{Bj} (mew sub b j): the population factor mean for the jth level of Factor B

μ_i (mew sub i): the mean of the ith population

μ_0 (mew nought): the hypothesized value of the population mean

MW: the Mann-Whitney test statistic

MW_{calc} (m w calc): the calculated value of the Mann-Whitney test statistic

n: the number of observations

n_{AiBj} (n sub a i b j): the number of observations in the cell for the ith level of Factor A and the jth level of Factor B

n_D (n sub d): in the McNemar test, the number of subjects with discrepant responses; in the Wilcoxon signed rank test or the sign test, the number of nonzero observations or nonzero differences

n_i (n sub i): the number of observations in the ith sample

n_{Ii} (n sub i i): the initial sample size needed for the ith sample in order to obtain the desired final sample size after subjects drop out

n_T (n sub t): the total number of observations when all samples are combined

O_i (o sub i): the sample frequency for the ith category of a variable

O_{ij} (o sub i j): the expected frequency for the ith category of the row variable and the jth category of the column variable of a contingency table

$100(1 - \alpha)\%$ (one hundred times one minus alpha per cent):   the confidence level for a confidence interval

p: a population proportion

p_{Di} (p sub d i):   the proportion of subjects who will drop out of the ith sample

$P(\text{Event})$:   the probability of an event

$P(\text{Event} | \text{Conditioning event})$:   the conditional probability of an event, given the conditioning event

$\hat{p}$ (p hat):   a sample proportion

p_i (p sub i):   a proportion for the ith population; or the population proportion for the ith category of a variable

$\hat{p}_i$ (p sub i hat):   a proportion for the ith sample; or the sample proportion for the ith category of a variable

p_{i0} (p sub i nought):   the hypothesized value of the population proportion for the ith category

p_0 (p nought):   the hypothesized value of a population proportion

q_{α, d_1, d_2} (q sub alpha d one d two):   the α upper percentage point of the studentized range distribution with d_1 numerator degrees of freedom and d_2 denominator degrees of freedom

r: the sample Pearson correlation coefficient

ρ (rō):   the population Spearman rank correlation coefficient

row pct$_{ij}$ (row per cent i j):   the row percentage for category i of the row variable and category j of the column variable of a contingency table

r_s (r sub s):   the sample Spearman rank correlation coefficient

r^2 (r squared):   the squared sample Pearson correlation coefficient

s: the sample standard deviation

S: the sign test statistic

s_{AiBj} (s sub a i b j):   the standard deviation of the cell for the ith level of Factor A and the jth level of Factor B

S_{calc} (s calc):   the calculated value of the sign test statistic

s_d (s sub d):   the standard deviation of a sample of differences

SD: standard deviation

s_{diff} (s diff):   the estimated standard deviation of $\hat{p}_1 - \hat{p}_2$

$\text{se}(b_0)$ (s e b nought):   the estimated standard error of the sample regression intercept

$\text{se}(b_1)$ (s e b sub one):   the estimated standard error of the sample regression slope

s_i (s sub i):   the standard deviation of the ith sample

σ (sigma):   the population standard deviation; or the standard deviation of a random variable

Σ (sigma):   sum

σ^2 (sigma squared):   the population variance; or the variance of a random variable

s_{pool} (s pool):   a pooled estimate of a common population standard deviation used for the separate-variance confidence interval and the separate-variance t test

s_{prop} (s prop):   the estimated standard deviation of $\hat{p}$

s^2 (s squared):   the sample variance

$s_{\text{subject}j}$ (s subject j):   the standard deviation of all the observations for the jth subject

SSA: the Factor A sum of squares in two-way analysis of variance

SSAB: the interaction sum of squares in two-way analysis of variance

SSB: the between-groups sum of squares in one-way analysis of variance; or the Factor B sum of squares in two-way analysis of variance

SSBS: the between-subjects sum of squares in one-factor repeated-measures analysis of variance

SSE: the error sum of squares in analysis of variance

SSF: the factor sum of squares in one-factor repeated-measures analysis of variance

SST: the total sum of squares in analysis of variance

SSW: the within-groups sum of squares in one-way analysis of variance

SSWS: the within-subjects sum of squares in one-factor repeated-measures analysis of variance

t: a random variable with a t distribution

$t_{\alpha, d}$ (t sub alpha d):   the α upper percentage point for the t distribution with d degrees of freedom

t_{calc} (t calc):   the calculated value of a t statistic

t_d (t sub d):   a random variable having a t distribution with d degrees of freedom

$\text{var}(\bar{x}_{Ai})$ (var x sub a i bar):   the estimated variance of the sample factor mean for the ith level of Factor A

$\text{var}(\bar{x}_{AiBj})$ (var x sub a i b j bar):   the estimated variance of the sample cell mean for the ith level of Factor A and the jth level of Factor B

$\text{var}(\bar{x}_{Bj})$ (var x sub b j bar):   the estimated variance of the sample factor mean for the jth level of Factor B

$\text{var}(\bar{x}_i)$ (var x sub i bar):   the estimated variance of the ith sample mean

W: the Wilcoxon signed rank test statistic

W_{calc} (w calc):   the calculated value of the Wilcoxon signed rank test statistic

X: random variable; or the independent variable in bivariate regression

$\bar{x}$ (x bar):   the sample mean

$\bar{x}_{Ai}$ (x sub a i bar):   the sample factor mean for the ith level of Factor A

$\bar{x}_{AiBj}$ (x sub a i b j bar):   the sample cell mean for the ith level of Factor A and the jth level of Factor B

$\bar{x}_{Bj}$ (x sub b j bar):   the sample factor mean for the jth level of Factor B

$\bar{x}_i$ (x sub i bar):   the mean of the ith sample

x_i (x sub i):   the ith observation

X_i (x sub i):   the ith random variable; or the ith independent variable in multiple regression

x_{ij} (x sub i j):   the jth observation in the ith sample

$\bar{x}_{\text{subject}j}$ (x subject j bar):   the mean of all the observations for the jth subject

Y: a random variable; or the dependent variable in bivariate regression

$\hat{Y}$ (y hat):   the estimated value of the dependent variable in regression analysis

Z: a random variable, usually with a standard normal distribution

z_α (z sub alpha):   the α upper percentage point of the standard normal distribution

z_{calc} (z calc):   the calculated value of a Z statistic

In Chapter 7, we discussed two mistakes you can make when carrying out a hypothesis test. You can reject the null hypothesis when it is true (Type I error), or you can fail to reject the null hypothesis when it is false (Type II error). The significance level is the probability of making a Type I error. Since the researcher chooses the significance level, she controls the probability of making a Type I error. She would also like to control the probability of making a Type II error. Once the significance level has been set, the probability of making a Type II error can be controlled only by changing the sample size.

Since the probability of a Type II error decreases as the sample size increases, it might seem that the best strategy is to obtain the largest possible sample. But increasing the sample size is time consuming and expensive. We do not want a sample size that is larger than the minimum necessary for a small probability of a Type II error. How can we determine the minimum size needed?

A very useful reference called *Statistical Power Analysis for the Behavioral Sciences*[1] can often be used to obtain minimum sample sizes. This book contains tables of the sample sizes needed to obtain small probabilities of a Type II error for various statistical procedures. To use these tables, we work with *power* instead of the probability of a Type II error. Power is the probability of *rejecting* the null hypothesis when it is false. In other words,

$$\text{power} = 1 - P(\text{Type II error})$$

We want to make the power as large as possible, given practical limitations on the sample size. This is equivalent to making the probability of a Type II error as small as possible.

Power depends not only on the sample size, but also on the discrepancy between the hypothesized population parameters and the actual population parameters. The greater the discrepancy, the larger the power. Let us consider the two-sample Z test of the null hypothesis

$$H_0: p_1 = p_2 \qquad (A.1)$$

Suppose the population proportions p_1 and p_2 are not equal, but the difference between them is extremely small. Unless our samples are very large, we have little chance of detecting the difference between p_1 and p_2 and rejecting the null hypothesis (A.1). In other words, our power is low for all but very large samples. Now suppose that the difference between p_1 and p_2 is extremely large. Even if our samples are small, we have a good chance of detecting the difference between p_1 and p_2 and rejecting the null hypothesis (A.1). Our power is high even for small samples.

Table A.1 shows the sample sizes needed to obtain various power values for the two-sided two-sample Z test. To use this table, we need to specify the desired power, our significance level, and the size of the difference between p_1 and p_2 that we are interested in detecting. For example, we might not care about detecting a small difference between p_1 and p_2, but we might want to detect a moderate difference. Or we might be interested only in detecting a large difference.

To use Table A.1, we first find the block in the table that corresponds to our significance level. We then find the row for our power and the column for the size of the difference of interest. The sample size in this row and column is the sample size *for each group*. The *total* sample size ($n_1 + n_2$) is equal to *twice* this sample size. When we use Table A.1 in this way, we assume that equal sample sizes will be used in each group.* Let us consider an example that illustrates the use of this table.

Example A.1 _____

A nurse wants to study the effectiveness of transcutaneous nerve stimulation (TENS) for the relief of postsurgical pain. Patients are to be randomly assigned to receive either analgesic drugs p.r.n. or TENS plus analgesic drugs p.r.n. He wants to use a two-sided two-sample Z test of the hypothesis that the population proportion of TENS patients who complain of unsatisfactory pain relief is the same as the population proportion of non-TENS patients who complain of unsatisfactory pain relief. His significance level is 0.01 and his desired power is 0.99. He is interested in detecting a small difference between the population proportions.

In the block for a 0.01 significance level in Table A.1, we find the row for power = 0.99 and the column for a small difference. The sample size for each sample is 1202, producing a total sample size

_____

*If different sample sizes are desired, Table A.1 can be used differently to take this into account. Cohen describes the use of tables like Table A.1 to obtain unequal sample sizes.[1]

TABLE A.1   SAMPLE SIZES FOR TWO-SIDED TWO-SAMPLE Z TEST*

| | Significance Level = 0.01 | | | Significance Level = 0.05 | | |
| | Size of Difference between p_1 and p_2 | | | Size of Difference between p_1 and p_2 | | |
Power	SMALL	MODERATE	LARGE	SMALL	MODERATE	LARGE
0.80	584	93	36	392	63	25
0.85	652	104	41	449	72	28
0.90	744	119	46	525	84	33
0.95	891	143	56	650	104	41
0.99	1202	192	75	919	147	57

*Cohen, J. *Statistical power analysis for the behavioral sciences* (rev. ed.). Hillsdale: Erlbaum, 1977.

of $2 \times 1202 = 2404$. This sample size is so large that it is completely impractical. Why did we get such a large sample size? How can we reduce it?

It can be shown that the required sample size is affected by the significance level, the power, and the size of the difference as follows:

1. The *smaller* the significance level, the larger the sample size needed.
2. The *larger* the power, the larger the sample size needed.
3. The *smaller* the difference of interest, the larger the sample size needed.

Given these relationships, the nurse was too ambitious when he specified his significance level, power, and difference size. In general, power values of 0.95 or higher produce unacceptably large sample sizes when small or moderate differences are of interest. The nurse should first reduce his desired power. In most cases, the minimum acceptable power is 0.80.

Let us see what his required sample size would be if he decided to settle for a power of 0.80, again using a 0.01 significance level and a small difference size. From Table A.1, we obtain a sample size of 584, resulting in a total sample size of $2 \times 584 = 1168$. This is better than a total sample size of 2404, but it is still quite large. Let us try increasing the significance level to 0.05, keeping the power of 0.80 and the small difference size. From the block for the 0.05 significance level in Table A.1, we obtain the total sample size $2 \times 392 = 784$. Again, the total sample size is quite large.

The only specification left to change is the size of the difference. Suppose the nurse decides that he is interested only in detecting a moderate difference between the population proportions. Using a 0.05 significance level and a power of 0.80, we get a total sample size of $2 \times 63 = 126$ from Table A.1. By reducing the desired power, increasing the significance level, and increasing the size of the difference of interest, we have obtained a manageable sample size.

Many studies have fairly high dropout rates, and anticipated dropout rates must be taken into account when selecting sample sizes. Suppose p_{D1} is

the proportion of subjects who will drop out of the first sample and p_{D2} is the proportion of subjects who will drop out of the second sample. Let n_1 be the sample size needed for the first sample and let n_2 be the sample size needed for the second sample. We need to determine the *initial* sample sizes n_{I1} and n_{I2} needed to ensure that the final sample sizes after losing subjects are equal to n_1 and n_2. It can be shown that the required initial sample sizes are

$$n_{I1} = \frac{n_1}{1 - p_{D1}} \qquad n_{I2} = \frac{n_2}{1 - p_{D2}} \qquad (A.2)$$

When formula (A.2) is used, noninteger sample sizes often result. Noninteger sample sizes should be rounded *up* to the nearest integer. For example, the sample size 41.3 should be rounded up to 42.

Let us consider the TENS example again. Suppose the nurse expects 15% of the TENS patients to drop out of the study and 10% of the non-TENS patients to drop out of the study. If we consider the TENS group to be the first sample and the non-TENS group to be the second sample, $p_{D1} = 0.15$ and $p_{D2} = 0.10$. If he uses a 0.05 significance level, power equal to 0.80, and a moderate difference size, the final sample sizes should be $n_1 = n_2 = 63$. Using formula (A.2), we can obtain the initial sample sizes needed:

$$n_{I1} = \frac{63}{1 - 0.15} = \frac{63}{0.85} = 74.1$$

$$n_{I2} = \frac{63}{1 - 0.10} = \frac{63}{0.90} = 70$$

Rounding up to get n_{I1}, we obtain $n_{I1} = 75$ and $n_{I2} = 70$. The nurse should begin his study with 75 TENS patients and 70 non-TENS patients.

How do we estimate the dropout rates p_{D1} and p_{D2}? Dropout rates must be determined from experience and cannot be calculated from a statistical formula. Previous research in the area you are studying may give you some idea of the dropout rates to expect. Researchers who have done similar studies can tell you the dropout rates for their studies. In many cases, anticipated dropout rates are no more than educated guesses. If you must guess, it is better to overestimate dropout rates than to underestimate them. Having slightly more subjects than necessary is not a problem, but having too few subjects can greatly reduce power.

Sample-size tables can be used for a wide variety of statistical procedures, including t tests for hypotheses about means, one-way and two-way analysis of variance, chi-square tests of association, and regression and correlation. Such tables can be found in Cohen.[1] In addition, power tables can be used to determine the power of a test, given a specific sample size, significance level, and difference size.[1] Power tables are quite useful for evaluating studies that fail to reject null hypotheses. If the power for such a study is small, the nonsignificant results may be due to low power rather than a true null hypothesis. If you are designing a study, however, it is best to start with the desired power and select an appropriate sample size, rather than beginning with the sample size and looking up the resulting power.

REFERENCE

1. Cohen J: Statistical Power Analysis for the Behavioral Sciences. 2nd ed. Hillsdale: Erlbaum, 1988.

Appendix B

Summarizing Statistical Results for Publication

Many health professionals have difficulty summarizing statistical results when writing for publication. This is not surprising, since statistics texts do not usually discuss appropriate ways to describe statistical results. We will consider some common errors in summarizing statistical results and suggest some guidelines for reporting statistical results.

Consider the following sentences, which are typical of many statistical summaries in the medical and health care literature.

> The data were analyzed using the SAS data analysis program. The analysis demonstrated that women who became pregnant had significantly lower biopsy scores ($p < 0.05$) than women who did not become pregnant.

What is wrong with this summary? There are so many problems that we need to list them separately.

1. The meaning of the second sentence is not clear. Do the authors mean that the proportion of pregnant women with low biopsy scores is higher than the proportion of nonpregnant women with low biopsy scores? Or that the mean biopsy score for pregnant women is lower than the mean biopsy score for nonpregnant women? Or that all pregnant women have lower biopsy scores than all nonpregnant women?
2. The method used to determine statistical significance is not described.
3. The phrase "significantly lower" is used, suggesting that the difference between pregnant and nonpregnant women is clinically significant. This difference may be statistically significant but not clinically significant.
4. The term "demonstrated" is used. Statistical analyses cannot demonstrate or prove anything. They only allow the researcher to evaluate evidence for or against a hypothesis.
5. The exact p-value is not given.

How can we rewrite this summary so that the statistical results are described accurately and clearly? Suppose the authors used the separate-variance t test to compare the population mean biopsy scores for pregnant and nonpregnant women, and they obtained a p-value of 0.026. Their results can be summarized as follows:

> We concluded that the population mean biopsy score for pregnant women differs from the population mean biopsy score for nonpregnant women (separate-variance t test, $p = 0.026$).

If the authors want to say something about the clinical significance of the difference between the population mean biopsy scores, they need to obtain a confidence interval for this difference. Suppose that a 95% separate-variance confidence interval for the difference between the population mean biopsy score for pregnant women and the population mean biopsy score for nonpregnant women is (-34.7, -11.7). Suppose also that a difference of 10 or more is considered clinically significant. The authors could then summarize their results as follows:

> We concluded that the population mean biopsy score for pregnant women differs from the population mean biopsy score for nonpregnant women (separate-variance t test, $p = 0.026$). A 95% separate-variance confidence interval for the difference between the population mean biopsy score for pregnant women and the population mean biopsy score for nonpregnant women is (-34.7, -11.7). We are 95% sure that the population mean biopsy score for pregnant women is lower than the population mean biopsy score for nonpregnant women. We are also 95% sure that the difference is clinically significant.

The following guidelines may help you summarize statistical results correctly.

1. Specify the exact statistical procedures used. If more than one procedure was used, clearly indicate which procedure was used to obtain each result.
2. If groups are compared, clearly specify what was compared (e.g., proportions, means, medians).
3. Whenever possible, state the exact p-value. Before the use of computers, approximate p-values were reported because exact p-values could not be obtained from tables. The widespread use of statistical software now makes the reporting of exact p-values possible.
4. If you want to make statements about clinical significance, include descriptions of appropriate statistics (e.g, confidence intervals, squared correlation coefficients).
5. If your results are nonsignificant, include a description of the power of your statistical methods whenever possible. Failure to reject the null hypothesis can occur for two reasons: (1) the null hypothesis is actually correct or nearly correct, or (2) the null hypothesis is false but the study failed to detect this. By including power calculations, you allow the reader to determine whether your study had a reasonable chance of rejecting a false null hypothesis.

A discussion of the importance of power calculations in nonsignificant studies is provided by Freiman et al.[1]

To illustrate the application of these guidelines, let us consider good and bad examples of statistical reporting for some of the statistical methods described in this text.

1. Two-Sample Z-Test

Obscure Version. Cats treated with taurine showed significant improvement ($p < 0.01$) over cats treated with placebo.

Corrected Version. Eighty-two percent of the taurine-treated cats improved and 11% of the placebo-treated cats improved. We concluded that the population proportion of taurine-treated cats that improve is different from the population proportion of placebo-treated cats that improve (two-sample Z test, p-value = 0.0004). A 99% confidence interval for the difference between the population proportion of taurine-treated cats that improve and the population proportion of placebo-treated cats that improve is (0.51, 0.91). We are 99% sure that the population proportion of taurine-treated cats that improve is greater than the population proportion of placebo-treated cats that improve. We are also 99% sure that the difference is clinically important.

2. Separate-Variance t Test

Obscure Version. A t test was used to compare the means of the groups. The mean job satisfaction score for pediatric nurses was significantly lower ($p < 0.05$) than the mean job satisfaction score for surgical nurses.

Corrected Version. We concluded that the population mean job satisfaction score for pediatric nurses differs from the population mean job satisfaction score for surgical nurses (separate-variance t test, $p = 0.041$). A 95% confidence interval for the difference between the population mean job satisfaction score for pediatric nurses and the population mean job satisfaction score for surgical nurses is (-1.1, -8.9). We are 95% sure that the population mean job satisfaction score for pediatric nurses is less than the population mean job satisfaction score for surgical nurses. We are also 95% sure that the difference is small, with little if any practical importance.

3. One-Way Analysis of Variance

Obscure Version. The data were analyzed according to methods described in Sneaky and Cockroach. All of the groups were significantly different ($p < 0.05$).

Corrected Version. One-way analysis of variance, followed by the Tukey method of multiple comparisons, was used to compare group means. A 0.05 significance level was used for the analysis of variance and a 90% overall confidence level was used for the Tukey comparisons. Based on this analysis, we are 90% sure that all of the population group means are different.

4. One-Factor Repeated-Measures Analysis of Variance

Obscure Version. ANOVA was used to analyze the data. No significant differences ($p > 0.10$) between the baseline estradiol levels and the three postdrug estradiol levels were found.

Corrected Version. Multivariate one-factor repeated-measures analysis of variance was used to compare the population baseline estradiol mean and the population postdrug estradiol means. On the basis of this analysis, we cannot conclude that any of the population means are different ($p = 0.381$).

5. Chi-Square Test of Association

Obscure Version. A chi-square test was used to analyze the data. The relationship between sex and postsurgical pain was significant ($p < 0.01$).

Corrected Version. We concluded that sex and postsurgical pain are associated (chi-square test of association, $p = 0.006$). The percentages shown in Table 2 suggest that men are more likely than women to complain of severe postsurgical pain.

6. Sign Test

Obscure Version. Acupuncture had no significant effect on tension scores ($p > 0.05$).

Corrected Version. The sign test was used to test the hypothesis that the population median difference between the postacupuncture tension scores and the preacupuncture tension scores is 0. We were unable to reject this hypothesis ($p = 0.083$). Because the sample was small, however, the power of the sign test is very low even if the population median difference is quite different from 0 (power = 0.28).

7. Kruskal-Wallis Test

Obscure Version. The Kruskal-Wallis test showed that the glomerular filtration rates for the three disease groups were significantly different ($p < 0.005$).

Corrected Version. We concluded that not all of the three disease populations of glomerular filtration rates are identical (Kruskal-Wallis test, $p = 0.0032$).

8. Test of the Hypothesis That the Population Pearson Correlation Coefficient is 0

Obscure Version. A significant correlation ($p < 0.001$) was found between duration of nausea and dose/kg.

Corrected Version. We concluded that the population Pearson correlation coefficient for duration of nausea and dose/kg is not zero ($p = 0.0002$). A scatterplot of duration of nausea and dose/kg is consistent with a linear relationship between these variables (Figure 4). The r^2 value is only 0.09, however, indicating a very weak relationship with little clinical importance.

9. Two-Way Analysis of Variance

Obscure Version. The SPSS/PC software system was used to analyze the data. Although race did not significantly affect depression scores ($p > 0.05$), previous hospitalization had a significant effect on depression scores ($p < 0.05$).

Corrected Version. Two-way analysis of variance was used to determine whether the population mean depression scores are related to race and previous hospitalization. We could not reject the hypothesis of no interaction between race and pre-vious hospitalization ($p = 0.812$). We also could not reject the hypothesis that the population race factor means are equal ($p = 0.361$). We did reject the hypothesis that the population previous hospitalization factor means are equal ($p = 0.038$).

These examples should give you some idea of the format to use and the mistakes to avoid when reporting statistical results. If you are not sure whether a statistical summary is correct, ask a statistician to evaluate it before publication.

REFERENCE

1. Freiman JA, Chalmers TC, Smith H, et al: The impor-tance of beta, the Type II error and sample size in the design and interpretation of the randomized control trial. N Engl J Med 299:690–694, 1978.

Appendix C
Consulting a Statistician

Although you have learned how to obtain many statistical analyses on your own, you will probably need to consult a statistician if you carry out medical or health care research. Statistical knowledge fades quickly if not used regularly. In a few years, you may find that your statistical skills have become a bit feeble. Or you may encounter an unusual data set that cannot be analyzed with standard statistical methods.

Health professionals usually consult statisticians for information about one or more of the following.

1. Study design and sample size
2. Appropriate statistical procedures
3. Use of computer programs
4. Interpretation of statistical results

We will discuss four aspects of statistical consulting: timing of statistical consultation, selection of a statistician, working with a statistician, and resolution of consulting problems.

When should you see a statistician? If you know that statistical consultation will be necessary at some point, you should see a statistician as soon as possible. Ideally, a statistician should be consulted *before* collecting data. Design problems can then be corrected before they sink the entire study. A statistician can also help you prepare data collection forms and select appropriate sample sizes. It is not very helpful to find out *after* completing a study that the data collection form is a mess and the sample size is much too small.

Once you have decided on statistical consultation, how do you select a statistician? To find a statistician, you first need to know what a statistician is. This is not as obvious as it may seem. Anyone who has taken one or two statistics courses can legally but incorrectly call herself a statistician. In fact, a statistician is a person with a master's or Ph.D. degree in statistics. (A degree in mathematics or methodology is *not* equivalent to a degree in statistics.) Asking a nonstatistician for statistical advice is as risky as asking a non-health professional for medical advice. In both cases, it is possible to get sound information but the odds are against it. You would not ask a statistician to treat your medical problems, and it makes no more sense to ask a nonstatistician to interpret your data.

If you live in an isolated rural area, you may have few options when seeking a statistician. If you live in a large city or work at a university, you should have a much better selection. University statistics departments often provide consulting services for faculty and students. In addition, medical and nursing departments sometimes hire their own statisti-

cians. Private statistical consulting firms and free-lance statistical consultants are also available.

After you have found a statistician, you can take certain steps to help the consultation procede smoothly. First, you should be able to tell the statistician exactly what the purpose of your study is. If you are not sure yet, postpone the consultation. The statistician cannot help you answer clinical questions. You should also give the statistician information about the following.

1. The subjects available for sampling
2. The maximum number of subjects you could reasonably study
3. The estimated percentage of subjects who will drop out
4. The types of variables of interest (discrete or continuous)
5. The presence or absence of repeated measurements

If further detail is requested, you should be ready to provide it.

The most commonly encountered difficulties in statistical consultation seem to be (1) incomprehensible advice and (2) conflicting advice.* Let us consider the problem of unintelligible advice first. Some statisticians tend to use an esoteric language understood only by other statisticians. If your statistician begins slipping into jargon, a gentle reminder (such as "Toto, I don't think we're in Kansas anymore") is often sufficient. Persist in asking questions until the information is reasonably clear. You cannot expect to comprehend the theoretical underpinnings of statistical methods, but the statistician should be willing to explain as much as you can understand. In rare instances, you may encounter a statistician who refuses to speak English. If this occurs, your only recourse is to find another statistician.

If you see more than one statistician, they may suggest different methods for analyzing your data. This does not necessarily mean that one of them is wrong. In many cases, more than one statistical procedure is appropriate and no method is best. You should discuss the advantages and disadvantages of different procedures and then select the one that seems most appropriate. To a large extent, the problem of conflicting advice can be avoided by

---

*These also seem to be the most commonly encountered problems in medical consultations. If you are unfortunate enough to have these difficulties with a statistician, the experience may at least help you sympathize with patients who have similar problems with physicians.

collecting data that can be analyzed with standard statistical methods. If your data are out of the ordinary, it may not be clear which statistical procedures are appropriate. Giving statisticians an unusual data set is like showing health professionals an unusual patient. In both cases, you are likely to get conflicting opinions.

Few medical or health care researchers would start a study without arranging for appropriate laboratory and clinical assistance. Yet researchers often fail to seek statistical consultation until a study is completed. By choosing a statistician as a research partner at the beginning of a study, you can greatly increase your chances of successful research.

Appendix D
Answers to Problems

CHAPTER 1

1. No control group was used. It seems unlikely that close medical supervision or a placebo effect could account for the achievement of normocalcemia by 69% of the patients, but this cannot be ruled out.

3. Patients were randomly assigned to treatment groups, and neither the surgeon nor the data collector knew the treatment status of patients. Since acetaminophen and the placebo looked identical, it seems reasonable to assume that patients did not know what they were given. The authors do not state that this was the case, however. If patients were unaware of their drug status, the design is excellent. (Readers facing a third-molar extraction may be interested in the results: Patients preferred the regimen of acetaminophen before surgery, followed by acetaminophen as needed after surgery.)

5. The assignment of Ward A patients to the experimental group and Ward B patients to the control group ensures that the effects of the lactation suppression method are confounded with ward effects. Hospital environments often affect the amount of pain experienced and expressed. If Ward A is more pleasant than Ward B, a bias favoring the experimental method would have resulted. Perhaps patients were assigned by ward because of contact between patients within wards. If two methods were used simultaneously in a ward, patients could have discussed different methods with each other, and some patients might have insisted on changing to the other method. This problem could have been resolved with less risk of confounding. Assignment of Ward A patients to the experimental group and Ward B patients to the control group could have been done for only the first half of the patients in the study. After all of these patients had left the hospital, the rest of the patients could have been assigned in the opposite fashion (Ward A patients to the control group and Ward B patients to the experimental group). In this way, patients from both wards would have been assigned to both experimental and control groups. The effects of the lactation suppression method could have been distinguished from ward effects.

6. The study is single blind, which presumably means that the physicians caring for the patients, but not the patients, were aware of treatment status. If the person asking patients about adverse reactions knew which drugs the patients received, the chance of bias was quite high. The manner in which a question is asked can greatly influence the answer given. If the questioner knew that a patient received a drug that often causes dizziness, she might have phrased her questions in a way that led many patients to report this symptom. Double-blind procedures would have been unethical in this study, since physicians needed to know the drugs received in order to evaluate possible adverse reactions. If patients had been given a list of symptoms to check off, the potential for bias would have been reduced.

9. Patients were not randomly assigned to experimental and control groups. It appears that the experimental and control patients were at different health care facilities. If so, the effect of sensory simulation is confounded with the effect of health care facility. Differences between the groups could be due to differences in care other than sensory stimulation. It is also not clear whether observers who measured cognitive function knew the patients' treatment status. If the study was not single blind, observers' opinions of sensory stimulation could have affected their ratings of cognitive function.

CHAPTER 2

1. a.

FREQUENCY DISTRIBUTION AND CUMULATIVE FREQUENCY DISTRIBUTION OF WBC

WBC ($\times 10^3/mm^3$)	No. of Dogs	Cumulative No. of Dogs
10.0–19.9	3	3
20.0–29.9	2	5
30.0–39.9	3	8
40.0–49.9	2	10

Quick histogram of WBC

```
10.0 – 19.9 | XXX
20.0 – 29.9 | XX
30.0 – 39.9 | XXX
40.0 – 49.9 | XX
```

The histogram is neither symmetric nor skewed.

b. $\bar{x} = 28.9$, median $= 30.2$, $s^2 = 122.4$, $s = 11.1$. The mean and median are quite similar. The data are only moderately variable. There is no mode, since each WBC is different.

2. Nominal data: sex, source of admission
Ordinal data: decubitis ulcer stage

Ratio data: age, number of medications, size of ulcer

4. No. Two of the survival times are censored.

6. The nurses would use the median salary, which would accurately reflect the low salaries of most of the staff. The administration would use the mean salary, which would be high because of the large salary.

9. a.

FREQUENCY DISTRIBUTION AND CUMULATIVE FREQUENCY DISTRIBUTION FOR DEPRESSION-PSYCHOSIS GROUP

Cortisol (μg/dl)	No. of Patients	Cumulative No. of Patients
5.0–7.9	2	2
8.0–10.9	1	3
11.0–13.9	1	4
14.0–16.9	2	6

FREQUENCY DISTRIBUTION AND CUMULATIVE FREQUENCY DISTRIBUTION FOR SCHIZOPHRENIA GROUP

Cortisol (μg/dl)	No. of Patients	Cumulative No. of Patients
0.6–0.9	9	9
1.0–1.3	4	13
1.4–1.7	2	15
1.8–2.1	3	18
2.2–2.5	0	18
2.6–2.9	0	18
3.0–3.3	1	19
3.4–3.7	0	19
3.8–4.1	1	20

Quick histogram for depression-psychosis group

```
5.0 – 7.9 | XX
8.0 – 10.9 | X
11.0 – 13.9 | X
14.0 – 16.9 | XX
```

Quick histogram for schizophrenia group

```
0.6 – 0.9 | XXXXXXXXX
1.0 – 1.3 | XXXX
1.4 – 1.7 | XX
1.8 – 2.1 | XXX
2.2 – 2.5 |
2.6 – 2.9 |
3.0 – 3.3 | X
3.4 – 3.7 |
3.8 – 4.1 | X
```

The depression-psychosis group histogram is symmetric, with data clumped at both ends of the histogram. The schizophrenia group histogram is markedly skewed to the right. (Other interval lengths and starting points could be used, resulting in slightly different interpretations of the histograms.) All of the patients with chronic schizophrenia (100%) have cortisol levels below 5 μg/dl, and none of the patients with major depression with psychosis (0%) have cortisol levels below 5 μg/dl. For this sample of 26 patients, there is no overlap in the cortisol levels for the two groups. Since the DST discriminates perfectly between these two groups, the data support the author's statement.

b. Depression-psychosis group: $\bar{x} = 10.4$, median = 10.8, no mode, $s = 3.6$. Schizophrenia group: $\bar{x} = 1.4$, median = 1.05, mode = 0.9, $s = 0.8$. The large difference between the group means suggests that patients with chronic schizophrenia have lower DST cortisol levels, on average, than patients with major depression with psychosis when both types of patients are in a drug-free acute exacerbation phase of illness.

10. a.

FREQUENCY DISTRIBUTION AND CUMULATIVE FREQUENCY DISTRIBUTION FOR GROUP 1

Antithrombin Percentage	No. of Horses	Cumulative No. of Horses
50–69	5	5
70–89	0	5
90–109	2	7
110–129	1	8

FREQUENCY DISTRIBUTION AND CUMULATIVE FREQUENCY DISTRIBUTION FOR GROUP 2

Antithrombin Percentage	No. of Horses	Cumulative No. of Horses
70–89	4	4
90–109	2	6
110–129	4	10
130–149	2	12

FREQUENCY DISTRIBUTION AND CUMULATIVE FREQUENCY DISTRIBUTION FOR GROUP 3

Antithrombin Percentage	No. of Horses	Cumulative No. of Horses
80–89	2	2
90–99	1	3
100–109	6	9
110–119	1	10

Quick histogram for Group 1

```
50 – 69 | XXXXX
70 – 89 |
90 – 109 | XX
110 – 129 | X
```

Quick histogram for Group 2

```
 70 – 89 | XXXX
 90 – 109 | XX
110 – 129 | XXXX
130 – 149 | XX
```

Quick histgram for Group 3

```
 80 – 89 | XX
 90 – 99 | X
100 – 109 | XXXXX
110 – 119 | X
```

The Group 1 histogram is skewed to the right, with antithrombin percentages clumped at below-normal values. The Group 2 histogram is neither skewed nor symmetric, with antithrombin percentages clumped at below-normal values and above-normal values. The Group 3 histogram is slightly skewed to the left, with antithrombin percentages clumped at normal and near-normal values.

b. Group 1: $\bar{x} = 73.9$, median = 58, no mode, $s = 28.4$

Group 2: $\bar{x} = 106.6$, median = 106.5, mode = 100, $s = 20.7$

Group 3: $\bar{x} = 100.8$, median = 105, mode = 105, $s = 8.9$

The antithrombin percentages for Groups 1 and 2 are similar in variability, since their standard deviations are fairly close. The antithrombin percentages for Group 3 are much less variable than those for Groups 1 or 2, since the Group 3 standard deviation is much smaller. The means suggest that (1) horses with clinical colic associated with colitis or severe diarrhea tend to have antithrombin values below normal, on average; (2) horses with clinical colic associated with torsion or obstruction of the intestine tend to have antithrombin values slightly above normal, on average; and (3) horses with clinical colic associated with impaction of the intestine tend to have normal antithrombin values, on average.

CHAPTER 3

1. General physical condition, movement of limb, drainage at pin.

3. The events are not disjoint, so formula (3.6) cannot be used for part c.
a. P(Tearing) = 0.38
b. P(Itching) = 0.10
c. P(Tearing or itching) cannot be calculated. Since formula (3.4) must be used, we need to know P(Both tearing and itching) to calculate this probability.

5. The events are not disjoint, so formula (3.4) must be used.
a. P(Edema and swelling in jaw or neck) = 0.90
b. P(Edema and swelling in jaw or brisket) = 0.90
c. P(Edema and swelling in neck or brisket) = 0.90

7. a. P(ST depression|Cardiac disease) = 0.63
P(ST depression|No cardiac disease) = 0.11
In this sample, cardiac patients are much more likely than noncardiac patients to have ECGs with ST-segment depression.
b. Yes.

9. a. P(Headaches|No VDT use) = 0.08
P(Headaches|7 or more hours of VDT use) = 0.15
In this sample, heavy VDT users are almost twice as likely as non-VDT users to complain of headaches.
b. P(Headaches|No VDT use) = 0.13
P(Headaches|7 or more hours of VDT use) = 0.09
In this sample, heavy VDT users are slightly less likely than non-VDT users to complain of headaches.
c. Yes. The type of industry matters. The data suggest that (1) the risk of headache for heavy VDT users is higher than the risk of headache for non-VDT users in computer and data processing industries, public utilities, and state departments; and (2) the risk of headache for heavy VDT users is slightly lower than the risk of headache for non-VDT users in banks, communications industries, and hospitals.

11. a. P(Death|Treatment with streptokinase) = 0.06
P(Death) = 0.07
Since P(Death|Treatment with streptokinase) does not equal P(Death), the events "death" and "treatment with streptokinase" are not independent for this sample.
b. P(Death|Treatment with streptokinase) = 0.06
P(Death|Treatment with placebo) = 0.07
The chances of dying within 21 days are nearly the same for the streptokinase group and the placebo group.
c. No.

13. a. P(Death|Restraint) = 0.0004
P(Death) = 0.002
Since P(Death|Restraint) does not equal P(Death), the events "death" and "restraint" are not independent for this sample.
b. P(Death|Restraint) = 0.0004
P(Death|No restraint) = 0.002

In this sample, children who were not restrained were five times more likely to die than children who were restrained.

c. P(Non-fatal injury|Restraint) = 0.07
P(Non-fatal injury) = 0.12
Since P(Non-fatal injury|Restraint) does not equal P(Non-fatal injury), the events "non-fatal injury" and "restraint" are not independent for this sample.

d. P(Non-fatal injury|Restraint) = 0.07
P(Non-fatal injury|No restraint) = 0.14
In the sample of children who were not killed, children who were not restrained were twice as likely to be non-fatally injured as children who were restrained.

e. Yes.

15. a. P(Both Asian Indian and affected by bloating) = 0.55
b. P(Both black and affected by cramping) = 0.02
c. P(Both white and affected by diarrhea) = 0.08
d. P(Affected by both bloating and cramping) cannot be calculated from Table 3.19. The number of subjects with both bloating and cramping is not given, and we cannot calculate this number from the table.

17. a. P(Thickened bowel wall and thickened mesentery) = 0.60
b. P(Thickened bowel wall and peritoneal fluid) = 0.67
c. P(Thickened mesentery and free air) = 0.13
d. P(Peritoneal fluid and free air) = 0.20

19. a. P(Phlebitis|Filter) = 0.30
b. P(Phlebitis|No filter) = 0.26
c. No.

21. a. P(Total obstruction|Nonvisualization) = 0.93
b. P(Partial or no obstruction|Visualization) = 1
c. Yes.

CHAPTER 4

1. The minimum and maximum IgG levels for the same patient are not independent. The IgG levels for different patients are independent.

3. The exposure values are independent.

5. a. $P(Z \geq 0.45) = 0.3264$
b. $P(Z \geq 2.59) = 0.0048$
c. $P(Z \geq 3.98) < 0.0001$
d. $P(Z \geq 2.67) \cong 0.0040$

7. a. $P(Z \leq -0.21$ or $Z \geq 0.21) = 0.8337$
b. $P(Z \leq -2.00$ or $Z \geq 2.00) = 0.0455$
c. $P(Z \leq -2.81$ or $Z \geq 2.81) \cong 0.0051$
d. $P(Z \leq -4.72$ or $Z \geq 4.72) < 0.0001$

9. Only X_1 and X_2 could have normal or approximately normal distributions. X_3 is discrete, with a limited range of values.

11. Y does not have a binomial distribution since the independence condition (4.2) does not hold.

13. Y has a binomial distribution with parameters $n = 3$ and $p = 0.10$.
a. P(3 patients have a second stroke) = 0.0010
b. P(1 or 2 patients have a second stroke) = 0.2700
c. P(No patients have a second stroke) = 0.7290

15. Y does not have a binomial distribution since the independence condition (4.2) does not hold.

CHAPTER 5

1. Patients in sample: G. Hoogenboom, J. Mudge, T. Dreeze, T. Zych, W. Wenckus, T. Leeth, L. Nazey, F. Junkroski, C. Crater, C. Pflugel, B. Osnoss, M. Eidlhuber, E. Beasley, E. Scheib, J. Unfried.

3. Patients in Group 1: C. Crater, T. Dreeze, J. Mudge, L. Nazey, G. Hoogenboom, W. Wenckus.
Patients in Group 2: H. Kwartowski, C. Pflugel, T. Leeth, J. Unfried, E. Scheib, S. Ribstein.
Patients in Group 3: Rest of patients.

5. No. The histogram is quite skewed.

7. Yes. The histogram is symmetric and unimodal.

9. No. The histogram is extremely skewed.

CHAPTER 6

2. Yes. The 95% confidence interval for $p_1 - p_2$ is (0.08, 0.70). We are 95% sure that the difference between the malnourished population morbidity and the well-nourished population morbidity is between 0.08 and 0.70. We are 95% sure that the malnourished population morbidity is higher than the well-nourished population morbidity. The difference might be small (as low as 0.08), large (as high as 0.70), or moderate.

4. No. The 90% paired-samples confidence interval for $\mu_1 - \mu_2$ is (−49.9, 57.9). Since 0 is included in the confidence interval, we cannot say that the lorcainide population mean number of PVDs per hour differs from the placebo population mean number of PVDs per hour.

7. No. Since there are two more eyes than patients, two patients had surgery on both eyes. Each of these patients has repeated measurements, one for each eye. Repeated measurements are not independent, and the independence assumption is vio-

lated. If we knew the surgical outcome for each eye and the patient associated with each eye, we could discard the second-surgery outcome for each patient with two surgeries. We would then have 25 independent observations and could obtain a confidence interval for the population proportion of successes.

8. No. The 95% confidence interval for $p_1 - p_2$ is $(-0.54, 0.04)$. Since 0 is included in the confidence interval, we cannot say that the zearalenone population conception rate differs from the placebo population conception rate.

9. No. The 90% separate-variance confidence for $\mu_1 - \mu_2$ is $(-0.7, 16.9)$ ($f = 10$). Since 0 is included in the confidence interval, we cannot say that the day population nausea score mean differs from the night population nausea score mean.

12. The ratings are so nonnormal that we cannot obtain a pooled-variance confidence interval for $\mu_1 - \mu_2$.

13. No. The 95% separate-variance confidence interval for $\mu_1 - \mu_2$ is $(-117.7, 24.5)$ ($f = 6$). Since 0 is included in the confidence interval, we cannot say that the SSS-dip population flea count mean differs from the water-dip population flea count mean.

14. Yes. The 90% pooled-variance confidence interval for $\mu_1 - \mu_2$ is $(-28.6, -2.6)$. We are 90% sure that the difference between the asthma population FEV_1 mean and the nonasthma population FEV_1 mean is between -28.6 and -2.6. We are 90% sure that the asthma population FEV_1 mean is less than the nonasthma population FEV_1 mean. The difference might be small (as low as 2.6), large (as high as 28.6), or moderate.

17. Yes. The 90% confidence interval for the population mean is $(9.3, 10.1)$. We are 90% sure that the population patient–average hemoglobin mean is between 9.3 and 10.1.

19. Yes. The 99% confidence interval for $\mu_1 - \mu_2$ is $(-58.2, -10.2)$. We are 99% sure that the difference between the population test score mean before the educational program and the population test score mean after the program is between -58.2 and -10.2. We are 99% sure that the population test score mean is lower before the program than after the program. The difference might be small (as low as 10.2), extremely large (as high as 58.2), or somewhere in between.

21. The data are so nonnormal that we cannot obtain a separate-variance confidence interval for $\mu_1 - \mu_2$.

23. Yes. The 95% confidence interval for p is $(0.61, 0.77)$. We are 95% sure that the population proportion of bovine/equine trauma patients with orthopedic injuries is between 0.61 and 0.77.

25. Since there are 30 eyes and 25 patients, five patients had surgery on both eyes. Each of these

patients has repeated IOP differences, one for each eye. Repeated measurements are not independent, and the independence assumption is violated. If we knew the patient associated with each eye, we could discard the second-surgery IOP difference for each patient with two surgeries. We would then have 25 independent IOP differences and could obtain a paired-samples confidence interval for $\mu_1 - \mu_2$.

CHAPTER 7

2. The data are so extremely nonnormal that we cannot use the pooled-variance t test of H_0: $\mu_1 = \mu_2$.

4. Since 40 operations were performed on 32 patients, some patients had more than one operation. Surgery results from the same patient cannot be considered independent, so we cannot use a one-sample Z test of H_0: $p = 0.65$. If we knew which operations were associated with each patient, we could calculate the sample proportion of first operations that were successful. A one-sample Z test could be based on this proportion since the results of the 32 first operations should be independent.

7. Yes. H_0: $p_1 = p_2$, H_A: $p_1 \neq p_2$, two-sample $Z = -2.64$, two-tailed p-value = 0.0083. If the two population proportions are equal, the probability of getting a two-sample Z statistic at least as extreme as -2.64 is 0.0083. We reject the hypothesis of equal population proportions at the 0.01 significance level and conclude that the IDP population proportion with developmental delay does not equal the traditional-care population proportion with developmental delay.

9. Yes. H_0: $p = 0.25$, H_A: $p \neq 0.25$, one-sample $Z = -2.56$, two-tailed p-value = 0.0105. If the population proportion p is 0.25, the probability of getting a one-sample Z statistic at least as extreme as -2.56 is 0.0105. We reject the hypothesis that the population proportion is 0.25 at the 0.10 significance level and conclude that the population proportion of children who remain in a persistent vegetative state is not equal to 0.25.

10. No. H_0: $\mu_1 = \mu_2$, H_A: $\mu_1 \neq \mu_2$, pooled-variance $t = -1.47$, 24 df, $0.10 <$ two-tailed p-value < 0.20. If the two population means are equal, the probability of getting a pooled-variance t statistic at least as extreme as -1.47 is between 0.10 and 0.20. We cannot reject the hypothesis of equal population means at any reasonable significance level, so we cannot say that the population mean platelet count for healthy cats differs from the population mean platelet count for cats with cardiomyopathy.

11. No. H_0: $\mu_1 - \mu_2 = 35$, H_A: $\mu_1 - \mu_2 \neq 35$, paired $t = 0.24$, 7 df, two-tailed p value > 0.80. If the difference between the two population means is 35, the probability of getting a paired t statistic at least as extreme as 0.24 is greater than 0.80. We cannot reject the hypothesis that the difference between the two population means is 35 at any reasonable significance level.

13. No. H_0: $\mu_1 - \mu_2 = -1005$, H_A: $\mu_1 - \mu_2 \neq -1005$, separate-variance $t = -0.22$, 5 df, two-tailed p-value > 0.80. If the difference between the population means is -1005, the probability of getting a separate-variance t statistic at least as extreme as -0.22 is greater than 0.80. We cannot reject the hypothesis that the difference between the two population means is -1005 at any reasonable significance level.

14. No. H_0: $p_1 = p_2$, H_A: $p_1 \neq p_2$, two-sample $Z = -0.78$, two-tailed p-value $= 0.4354$. If the two population proportions are equal, the probability of getting a two-sample Z statistic at least as extreme as -0.78 is 0.4354. We cannot reject the hypothesis of equal population proportions at any reasonable significance level.

16. No. H_0: $\mu = -3$, H_A: $\mu \neq -3$, one-sample $t = 1.74$, 17 df, two-tailed p-value $= 0.10$. If the population mean discrepancy is -3, the probability of getting a one-sample t statistic at least as extreme as 1.74 is 0.10. We cannot reject the hypothesis that the population mean is -3 at any reasonable significance level.

17. The data are so nonnormal that we cannot use the paired t test of H_0: $\mu_1 - \mu_2 = 2.5$.

24. Yes. H_0: $\mu_1 = \mu_2$, H_A: $\mu_1 \neq \mu_2$, separate-variance $t = 5.57$, 7 df, two-tailed p-value < 0.001. If the two population means are equal, the probability of getting a separate-variance t statistic at least as extreme as 5.57 is less than 0.001. We reject the hypothesis of equal population means at any reasonable significance level and conclude that the population MUCP mean for normal mares does not equal the population MUCP mean for incontinent mares.

25. Yes. H_0: $p = 0.50$, H_A: $p \neq 0.50$, one-sample $Z = 2.01$, two-tailed p-value $= 0.0444$. If the population proportion p is 0.50, the probability of getting a one-sample Z statistic at least as extreme as 2.01 is 0.0444. We reject the hypothesis that the population proportion is 0.50 at the 0.05 significance level and conclude that the population proportion of hypertensive patients who would show positive changes after group education is not equal to 0.50.

CHAPTER 8

3. Since repeated measurements were obtained, the independent-samples assumption is violated. In addition, the data are extremely nonnormal, taking only a few values. One-way ANOVA is not appropriate.

4. Yes. H_0: $\mu_1 = \mu_2 = \mu_3 = \mu_4$, H_A: At least one population mean does not equal another population mean, $F = 16.71$, 3 and 31 df, p-value $<$

0.001. If all four population log SI means are equal, the probability of getting an F statistic at least as extreme as 16.71 is less than 0.001. We reject the hypothesis that all four population log SI means are equal at any reasonable significance level and conclude that at least one population mean does not equal another population mean.

Since $q_{.01, 4, 31}/\sqrt{2} \cong 4.80/\sqrt{2} = 3.39$ and $t_{.0017, 31} \cong t_{.0025, 30} = 3.030$, we will use the Bonferroni procedure to make the three comparisons selected before examining the sample means. The 99% Bonferroni confidence intervals are as follows:

$\mu_4 - \mu_1$ (*work applicant versus allergic and employed in bacampicillin production*): $(-1.71, -0.43)$

$\mu_4 - \mu_2$ (*work applicant versus allergic with negative skin test and employed in bacampicillin production*): $(-1.45, -0.11)$

$\mu_4 - \mu_3$ (*work applicant versus healthy and handling drugs*): $(-0.33, 0.91)$

We are 99% sure that the following is true.

1. The population log SI mean for work applicants is lower than the population log SI mean for allergic workers employed in bacampicillin production. The difference might be moderate (no less than 0.43) or large (as high as 1.71).

2. The population log SI mean for work applicants is lower than the population log SI mean for allergic workers with negative skin tests employed in bacampicillin production. The difference might be small (as low as 0.11), large (as high as 1.45), or moderate.

3. We cannot say that the population log SI mean for work applicants differs from the population log SI mean for healthy workers who have handled drugs for several years.

5. Yes. H_0: $\mu_1 = \mu_2 = \mu_3$, H_A: At least one population mean does not equal another population mean, $F = 14.79$, 2 and 21 df, p-value < 0.001. If all three population FEV_1 means are equal, the probability of getting an F statistic at least as extreme as 14.79 is less than 0.001. We reject the hypothesis that all three population FEV_1 means are equal at any reasonable significance level and conclude that at least one population mean does not equal another population mean.

Since $q_{.05, 3, 21}/\sqrt{2} \cong 3.58/\sqrt{2} = 2.53$ and $t_{.0083, 21} \cong t_{.0075, 21} = 2.649$, we will use the Tukey procedure to make all three possible comparisons. The 95% Tukey confidence intervals are as follows:

$\mu_1 - \mu_2$ (*tracheostomy and lung disease versus lung disease and no tracheostomy*): $(-15.7, 12.9)$

$\mu_1 - \mu_3$ (*tracheostomy and lung disease versus tracheostomy and no lung disease*): $(-51.8, -17.0)$

$\mu_2 - \mu_3$ (*lung disease and no tracheostomy versus tracheostomy and no lung disease*): $(-50.1, -15.9)$

We are 95% sure that the following is true.

1. We cannot say that the population FEV_1 mean for patients with tracheostomies and lung

disease is different from the population FEV_1 mean for patients with parenchymal lung disease but no tracheostomy.

2. The population FEV_1 mean for patients with tracheostomies and lung disease is smaller than the population FEV_1 mean for patients with tracheostomies but no clinically obvious lung disease. The difference might be small (as low as 17.0), large (as high as 51.8), or moderate.

3. The population FEV_1 mean for patients with parenchymal lung disease but no tracheostomy is smaller than the population FEV_1 mean for patients with tracheostomies but no clinically obvious lung disease. The difference might be small (as low as 15.9), large (as high as 50.1), or moderate.

9. No. H_0: $\mu_1 = \mu_2 = \mu_3$, H_A: At least one population mean does not equal another population mean, $F = 0.13$, 2 and 25 df, p-value > 0.50. If all three population square-root LOS means are equal, the probability of getting an F statistic at least as extreme as 0.13 is greater than 0.50. We cannot reject the hypothesis that all three population square-root LOS means are equal at any reasonable significance level. Multiple comparisons are not needed.

13. Yes. H_0: $\mu_1 = \mu_2 = \mu_3$, H_A: At least one population mean does not equal another population mean, $F = 41.62$, 2 and 23 df, p-value < 0.001. If all three population PI_{max} means are equal, the probability of getting an F statistic at least as extreme as 41.62 is less than 0.001. We reject the hypothesis that all three population PI_{max} means are equal at any reasonable significance level and conclude that at least one population mean does not equal another population mean.

Since $q_{.05, 3, 23}/\sqrt{2} \cong 3.53/\sqrt{2} = 2.50$ and $t_{.0083, 23} \cong t_{.0075, 23} = 2.629$ we will use the Tukey procedure to make all three possible comparisons. The 95% Tukey confidence intervals are as follows:

$\mu_1 - \mu_2$ (*UDP only versus UDP and cardiopulmonary disease*): (5.6, 59.2)

$\mu_1 - \mu_3$ (*UDP only versus normal*): (-79.8, -31.6)

$\mu_2 - \mu_3$ (*UDP and cardiopulmonary disease versus normal*): (-113.1, -63.1)

We are 95% sure that the following is true.

1. The population PI_{max} mean for patients with UDP only is larger than the population PI_{max} mean for patients with UDP and cardiopulmonary disease. The difference might be quite small (as low as 5.6), large (as high as 59.2), or moderate.

2. The population PI_{max} mean for patients with UDP only is smaller than the population PI_{max} mean for normal people. The difference might be moderate (no less than 31.6) or large (as high as 79.8).

3. The population PI_{max} mean for patients with UDP and cardiopulmonary disease is smaller than the population PI_{max} mean for normal people. The difference might be large (no less than 63.1) or extremely large (as high as 113.1).

15. No. H_0: $\mu_1 = \mu_2 = \mu_3$, H_A: At least one population mean does not equal another population mean, $F = 0.58$, 2 and 58 df, p-value > 0.50. If all three population square-root gastric volume means are equal, the probability of getting an F statistic at least as extreme as 0.58 is greater than 0.50. We cannot reject the hypothesis that all three population square-root gastric volume means are equal at any reasonable significance level. Multiple comparisons are not needed.

16. Yes. H_0: $\mu_1 = \mu_2 = \mu_3$, H_A: At least one population mean does not equal another population mean, $F = 5.46$, 2 and 40 df, $0.005 < p$-value < 0.01. If all three population sulphoxidation score means are equal, the probability of getting an F statistic at least as extreme as 5.46 is between 0.005 and 0.01. We reject the hypothesis that all three population sulphoxidation score means are equal at the 0.05 significance level and conclude that at least one population mean does not equal another population mean.

Since $q_{.10, 3, 40}/\sqrt{2} = 2.99/\sqrt{2} = 2.11$ and $t_{.017, 40} \cong t_{.015, 40} = 2.250$, we will use the Tukey procedure to make all three possible comparisons. The 90% Tukey confidence intervals are as follows:

$\mu_1 - \mu_2$ (*no major adverse reactions versus major adverse renal reactions*): (-0.80, -0.12)

$\mu_1 - \mu_3$ (*no major adverse reactions versus major adverse dermatological reactions*): (-0.82, -0.06)

$\mu_2 - \mu_3$ (*major adverse renal reactions versus major adverse dermatological reactions*): (-0.41, 0.45)

We are 90% sure that the following is true.

1. The population mean sulphoxidation score for RA patients without major adverse reactions to SA is smaller than the population mean sulphoxidation score for RA patients with major adverse renal reactions to SA. The difference might be small (as low as 0.12), large (as high as 0.80), or moderate.

2. The population mean sulphoxidation score for RA patients without major adverse reactions to SA is smaller than the population mean sulphoxidation score for RA patients with major adverse dermatological reactions to SA. The difference might be small (as low as 0.06), large (as high as 0.82), or moderate.

3. We cannot say that the population mean sulphoxidation score for RA patients with major adverse renal reactions to SA differs from the population mean sulphoxidation score for RA patients with major adverse dermatological reactions to SA.

The results indicate that RA patients without major adverse reactions to SA have better sulphoxidation capacities, on average, than RA patients with major adverse renal or dermatological reactions to SA.

17. Yes, H_0: $\mu_1 = \mu_2 = \mu_3 = \mu_4$, H_A: At least one population mean does not equal another population mean, $F = 8.52$, 3 and 34 df, p-value < 0.001. If all four population square-root VPA clearance means are equal, the probability of getting an F

statistic at least as extreme as 8.52 is less than 0.001. We reject the hypothesis that all four population square-root VPA clearance means are equal at any reasonable significance level and conclude that at least one population mean does not equal another population mean.

Since $q_{.05, 4, 34}/\sqrt{2} \cong 3.85/\sqrt{2} = 2.72$ and $t_{.0083, 34} \cong t_{.0075, 30} = 2.581$, we will use the Bonferroni procedure to make our three comparisons. The 95% Bonferroni confidence intervals are as follows:

$\mu_1 - \mu_2$ (*no concurrent anticonvulsants versus phenytoin*): $(-0.16, 0.10)$
$\mu_1 - \mu_3$ (*no concurrent anticonvulsants versus phenobarbital*): $(-0.37, -0.09)$
$\mu_1 - \mu_4$ (*no concurrent anticonvulsants versus phenytoin and phenobarbital*): $(-0.27, -0.05)$

We are 95% sure that the following is true.

1. We cannot say that the population mean square-root VPA clearance for children with seizure disorders who are not taking concurrent anticonvulsants differs from the population mean square-root VPA clearance for children with seizure disorders who are taking phenytoin.

2. The population mean square-root VPA clearance for children with seizure disorders who are not taking concurrent anticonvulsants is lower than the population mean square-root VPA clearance for children with seizure disorders who are taking phenobarbital. The difference might be small (as low as 0.09), large (as high as 0.37), or moderate.

3. The population mean square-root VPA clearance for children with seizure disorders who are not taking concurrent anticonvulsants is lower than the population mean square-root VPA clearance for children with seizure disorders who are taking phenytoin and phenobarbital. The difference might be small (as low as 0.05) or moderate (no more than 0.27).

CHAPTER 9

1. No. H_0: $\mu_1 = \mu_2 = \mu_3$, H_A: At least one population mean does not equal another population mean. The *p*-value for Mauchly's test is 0.103, so we will use the univariate approach. Since the univariate *p*-value for testing the hypothesis of equal population means is 0.985, we cannot reject this hypothesis at any reasonable significance level. If all three population T helper means are equal, the probability of getting a univariate *F* statistic at least as extreme as 0.02 is 0.985. Multiple comparisons are not needed.

3. Yes, according to the multivariate approach; no, according to the HF adjusted univariate approach. H_0: $\mu_1 = \mu_2 = \mu_3$, H_A: At least one population mean does not equal another population mean. Since the *p*-value for Mauchly's test is less than or equal to 0.0005, we cannot use the univariate approach. The multivariate *p*-value for testing

the hypothesis of equal population means is less than or equal to 0.0005, and the HF adjusted univariate *p*-value for testing this hypothesis is between 0.025 and 0.05 (1 and 12 df). If all three population square-root testosterone means are equal, the probability of getting multivariate test statistics at least as extreme as the calculated test statistics is less than or equal to 0.0005 and the probability of getting an HF adjusted univariate *F* statistic at least as extreme as 5.62 is between 0.025 and 0.05. The HF adjusted univariate approach does not allow us to reject the hypothesis that all three population square-root testosterone means are equal at the 0.01 significance level. The multivariate approach allows us to reject this hypothesis at any reasonable significance level. Using $t_{.0083, 11} \cong t_{.0075, 11} = 2.879$, the means in Table 9.12, and the standard deviations of the differences in Table 9.13, we apply formula (9.14) to obtain 95% Bonferroni confidence intervals for all three possible comparisons.

$\mu_1 - \mu_2$ (*peripheral vein versus adrenal vein*): $(-1.03, -0.29)$
$\mu_1 - \mu_3$ (*peripheral vein versus ovarian vein*): $(-2.23, -0.07)$
$\mu_2 - \mu_3$ (*adrenal vein versus ovarian vein*): $(-1.78, 0.80)$

We are 95% sure that the following is true.

1. The population mean square-root testosterone concentration is lower for peripheral veins than for adrenal veins. The difference might be moderate (no less than 0.29) or large (as high as 1.03).

2. The population mean square-root testosterone concentration is lower for peripheral veins than for ovarian veins. The difference might be quite small (as low as 0.07), quite large (as high as 2.23), or somewhere in between.

3. We cannot say that the population mean square-root testosterone concentration for adrenal veins differs from the population mean square-root testosterone concentration for ovarian veins.

4. No. H_0: $\mu_1 = \mu_2 = \mu_3$, H_A: At least one population mean does not equal another population mean. The *p*-value for Mauchly's test is 0.116, so we will use the univariate approach. Since the univariate *p*-value for testing the hypothesis of equal population means is 0.381, we cannot reject the hypothesis that all three population percentage overweight means are equal at any reasonable significance level. If all three population percentage overweight means are equal, the probability of getting a univariate *F* statistic at least as extreme as 1.09 is 0.381. Multiple comparisons are not needed.

6. The umbilicus and liver percentages are extremely nonnormal, with most of the values equal to 0. The multivariate normality assumption is not reasonable for these data, and one-factor repeated-measures ANOVA is not appropriate.

10. The within-samples independence assumption is violated, since three assays were done for each patient after each diet. If we use only the results of one assay per patient after each diet, it can be shown that there are not enough subjects to carry out Mauchly's test or multivariate one-factor repeated-measures ANOVA. Although univariate one-factor repeated-measures ANOVA could be done with one assay from each patient, we cannot use Mauchly's test to determine whether the univariate approach is appropriate. One-factor repeated-measures ANOVA cannot be used to analyze these data.

12. Yes. H_0: $\mu_1 = \mu_2 = \mu_3 = \mu_4$, H_A: At least one population mean does not equal another population mean. Since the p-value for Mauchly's test is 0.057, we cannot use the univariate approach. The multivariate p-value for testing the hypothesis of equal population means is 0.002, and the HF adjusted univariate p-value for testing this hypothesis is less than 0.001 (2 and 35 df). If all four population log provocation dose means are equal, the probability of getting multivariate test statistics at least as extreme as the calculated test statistics is 0.002 and the probability of getting an HF adjusted univariate F statistic at least as extreme as 9.26 is less than 0.001. Both the multivariate approach and the HF adjusted univariate approach allow us to reject the hypothesis that all four population log provocation dose means are equal at the 0.05 significance level.

Since our comparisons were selected after examining the sample means, $c = 6$. Using $t_{.0042, 14} \cong t_{.005, 14} = 2.977$, the means in Table 9.26, and the standard deviations of the differences in Table 9.27, we apply formula (9.14) to obtain 95% Bonferroni confidence intervals for our three comparisons.

$\mu_1 - \mu_2$ (*baseline versus saline*): $(-1.33, -0.17)$
$\mu_1 - \mu_3$ (*baseline versus verapamil*): $(-1.88, -0.58)$
$\mu_1 - \mu_4$ (*baseline versus sodium cromoglycate*): $(-1.59, 0.11)$

We are 95% sure that the following is true.

1. The population log provocation dose mean is smaller at baseline than after saline administration. The difference might be quite small (as low as 0.17) or moderate (no more than 1.33).
2. The population log provocation dose mean is smaller at baseline than after verapamil administration. The difference might be small (as low as 0.58), large (as high as 1.88), or moderate.
3. We cannot say that the population log provocation dose mean at baseline differs from the population log provocation dose mean after sodium cromoglycate administration.

14. Yes. H_0: $\mu_1 = \mu_2 = \mu_3$, H_A: At least one population mean does not equal another population mean. The p-value for Mauchly's test is 0.555, so we will use the univariate approach. Since the univariate p-value for testing the hypothesis of equal population means is less than or equal to 0.0005, we reject the hypothesis that all three population exer-

cise duration means are equal at any reasonable significance level. If all three population exercise duration means are equal, the probability of getting a univariate F statistic at least as extreme as 16.00 is less than or equal to 0.0005. Using $t_{.017, 14} \cong t_{.015, 14} = 2.415$, the means in Table 9.29, and the standard deviations of the differences in Table 9.30, we apply formula (9.14) to obtain 90% Bonferroni confidence intervals for all three possible comparisons.

$\mu_1 - \mu_2$ (*placebo versus propranolol*): $(0.0, 3.4)$
$\mu_1 - \mu_3$ (*placebo versus nifedipine*): $(-3.3, -0.3)$
$\mu_2 - \mu_3$ (*propranolol versus nifedipine*): $(-4.8, -2.2)$

We are 90% sure that the following is true.

1. We cannot say that the population mean exercise duration after taking the placebo differs from the population mean exercise duration after taking propanolol.
2. The population mean exercise duration is smaller after taking the placebo than after taking nifedipine. The difference might be quite small (as low as 0.3), quite large (as high as 3.3), or somewhere in between.
3. The population mean exercise duration is smaller after taking propranolol than after taking nifedipine. The difference might be large (no less than 2.2) or extremely large (as high as 4.8).

16. Yes. H_0: $\mu_1 = \mu_2 = \mu_3 = \mu_4$, H_A: At least one population mean does not equal another population mean. Since the p-value for Mauchly's test is 0.014, we cannot use the univariate approach. The multivariate p-value for testing the hypothesis of equal population means is 0.001, and the HF adjusted univariate p-value for testing this hypothesis is less than 0.001 (2 and 13 df). If all four population square-root clearance means are equal, the probability of getting multivariate statistics at least as extreme as the calculated test statistics is 0.001 and the probability of getting an HF adjusted univariate F statistic at least as extreme as 17.28 is less than 0.001. Both the multivariate approach and the HF adjusted univariate approach allow us to reject the hypothesis that all four population square-root clearance means are equal at the 0.01 significance level. Using $t_{.0083, 8} \cong t_{.0075, 8} = 3.085$, the means in Table 9.33, and the standard deviations of the differences in Table 9.34, we apply formula (9.14) to obtain 95% Bonferroni confidence intervals for our three comparisons.

$\mu_1 - \mu_2$ (*0–6-hour interval versus 6–12-hour interval*): $(0.22, 3.14)$
$\mu_1 - \mu_3$ (*0–6-hour interval versus 12–18-hour interval*): $(0.42, 4.08)$
$\mu_1 - \mu_4$ (*0–6-hour interval versus 18–24-hour interval*): $(1.28, 4.04)$

We are 95% sure that the following is true.

1. The population mean square-root renal platinum clearance is larger during the zero- to six-hour interval than during the six- to 12-hour interval. The

difference might be quite small (as low as 0.22), quite large (as high as 3.14), or somewhere in between.

2. The population mean square-root renal platinum clearance is larger during the zero- to six-hour interval than during the 12- to 18-hour interval. The difference might be small (as low as 0.42), extremely large (as high as 4.08), or somewhere in between.

3. The population mean square-root renal platinum clearance is larger during the zero- to six-hour interval than during the 18- to 24-hour interval. The difference might be moderate (no less than 1.28) or extremely large (as high as 4.04).

CHAPTER 10

1. No. H_0: There is no association between needle strategy and tenderness, H_A: There is an association between needle strategy and tenderness, $\chi^2 = 0.476$, 1 df, $0.40 < p$-value < 0.50. If there is no association between needle strategy and tenderness, the probability of getting a χ^2 statistic at least as extreme as 0.476 is between 0.40 and 0.50. We cannot reject the hypothesis of no association at any reasonable significance level.

3. No. H_0: $p_1 = p_2$, H_A: $p_1 \neq p_2$, $M = 0$, $n_D = 3$, two-tailed p-value > 0.10. If the paired population proportions are equal, the probability of getting an M statistic at least as extreme as 0 is greater than 0.10. We cannot reject the hypothesis that the population proportion of pregnant diabetic women with retinopathy is the same before and after delivery at any reasonable significance level.

5. No. H_0: $p_1 = 0.333$, $p_2 = 0.333$, $p_3 = 0.333$, H_A: At least one of the hypothesized population proportions is wrong, $\chi^2 = 2.988$, 2 df, $0.20 < p$-value < 0.30. If all of the hypothesized population proportions are correct, the probability of getting a χ^2 statistic at least as extreme as 2.988 is between 0.20 and 0.30. We cannot reject the hypothesis that the population proportions are equal to the hypothesized population proportions at any reasonable significance level.

9. Yes. H_0: There is no association between number of clams eaten and illness, H_A: There is an association between number of clams eaten and illness, $\chi^2 = 74.150$, 5 df, p-value < 0.0005. If there is no association between number of clams eaten and illness, the probability of getting a χ^2 statistic at least as extreme as 74.150 is less than 0.0005. We reject the hypothesis of no association at any reasonable significance level.

Since illness can be considered a response variable and number of clams eaten a nonresponse variable, we will examine the row percentages shown in the following table. These percentages suggest that (1) people who ate clams are much more likely to become ill than people who did not eat clams and (2) people who ate more than six clams are more

likely to become ill than people who ate one to six clams.

ROW PERCENTAGES FOR TABLE 10.20

Number of Clams Eaten	Illness	
	PRESENT	NOT PRESENT
0	2.2%	97.8%
1–6	21.1%	78.9%
7–12	62.5%	37.5%
13–24	73.1%	26.9%
25–36	80.0%	20.0%
37–102	85.0%	15.0%

10. Yes. H_0: $p_1 = p_2$, H_A: $p_1 \neq p_2$, $M = 0$, $n_D = 7$, $0.01 <$ two-tailed p-value < 0.02. If the paired population proportions are equal, the probability of getting an M statistic at least as extreme as 0 is between 0.01 and 0.02. Using a 0.10 significance level, we reject the hypothesis that the population proportion of normal X-ray CT diagnoses is the same as the population proportion of normal MRI diagnoses.

12. Yes. H_0: There is no association between type of insurance and tooth extraction, H_A: There is an association between type of insurance and tooth extraction, $\chi^2 = 7.517$, 2 df, $0.01 < p$-value < 0.025. If there is no association between type of insurance and tooth extraction, the probability of getting a χ^2 statistic at least as extreme as 7.517 is between 0.01 and 0.025. We reject the hypothesis of no association at the 0.05 significance level. Since type of insurance is the independent variable, we will examine the column percentages shown in the following table. These percentages suggest that people with the stingy plan are less likely to have tooth extractions than people with the free plan.

COLUMN PERCENTAGES FOR TABLE 10.23

Tooth Extraction	Type of Insurance		
	FREE	INTERMEDIATE	STINGY
One or more	35.1%	30.1%	26.9%
None	64.9%	69.9%	73.1%

16. Yes. H_0: There is no association between specialty and back injury status, H_A: There is an association between specialty and back injury status, $\chi^2 = 12.433$, 3 df, $0.005 < p$-value < 0.01. If there is no association between specialty and back injury status, the probability of getting a χ^2 statistic at least as extreme as 12.433 is between 0.005 and 0.01. We reject the hypothesis of no association at the 0.01 significance level.

Although back injury status can be considered a response variable and specialty a nonresponse variable, samples of back-injured nursing personnel and non-back-injured nursing personnel were selected rather than samples of nursing personnel in the four specialties. For this reason, we will examine the row percentages shown in the following table. These percentages suggest that nursing personnel with back injuries are more likely than nursing personnel without back injuries to be in medicine and less likely to be in psychiatry or long-term care.

ROW PERCENTAGES FOR TABLE 10.27

Back Injury Status	Specialty			
	MEDICINE	SURGERY	PSYCHIATRY	LONG-TERM CARE
Injured	54.5%	12.2%	18.7%	14.6%
Not injured	40.3%	8.8%	28.4%	22.6%

18. Yes. H_0: There is no association between protocol and frequency of bruising, H_A: There is an association between protocol and frequency of bruising, $\chi^2 = 10.010$, 2 df, $0.005 < p\text{-value} < 0.01$. If there is no association between protocol and frequency of bruising, the probability of getting a χ^2 statistic at least as extreme as 10.010 is between 0.005 and 0.01. We reject the hypothesis of no association at the 0.01 significance level.

Since frequency of bruising can be considered a response variable and protocol a nonresponse variable, we will examine the row percentages shown in the following table. These percentages suggest that (1) heart-transplant recipients on an azathioprine-based protocol are more likely than heart-transplant recipients on a cyclosporine-based protocol to report that bruising occurs often or always, (2) heart-transplant recipients on an azathioprine-based protocol are less likely than heart-transplant recipients on a cyclosporine-based protocol to report that bruising occurs rarely or sometimes, and (3) heart-transplant recipients on an azathioprine-based protocol are less likely than heart-transplant recipients on a cyclosporine-based protocol to report that bruising never occurs.

ROW PERCENTAGES FOR TABLE 10.29

Protocol	Frequency of Bruises		
	NEVER	RARELY OR SOMETIMES	OFTEN OR ALWAYS
Azathioprine	12.9%	25.8%	61.3%
Cyclosporine	22.7%	52.3%	25.0%

20. Since 41 BAL specimens were obtained from 30 patients, some of the BAL results are repeated measurements. The within-samples independence assumption does not hold, and the McNemar test cannot be done.

21. Forty per cent of the expected frequencies are less than 5 ($E_4 = E_5 = 3.225$). The chi-square test of hypothesized proportions cannot be done unless the agonal respiration and apneic respiration categories are combined. If this is done, the hypothesized proportions are as follows:

$P(\text{Eupnea}) = 0.40$
$P(\text{Tachypnea}) = 0.40$
$P(\text{Dyspnea}) = 0.15$
$P(\text{Agonal respiration or apnea}) = 0.05$

All of the expected frequencies are now at least 5. H_0: $p_1 = 0.40$, $p_2 = 0.40$, $p_3 = 0.15$, $p_4 = 0.05$, H_A: At least one of the hypothesized population proportions is wrong, $\chi^2 = 2.408$, 3 df, $0.40 < p\text{-value} < 0.50$. If all of the hypothesized population proportions are correct, the probability of getting a χ^2 statistic at least as extreme as 2.408 is between 0.40 and 0.50. We cannot reject the hypothesis that the population proportions are equal to the hypothesized population proportions at any reasonable significance level.

22. Yes. H_0: $p_1 = p_2$, H_A: $p_1 \neq p_2$, $M = 12$, $n_D = 12$, two-tailed $p\text{-value} < 0.01$. If the paired population proportions are equal, the probability of getting an M statistic at least as extreme as 12 is less than 0.01. Using a 0.05 significance level, we reject the hypothesis that the population proportion of patients with night and rest pain is the same before and after surgery.

25. Yes. H_0: There is no association between disease and fatigue on awakening, H_A: There is an association between disease and fatigue on awakening, $\chi^2 = 5.933$, 1 df, $0.01 < p\text{-value} < 0.025$. If there is no association between disease and fatigue on awakening, the probability of getting a χ^2 statistic at least as extreme as 5.933 is between 0.01 and 0.025. We reject the hypothesis of no association at the 0.05 significance level.

Since fatigue on awakening can be considered a response variable and disease a nonresponse variable, we will examine the column percentages shown in the following table. These percentages suggest that COPD patients are more likely to experience fatigue on awakening than PVD patients.

COLUMN PERCENTAGES FOR TABLE 10.36

Fatigue on Awakening	Disease	
	COPD	PVD
Present	66.7%	33.3%
Not Present	33.3%	66.7%

28. Since 70 patients had 173 grafts, repeated measurements were obtained. The independence assumption does not hold, and the chi-square test of hypothesized proportions cannot be used.

CHAPTER 11

5. No. A histogram of the days since last transfusion is consistent with an approximately symmetric population, so we will use the Wilcoxon signed rank test.

Quick histogram of days since last transfusion

```
0 – 4 | XX
5 – 9 | XXX
10 – 14 | XXXXXX
15 – 19 | X
20 – 24 | X
```

H_0: Population median = 10, H_A: Population median $\neq$ 10, $W = 19.5$, $n_D = 9$, two-tailed p-value > 0.10. If the population median is 10, the probability of getting a W statistic at least as extreme as 19.5 is greater than 0.10. We cannot reject the hypothesis that the population median number of days since the last transfusion is 10 at any reasonable significance level.

6. Yes. H_0: The two populations are identical, H_A: One population tends to produce larger IRI values than the other population, $MW = 45$, $n_1 = 6$, $n_2 = 4$, $0.002 <$ two-tailed p-value < 0.01. If the two populations of IRI values are identical, the probability of getting an MW statistic at least as extreme as 45 is between 0.002 and 0.01. We reject the hypothesis that the insulin autoimmune population of IRI values and the insulin-treated diabetes population of IRI values are identical at the 0.05 significance level.

9. Yes. Since the following histogram of the times is fairly skewed, we will use the sign test instead of the Wilcoxon signed rank test to test the hypothesis that the population median is 6.

Quick histogram of time

```
2 | XXX
3 | XXXXXXXX
4 | XXXXXX
5 | XXXXXX
6 | XXXXX
7 | X
8 |
9 | X
```

H_0: Population median = 6, H_A: Population median $\neq$ 6, $S = 2$, $n_D = 25$, two-tailed p-value < 0.01. If the population median is 6, the probability of getting an S statistic at least as extreme as 2 is less than 0.01. We reject the hypothesis that the population median time from AMI onset to SICT is 6 hours at the 0.05 significance level.

10. Because more than one specimen was obtained from four of the six infants, repeated measurements were obtained. The within-samples independence assumption is not reasonable for these data, and the Spearman rank correlation coefficient cannot be used to test the hypothesis of no correlation. If one specimen of the same type is selected from each infant with more than one specimen, the resulting independent observations can be used to test the hypothesis of no correlation.

13. No. Since the following histogram of the differences is consistent with an approximately symmetric population, we can use the Wilcoxon signed rank test instead of the sign test to test the hypothesis that the population median difference is 0.

Quick histogram of difference

```
– 8 – – 5 | X
– 4 – – 1 | XXXX
0 – 3 | XXX
4 – 7 | X
8 – 11 | X
```

H_0: Population median difference = 0, H_A: Population median difference $\neq$ 0, $W = 31.5$, $n_D = 10$, two-tailed p-value > 0.10. If the population median difference is 0, the probability of getting a W statistic at least as extreme as 31.5 is greater than 0.10. We cannot reject the hypothesis that the population median difference between the movement percentage before sampling and the movement percentage after sampling is 0 at any reasonable significance level.

14. Yes. H_0: All possible rankings of the percentages for any patient are equally likely, H_A: At least one population tends to produce larger percentages than another population, Friedman $\chi^2 = 6.1000$, 2 df, $0.025 < p$-value < 0.05. If all possible rankings of the percentages for any patient are equally likely, the probability of getting a Friedman χ^2 statistic at least as extreme as 6.1000 is between 0.025 and 0.05. We reject the hypothesis that all possible rankings of the percentages are equally likely at the 0.05 significance level.

There are three possible comparisons (myelomonocytic population versus granulocytic population, myelomonocytic population versus monocytic population, and granulocytic population versus monocytic population), so $c = 3$. The overall significance level is 0.10, so we will use a significance level of $0.10/3 = 0.033 \cong 0.02$ for each Wilcoxon signed rank test or sign test.

Myelomonocytic Population Versus Granulocytic Population. The following figure is a histogram of the difference between the myelomonocytic percentage and the granulocytic percentage. This histogram is so skewed that the Wilcoxon signed rank test cannot be used. There is no point in carrying out the sign test since no S statistic will produce a two-tailed p-value less than 0.02 when $n_D = 5$. We cannot use any method described in this chapter to compare the myelomonocytic population and the granulocytic population with a 0.02 significance level. Additional data are needed.

Quick histogram of myelomonocytic – granulocytic difference

```
 - 30 - - 1 | XXX
    0 - 29 | X
   30 - 59 |
   60 - 89 | X
```

Myelomonocytic Population Versus Monocytic Population. The following figure is a histogram of the difference between the myelomonocytic percentage and the monocytic percentage. This histogram is so skewed that the Wilcoxon signed rank test cannot be used. There is no point in carrying out the sign test, since no S statistic will produce a two-tailed p-value less than 0.02 when $n_D = 5$. We cannot use any method described in this chapter to compare the myelomonocytic population and the monocytic population with a 0.02 significance level. Additional data are needed.

Quick histogram of myelomonocytic – monocytic difference

```
 10 - 29 | XXXX
 30 - 49 |
 50 - 69 |
 70 - 89 | X
```

Granulocytic Population Versus Monocytic Population. The following figure is a histogram of the difference between the granulocytic percentage and the monocytic percentage. This histogram is consistent with an approximately symmetric population, so the Wilcoxon signed rank test could be used. There is no point in carrying out this test, however, since no W statistic will produce a two-tailed p-value less than 0.02 when $n_D = 5$. We cannot use any method described in this chapter to compare the granulocytic population and the monocytic population with a 0.02 significance level. Additional data are needed.

Quick histogram of granulocytic – monocytic difference

```
  0 - 10 | X
 11 - 21 | XX
 22 - 32 | X
 33 - 43 | X
```

15. Yes. H_0: The three populations are identical, H_A: At least one population tends to produce larger numbers of antigen-presenting dendritic cells than another population, KW $\chi^2 = 22.9542$, 2 df, p-value < 0.0005. If the three populations of cell numbers are identical, the probability of getting a KW χ^2 statistic at least as extreme as 22.9542 is less than 0.0005. We reject the hypothesis that all three populations of numbers of antigen-presenting dendritic cells are identical at any reasonable significance level.

There are three possible comparisons (no-thyroid-disease population versus nontoxic goiter population, no-thyroid-disease population versus Graves' disease population, and nontoxic goiter population versus Graves' disease population), so $c = 3$. The overall significance level is 0.10, so we will use a significance level of $0.10/3 = 0.033 \cong 0.02$ for each Mann–Whitney test.

No-Thyroid-Disease Population Versus Nontoxic Goiter Population. H_0: The two populations are identical, H_A: One population tends to produce larger numbers of antigen-presenting dendritic cells than the other population, $MW = 45$, $n_1 = 9$, $n_2 = 10$, two-tailed p-value < 0.002. If the two populations of cell numbers are identical, the probability of getting an MW statistic at least as extreme as 45 is less than 0.002. We reject the hypothesis that the no-thyroid-disease and nontoxic goiter populations of numbers of antigen-presenting dendritic cells are identical at the 0.02 significance level.

No-Thyroid-Disease Population Versus Graves' Disease Population. H_0: The two populations are identical, H_A: One population tends to produce larger numbers of antigen-presenting dendritic cells than the other population, $MW = 45$, $n_1 = 9$, $n_2 = 12$, two-tailed p-value < 0.002. If the two populations of cell numbers are identical, the probability of getting an MW statistic at least as extreme as 45 is less than 0.002. We reject the hypothesis that the no-thyroid-disease and Graves' disease populations of numbers of antigen-presenting dendritic cells are identical at the 0.02 significance level.

Nontoxic Goiter Population Versus Graves' Disease Population. H_0: The two populations are identical, H_A: One population tends to produce larger numbers of antigen-presenting dendritic cells than the other population, $MW = 70.5$, $n_1 = 10$, $n_2 = 12$, $0.002 <$ two-tailed p-value < 0.01. If the two populations of cell numbers are identical, the probability of getting an MW statistic at least as extreme as 70.5 is between 0.002 and 0.01. We reject the hypothesis that the nontoxic goiter and Graves' disease populations of numbers of antigen-presenting dendritic cells are identical at the 0.02 significance level.

16. Yes. Since the histogram of the difference between the lidocaine KCl infusion and the placebo KCl infusion is fairly skewed, we will use the sign test instead of the Wilcoxon signed rank test to test the hypothesis that the population median difference is 0.

Quick histogram of lidocaine – placebo difference

```
-5 - -4 | XXXX
-3 - -2 |
-1 - 0 | XX
```

H_0: Population median difference = 0, H_A: Population median difference ≠ 0, $S = 0$, $n_D = 5$, 0.05 < two-tailed p-value < 0.10. If the population median difference is 0, the probability of getting an S statistic at least as extreme as 0 is between 0.05 and 0.10. We reject the hypothesis that the population median difference between the lidocaine KCl infusion and the placebo KCl infusion is 0 at the 0.10 significance level.

18. Since 40 specimens were obtained from 36 patients, repeated measurements were obtained for at least one patient. The independence assumption required for the Wilcoxon signed rank test and the sign test is not reasonable for these data. We cannot use either test to test the hypothesis that the population median rating is 2. If we knew which specimens belonged to each patient, we could randomly select one of the specimens for each of the patients with more than one specimen. The Wilcoxon signed rank test or the sign test could then be used to analyze the resulting 36 independent ratings.

19. No. H_0: The three populations are identical, H_A: At least one population tends to produce larger test scores than another population, KW $\chi^2 = 0.5878$, 2 df, 0.70 < p-value < 0.80. If the three populations of test scores are identical, the probability of getting a KW χ^2 statistic at least as extreme as 0.5878 is between 0.70 and 0.80. We cannot reject the hypothesis that all three populations of test scores are identical at any reasonable significance level.

20. No. H_0: Spearman's $\rho = 0$, H_A: Spearman's $\rho \neq 0$, two-tailed p-value = 0.613. We cannot reject the hypothesis that Spearman's ρ is equal to 0 at any reasonable significance level. If Spearman's ρ is equal to 0, the probability of getting an r_s statistic at least as extreme as 0.2342 is 0.613. To determine whether a nonlinear relationship exists between the presplenectomy ranks and the postsplenectomy ranks, we examine the scatterplot of the ranks in Figure 11.32. No relationship of any kind is evident in this scatterplot.

22. No. Since the following histogram of the difference between the 24-hour diameter and the 48-hour diameter is quite skewed, we will use the sign test instead of the Wilcoxon signed rank test to test the hypothesis that the population median difference is 0.

Quick histogram of 24-hour – 48-hour difference

```
-16 - -13 | X
-12 - -9 |
 -8 - -5 | X
 -4 - -1 | XXX
  0 - 3 | XXXX
  4 - 7 | XX
```

H_0: Population median difference = 0, H_A: Population median difference ≠ 0, $S = 3$, $n_D = 8$, two-tailed p-value > 0.10. If the population median difference is 0, the probability of getting an S statistic at least as extreme as 3 is greater than 0.10. We cannot reject the hypothesis that the population median difference between the 24-hour diameter and the 48-hour diameter is 0 at any reasonable significance level.

23. Duration of gestation was recorded for 23 pregnancies in 15 women, so repeated measurements were obtained. Since the independence assumptions required for the Kruskal-Wallis test are not reasonable for these data, this test cannot be used to test the hypothesis of identical populations. If we knew which pregnancies were associated with each subject, we could select the weeks of gestation for the first pregnancies. The resulting observations would be independent and the Kruskal-Wallis test could be used.

27. No. Since the following histogram of years of infertility is consistent with an approximately symmetric population, we can use the Wilcoxon signed rank test instead of the sign test to test the hypothesis that the population median is 2.

Quick histogram of years of infertility

```
0 - 1 | X
2 - 3 | XXX
4 - 5 | XX
6 - 7 | XX
```

H_0: Population median = 2, H_A: Population median ≠ 2, $W = 19.5$, $n_D = 6$, 0.05 < two-tailed p-value < 0.10. If the population median is 2, the probability of getting a W statistic at least as extreme as 19.5 is between 0.05 and 0.10. We cannot reject the hypothesis that the population median duration of infertility is 2 at the 0.01 significance level.

29. Yes. H_0: All possible rankings of the numbers of reported changes for any patient are equally likely, H_A: At least one population tends to produce larger numbers of reported changes than another population, Friedman $\chi^2 = 43.9100$, 3 df, p-value < 0.0005. If all possible rankings of the numbers of reported changes for any patient are equally likely, the probability of getting a Friedman χ^2 statistic at least as extreme as 43.9100 is less than 0.0005. We reject the hypothesis that all possible rankings of the numbers of reported changes are equally likely at any reasonable significance level.

There are three comparisons of interest (social interaction population versus food-and-water population, social interaction population versus hazards population, and social interaction population versus normality population). Since these comparisons were selected before examining the data, $c = 3$. The overall significance level is 0.05, so we will use a significance level of $0.05/3 = 0.017 \cong 0.02$ for each Wilcoxon signed rank test or sign test.

Social Interaction Population Versus Food-and-Water Population. The following figure is a histogram of the difference between the number of reported changes related to social interaction and

Quick histogram of social interaction – food-and-water difference

```
 −7 | XX
 −6 | X
 −5 |
 −4 | X
 −3 | XXXXXXXXXX
 −2 | XXXXXXXXX
 −1 | XXX
  0 | XXX
```

the number of reported changes related to food and water. Since this histogram suggests a nonsymmetric population, we will use the sign test instead of the Wilcoxon signed rank test to compare the social interaction and food-and-water populations.

H_0: Population median difference $= 0$, H_A: Population median difference $\neq 0$, $S = 0$, $n_D = 27$, two-tailed p-value < 0.01. If the population median difference is 0, the probability of getting an S statistic at least as extreme as 0 is less than 0.01. We reject the hypothesis that the population median difference is 0 at the 0.02 significance level.

Social Interaction Population Versus Hazards Population. The following figure is a histogram of the difference between the number of reported changes related to social interaction and the number of reported changes related to hazards. Since this histogram suggests a nonsymmetric population, we will use the sign test instead of the Wilcoxon signed rank test to compare the social interaction and hazards populations.

Quick histogram of social interaction – hazards difference

```
 −8 | X
 −7 |
 −6 | X
 −5 | XXXX
 −4 | XXX
 −3 | XXXXXX
 −2 | XXXXXXX
 −1 | XXXX
  0 | XXXX
```

H_0: Population median difference $= 0$, H_A: Population median difference $\neq 0$, $S = 0$, $n_D = 26$, two-tailed p-value < 0.01. If the population median difference is 0, the probability of getting an S statistic at least as extreme as 0 is less than 0.01. We reject the hypothesis that the population median difference is 0 at the 0.02 significance level.

Social Interaction Population Versus Normal Population. The following figure is a histogram of the difference between the number of reported changes related to social interaction and the number of reported changes related to normality. Since this histogram suggests a nonsymmetric population, we will use the sign test instead of the Wilcoxon signed rank test to compare the social interaction and normality populations.

H_0: Population median difference $= 0$, H_A: Population median difference $\neq 0$, $S = 0$, $n_D = 26$, two-tailed p-value < 0.01. If the population median difference is 0, the probability of getting an S statistic at least as extreme as 0 is less than 0.01. We reject the hypothesis that the population median difference is 0 at the 0.02 significance level.

Quick histogram of social interaction – normality difference

```
 −6 | X
 −5 | X
 −4 | XX
 −3 | XXXXX
 −2 | XXXXXXXXXX
 −1 | XXXXXX
  0 | XXXX
```

CHAPTER 12

1. The scatterplot of the data suggests a pattern of decreasing variance as the postdischarge scores increase. This is confirmed by the funnel pattern in the scatterplot of the residuals and the estimated values. The scores should be transformed to obtain constant variance before obtaining regression hypothesis tests or confidence intervals.

3. Both the scatterplot of the data and the scatterplot of the residuals and estimated values suggest a nonlinear relationship between creatinine clearance and serum creatinine. The data should be transformed to obtain a linear relationship before obtaining regression hypothesis tests or confidence intervals.

5. Yes. a. H_0: Population Pearson correlation coefficient = 0, H_A: Population Pearson correlation coefficient ≠ 0, $t = -2.80$, 10 df, $0.015 <$ two-tailed p-value < 0.02. If the population Pearson correlation coefficient is 0, the probability of getting a t statistic at least as extreme as -2.80 is between 0.015 and 0.02. We reject the hypothesis that the population Pearson correlation coefficient for CI and Rs is 0 at the 0.10 significance level.

b. Since the 90% confidence interval for β_1 is $(-0.39, -0.09)$, we are 90% sure that the population regression slope is between -0.39 and -0.09.

c. and d. Since Rs values cannot equal 0, inferences about β_0 are not appropriate.

7. No. a. H_0: $\beta_1 = 0$, H_A: $\beta_1 \neq 0$, $t = 16.39$, 13 df, two-tailed p-value < 0.001. If the population regression slope is 0, the probability of getting a t statistic at least as extreme as 16.39 is less than 0.001. We reject the hypothesis that the population regression slope is 0 at any reasonable significance level.

b. H_0: $\beta_1 = 1$, H_A: $\beta_1 \neq 1$, $t = -0.68$, 13 df, $0.40 <$ two-tailed p-value < 0.60. If the population regression slope is 1, the probability of getting a t statistic at least as extreme as -0.68 is between 0.40 and 0.60. We cannot reject the hypothesis that the population regression slope is 1 at any reasonable significance level.

c. and d. Since cardiac output values cannot equal 0, inferences about β_0 are not appropriate.

8. The scatterplot of the data suggests a pattern of increasing variance as the BUN increases. This is confirmed by the funnel shape in the scatterplot of the residuals and the estimated values. The data should be transformed to obtain constant variance before obtaining regression hypothesis tests or confidence intervals.

11. Yes. a. H_0: Population Pearson correlation coefficient = 0, H_A: Population Pearson correlation coefficient ≠ 0, $t = 8.91$, 26 df, two-tailed p-value < 0.001. If the population Pearson correlation coefficient is 0, the probability of getting a t statistic at least as extreme as 8.91 is less than 0.001. We reject the hypothesis that the population Pearson correlation coefficient for the posthemorrhage score and the prehemorrhage score is 0 at any reasonable significance level.

b. Since the 99% confidence interval for β_1 is $(0.74, 1.40)$, we are 99% sure that the population regression slope is between 0.74 and 1.40.

c. and d. Since symptom scores cannot equal 0, inferences about β_0 are not appropriate.

14. Since the 32 episodes were based on 21 patients, some patients had multiple episodes of acute pancreatitis. The independence assumption for the dependent variable is not reasonable, and we cannot make inferences about the population Pearson correlation coefficient or the population regression equation. If we knew which episodes belonged to each patient, we could select the serum amylase values for the first episodes. The resulting 21 pairs of observations would satisfy the independence assumption and could be used to obtain correlation and regression hypothesis tests and confidence intervals.

16. Both the scatterplot of the data and the scatterplot of the residuals and estimated values suggest a nonlinear relationship between daily fluid intake and urine pH. The data should be transformed to obtain a linear relationship before obtaining correlation or regression hypothesis tests or confidence intervals.

17. No. a. H_0: $\beta_1 = 0$, H_A: $\beta_1 \neq 0$, $t = 28.15$, 12 df, two-tailed p-value < 0.001. If the population regression slope is 0, the probability of getting a t statistic at least as extreme as 28.15 is less than 0.001. We reject the hypothesis that the population regression slope is 0 at any reasonable significance level.

b. H_0: $\beta_1 = 1$, H_A: $\beta_1 \neq 1$, $t = -1.86$, 12 df, $0.05 <$ two-tailed p-value < 0.10. If the population regression slope is 1, the probability of getting a t statistic at least as extreme as -1.86 is between 0.05 and 0.10. We cannot reject the hypothesis that the population regression slope is 1 at the 0.05 significance level.

c. and d. Since prosthetic annulus diameters cannot equal 0, inferences about β_0 are not appropriate.

CHAPTER 13

2. Yes. H_0: No interaction, H_A: Interaction present, $F = 2.50$, 2 and 47 df, $0.05 < p$-value < 0.10. If interaction is not present, the probability of getting an interaction F statistic at least as extreme as 2.50 is between 0.05 and 0.10. We reject the hypothesis of no interaction at the 0.10 significance level. No further tests for factor effects are done.

Comparison of cell means is appropriate. Let morphology be Factor A and age be Factor B. The estimated variances for the sample cell means of interest to us are

$$\mathrm{var}(\bar{x}_{A2B1}) = 9.97 \qquad \mathrm{var}(\bar{x}_{A1B2}) = 3.32$$
$$\mathrm{var}(\bar{x}_{A1B1}) = 7.12 \qquad \mathrm{var}(\bar{x}_{A1B3}) = 5.54$$

There are 15 possible cell mean comparisons, and we selected our three comparisons after examining the sample means, so $c = 15$. Since $q_{.10, 6, 47}/\sqrt{2} \cong 3.80/\sqrt{2} = 2.69$ and $t_{.0033, 47} \cong t_{.0025, 40} = 2.971$, we will use the Tukey procedure to make our three comparisons. Applying formula (13.13), we obtain the following 90% Tukey confidence intervals.

$\mu_{A2B1} - \mu_{A1B1}$ (*normal morphology and age one year or less versus toxic vacuolation and age one year or less*): $(-0.3, 21.9)$

$\mu_{A2B1} - \mu_{A1B2}$ (*normal morphology and age one year or less versus toxic vacuolation and age between one and five years*): $(4.6, 24.2)$

$\mu_{A2B1} - \mu_{A1B3}$ (*normal morphology and age one year or less versus toxic vacuolation and age at least five years*): $(-0.9, 20.3)$

We are 90% sure that the following is true.

1. We cannot say that the population PCV mean for neutropenic cats one year old or less with normal neutrophil morphology differs from the population PCV mean for neutropenic cats one year old or less with toxic vacuolation.
2. The population PCV mean for neutropenic cats one year old or less with normal neutrophil morphology is larger than the population PCV mean for neutropenic cats more than one year old but less than five years old with toxic vacuolation. The difference might be small (as low as 4.6), large (as high as 24.2), or moderate.
3. We cannot say that the population PCV mean for neutropenic cats one year old or less with normal neutrophil morphology differs from the population PCV mean for neutropenic cats at least five years old with toxic vacuolation.

3. Three-fourths of the eight patients without COPD who were successfully weaned have two days of previous support, so the data for this cell appear extremely nonnormal. In addition, the ratio of the largest sample cell variance to the smallest sample cell variance is 955.4. The equal-variance assumption is not reasonable for these data. Data transformation might make the variances less different but the data for the COPD patients who were successfully weaned would still be extremely nonnormal. Two-way ANOVA is not appropriate.

4. Yes. H_0: No interaction, H_A: Interaction present, $F = 1.98$, 2 and 27 df, $0.10 < p$-value < 0.50. If interaction is not present, the probability of getting an F statistic at least as extreme as 1.98 is between 0.10 and 0.50. We cannot reject the hypothesis of no interaction at any reasonable significance level. Let mood change be Factor A and diagnosis be Factor B.

H_0: $\mu_{A1} = \mu_{A2}$, H_A: $\mu_{A1} \neq \mu_{A2}$, $F = 2.73$, 1 and 27 df, $0.10 < p$-value < 0.50. If the two population mood-change factor means are equal, the probability of getting an F statistic at least as extreme as 2.73 is between 0.10 and 0.50. We cannot reject the

hypothesis of equal population mood-change factor means at any reasonable significance level.

H_0: $\mu_{B1} = \mu_{B2} = \mu_{B3}$, H_A: At least one population diagnosis factor mean does not equal another population diagnosis factor mean, $F = 18.18$, 2 and 27 df, p-value < 0.001. If all three population diagnosis factor means are equal, the probability of getting an F statistic at least as extreme as 18.18 is less than 0.001. We reject the hypothesis of equal population diagnosis factor means at any reasonable significance level.

Comparison of the diagnosis factor means is appropriate. The sample diagnosis factor means and their estimated variances are

$$\bar{x}_{B1} = 19.9 \qquad \text{var}(\bar{x}_{B1}) = 16.5$$
$$\bar{x}_{B2} = 21.2 \qquad \text{var}(\bar{x}_{B2}) = 12.9$$
$$\bar{x}_{B3} = 44.6 \qquad \text{var}(\bar{x}_{B3}) = 8.6$$

Since $q_{.10, 3, 27}/\sqrt{2} \cong 3.05/\sqrt{2} = 2.16$ and $t_{.025, 27} = 2.052$, we will use the Bonferroni procedure to make the two comparisons of interest to us. Applying formula (13.18), we obtain the following 90% Bonferroni confidence intervals.

$\mu_{B3} - \mu_{B1}$ (*autistic versus language disorder*): $(14.4, 35.0)$

$\mu_{B3} - \mu_{B2}$ (*autistic versus developmental disorder*): $(13.9, 32.9)$

We are 90% sure that the following is true.

1. The population mean BCDP score for autistic children is larger than the population mean BCDP score for children with developmental language disorder. The difference might be large (no less than 14.4) or extremely large (as high as 35.0).
2. The population mean BCDP score for autistic children is larger than the population mean BCDP score for children with atypical pervasive developmental disorder. The difference might be large (no less than 13.9) or extremely large (as high as 32.9).

9. Since the data consist of repeated measurements, the independence assumption is violated. In addition, the data for some of the cells appear extremely nonnormal. Two-way ANOVA is not appropriate.

10. No. Interaction $F = 0.24$, 1 and 36 df, p-value > 0.50. If interaction is not present, the probability of getting an F statistic at least as extreme as 0.24 is greater than 0.50. We cannot reject the hypothesis of no interaction at any reasonable significance level. Let DST result be Factor A and previous episode be Factor B.

H_0: $\mu_{A1} = \mu_{A2}$, H_A: $\mu_{A1} \neq \mu_{A2}$, $F = 0.16$, 1 and 36 df, p-value > 0.50. If the two population DST result factor means are equal, the probability of getting an F statistic at least as extreme as 0.16 is greater than 0.50. We cannot reject the hypothesis of equal population DST result factor means at any reasonable significance level.

H_0: $\mu_{B1} = \mu_{B2}$, H_A: $\mu_{B1} \neq \mu_{B2}$, $F = 0.40$, 1 and 36 df, p-value > 0.50. If the two population previous-episode factor means are equal, the probability of getting an F statistic at least as extreme as 0.40 is greater than 0.50. We cannot reject the hypothesis of equal population previous episode factor means at any reasonable significance level.

Multiple comparisons are not needed.

11. Yes. Interaction $F = 0.09$, 2 and 34 df, p-value > 0.50. If interaction is not present, the probability of getting an F statistic at least as extreme as 0.09 is greater than 0.50. We cannot reject the hypothesis of no interaction at any reasonable significance level. Let starting height be Factor A and pubertal rating be Factor B.

H_0: $\mu_{A1} = \mu_{A2}$, H_A: $\mu_{A1} \neq \mu_{A2}$, $F = 25.44$, 1 and 34 df, p-value < 0.001. If the two population starting-height factor means are equal, the probability of getting an F statistic at least as extreme as 25.44 is less than 0.001. We reject the hypothesis of equal population starting height factor means at any reasonable significance level.

H_0: $\mu_{B1} = \mu_{B2} = \mu_{B3}$, H_A: At least one population pubertal rating factor mean does not equal another population pubertal rating factor mean, $F = 0.51$, 2 and 34 df, p-value > 0.50. If all three population pubertal rating factor means are equal, the probability of getting an F statistic at least as extreme as 0.51 is greater than 0.50. We cannot reject the hypothesis of equal population pubertal rating factor means at any reasonable significance level.

Since the starting-height factor has only two levels, there are only two starting-height factor means. We do not need confidence intervals to determine which population factor means are different, but a confidence interval is useful for estimating the magnitude of the difference between the two population starting-height factor means. The sample starting-height factor means and their estimated variances are

$$\bar{x}_{A1} = -0.46 \qquad \text{var}(\bar{x}_{A1}) = 0.048$$
$$\bar{x}_{A2} = 0.83 \qquad \text{var}(\bar{x}_{A2}) = 0.018$$

Since $q_{.05,2,34}/\sqrt{2} \cong 2.89/\sqrt{2} = 2.044$ and $t_{.025,34} \cong t_{.025,30} = 2.042$, there is no practical difference between the Tukey and Bonferroni confidence intervals in this case. (For the Bonferroni procedure, c is 1 because only one comparison between the starting height factor means is possible.) Applying the Bonferroni formula (13.17), we obtain the following 95% Bonferroni confidence interval.

$\mu_{A1} - \mu_{A2}$ (*starting height less than mean for age versus starting height greater than or equal to mean for age*): $(-1.81, -0.77)$

We are 95% sure that the population mean square-root height deviate for girls whose starting height was less than the mean for their age is smaller than the population mean square-root height deviate for girls whose starting height was greater than or equal to the mean for their age. The difference might be large (no less than 0.77) or extremely large (as high as 1.81).

12. Yes. H_0: No interaction, H_A: Interaction present, $F = 5.99$, 2 and 48 df, $0.001 < p$-value < 0.005. If interaction is not present, the probability of getting an interaction F statistic at least as extreme as 5.99 is between 0.001 and 0.005. We reject the hypothesis of no interaction at the 0.01 significance level. No further tests for factor effects are done.

Comparison of cell means is appropriate. Let treatment be Factor A and number of vertebrae be Factor B. The estimated variances of the sample cell means are

$$\text{var}(\bar{x}_{A1B1}) = 0.028 \qquad \text{var}(\bar{x}_{A2B1}) = 0.106$$
$$\text{var}(\bar{x}_{A1B2}) = 0.028 \qquad \text{var}(\bar{x}_{A2B2}) = 0.132$$
$$\text{var}(\bar{x}_{A1B3}) = 0.132 \qquad \text{var}(\bar{x}_{A2B3}) = 0.176$$

There are 15 possible cell mean comparisons, and we selected our three comparisons after examining the sample means, so $c = 15$. Since $q_{.10,6,48}/\sqrt{2} \cong 3.80/\sqrt{2} = 2.69$ and $t_{.0033,48} \cong t_{.0025,40} = 2.971$, we will use the Tukey procedure to make our three comparisons. Applying formula (13.13), we obtain the following 90% Tukey confidence intervals.

$\mu_{A1B1} - \mu_{A2B1}$ (*no treatment with three to seven vertebrae versus brace with three to seven vertebrae*): $(-0.14, 1.82)$

$\mu_{A1B2} - \mu_{A2B2}$ (*no treatment with eight to 13 vertebrae versus brace with eight to 13 vertebrae*): $(-1.64, 0.52)$

$\mu_{A1B3} - \mu_{A2B3}$ (*no treatment with 14 to 16 vertebrae versus brace with 14 to 16 vertebrae*): $(0.14, 3.12)$

We are 90% sure that the following is true.

1. We cannot say that the population mean square-root kyphosis for untreated patients with three to seven vertebrae in the curve differs from the population mean square-root kyphosis for brace-treated patients with three to seven vertebrae in the curve.

2. We cannot say that the population mean square-root kyphosis for untreated patients with eight to 13 vertebrae in the curve differs from the population mean square-root kyphosis for brace-treated patients with eight to 13 vertebrae in the curve.

3. The population mean square-root kyphosis for untreated patients with 14 to 16 vertebrae in the curve is larger than the population mean square-root kyphosis for brace-treated patients with 14 to 16 vertebrae in the curve. The difference might be extremely small (as low as 0.14), large (as high as 3.12), or somewhere in between.

TABLE E.1   RANDOM NUMBERS*

53872	34774	19087	81775	71440	12082	75092	34608	75448	13148
04226	62404	71577	00984	56056	32404	87641	53392	92561	33388
28666	44190	75524	62038	21423	46281	92238	96306	72606	80601
63817	30279	14088	86434	16183	06401	90586	80292	54555	47371
22359	16442	83879	47486	19838	32252	39560	95851	36758	36141
50968	28728	83525	16031	77583	65578	84794	51367	32535	83834
39652	24248	96617	91200	10769	52386	39559	75921	49375	22847
35493	00529	69632	29684	80284	87828	72418	80950	86311	34016
75687	53919	80439	20534	96185	72345	96391	52625	50866	45132
31509	93521	10681	44124	88345	84969	88768	48819	22311	41235
40389	76282	37506	60661	23295	67357	95419	10864	87833	09152
59244	54664	63424	97899	44153	69251	08781	18604	02312	21658
99876	17075	40934	08912	96196	58503	63613	24486	98092	45672
06457	50072	18060	71023	84349	40984	59487	77782	32107	53770
14297	07687	05517	10362	35783	62236	63764	45542	68889	03862
51661	57130	97442	29590	21634	79772	73801	70122	46467	47152
53455	41788	16117	09698	24409	05079	76603	57563	33461	46791
48086	31512	62819	27689	63744	11023	11184	87679	22218	70139
19108	01602	96950	41536	39974	88287	83546	69187	45539	78263
39001	77727	33095	58785	29179	45421	71416	20418	38558	78700
72346	55617	14714	21930	14851	38209	52202	03979	05970	74483
19094	64359	89829	10942	53101	37758	29583	26792	42840	45872
82247	77127	01652	50774	04970	83300	33760	22172	67516	62135
75968	18386	31874	52249	21015	20365	57475	32756	58268	75739
01963	38095	99960	91307	99654	74279	80145	53303	11870	50485
64828	15817	80923	55226	51893	93362	15757	47430	84855	95822
64347	61578	44160	06266	35118	52558	56436	96155	10293	67506
54746	52337	84826	39012	59118	19851	10156	78167	41473	99025
22241	41501	02993	99340	91044	67268	51088	12751	74008	33773
11906	20043	10415	44425	31712	54831	85591	62237	88797	14382
76637	07609	95378	95580	86909	50609	99008	99042	50364	36664
93896	47120	98926	30636	28136	49458	84145	79205	79517	93446
75292	88232	14360	12455	13656	65736	70428	66917	64412	38502
98792	29828	10577	48184	29433	98278	22543	76155	82107	22066
65751	91049	94127	47558	99880	79667	86254	72797	67117	44699
72064	62102	39155	79462	82975	02638	00302	79476	72656	84003
01227	35821	80607	61734	02600	45564	72344	71034	48370	96826
44768	56504	13993	59701	88238	92483	09497	66058	36651	37927
69838	91226	85736	72247	64099	86305	49877	76215	66980	30228
01800	39313	57730	84410	47637	81369	51830	43536	58937	91901
11756	45441	59948	57975	92422	70057	50210	30345	55912	31638
39056	86614	53643	62909	27198	04454	33789	86463	66603	48083
88086	93172	68311	39164	42012	10447	45933	28844	36844	57684
12648	27948	76750	19915	34015	66815	43011	27150	94264	89516
16254	87661	66181	68609	58626	58428	75051	27558	49463	66646
69682	19109	94189	94626	09299	10649	55405	54571	57855	54921
61336	86663	13010	40412	50139	30769	13048	61407	41056	60510
65727	66488	12304	70011	93324	58764	87274	43103	96002	06984
55705	34418	99410	32635	42984	40981	91750	27431	05142	77950
95402	51746	98184	38830	97590	00066	82770	42325	28778	83571
79228	94510	57711	64366	89040	43278	69072	22003	89465	61483
48103	56760	82564	33649	35176	32278	51357	05489	47462	55931
70969	27677	99621	63065	73194	70462	19316	77945	45004	39895
69931	20237	75246	59124	12484	22012	79731	82435	56301	99752
37208	22741	41946	74109	03760	24094	40210	76617	52317	50643
60151	92327	85150	27728	64813	47667	66078	03628	95240	03808
46210	47674	53747	95354	67757	75477	26396	09592	96239	50854
55399	48142	12284	95298	56399	61358	87541	12998	79639	63633
23677	64950	97041	43088	80143	34294	91468	01066	90350	78891
41947	70066	90311	17133	11674	00826	75760	37586	33621	14199

TABLE E.1   RANDOM NUMBERS (CONT.)

16972	42181	87945	94104	95701	00743	75411	51930	54869	98991
74938	79042	38473	89672	45752	35715	89537	78155	09851	24983
78075	53671	81047	92759	94519	59473	91679	90536	41676	35230
76744	26190	21649	79753	21287	17698	39490	00533	34823	08134
82273	69293	23383	59365	18258	54530	47274	69686	55081	28731
30239	23081	09526	26055	87099	41372	55542	32754	87317	94638
41177	77163	38252	10349	49511	17540	61781	32769	51662	55606
07715	88600	69730	78912	19642	39764	47146	19472	84012	08887
16855	47454	98638	15189	87345	80509	33392	50866	17629	28208
27985	61979	02979	98092	41184	73815	57939	91057	04860	66667
77411	98433	42302	86602	26596	64175	64359	97570	64437	55592
19453	18731	01039	18933	92188	83767	56148	56261	79920	78514
03381	35119	30355	08287	00448	32800	24106	04054	70572	71063
11659	27315	09204	26213	57325	51470	56108	23141	16121	53925
35032	14283	20642	15311	36238	12079	67596	00017	51789	90737
32061	51250	39825	08554	88716	40945	68579	33784	62025	32535
81855	16888	24630	15077	47256	08529	54837	24161	95621	53483
48422	09247	43406	16093	01168	28523	31406	49360	99243	85090
86190	56195	31409	88248	52436	70161	98500	74702	99546	74570
90627	37048	50285	69189	97489	83007	31477	13908	97472	74448
60103	76739	57644	56746	63005	08804	47081	65928	65045	58629
09606	69465	16536	94055	86328	56533	16670	57295	26249	18524
62479	29610	03235	51050	15855	66828	08115	16166	32854	74206
40232	52840	02512	99258	09327	55073	86030	29933	00528	67359
10690	55550	81275	78369	33658	47000	89425	60573	81137	25474
73958	38949	99568	72713	22665	03244	17399	83950	66820	08704
56554	57926	41529	00619	51972	09442	60298	81066	28362	41165
35676	20333	77622	93718	57255	09780	26798	60083	58959	45691
01383	85677	96572	16401	31379	88519	41325	33938	36342	03327
29448	88487	05814	82402	42132	85708	89754	57495	57655	78644
56863	94737	68661	43498	33376	81659	07422	58435	24855	15523
20269	34456	48608	11787	86056	88290	17463	66628	03033	80771
06790	99803	86439	94235	48560	62912	82302	43198	97087	97104
73690	79726	06492	77431	49864	69775	46450	02122	09083	92746
76222	20006	98660	88690	01190	05588	76651	03461	11987	80756
18434	21893	80472	19499	80423	58643	27088	66458	78358	56606
20463	75133	41713	84279	56045	79079	20212	91560	60548	95128
27105	77095	72016	23683	01386	40381	74673	11811	36625	62958
47736	56338	07546	36084	73126	33364	78730	47282	76795	95719
60938	13970	90288	79457	50343	92054	12541	93216	58624	37392
02743	59982	92806	62853	39755	42550	31081	38860	35712	78632
74802	59354	91213	26293	18112	93831	01473	10798	18229	18642
06933	78651	45636	77509	28610	34307	68045	15107	62935	34149
40345	80092	50587	18535	19001	82179	12572	77589	33459	35130
70055	98685	10244	11760	21952	73985	68903	66934	42442	07608
34552	76373	40928	93696	97711	15818	31004	03263	05626	07460
45253	86947	42417	28778	14936	94099	90775	42001	86675	62770
71558	21692	84077	17814	33316	49494	31817	90127	39485	92302
95474	76468	12019	04274	01893	23930	88771	31142	65859	28948
34619	91898	28499	00279	35351	87736	83909	43736	19258	95068
44546	75524	68535	77434	18543	15479	58850	73802	10636	82735
22917	96024	04784	05809	52788	83577	02269	68632	23310	46261
33043	31433	47833	75234	74539	38529	57893	45997	71749	28666
99357	54593	21688	64216	85938	51742	12898	09737	61504	18946
01072	31679	80961	34029	56463	09594	11939	51777	64796	52452
90838	50179	42064	62987	13072	84227	24060	59438	05695	38136
35914	39441	90149	67957	16955	39960	26142	45600	75486	74103
87047	77284	12753	45644	47843	55781	06672	57548	84706	25453
93727	46613	48045	49685	28385	37200	98473	56808	86774	07305
37439	50362	44171	18495	57370	77691	28006	55318	39723	25299

TABLE E.1   RANDOM NUMBERS (CONT.)

98892	53633	33909	81674	91956	84531	60422	55574	31670	61059
95398	77381	21912	24873	26372	12044	43234	08503	86716	08095
28982	24589	88896	31137	87512	33216	29665	26014	02919	17639
31303	70209	42174	10757	98531	35725	68208	61239	26705	43916
08457	10085	35741	79416	72457	59502	46986	09051	70963	19759
30698	80818	90073	78320	83675	78361	49929	70495	92247	04318
27142	41186	52273	81087	67396	16795	98542	83820	48765	24164
36775	63628	70856	43164	88426	51415	37514	24870	55665	05311
02560	51679	79600	23297	36434	17174	00109	02731	05909	58959
36744	66697	08331	50201	56303	09171	55995	60232	31305	30689
66482	04302	29770	46201	04588	42575	99318	84406	83405	21186
76375	41539	65940	57820	29283	94564	96598	00619	60468	97375
95772	72925	19454	63712	21401	96665	77750	21218	02990	50796
59013	81632	85000	39180	99975	73253	46534	59083	60243	27664
52392	04440	45628	34976	92012	16596	28596	15493	80754	48760
08027	07629	04339	77570	47155	77128	24498	67455	06320	82004
27284	39416	57313	03508	71443	42543	73335	68620	87559	77927
20513	38581	82309	69951	82658	60958	18290	60534	30741	89647
36076	12821	68723	37934	62818	64157	54590	98263	70109	06755
60679	43862	43675	03653	21060	81096	71332	28930	44207	08354
49416	58370	63738	87515	39290	87656	36130	23490	30963	57350
65757	39149	11780	92494	41335	35835	69882	56431	08091	01981
17379	77731	65133	44979	90939	29184	76634	58007	34873	83816
00757	13129	09648	07644	81689	68088	34882	04971	27565	66577
68276	79035	78273	83412	97328	81003	65938	85510	78367	29316
64716	91696	45448	92281	73854	67452	52145	41582	81549	82434
83695	11496	57066	48153	74754	56383	09253	65456	32438	96357
58275	66797	35380	41155	44389	94860	42074	31178	27967	12666
58005	84170	29999	23631	93032	41592	55688	78599	59902	21568
99993	80083	08810	07244	42067	76669	19686	64064	67141	80520
31692	51607	89056	74472	91284	20263	16039	94491	33767	73915
82997	58320	04852	52595	95514	56543	06636	61291	67504	57205
05043	40582	46051	60261	04996	82256	47375	87507	05112	88489
75781	38768	70475	00601	18378	32077	36523	30843	07057	78326
21033	15175	30741	45814	92222	16704	00197	51267	33224	40276
99092	60991	12571	71753	65214	33885	82939	50723	88987	69761
07204	93373	85112	29610	30375	64836	18459	08235	67650	72930
88859	97254	07771	21393	64657	42013	12753	03028	24224	24918
30497	91407	72900	15699	58653	38063	25072	48698	88083	48040
09726	18075	45852	54968	43743	82050	78412	79456	95032	10984
95330	01985	24128	60514	42539	91907	25694	37097	39566	24043
09760	32388	05601	49923	66126	54146	67213	52234	48381	89442
01534	81967	15337	95831	84643	40792	47562	95494	62087	18064
11234	59350	48368	57195	36287	03046	87136	36057	93913	70080
71056	48762	80221	59683	27504	21121	94711	11807	80882	48359
34208	05374	60304	43178	97247	24875	26259	67622	14657	80354
47132	62839	82198	92445	60650	76219	02772	48651	66449	89213
55685	93302	43019	45861	95493	16106	12783	37248	83533	25440
17803	18184	10510	27159	83008	20544	41665	99439	70606	28974
55045	17219	66737	59080	78489	12626	60661	53733	70062	14289
01923	33647	98442	59293	83318	33425	76412	87062	01295	11083
07202	76476	71888	54845	17468	41964	68694	59662	55905	26898
68825	68242	95750	11033	58634	78411	08523	19313	29327	47526
68525	06496	17446	41378	32368	82019	66101	56733	43308	82641
80819	33515	97373	43064	16221	99697	37951	07947	12935	49391
64200	96929	26044	49283	56545	67200	21325	85056	51345	06309
30156	29121	75874	42399	41121	90643	19585	06364	47203	19679
50467	14282	89098	66717	14753	73356	47781	34165	82842	00121
53764	83212	26675	64184	64455	29023	03181	13674	08838	83829
81727	35572	95469	36825	81882	95083	68323	14965	34166	32351

TABLE E.1   RANDOM NUMBERS (CONT.)

30807	55558	96026	97398	21723	86560	52617	07771	61886	48234
75104	23682	78756	72728	85940	57290	75507	78715	01426	02310
06180	62724	36835	80288	25075	32609	33312	21348	87710	55457
22098	34834	66117	36252	82717	50585	43639	79999	07414	84003
13173	64783	20984	11929	18849	26211	77375	49561	96747	67007
75273	36108	55265	15653	82270	99216	27805	60088	06056	97377
89849	65756	44454	04602	14292	74458	57777	35934	05160	26359
91108	43562	18883	16569	49599	73871	67101	12054	56492	15981
51843	01542	17881	12954	94913	39583	94969	61146	35907	72184
02644	23564	85464	62947	92571	89377	85004	84654	20465	86212
38608	83374	74032	62183	08740	05279	30455	31032	71512	16476
43164	28909	88624	14992	85359	10193	32491	14769	63694	92640
80933	52950	45646	36636	05085	28053	27596	54873	68476	65823
67690	96766	69250	19344	47855	43489	77479	62418	54079	40069
68579	17014	25362	15114	30982	27250	29052	71115	83369	46776
46353	39733	44677	50133	26623	15979	10651	04263	34087	67005
30039	09532	52215	09164	20930	88230	43403	63230	83525	93550
89200	92772	42195	91634	39272	46462	76835	27755	03151	75692
58118	57942	14807	68214	76093	47484	24468	91764	52907	16675
97230	33027	70166	43232	98802	70715	30216	35586	18909	79658

TABLE E.2   STANDARD NORMAL-TAIL PROBABILITIES

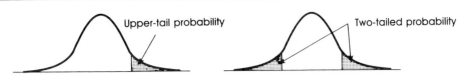

z	Upper-tail Prob.	Two-tailed Prob.	z	Upper-tail Prob.	Two-tailed Prob.
0.00	0.5000	1.0000	0.36	0.3594	0.7188
0.01	0.4960	0.9920	0.37	0.3557	0.7114
0.02	0.4920	0.9840	0.38	0.3520	0.7039
0.0251	0.49	0.98	0.3853	0.35	0.70
0.03	0.4880	0.9761	0.39	0.3483	0.6965
0.04	0.4840	0.9681	0.40	0.3446	0.6892
0.05	0.4801	0.9601	0.41	0.3409	0.6818
0.0502	0.48	0.96	0.4125	0.34	0.68
0.06	0.4761	0.9522	0.42	0.3372	0.6745
0.07	0.4721	0.9442	0.43	0.3336	0.6672
0.0753	0.47	0.94	0.4399	0.33	0.66
0.08	0.4681	0.9362	0.44	0.3300	0.6599
0.09	0.4641	0.9283	0.45	0.3264	0.6527
0.10	0.4602	0.9203	0.46	0.3228	0.6455
0.1004	0.46	0.92	0.4677	0.32	0.64
0.11	0.4562	0.9124	0.47	0.3192	0.6384
0.12	0.4522	0.9045	0.48	0.3156	0.6312
0.1257	0.45	0.9	0.49	0.3121	0.6241
0.13	0.4483	0.8966	0.4959	0.31	0.62
0.14	0.4443	0.8887	0.50	0.3085	0.6171
0.15	0.4404	0.8808	0.51	0.3050	0.6101
0.1510	0.44	0.88	0.52	0.3015	0.6031
0.16	0.4364	0.8729	0.5244	0.3	0.6
0.17	0.4325	0.8650	0.53	0.2981	0.5961
0.1764	0.43	0.86	0.54	0.2946	0.5892
0.18	0.4286	0.8571	0.55	0.2912	0.5823
0.19	0.4247	0.8493	0.5534	0.29	0.58
0.20	0.4207	0.8415	0.56	0.2877	0.5755
0.2019	0.42	0.84	0.57	0.2843	0.5687
0.21	0.4168	0.8337	0.58	0.2810	0.5619
0.22	0.4129	0.8259	0.5828	0.28	0.56
0.2275	0.41	0.82	0.59	0.2776	0.5552
0.23	0.4090	0.8181	0.60	0.2743	0.5485
0.24	0.4052	0.8103	0.61	0.2709	0.5419
0.25	0.4013	0.8026	0.6128	0.27	0.54
0.2533	0.40	0.80	0.62	0.2676	0.5353
0.26	0.3974	0.7949	0.63	0.2643	0.5287
0.27	0.3936	0.7872	0.64	0.2611	0.5222
0.2793	0.39	0.78	0.6433	0.26	0.52
0.28	0.3897	0.7795	0.65	0.2578	0.5157
0.29	0.3859	0.7718	0.66	0.2546	0.5093
0.30	0.3821	0.7642	0.67	0.2514	0.5029
0.3055	0.38	0.76	0.6745	0.25	0.50
0.31	0.3783	0.7566	0.68	0.2483	0.4965
0.32	0.3745	0.7490	0.69	0.2451	0.4902
0.33	0.3707	0.7414	0.70	0.2420	0.4839
0.3319	0.37	0.74	0.7063	0.24	0.48
0.34	0.3669	0.7339	0.71	0.2389	0.4777
0.35	0.3632	0.7263	0.72	0.2358	0.4715
0.3585	0.36	0.72	0.73	0.2327	0.4654

TABLE E.2   STANDARD NORMAL-TAIL PROBABILITIES (CONT.)

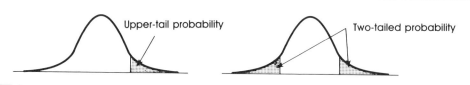

z	Upper-tail Prob.	Two-tailed Prob.	z	Upper-tail Prob.	Two-tailed Prob.
0.7388	0.23	0.46	1.13	0.1292	0.2585
0.74	0.2296	0.4593	1.14	0.1271	0.2543
0.75	0.2266	0.4533	1.15	0.1251	0.2501
0.76	0.2236	0.4473	1.16	0.1230	0.2460
0.77	0.2206	0.4413	1.17	0.1210	0.2420
0.7722	0.22	0.44	1.175	0.12	0.24
0.78	0.2177	0.4354	1.18	0.1190	0.2380
0.79	0.2148	0.4295	1.19	0.1170	0.2340
0.80	0.2119	0.4237	1.20	0.1151	0.2301
0.8064	0.21	0.42	1.21	0.1131	0.2263
0.81	0.2090	0.4179	1.22	0.1112	0.2225
0.82	0.2061	0.4122	1.227	0.11	0.22
0.83	0.2033	0.4065	1.23	0.1093	0.2187
0.84	0.2005	0.4009	1.24	0.1075	0.2150
0.8416	0.20	0.40	1.25	0.1056	0.2113
0.85	0.1977	0.3953	1.26	0.1038	0.2077
0.86	0.1949	0.3898	1.27	0.1020	0.2041
0.87	0.1922	0.3843	1.28	0.1003	0.2005
0.8779	0.19	0.38	1.282	0.10	0.20
0.88	0.1894	0.3789	1.29	0.0985	0.1971
0.89	0.1867	0.3735	1.30	0.0968	0.1936
0.90	0.1841	0.3681	1.31	0.0951	0.1902
0.91	0.1814	0.3628	1.32	0.0934	0.1868
0.9154	0.18	0.36	1.33	0.0918	0.1835
0.92	0.1788	0.3576	1.34	0.0901	0.1802
0.93	0.1762	0.3524	1.341	0.09	0.18
0.94	0.1736	0.3472	1.35	0.0885	0.1770
0.95	0.1711	0.3421	1.36	0.0869	0.1738
0.9542	0.17	0.34	1.37	0.0853	0.1707
0.96	0.1685	0.3371	1.38	0.0838	0.1676
0.97	0.1660	0.3320	1.39	0.0823	0.1645
0.98	0.1635	0.3271	1.40	0.0808	0.1615
0.99	0.1611	0.3222	1.405	0.08	0.16
0.9945	0.16	0.32	1.41	0.0793	0.1585
1.00	0.1587	0.3173	1.42	0.0778	0.1556
1.01	0.1562	0.3125	1.43	0.0764	0.1527
1.02	0.1539	0.3077	1.44	0.0749	0.1499
1.03	0.1515	0.3030	1.45	0.0735	0.1471
1.036	0.15	0.3	1.46	0.0721	0.1443
1.04	0.1492	0.2983	1.47	0.0708	0.1416
1.05	0.1469	0.2937	1.476	0.07	0.14
1.06	0.1446	0.2891	1.48	0.0694	0.1389
1.07	0.1423	0.2846	1.49	0.0681	0.1362
1.08	0.1401	0.2801	1.50	0.0668	0.1336
1.080	0.14	0.28	1.51	0.0655	0.1310
1.09	0.1379	0.2757	1.52	0.0643	0.1285
1.10	0.1357	0.2713	1.53	0.0630	0.1260
1.11	0.1335	0.2670	1.54	0.0618	0.1236
1.12	0.1314	0.2627	1.55	0.0606	0.1211
1.1264	0.13	0.26	1.555	0.06	0.12

TABLE E.2 STANDARD NORMAL-TAIL PROBABILITIES (CONT.)

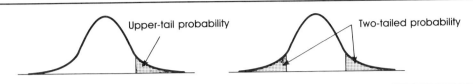

z	Upper-tail Prob.	Two-tailed Prob.	z	Upper-tail Prob.	Two-tailed Prob.
1.56	0.0594	0.1188	2.03	0.0212	0.0424
1.57	0.0582	0.1164	2.04	0.0207	0.0414
1.58	0.0571	0.1141	2.05	0.0202	0.0404
1.59	0.0559	0.1118	2.054	0.02	0.04
1.60	0.0548	0.1096	2.06	0.0197	0.0394
1.61	0.0537	0.1074	2.07	0.0192	0.0385
1.62	0.0526	0.1052	2.08	0.0188	0.0375
1.63	0.0516	0.1031	2.09	0.0183	0.0366
1.64	0.0505	0.1010	2.10	0.0179	0.0357
1.645	0.05	0.10	2.11	0.0174	0.0349
1.65	0.0495	0.0989	2.12	0.0170	0.0340
1.66	0.0485	0.0969	2.13	0.0166	0.0332
1.67	0.0475	0.0949	2.14	0.0162	0.0324
1.68	0.0465	0.0930	2.15	0.0158	0.0316
1.69	0.0455	0.0910	2.16	0.0154	0.0308
1.70	0.0446	0.0891	2.17	0.0150	0.0300
1.71	0.0436	0.0873	2.18	0.0146	0.0293
1.72	0.0427	0.0854	2.19	0.0143	0.0285
1.73	0.0418	0.0836	2.20	0.0139	0.0278
1.74	0.0409	0.0819	2.21	0.0136	0.0271
1.75	0.0401	0.0801	2.22	0.0132	0.0264
1.751	0.04	0.08	2.23	0.0129	0.0257
1.76	0.0392	0.0784	2.24	0.0125	0.0251
1.77	0.0384	0.0767	2.25	0.0122	0.0244
1.78	0.0375	0.0751	2.26	0.0119	0.0238
1.79	0.0367	0.0734	2.27	0.0116	0.0232
1.80	0.0359	0.0719	2.28	0.0113	0.0226
1.81	0.0352	0.0703	2.29	0.0110	0.0220
1.82	0.0344	0.0688	2.30	0.0107	0.0214
1.83	0.0336	0.0672	2.31	0.0104	0.0209
1.84	0.0329	0.0658	2.32	0.0102	0.0203
1.85	0.0322	0.0643	2.326	0.01	0.02
1.86	0.0314	0.0629	2.33	0.0099	0.0198
1.87	0.0307	0.0615	2.34	0.0096	0.0193
1.88	0.0301	0.0601	2.35	0.0094	0.0188
1.881	0.03	0.06	2.36	0.0091	0.0183
1.89	0.0294	0.0588	2.37	0.0089	0.0178
1.90	0.0287	0.0574	2.38	0.0087	0.0173
1.91	0.0281	0.0561	2.39	0.0084	0.0168
1.92	0.0274	0.0549	2.40	0.0082	0.0164
1.93	0.0268	0.0536	2.41	0.0080	0.0160
1.94	0.0262	0.0524	2.42	0.0078	0.0155
1.95	0.0256	0.0512	2.43	0.0075	0.0151
1.960	0.025	0.05	2.44	0.0073	0.0147
1.97	0.0244	0.0488	2.45	0.0071	0.0143
1.98	0.0239	0.0477	2.46	0.0069	0.0139
1.99	0.0233	0.0466	2.47	0.0068	0.0135
2.00	0.0228	0.0455	2.48	0.0066	0.0131
2.01	0.0222	0.0444	2.49	0.0064	0.0128
2.02	0.0217	0.0434	2.50	0.0062	0.0124

TABLE E.2   STANDARD NORMAL-TAIL PROBABILITIES (CONT.)

z	Upper-tail Prob.	Two-tailed Prob.	z	Upper-tail Prob.	Two-tailed Prob.
2.51	0.0060	0.0121	2.90	0.0019	0.0037
2.52	0.0059	0.0117	2.95	0.0016	0.0032
2.53	0.0057	0.0114	3.00	0.0013	0.0027
2.54	0.0055	0.0111	3.05	0.0011	0.0023
2.55	0.0054	0.0108	3.090	0.001	0.002
2.56	0.0052	0.0105	3.10	0.0010	0.0019
2.57	0.0051	0.0102	3.15	0.0008	0.0016
2.576	0.005	0.01	3.20	0.0007	0.0014
2.58	0.0049	0.0099	3.25	0.0006	0.0012
2.59	0.0048	0.0096	3.291	0.0005	0.001
2.60	0.0047	0.0093	3.30	0.0005	0.0010
2.61	0.0045	0.0091	3.35	0.0004	0.0008
2.62	0.0044	0.0088	3.40	0.0003	0.0007
2.63	0.0043	0.0085	3.45	0.0003	0.0006
2.64	0.0041	0.0083	3.50	0.0002	0.0005
2.65	0.0040	0.0080	3.55	0.0002	0.0004
2.70	0.0035	0.0069	3.60	0.0002	0.0003
2.75	0.0030	0.0060	3.65	0.0001	0.0003
2.80	0.0026	0.0051	3.70	0.0001	0.0002
2.85	0.0022	0.0044	3.75	0.0001	0.0002
			3.80	0.0001	0.0001

*Abstracted from *National Bureau of Standards—Applied Mathematics Series—23*, U.S. Government Printing Office, Washington, D.C., 1953.

n	k	0.01	0.05	0.10	0.15	0.20	0.25	0.30	1/3	0.35	0.40	0.45	0.50
							p						
1	0	0.9900	0.9500	0.9000	0.8500	0.8000	0.7500	0.7000	0.6667	0.6500	0.6000	0.5500	0.5000
	1	0.0100	0.0500	0.1000	0.1500	0.2000	0.2500	0.3000	0.3333	0.3500	0.4000	0.4500	0.5000
2	0	0.9801	0.9025	0.8100	0.7225	0.6400	0.5625	0.4900	0.4444	0.4225	0.3600	0.3025	0.2500
	1	0.0198	0.0950	0.1800	0.2550	0.3200	0.3750	0.4200	0.4444	0.4550	0.4800	0.4950	0.5000
	2	0.0001	0.0025	0.0100	0.0225	0.0400	0.0625	0.0900	0.1111	0.1225	0.1600	0.2025	0.2500
3	0	0.9703	0.8574	0.7290	0.6141	0.5120	0.4219	0.3430	0.2963	0.2746	0.2160	0.1664	0.1250
	1	0.0294	0.1354	0.2430	0.3251	0.3840	0.4219	0.4410	0.4444	0.4436	0.4320	0.4084	0.3750
	2	0.0003	0.0071	0.0270	0.0574	0.0960	0.1406	0.1890	0.2222	0.2389	0.2880	0.3341	0.3750
	3	0.0000	0.0001	0.0010	0.0034	0.0080	0.0156	0.0270	0.0370	0.0429	0.0640	0.0911	0.1250
4	0	0.9606	0.8145	0.6561	0.5220	0.4096	0.3164	0.2401	0.1975	0.1785	0.1296	0.0915	0.0625
	1	0.0388	0.1715	0.2916	0.3685	0.4096	0.4219	0.4116	0.3951	0.3845	0.3456	0.2995	0.2500
	2	0.0006	0.0135	0.0486	0.0975	0.1536	0.2109	0.2646	0.2963	0.3105	0.3456	0.3675	0.3750
	3	0.0000	0.0005	0.0036	0.0115	0.0256	0.0469	0.0756	0.0988	0.1115	0.1536	0.2005	0.2500
	4	0.0000	0.0000	0.0001	0.0005	0.0016	0.0039	0.0081	0.0123	0.0150	0.0256	0.0410	0.0625
5	0	0.9510	0.7738	0.5905	0.4437	0.3277	0.2373	0.1681	0.1317	0.1160	0.0778	0.0503	0.0312
	1	0.0480	0.2036	0.3280	0.3915	0.4096	0.3955	0.3601	0.3292	0.3124	0.2592	0.2059	0.1563
	2	0.0010	0.0214	0.0729	0.1382	0.2048	0.2637	0.3087	0.3292	0.3364	0.3456	0.3369	0.3125
	3	0.0000	0.0012	0.0081	0.0244	0.0512	0.0879	0.1323	0.1646	0.1812	0.2304	0.2757	0.3125
	4	0.0000	0.0000	0.0005	0.0021	0.0064	0.0146	0.0284	0.0412	0.0487	0.0768	0.1127	0.1563
	5	0.0000	0.0000	0.0000	0.0001	0.0003	0.0010	0.0024	0.0041	0.0053	0.0102	0.0185	0.0312
6	0	0.9145	0.7351	0.5314	0.3771	0.2621	0.1780	0.1176	0.0878	0.0754	0.0467	0.0277	0.0156
	1	0.0570	0.2321	0.3543	0.3994	0.3932	0.3559	0.3026	0.2634	0.2437	0.1866	0.1359	0.0938
	2	0.0015	0.0306	0.0984	0.1762	0.2458	0.2967	0.3241	0.3292	0.3280	0.3110	0.2779	0.2344
	3	0.0000	0.0021	0.0146	0.0414	0.0819	0.1318	0.1852	0.2195	0.2355	0.2765	0.3032	0.3125
	4	0.0000	0.0001	0.0012	0.0055	0.0154	0.0330	0.0596	0.0823	0.0951	0.1382	0.1861	0.2344
	5	0.0000	0.0000	0.0001	0.0004	0.0015	0.0044	0.0102	0.0165	0.0205	0.0369	0.0609	0.0938
	6	0.0000	0.0000	0.0000	0.0000	0.0001	0.0002	0.0007	0.0014	0.0018	0.0041	0.0083	0.0156
7	0	0.9321	0.6983	0.4783	0.3206	0.2097	0.1335	0.0824	0.0585	0.0490	0.0280	0.0152	0.0078
	1	0.0659	0.2573	0.3720	0.3960	0.3670	0.3114	0.2470	0.2048	0.1848	0.1306	0.0872	0.0547
	2	0.0020	0.0406	0.1240	0.2096	0.2753	0.3115	0.3177	0.3073	0.2985	0.2613	0.2140	0.1641
	3	0.0000	0.0036	0.0230	0.0617	0.1147	0.1730	0.2269	0.2561	0.2679	0.2903	0.2919	0.2734
	4	0.0000	0.0002	0.0025	0.0109	0.0286	0.0577	0.0972	0.1280	0.1442	0.1935	0.2388	0.2734
	5	0.0000	0.0000	0.0002	0.0011	0.0043	0.0116	0.0250	0.0384	0.0466	0.0775	0.1172	0.1641
	6	0.0000	0.0000	0.0000	0.0001	0.0004	0.0012	0.0036	0.0064	0.0084	0.0172	0.0320	0.0547
	7	0.0000	0.0000	0.0000	0.0000	0.0000	0.0001	0.0002	0.0005	0.0006	0.0016	0.0037	0.0078
8	0	0.9227	0.6634	0.4305	0.2725	0.1678	0.1001	0.0576	0.0390	0.0319	0.0168	0.0084	0.0039
	1	0.0746	0.2794	0.3826	0.3847	0.3355	0.2670	0.1977	0.1561	0.1372	0.0896	0.0548	0.0313
	2	0.0026	0.0514	0.1488	0.2376	0.2936	0.3114	0.2965	0.2731	0.2587	0.2090	0.1570	0.1093
	3	0.0001	0.0054	0.0331	0.0838	0.1468	0.2077	0.2541	0.2731	0.2786	0.2787	0.2569	0.2188
	4	0.0000	0.0004	0.0046	0.0185	0.0459	0.0865	0.1361	0.1707	0.1875	0.2322	0.2626	0.2734
	5	0.0000	0.0000	0.0004	0.0027	0.0092	0.0231	0.0467	0.0683	0.0808	0.1239	0.1718	0.2188
	6	0.0000	0.0000	0.0000	0.0002	0.0011	0.0038	0.0100	0.0171	0.0217	0.0413	0.0704	0.1093
	7	0.0000	0.0000	0.0000	0.0000	0.0001	0.0004	0.0012	0.0024	0.0034	0.0078	0.0164	0.0313
	8	0.0000	0.0000	0.0000	0.0000	0.0000	0.0000	0.0001	0.0002	0.0002	0.0007	0.0017	0.0039
9	0	0.9135	0.6302	0.3874	0.2316	0.1342	0.0751	0.0404	0.0260	0.0207	0.0101	0.0046	0.0020
	1	0.0831	0.2986	0.3874	0.3678	0.3020	0.2252	0.1556	0.1171	0.1004	0.0604	0.0339	0.0175
	2	0.0033	0.0628	0.1722	0.2597	0.3020	0.3004	0.2668	0.2341	0.2162	0.1613	0.1110	0.0703
	3	0.0001	0.0078	0.0447	0.1070	0.1762	0.2336	0.2669	0.2731	0.2716	0.2508	0.2119	0.1641
	4	0.0000	0.0006	0.0074	0.0283	0.0660	0.1168	0.1715	0.2048	0.2194	0.2508	0.2600	0.2461
	5	0.0000	0.0000	0.0008	0.0050	0.0165	0.0389	0.0735	0.1024	0.1181	0.1672	0.2128	0.2461
	6	0.0000	0.0000	0.0001	0.0006	0.0028	0.0087	0.0210	0.0341	0.0424	0.0744	0.1160	0.1641
	7	0.0000	0.0000	0.0000	0.0000	0.0003	0.0012	0.0039	0.0073	0.0098	0.0212	0.0407	0.0703
	8	0.0000	0.0000	0.0000	0.0000	0.0000	0.0001	0.0004	0.0009	0.0013	0.0035	0.0083	0.0175
	9	0.0000	0.0000	0.0000	0.0000	0.0000	0.0000	0.0000	0.0001	0.0001	0.0003	0.0008	0.0020
10	0	0.9044	0.5987	0.3487	0.1969	0.1074	0.0563	0.0282	0.0173	0.0135	0.0060	0.0025	0.0010
	1	0.0913	0.3152	0.3874	0.3474	0.2684	0.1877	0.1211	0.0867	0.0725	0.0404	0.0208	0.0097
	2	0.0042	0.0746	0.1937	0.2759	0.3020	0.2816	0.2335	0.1951	0.1756	0.1209	0.0763	0.0440
	3	0.0001	0.0105	0.0574	0.1290	0.2013	0.2503	0.2668	0.2601	0.2522	0.2150	0.1664	0.1172
	4	0.0000	0.0009	0.0112	0.0401	0.0881	0.1460	0.2001	0.2276	0.2377	0.2508	0.2384	0.2051
	5	0.0000	0.0001	0.0015	0.0085	0.0264	0.0584	0.1030	0.1366	0.1536	0.2007	0.2340	0.2460
	6	0.0000	0.0000	0.0001	0.0013	0.0055	0.0162	0.0367	0.0569	0.0689	0.1114	0.1596	0.2051
	7	0.0000	0.0000	0.0000	0.0001	0.0008	0.0031	0.0090	0.0163	0.0212	0.0425	0.0746	0.1172

n	k						p						
		0.01	0.05	0.10	0.15	0.20	0.25	0.30	1/3	0.35	0.40	0.45	0.50
10	8	0.0000	0.0000	0.0000	0.0000	0.0001	0.0004	0.0015	0.0030	0.0043	0.0106	0.0229	0.0440
	9	0.0000	0.0000	0.0000	0.0000	0.0000	0.0000	0.0001	0.0003	0.0005	0.0016	0.0042	0.0097
	10	0.0000	0.0000	0.0000	0.0000	0.0000	0.0000	0.0000	0.0000	0.0000	0.0001	0.0003	0.0010
11	0	0.8953	0.5688	0.3138	0.1673	0.0859	0.0422	0.0198	0.0116	0.0088	0.0036	0.0014	0.0005
	1	0.0995	0.3293	0.3836	0.3249	0.2362	0.1549	0.0932	0.0636	0.0518	0.0266	0.0125	0.0054
	2	0.0050	0.0867	0.2130	0.2866	0.2953	0.2581	0.1998	0.1590	0.1395	0.0887	0.0513	0.0268
	3	0.0002	0.0136	0.0711	0.1518	0.2215	0.2581	0.2568	0.2384	0.2255	0.1774	0.1259	0.0806
	4	0.0000	0.0015	0.0157	0.0535	0.1107	0.1721	0.2201	0.2384	0.2427	0.2365	0.2060	0.1611
	5	0.0000	0.0001	0.0025	0.0132	0.0387	0.0803	0.1321	0.1669	0.1830	0.2207	0.2360	0.2256
	6	0.0000	0.0000	0.0003	0.0024	0.0097	0.0267	0.0566	0.0835	0.0986	0.1471	0.1931	0.2256
	7	0.0000	0.0000	0.0000	0.0003	0.0018	0.0064	0.0173	0.0298	0.0379	0.0701	0.1128	0.1611
	8	0.0000	0.0000	0.0000	0.0000	0.0002	0.0011	0.0037	0.0075	0.0102	0.0234	0.0462	0.0806
	9	0.0000	0.0000	0.0000	0.0000	0.0000	0.0001	0.0006	0.0012	0.0018	0.0052	0.0126	0.0268
	10	0.0000	0.0000	0.0000	0.0000	0.0000	0.0000	0.0000	0.0001	0.0002	0.0007	0.0020	0.0054
	11	0.0000	0.0000	0.0000	0.0000	0.0000	0.0000	0.0000	0.0000	0.0000	0.0000	0.0002	0.0005
12	0	0.8864	0.5404	0.2824	0.1422	0.0687	0.0317	0.0138	0.0077	0.0057	0.0022	0.0008	0.0002
	1	0.1074	0.3412	0.3766	0.3013	0.2062	0.1267	0.0712	0.0462	0.0367	0.0174	0.0075	0.0030
	2	0.0060	0.0988	0.2301	0.2923	0.2834	0.2323	0.1678	0.1272	0.1089	0.0638	0.0338	0.0161
	3	0.0002	0.0174	0.0853	0.1720	0.2363	0.2581	0.2397	0.2120	0.1954	0.1419	0.0924	0.0537
	4	0.0000	0.0020	0.0213	0.0683	0.1328	0.1936	0.2312	0.2384	0.2366	0.2129	0.1700	0.1208
	5	0.0000	0.0002	0.0038	0.0193	0.0532	0.1032	0.1585	0.1908	0.2040	0.2270	0.2225	0.1934
	6	0.0000	0.0000	0.0004	0.0039	0.0155	0.0401	0.0792	0.1113	0.1281	0.1766	0.2124	0.2256
	7	0.0000	0.0000	0.0001	0.0006	0.0033	0.0115	0.0291	0.0477	0.0591	0.1009	0.1489	0.1934
	8	0.0000	0.0000	0.0000	0.0001	0.0005	0.0024	0.0078	0.0149	0.0199	0.0420	0.0761	0.1208
	9	0.0000	0.0000	0.0000	0.0000	0.0001	0.0004	0.0015	0.0033	0.0048	0.0125	0.0277	0.0537
	10	0.0000	0.0000	0.0000	0.0000	0.0000	0.0000	0.0002	0.0005	0.0007	0.0025	0.0068	0.0161
	11	0.0000	0.0000	0.0000	0.0000	0.0000	0.0000	0.0000	0.0000	0.0001	0.0003	0.0010	0.0030
	12	0.0000	0.0000	0.0000	0.0000	0.0000	0.0000	0.0000	0.0000	0.0000	0.0000	0.0001	0.0002
15	0	0.8601	0.4633	0.2059	0.0874	0.0352	0.0134	0.0047	0.0023	0.0016	0.0005	0.0001	0.0000
	1	0.1301	0.3667	0.3431	0.2312	0.1319	0.0668	0.0306	0.0171	0.0126	0.0047	0.0016	0.0005
	2	0.0092	0.1348	0.2669	0.2856	0.2309	0.1559	0.0915	0.0599	0.0475	0.0219	0.0090	0.0032
	3	0.0004	0.0307	0.1285	0.2185	0.2502	0.2252	0.1701	0.1299	0.1110	0.0634	0.0317	0.0139
	4	0.0000	0.0049	0.0429	0.1156	0.1876	0.2252	0.2186	0.1948	0.1792	0.1268	0.0780	0.0416
	5	0.0000	0.0005	0.0105	0.0449	0.1031	0.1651	0.2061	0.2143	0.2124	0.1859	0.1404	0.0917
	6	0.0000	0.0001	0.0019	0.0132	0.0430	0.0918	0.1473	0.1786	0.1905	0.2066	0.1914	0.1527
	7	0.0000	0.0000	0.0003	0.0030	0.0139	0.0393	0.0811	0.1148	0.1320	0.1771	0.2013	0.1964
	8	0.0000	0.0000	0.0000	0.0005	0.0034	0.0131	0.0348	0.0574	0.0710	0.1181	0.1657	0.1964
	9	0.0000	0.0000	0.0000	0.0001	0.0007	0.0034	0.0115	0.0223	0.0298	0.0612	0.1049	0.1527
	10	0.0000	0.0000	0.0000	0.0000	0.0001	0.0007	0.0030	0.0067	0.0096	0.0245	0.0514	0.0917
	11	0.0000	0.0000	0.0000	0.0000	0.0000	0.0001	0.0006	0.0015	0.0023	0.0074	0.0192	0.0416
	12	0.0000	0.0000	0.0000	0.0000	0.0000	0.0000	0.0001	0.0003	0.0004	0.0016	0.0052	0.0139
	13	0.0000	0.0000	0.0000	0.0000	0.0000	0.0000	0.0000	0.0000	0.0001	0.0003	0.0010	0.0032
	14	0.0000	0.0000	0.0000	0.0000	0.0000	0.0000	0.0000	0.0000	0.0000	0.0000	0.0001	0.0005
	15	0.0000	0.0000	0.0000	0.0000	0.0000	0.0000	0.0000	0.0000	0.0000	0.0000	0.0000	0.0000
20	0	0.8179	0.3585	0.1216	0.0388	0.0115	0.0032	0.0008	0.0003	0.0002	0.0000	0.0000	0.0000
	1	0.1652	0.3773	0.2701	0.1368	0.0577	0.0211	0.0068	0.0030	0.0019	0.0005	0.0001	0.0000
	2	0.0159	0.1887	0.2852	0.2293	0.1369	0.0670	0.0279	0.0143	0.0100	0.0031	0.0008	0.0002
	3	0.0010	0.0596	0.1901	0.2428	0.2053	0.1339	0.0716	0.0429	0.0323	0.0124	0.0040	0.0011
	4	0.0000	0.0133	0.0898	0.1821	0.2182	0.1896	0.1304	0.0911	0.0738	0.0350	0.0140	0.0046
	5	0.0000	0.0023	0.0319	0.1029	0.1746	0.2024	0.1789	0.1457	0.1272	0.0746	0.0364	0.0148
	6	0.0000	0.0003	0.0089	0.0454	0.1091	0.1686	0.1916	0.1821	0.1714	0.1244	0.0746	0.0370
	7	0.0000	0.0000	0.0020	0.0160	0.0546	0.1124	0.1643	0.1821	0.1844	0.1659	0.1221	0.0739
	8	0.0000	0.0000	0.0003	0.0046	0.0221	0.0609	0.1144	0.1480	0.1614	0.1797	0.1623	0.1201
	9	0.0000	0.0000	0.0001	0.0011	0.0074	0.0270	0.0653	0.0987	0.1158	0.1597	0.1771	0.1602
	10	0.0000	0.0000	0.0000	0.0002	0.0020	0.0100	0.0309	0.0543	0.0686	0.1172	0.1593	0.1762
	11	0.0000	0.0000	0.0000	0.0000	0.0005	0.0030	0.0120	0.0247	0.0336	0.0710	0.1185	0.1602
	12	0.0000	0.0000	0.0000	0.0000	0.0001	0.0007	0.0038	0.0092	0.0136	0.0355	0.0728	0.1201
	13	0.0000	0.0000	0.0000	0.0000	0.0000	0.0002	0.0010	0.0028	0.0045	0.0145	0.0366	0.0739
	14	0.0000	0.0000	0.0000	0.0000	0.0000	0.0000	0.0003	0.0007	0.0012	0.0049	0.0150	0.0370
	15	0.0000	0.0000	0.0000	0.0000	0.0000	0.0000	0.0000	0.0001	0.0003	0.0013	0.0049	0.0148
	16	0.0000	0.0000	0.0000	0.0000	0.0000	0.0000	0.0000	0.0000	0.0000	0.0003	0.0012	0.0046
	17	0.0000	0.0000	0.0000	0.0000	0.0000	0.0000	0.0000	0.0000	0.0000	0.0000	0.0003	0.0011
	18	0.0000	0.0000	0.0000	0.0000	0.0000	0.0000	0.0000	0.0000	0.0000	0.0000	0.0000	0.0002
	19	0.0000	0.0000	0.0000	0.0000	0.0000	0.0000	0.0000	0.0000	0.0000	0.0000	0.0000	0.0000
	20	0.0000	0.0000	0.0000	0.0000	0.0000	0.0000	0.0000	0.0000	0.0000	0.0000	0.0000	0.0000

TABLE E.4 UPPER PERCENTAGE POINTS FOR _t_ DISTRIBUTIONS

Upper-Tail Probability

df	0.40	0.30	0.20	0.15	0.10	0.05	0.025
1	0.325	0.727	1.376	1.963	3.078	6.314	12.706
2	0.289	0.617	1.061	1.386	1.886	2.920	4.303
3	0.277	0.584	0.978	1.250	1.638	2.353	3.182
4	0.271	0.569	0.941	1.190	1.533	2.132	2.776
5	0.267	0.559	0.920	1.156	1.476	2.015	2.571
6	0.265	0.553	0.906	1.134	1.440	1.943	2.447
7	0.263	0.549	0.896	1.119	1.415	1.895	2.365
8	0.262	0.546	0.889	1.108	1.397	1.860	2.306
9	0.261	0.543	0.883	1.100	1.383	1.833	2.262
10	0.260	0.542	0.879	1.093	1.372	1.812	2.228
11	0.260	0.540	0.876	1.088	1.363	1.796	2.201
12	0.259	0.539	0.873	1.083	1.356	1.782	2.179
13	0.259	0.537	0.870	1.079	1.350	1.771	2.160
14	0.258	0.537	0.868	1.076	1.345	1.761	2.145
15	0.258	0.536	0.866	1.074	1.341	1.753	2.131
16	0.258	0.535	0.865	1.071	1.337	1.746	2.120
17	0.257	0.534	0.863	1.069	1.333	1.740	2.110
18	0.257	0.534	0.862	1.067	1.330	1.734	2.101
19	0.257	0.533	0.861	1.066	1.328	1.729	2.093
20	0.257	0.533	0.860	1.064	1.325	1.725	2.086
21	0.257	0.532	0.859	1.063	1.323	1.721	2.080
22	0.256	0.532	0.858	1.061	1.321	1.717	2.074
23	0.256	0.532	0.858	1.060	1.319	1.714	2.069
24	0.256	0.531	0.857	1.059	1.318	1.711	2.064
25	0.256	0.531	0.856	1.058	1.316	1.708	2.060
26	0.256	0.531	0.856	1.058	1.315	1.706	2.056
27	0.256	0.531	0.855	1.057	1.314	1.703	2.052
28	0.256	0.530	0.855	1.056	1.313	1.701	2.048
29	0.256	0.530	0.854	1.055	1.311	1.699	2.045
30	0.256	0.530	0.854	1.055	1.310	1.697	2.042
40	0.255	0.529	0.851	1.050	1.303	0.684	2.021
60	0.254	0.527	0.848	1.045	1.296	1.671	2.000
120	0.254	0.526	0.845	1.041	1.289	1.658	1.980
∞	0.253	0.524	0.842	1.036	1.282	1.645	1.960

TABLE E.4   UPPER PERCENTAGE POINTS FOR *t* DISTRIBUTIONS (CONT.)

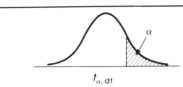

$t_{\alpha, df}$

Upper-Tail Probability

df	0.02	0.015	0.01	0.0075	0.005	0.0025	0.0005
1	15.895	21.205	31.821	42.434	63.657	127.322	636.590
2	4.849	5.643	6.965	8.073	9.925	14.089	31.598
3	3.482	3.896	4.541	5.047	5.841	7.453	12.924
4	2.999	3.298	3.747	4.088	4.604	5.598	8.610
5	2.757	3.003	3.365	3.634	4.032	4.773	6.869
6	2.612	2.829	3.143	3.372	3.707	4.317	5.959
7	2.517	2.715	2.998	3.203	3.499	4.029	5.408
8	2.449	2.634	2.896	3.085	3.355	3.833	5.041
9	2.398	2.574	2.821	2.998	3.250	3.690	4.781
10	2.359	2.527	2.764	2.932	3.169	3.581	4.587
11	2.328	2.491	2.718	2.879	3.106	3.497	4.437
12	2.303	2.461	2.681	2.836	3.055	3.428	4.318
13	2.282	2.436	2.650	2.801	3.012	3.372	4.221
14	2.264	2.415	2.624	2.771	2.977	3.326	4.140
15	2.249	2.397	2.602	2.746	2.947	3.286	4.073
16	2.235	2.382	2.583	2.724	2.921	3.252	4.015
17	2.224	2.368	2.567	2.706	2.898	3.222	3.965
18	2.214	2.356	2.552	2.689	2.878	3.197	3.922
19	2.205	2.346	2.539	2.674	2.861	3.174	3.883
20	2.197	2.336	2.528	2.661	2.845	3.153	3.849
21	2.189	2.328	2.518	2.649	2.831	3.135	3.819
22	2.183	2.320	2.508	2.639	2.819	3.119	3.792
23	2.177	2.313	2.500	2.629	2.807	3.104	3.768
24	2.172	2.307	2.492	2.620	2.797	3.091	3.745
25	2.167	2.301	2.485	2.612	2.787	3.078	3.725
26	2.162	2.296	2.479	2.605	2.779	3.067	3.707
27	2.158	2.291	2.473	2.598	2.771	3.057	3.690
28	2.154	2.286	2.467	2.592	2.763	3.047	3.674
29	2.150	2.282	2.462	2.586	2.756	3.038	3.659
30	2.147	2.278	2.457	2.581	2.750	3.030	3.646
40	2.123	2.250	2.423	2.542	2.704	2.971	3.551
60	2.099	2.223	2.390	2.504	2.660	2.915	3.460
120	2.076	2.196	2.358	2.468	2.617	2.860	3.373
∞	2.054	2.170	2.326	2.432	2.576	2.807	3.291

TABLE E.5   UPPER PERCENTAGE POINTS FOR *F* DISTRIBUTIONS*

$$F_{\alpha, d_1, d_2}$$

Denom. df	Upper-tail Prob.	Numerator df								
		1	2	3	4	5	6	7	8	9
1	0.50	1.00	1.50	1.71	1.82	1.89	1.94	1.98	2.00	2.03
	0.10	39.9	49.5	53.6	55.8	57.2	58.2	58.9	59.4	59.9
	0.05	161	200	216	225	230	234	237	239	241
	0.025	648	800	864	900	922	937	948	957	963
	0.01	4,052	5,000	5,403	5,625	5,764	5,859	5,928	5,981	6,022
	0.005	16,211	20,000	21,615	22,500	23,056	23,437	23,715	23,925	24,091
	0.001	405,280	500,000	540,380	562,500	576,400	585,940	592,870	598,140	602,280
2	0.50	0.667	1.00	1.13	1.21	1.25	1.28	1.30	1.32	1.33
	0.10	8.53	9.00	9.16	9.24	9.29	9.33	9.35	9.37	9.38
	0.05	18.5	19.0	19.2	19.2	19.3	19.3	19.4	19.4	19.4
	0.025	38.5	39.0	39.2	39.2	39.3	39.3	39.4	39.4	39.4
	0.01	98.5	99.0	99.2	99.2	99.3	99.3	99.4	99.4	99.4
	0.005	199	199	199	199	199	199	199	199	199
	0.001	998.5	999.0	999.2	999.2	999.3	999.3	999.4	999.4	999.4
3	0.50	0.585	0.881	1.00	1.06	1.10	1.13	1.15	1.16	1.17
	0.10	5.54	5.46	5.39	5.34	5.31	5.28	5.27	5.25	5.24
	0.05	10.1	9.55	9.28	9.12	9.01	8.94	8.89	8.85	8.81
	0.025	17.4	16.0	15.4	15.1	14.9	14.7	14.6	14.5	14.5
	0.01	34.1	30.8	29.5	28.7	28.2	27.9	27.7	27.5	27.3
	0.005	55.6	49.8	47.5	46.2	45.4	44.8	44.4	44.1	43.9
	0.001	167.0	148.5	141.1	137.1	134.6	132.8	131.6	130.6	129.9
4	0.50	0.549	0.828	0.941	1.00	1.04	1.06	1.08	1.09	1.10
	0.10	4.54	4.32	4.19	4.11	4.05	4.01	3.98	3.95	3.94
	0.05	7.71	6.94	6.59	6.39	6.26	6.16	6.09	6.04	6.00
	0.025	12.2	10.6	9.98	9.60	9.36	9.20	9.07	8.98	8.90
	0.01	21.2	18.0	16.7	16.0	15.5	15.2	15.0	14.8	14.7
	0.005	31.3	26.3	24.3	23.2	22.5	22.0	21.6	21.4	21.1
	0.001	74.1	61.2	56.2	53.4	51.7	50.5	49.7	49.0	48.5
5	0.50	0.528	0.799	0.907	0.965	1.00	1.02	1.04	1.05	1.06
	0.10	4.06	3.78	3.62	3.52	3.45	3.40	3.37	3.34	3.32
	0.05	6.61	5.79	5.41	5.19	5.05	4.95	4.88	4.82	4.77
	0.025	10.0	8.43	7.76	7.39	7.15	6.98	6.85	6.76	6.68
	0.01	16.3	13.3	12.1	11.4	11.0	10.7	10.5	10.3	10.2
	0.005	22.8	18.3	16.5	15.6	14.9	14.5	14.2	14.0	13.8
	0.001	47.2	37.1	33.2	31.1	29.8	28.8	28.2	27.6	27.2
6	0.50	0.515	0.780	0.886	0.942	0.977	1.00	1.02	1.03	1.04
	0.10	3.78	3.46	3.29	3.18	3.11	3.05	3.01	2.98	2.96
	0.05	5.99	5.14	4.76	4.53	4.39	4.28	4.21	4.15	4.10
	0.025	8.81	7.26	6.60	6.23	5.99	5.82	5.70	5.60	5.52
	0.01	13.7	10.9	9.78	9.15	8.75	8.47	8.26	8.10	7.98
	0.005	18.6	14.5	12.9	12.0	11.5	11.1	10.8	10.6	10.4
	0.001	35.5	27.0	23.7	21.9	20.8	20.0	19.5	19.0	18.7
7	0.50	0.506	0.767	0.871	0.926	0.960	0.983	1.00	1.01	1.02
	0.10	3.59	3.26	3.07	2.96	2.88	2.83	2.78	2.75	2.72
	0.05	5.59	4.74	4.35	4.12	3.97	3.87	3.79	3.73	3.68
	0.025	8.07	6.54	5.89	5.52	5.29	5.12	4.99	4.90	4.82
	0.01	12.2	9.55	8.45	7.85	7.46	7.19	6.99	6.84	6.72
	0.005	16.2	12.4	10.9	10.1	9.52	9.16	8.89	8.68	8.51
	0.001	29.2	21.7	18.8	17.2	16.2	15.5	15.0	14.6	14.3

TABLE E.5   UPPER PERCENTAGE POINTS FOR *F* DISTRIBUTIONS (CONT.)

F_{α, d_1, d_2}

Denom. df	Upper-tail Prob.	Numerator df								
		10	12	15	20	24	30	60	120	∞
1	0.50	2.04	2.07	2.09	2.12	2.13	2.15	2.17	2.18	2.20
	0.10	60.2	60.7	61.2	61.7	62.0	62.3	62.8	63.1	63.3
	0.05	242	244	246	248	249	250	252	253	254
	0.025	969	977	985	993	997	1,001	1,010	1,014	1,018
	0.01	6,056	6,106	6,157	6,209	6,235	6,261	6,313	6,339	6,366
	0.005	24,224	24,426	24,630	24,836	24,940	25,044	25,253	25,359	25,464
	0.001	605,620	610,670	615,760	620,910	623,500	626,100	631,340	633,970	636,620
2	0.50	1.34	1.36	1.38	1.39	1.40	1.41	1.43	1.43	1.44
	0.10	9.39	9.41	9.42	9.44	9.45	9.46	9.47	9.48	9.49
	0.05	19.4	19.4	19.4	19.4	19.5	19.5	19.5	19.5	19.5
	0.025	39.4	39.4	39.4	39.4	39.5	39.5	39.5	39.5	39.5
	0.01	99.4	99.4	99.4	99.4	99.5	99.5	99.5	99.5	99.5
	0.005	199	199	199	199	199	199	199	199	200
	0.001	999.4	999.4	999.4	999.4	999.5	999.5	999.5	999.5	999.5
3	0.50	1.18	1.20	1.21	1.23	1.23	1.24	1.25	1.26	1.27
	0.10	5.23	5.22	5.20	5.18	5.18	5.17	5.15	5.14	5.13
	0.05	8.79	8.74	8.70	8.66	8.64	8.62	8.57	8.55	8.53
	0.025	14.4	14.3	14.3	14.2	14.1	14.1	14.0	13.9	13.9
	0.01	27.2	27.1	26.9	26.7	26.6	26.5	26.3	26.2	26.1
	0.005	43.7	43.4	43.1	42.8	42.6	42.5	42.1	42.0	41.8
	0.001	129.2	128.3	127.4	126.4	125.9	125.4	124.5	124.0	123.5
4	0.50	1.11	1.13	1.14	1.15	1.16	1.16	1.18	1.18	1.19
	0.10	3.92	3.90	3.87	3.84	3.83	3.82	3.79	3.78	3.76
	0.05	5.96	5.91	5.86	5.80	5.77	5.75	5.69	5.66	5.63
	0.025	8.84	8.75	8.66	8.56	8.51	8.46	8.36	8.31	8.26
	0.01	14.5	14.4	14.2	14.0	13.9	13.8	13.7	13.6	13.5
	0.005	21.0	20.7	20.4	20.2	20.0	19.9	19.6	19.5	19.3
	0.001	48.1	47.4	46.8	46.1	45.8	45.4	44.7	44.4	44.1
5	0.50	1.07	1.09	1.10	1.11	1.12	1.12	1.14	1.14	1.15
	0.10	3.30	3.27	3.24	3.21	3.19	3.17	3.14	3.12	3.11
	0.05	4.74	4.68	4.62	4.56	4.53	4.50	4.43	4.40	4.37
	0.025	6.62	6.52	6.43	6.33	6.28	6.23	6.12	6.07	6.02
	0.01	10.1	9.89	9.72	9.55	9.47	9.38	9.20	9.11	9.02
	0.005	13.6	13.4	13.1	12.9	12.8	12.7	12.4	12.3	12.1
	0.001	26.9	26.4	25.9	25.4	25.1	24.9	24.3	24.1	23.8
6	0.50	1.05	1.06	1.07	1.08	1.09	1.10	1.11	1.12	1.12
	0.10	2.94	2.90	2.87	2.84	2.82	2.80	2.76	2.74	2.72
	0.05	4.06	4.00	3.94	3.87	3.84	3.81	3.74	3.70	3.67
	0.025	5.46	5.37	5.27	5.17	5.12	5.07	4.96	4.90	4.85
	0.01	7.87	7.72	7.56	7.40	7.31	7.23	7.06	6.97	6.88
	0.005	10.2	10.0	9.81	9.59	9.47	9.36	9.12	9.00	8.88
	0.001	18.4	18.0	17.6	17.1	16.9	16.7	16.2	16.0	15.7
7	0.50	1.03	1.04	1.05	1.07	1.07	1.08	1.09	1.10	1.10
	0.10	2.70	2.67	2.63	2.59	2.58	2.56	2.51	2.49	2.47
	0.05	3.64	3.57	3.51	3.44	3.41	3.38	3.30	3.27	3.23
	0.025	4.76	4.67	4.57	4.47	4.42	4.36	4.25	4.20	4.14
	0.01	6.62	6.47	6.31	6.16	6.07	5.99	5.82	5.74	5.65
	0.005	8.38	8.18	7.97	7.75	7.65	7.53	7.31	7.19	7.08
	0.001	14.1	13.7	13.3	12.9	12.7	12.5	12.1	11.9	11.7

TABLE E.5 UPPER PERCENTAGE POINTS FOR _F_ DISTRIBUTIONS (CONT.)

$$F_{\alpha, d_1, d_2}$$

Denom. df	Upper-tail prob.	Numerator df								
		1	2	3	4	5	6	7	8	9
8	0.50	0.499	0.757	0.860	0.915	0.948	0.971	0.988	1.00	1.01
	0.10	3.46	3.11	2.92	2.81	2.73	2.67	2.62	2.59	2.56
	0.05	5.32	4.46	4.07	3.84	3.69	3.58	3.50	3.44	3.39
	0.025	7.57	6.06	5.42	5.05	4.82	4.65	4.53	4.43	4.36
	0.01	11.3	8.65	7.59	7.01	6.63	6.37	6.18	6.03	5.91
	0.005	14.7	11.0	9.60	8.81	8.30	7.95	7.69	7.50	7.34
	0.001	25.4	18.5	15.8	14.4	13.5	12.9	12.4	12.0	11.8
9	0.50	0.494	0.749	0.852	0.906	0.939	0.962	0.978	0.990	1.00
	0.10	3.36	3.01	2.81	2.69	2.61	2.55	2.51	2.47	2.44
	0.05	5.12	4.26	3.86	3.63	3.48	3.37	3.29	3.23	3.18
	0.025	7.21	5.71	5.08	4.72	4.48	4.32	4.20	4.10	4.03
	0.01	10.6	8.02	6.99	6.42	6.06	5.80	5.61	5.47	5.35
	0.005	13.6	10.1	8.72	7.96	7.47	7.13	6.88	6.69	6.54
	0.001	22.9	16.4	13.9	12.6	11.7	11.1	10.7	10.4	10.1
10	0.50	0.490	0.743	0.845	0.899	0.932	0.954	0.971	0.983	0.992
	0.10	3.29	2.92	2.73	2.61	2.52	2.46	2.41	2.38	2.35
	0.05	4.96	4.10	3.71	3.48	3.33	3.22	3.14	3.07	3.02
	0.025	6.94	5.46	4.83	4.47	4.24	4.07	3.95	3.85	3.78
	0.01	10.0	7.56	6.55	5.99	5.64	5.39	5.20	5.06	4.94
	0.005	12.8	9.43	8.08	7.34	6.87	6.54	6.30	6.12	5.97
	0.001	21.0	14.9	12.6	11.3	10.5	9.93	9.52	9.20	8.96
12	0.50	0.484	0.735	0.835	0.888	0.921	0.943	0.959	0.972	0.981
	0.10	3.18	2.81	2.61	2.48	2.39	2.33	2.28	2.24	2.21
	0.05	4.75	3.89	3.49	3.26	3.11	3.00	2.91	2.85	2.80
	0.025	6.55	5.10	4.47	4.12	3.89	3.73	3.61	3.51	3.44
	0.01	9.33	6.93	5.95	5.41	5.06	4.82	4.64	4.50	4.39
	0.005	11.8	8.51	7.23	6.52	6.07	5.76	5.52	5.35	5.20
	0.001	18.6	13.0	10.8	9.63	8.89	8.38	8.00	7.71	7.48
15	0.50	0.478	0.726	0.826	0.878	0.911	0.933	0.949	0.960	0.970
	0.10	3.07	2.70	2.49	2.36	2.27	2.21	2.16	2.12	2.09
	0.05	4.54	3.68	3.29	3.06	2.90	2.79	2.71	2.64	2.59
	0.025	6.20	4.77	4.15	3.80	3.58	3.41	3.29	3.20	3.12
	0.01	8.68	6.36	5.42	4.89	4.56	4.32	4.14	4.00	3.89
	0.005	10.8	7.70	6.48	5.80	5.37	5.07	4.85	4.67	4.54
	0.001	16.6	11.3	9.34	8.25	7.57	7.09	6.74	6.47	6.26
20	0.50	0.472	0.718	0.816	0.868	0.900	0.922	0.938	0.950	0.959
	0.10	2.97	2.59	2.38	2.25	2.16	2.09	2.04	2.00	1.96
	0.05	4.35	3.49	3.10	2.87	2.71	2.60	2.51	2.45	2.39
	0.025	5.87	4.46	3.86	3.51	3.29	3.13	3.01	2.91	2.84
	0.01	8.10	5.85	4.94	4.43	4.10	3.87	3.70	3.56	3.46
	0.005	9.94	6.99	5.82	5.17	4.76	4.47	4.26	4.09	3.96
	0.001	14.8	9.95	8.10	7.10	6.46	6.02	5.69	5.44	5.24
24	0.50	0.469	0.714	0.812	0.863	0.895	0.917	0.932	0.944	0.953
	0.10	2.93	2.54	2.33	2.19	2.10	2.04	1.98	1.94	1.91
	0.05	4.26	3.40	3.01	2.78	2.62	2.51	2.42	2.36	2.30
	0.025	5.72	4.32	3.72	3.38	3.15	2.99	2.87	2.78	2.70
	0.01	7.82	5.61	4.72	4.22	3.90	3.67	3.50	3.36	3.26
	0.005	9.55	6.66	5.52	4.89	4.49	4.20	3.99	3.83	3.69
	0.001	14.0	9.34	7.55	6.59	5.98	5.55	5.23	4.99	4.80

TABLE E.5   UPPER PERCENTAGE POINTS FOR *F* DISTRIBUTIONS (CONT.)

$$F_{\alpha, d_1, d_2}$$

Denom. df	Upper-tail Prob.	Numerator df								
		10	12	15	20	24	30	60	120	∞
8	0.50	1.02	1.03	1.04	1.05	1.06	1.07	1.08	1.08	1.09
	0.10	2.54	2.50	2.46	2.42	2.40	2.38	2.34	2.32	2.29
	0.05	3.35	3.28	3.22	3.15	3.12	3.08	3.01	2.97	2.93
	0.025	4.30	4.20	4.10	4.00	3.95	3.89	3.78	3.73	3.67
	0.01	5.81	5.67	5.52	5.36	5.28	5.20	5.03	4.95	4.86
	0.005	7.21	7.01	6.81	6.61	6.50	6.40	6.18	6.06	5.95
	0.001	11.5	11.2	10.8	10.5	10.3	10.1	9.73	9.53	9.33
9	0.50	1.01	1.02	1.03	1.04	1.05	1.05	1.07	1.07	1.08
	0.10	2.42	2.38	2.34	2.30	2.28	2.25	2.21	2.18	2.16
	0.05	3.14	3.07	3.01	2.94	2.90	2.86	2.79	2.75	2.71
	0.025	3.96	3.87	3.77	3.67	3.61	3.56	3.45	3.39	3.33
	0.01	5.26	5.11	4.96	4.81	4.73	4.65	4.48	4.40	4.31
	0.005	6.42	6.23	6.03	5.83	5.73	5.62	5.41	5.30	5.19
	0.001	9.89	9.57	9.24	8.90	8.72	8.55	8.19	8.00	7.81
10	0.50	1.00	1.01	1.02	1.03	1.04	1.05	1.06	1.06	1.07
	0.10	2.32	2.28	2.24	2.20	2.18	2.16	2.11	2.08	2.06
	0.05	2.98	2.91	2.84	2.77	2.74	2.70	2.62	2.58	2.54
	0.025	3.72	3.62	3.52	3.42	3.37	3.31	3.20	3.14	3.08
	0.01	4.85	4.71	4.56	4.41	4.33	4.25	4.08	4.00	3.91
	0.005	5.85	5.66	5.47	5.27	5.17	5.07	4.86	4.75	4.64
	0.001	8.75	8.45	8.13	7.80	7.64	7.47	7.12	6.94	6.76
12	0.50	0.989	1.00	1.01	1.02	1.03	1.03	1.05	1.05	1.06
	0.10	2.19	2.15	2.10	2.06	2.04	2.01	1.96	1.93	1.90
	0.05	2.75	2.69	2.62	2.54	2.51	2.47	2.38	2.34	2.30
	0.025	3.37	3.28	3.18	3.07	3.02	2.96	2.85	2.79	2.72
	0.01	4.30	4.16	4.01	3.86	3.78	3.70	3.54	3.45	3.36
	0.005	5.09	4.91	4.72	4.53	4.43	4.33	4.12	4.01	3.90
	0.001	7.29	7.00	6.71	6.40	6.25	6.09	5.76	5.59	5.42
15	0.50	0.977	0.989	1.00	1.01	1.02	1.02	1.03	1.04	1.05
	0.10	2.06	2.02	1.97	1.92	1.90	1.87	1.82	1.79	1.76
	0.05	2.54	2.48	2.40	2.33	2.29	2.25	2.16	2.11	2.07
	0.025	3.06	2.96	2.86	2.76	2.70	2.64	2.52	2.46	2.40
	0.01	3.80	3.67	3.52	3.37	3.29	3.21	3.05	2.96	2.87
	0.005	4.42	4.25	4.07	3.88	3.79	3.69	3.48	3.37	3.26
	0.001	6.08	5.81	5.54	5.25	5.10	4.95	4.64	4.48	4.31
20	0.50	0.966	0.977	0.989	1.01	1.00	1.01	1.02	1.03	1.03
	0.10	1.94	1.89	1.84	1.79	1.77	1.74	1.68	1.64	1.61
	0.05	2.35	2.28	2.20	2.12	2.08	2.04	1.95	1.90	1.84
	0.025	2.77	2.68	2.57	2.46	2.41	2.35	2.22	2.16	2.09
	0.01	3.37	3.23	3.09	2.94	2.86	2.78	2.61	2.52	2.42
	0.005	3.85	3.68	3.50	3.32	3.22	3.12	2.92	2.81	2.69
	0.001	5.08	4.82	4.56	4.29	4.15	4.00	3.70	3.54	3.38
24	0.50	0.961	0.972	0.983	0.994	1.00	1.01	1.02	1.02	1.03
	0.10	1.88	1.83	1.78	1.73	1.70	1.67	1.61	1.57	1.53
	0.05	2.25	2.18	2.11	2.03	1.98	1.94	1.84	1.79	1.73
	0.025	2.64	2.54	2.44	2.33	2.27	2.21	2.08	2.01	1.94
	0.01	3.17	3.03	2.89	2.74	2.66	2.58	2.40	2.31	2.21
	0.005	3.59	3.42	3.25	3.06	2.97	2.87	2.66	2.55	2.43
	0.001	4.64	4.39	4.14	3.87	3.74	3.59	3.29	3.14	2.97

TABLE E.5 UPPER PERCENTAGE POINTS FOR *F* DISTRIBUTIONS (CONT.)

F_{α, d_1, d_2}

Denom. df	Upper-tail Prob.	Numerator df								
		1	2	3	4	5	6	7	8	9
30	0.50	0.466	0.709	0.807	0.858	0.890	0.912	0.927	0.939	0.948
	0.10	2.88	2.49	2.28	2.14	2.05	1.98	1.93	1.88	1.85
	0.05	4.17	3.32	2.92	2.69	2.53	2.42	2.33	2.27	2.21
	0.025	5.57	4.18	3.59	3.25	3.03	2.87	2.75	2.65	2.57
	0.01	7.56	5.39	4.51	4.02	3.70	3.47	3.30	3.17	3.07
	0.005	9.18	6.35	5.24	4.62	4.23	3.95	3.74	3.58	3.45
	0.001	13.3	8.77	7.05	6.12	5.53	5.12	4.82	4.58	4.39
60	0.50	0.461	0.701	0.798	0.849	0.880	0.901	0.917	0.928	0.937
	0.10	2.79	2.39	2.18	2.04	1.95	1.87	1.82	1.77	1.74
	0.05	4.00	3.15	2.76	2.53	2.37	2.25	2.17	2.10	2.04
	0.025	5.29	3.93	3.34	3.01	2.79	2.63	2.51	2.41	2.33
	0.01	7.08	4.98	4.13	3.65	3.34	3.12	2.95	2.82	2.72
	0.005	8.49	5.80	4.73	4.14	3.76	3.49	3.29	3.13	3.01
	0.001	12.0	7.77	6.17	5.31	4.76	4.37	4.09	3.86	3.69
120	0.50	0.458	0.697	0.793	0.844	0.875	0.896	0.912	0.923	0.932
	0.10	2.75	2.35	2.13	1.99	1.90	1.82	1.77	1.72	1.68
	0.05	3.92	3.07	2.68	2.45	2.29	2.18	2.09	2.02	1.96
	0.025	5.15	3.80	3.23	2.89	2.67	2.52	2.39	2.30	2.22
	0.01	6.85	4.79	3.95	3.48	3.17	2.96	2.79	2.66	2.56
	0.005	8.18	5.54	4.50	3.92	3.55	3.28	3.09	2.93	2.81
	0.001	11.4	7.32	5.78	4.95	4.42	4.04	3.77	3.55	3.38
∞	0.50	0.455	0.693	0.789	0.839	0.870	0.891	0.907	0.918	0.927
	0.10	2.71	2.30	2.08	1.94	1.85	1.77	1.72	1.67	1.63
	0.05	3.84	3.00	2.60	2.37	2.21	2.10	2.01	1.94	1.88
	0.025	5.02	3.69	3.12	2.79	2.57	2.41	2.29	2.19	2.11
	0.01	6.63	4.61	3.78	3.32	3.02	2.80	2.64	2.51	2.41
	0.005	7.88	5.30	4.28	3.72	3.35	3.09	2.90	2.74	2.62
	0.001	10.8	6.91	5.42	4.62	4.10	3.74	3.47	3.27	3.10

TABLE E.5 UPPER PERCENTAGE POINTS FOR *F* DISTRIBUTIONS (CONT.)

$$F_{\alpha, d_1, d_2}$$

Denom. df	Upper-tail Prob.	Numerator df								
		10	12	15	20	24	30	60	120	∞
30	0.50	0.955	0.966	0.978	0.989	0.994	1.00	1.01	1.02	1.02
	0.10	1.82	1.77	1.72	1.67	1.64	1.61	1.54	1.50	1.46
	0.05	2.16	2.09	2.01	1.93	1.89	1.84	1.74	1.68	1.62
	0.025	2.51	2.41	2.31	2.20	2.14	2.07	1.94	1.87	1.79
	0.01	2.98	2.84	2.70	2.55	2.47	2.39	2.21	2.11	2.01
	0.005	3.34	3.18	3.01	2.82	2.73	2.63	2.42	2.30	2.18
	0.001	4.24	4.00	3.75	3.49	3.36	3.22	2.92	2.76	2.59
60	0.50	0.945	0.956	0.967	0.978	0.983	0.989	1.00	1.01	1.01
	0.10	1.71	1.66	1.60	1.54	1.51	1.48	1.40	1.35	1.29
	0.05	1.99	1.92	1.84	1.75	1.70	1.65	1.53	1.47	1.39
	0.025	2.27	2.17	2.06	1.94	1.88	1.82	1.67	1.58	1.48
	0.01	2.63	2.50	2.35	2.20	2.12	2.03	1.84	1.73	1.60
	0.005	2.90	2.74	2.57	2.39	2.29	2.19	1.96	1.83	1.69
	0.001	3.54	3.32	3.08	2.83	2.69	2.55	2.25	2.08	1.89
120	0.50	0.939	0.950	0.961	0.972	0.978	0.983	0.994	1.00	1.01
	0.10	1.65	1.60	1.55	1.48	1.45	1.41	1.32	1.26	1.19
	0.05	1.91	1.83	1.75	1.66	1.61	1.55	1.43	1.35	1.25
	0.025	2.16	2.05	1.95	1.82	1.76	1.69	1.53	1.43	1.31
	0.01	2.47	2.34	2.19	2.03	1.95	1.86	1.66	1.53	1.38
	0.005	2.71	2.54	2.37	2.19	2.09	1.98	1.75	1.61	1.43
	0.001	3.24	3.02	2.78	2.53	2.40	2.26	1.95	1.77	1.54
∞	0.50	0.934	0.945	0.956	0.967	0.972	0.978	0.989	0.994	1.00
	0.10	1.60	1.55	1.49	1.42	1.38	1.34	1.24	1.17	1.00
	0.05	1.83	1.75	1.67	1.57	1.52	1.46	1.32	1.22	1.00
	0.025	2.05	1.94	1.83	1.71	1.64	1.57	1.39	1.27	1.00
	0.01	2.32	2.18	2.04	1.88	1.79	1.70	1.47	1.32	1.00
	0.005	2.52	2.36	2.19	2.00	1.90	1.79	1.53	1.36	1.00
	0.001	2.96	2.74	2.51	2.27	2.13	1.99	1.66	1.45	1.00

TABLE E.6   UPPER PERCENTAGE POINTS FOR STUDENTIZED RANGE DISTRIBUTIONS*

$\alpha = 0.10$

Denom. df	Numerator df																		
	2	3	4	5	6	7	8	9	10	11	12	13	14	15	16	17	18	19	20
1	8.93	13.4	16.4	18.5	20.2	21.5	22.6	23.6	24.5	25.2	25.9	26.5	27.1	27.6	28.1	28.5	29.0	29.3	29.7
2	4.13	5.73	6.77	7.54	8.14	8.63	9.05	9.41	9.72	10.0	10.3	10.5	10.7	10.9	11.1	11.2	11.4	11.5	11.7
3	3.33	4.47	5.20	5.74	6.16	6.51	6.81	7.06	7.29	7.49	7.67	7.83	7.98	8.12	8.25	8.37	8.48	8.58	8.68
4	3.01	3.98	4.59	5.03	5.39	5.68	5.93	6.14	6.33	6.49	6.65	6.78	6.91	7.02	7.13	7.23	7.33	7.41	7.50
5	2.85	3.72	4.26	4.66	4.98	5.24	5.46	5.65	5.82	5.97	6.10	6.22	6.34	6.44	6.54	6.63	6.71	6.79	6.86
6	2.75	3.56	4.07	4.44	4.73	4.97	5.17	5.34	5.50	5.64	5.76	5.87	5.98	6.07	6.16	6.25	6.32	6.40	6.47
7	2.68	3.45	3.93	4.28	4.55	4.78	4.97	5.14	5.28	5.41	5.53	5.64	5.74	5.83	5.91	5.99	6.06	6.13	6.19
8	2.63	3.37	3.83	4.17	4.43	4.65	4.83	4.99	5.13	5.25	5.36	5.46	5.56	5.64	5.72	5.80	5.87	5.93	6.00
9	2.59	3.32	3.76	4.08	4.34	4.54	4.72	4.87	5.01	5.13	5.23	5.33	5.42	5.51	5.58	5.66	5.72	5.79	5.85
10	2.56	3.27	3.70	4.02	4.26	4.47	4.64	4.78	4.91	5.03	5.13	5.23	5.32	5.40	5.47	5.54	5.61	5.67	5.73
11	2.54	3.23	3.66	3.96	4.20	4.40	4.57	4.71	4.84	4.95	5.05	5.15	5.23	5.31	5.38	5.45	5.51	5.57	5.63
12	2.52	3.20	3.62	3.92	4.16	4.35	4.51	4.65	4.78	4.89	4.99	5.08	5.16	5.24	5.31	5.37	5.44	5.49	5.55
13	2.50	3.18	3.59	3.88	4.12	4.30	4.46	4.60	4.72	4.83	4.93	5.02	5.10	5.18	5.25	5.31	5.37	5.43	5.48
14	2.49	3.16	3.56	3.85	4.08	4.27	4.42	4.56	4.68	4.79	4.88	4.97	5.05	5.12	5.19	5.26	5.32	5.37	5.43
15	2.48	3.14	3.54	3.83	4.05	4.23	4.39	4.52	4.64	4.75	4.84	4.93	5.01	5.08	5.15	5.21	5.27	5.32	5.38
16	2.47	3.12	3.52	3.80	4.03	4.21	4.36	4.49	4.61	4.71	4.81	4.89	4.97	5.04	5.11	5.17	5.23	5.28	5.33
17	2.46	3.11	3.50	3.78	4.00	4.18	4.33	4.46	4.58	4.68	4.77	4.86	4.93	5.01	5.07	5.13	5.19	5.24	5.30
18	2.45	3.10	3.49	3.77	3.98	4.16	4.31	4.44	4.55	4.65	4.75	4.83	4.90	4.98	5.04	5.10	5.16	5.21	5.26
19	2.45	3.09	3.47	3.75	3.97	4.14	4.29	4.42	4.53	4.63	4.72	4.80	4.88	4.95	5.01	5.07	5.13	5.18	5.23
20	2.44	3.08	3.46	3.74	3.95	4.12	4.27	4.40	4.51	4.61	4.70	4.78	4.85	4.92	4.99	5.05	5.10	5.16	5.20
24	2.42	3.05	3.42	3.69	3.90	4.07	4.21	4.34	4.44	4.54	4.63	4.71	4.78	4.85	4.91	4.97	5.02	5.07	5.12
30	2.40	3.02	3.39	3.65	3.85	4.02	4.16	4.28	4.38	4.47	4.56	4.64	4.71	4.77	4.83	4.89	4.94	4.99	5.03
40	2.38	2.99	3.35	3.60	3.80	3.96	4.10	4.21	4.32	4.41	4.49	4.56	4.63	4.69	4.75	4.81	4.86	4.90	4.95
60	2.36	2.96	3.31	3.56	3.75	3.91	4.04	4.16	4.25	4.34	4.42	4.49	4.56	4.62	4.67	4.73	4.78	4.82	4.86
120	2.34	2.93	3.28	3.52	3.71	3.86	3.99	4.10	4.19	4.28	4.35	4.42	4.48	4.54	4.60	4.65	4.69	4.74	4.78
∞	2.33	2.90	3.24	3.48	3.66	3.81	3.93	4.04	4.13	4.21	4.28	4.35	4.41	4.47	4.52	4.57	4.61	4.65	4.69

TABLE E.6 UPPER PERCENTAGE POINTS FOR STUDENTIZED RANGE DISTRIBUTIONS (CONT.)

α = 0.05

Denom. df	Numerator df																		
	2	3	4	5	6	7	8	9	10	11	12	13	14	15	16	17	18	19	20
1	18.0	27.0	32.8	37.1	40.4	43.1	45.4	47.4	49.1	50.5	52.0	53.2	54.3	55.4	56.3	57.2	58.0	58.8	59.6
2	6.08	8.33	9.80	10.9	11.7	12.4	13.0	13.5	14.0	14.4	14.7	15.1	15.4	15.7	15.9	16.1	16.4	16.6	16.8
3	4.50	5.91	6.82	7.50	8.04	8.48	8.85	9.18	9.46	9.72	9.95	10.2	10.3	10.5	10.7	10.8	11.0	11.1	11.2
4	3.93	5.04	5.76	6.29	6.71	7.05	7.35	7.60	7.83	8.03	8.21	8.37	8.52	8.66	8.79	8.91	9.03	9.13	9.23
5	3.64	4.60	5.22	5.67	6.03	6.33	6.58	6.80	6.99	7.17	7.32	7.47	7.60	7.72	7.83	7.93	8.03	8.12	8.21
6	3.46	4.34	4.90	5.30	5.63	5.90	6.12	6.32	6.49	6.65	6.79	6.92	7.03	7.14	7.24	7.34	7.43	7.51	7.59
7	3.34	4.16	4.68	5.06	5.36	5.61	5.82	6.00	6.16	6.30	6.43	6.55	6.66	6.76	6.85	6.94	7.02	7.10	7.17
8	3.26	4.04	4.53	4.89	5.17	5.40	5.60	5.77	5.92	6.05	6.18	6.29	6.39	6.48	6.57	6.65	6.73	6.80	6.87
9	3.20	3.95	4.41	4.76	5.02	5.24	5.43	5.59	5.74	5.87	5.98	6.09	6.19	6.28	6.36	6.44	6.51	6.58	6.64
10	3.15	3.88	4.33	4.65	4.91	5.12	5.30	5.46	5.60	5.72	5.83	5.93	6.03	6.11	6.19	6.27	6.34	6.40	6.47
11	3.11	3.82	4.26	4.57	4.82	5.03	5.20	5.35	5.49	5.61	5.71	5.81	5.90	5.98	6.06	6.13	6.20	6.27	6.33
12	3.08	3.77	4.20	4.51	4.75	4.95	5.12	5.27	5.39	5.51	5.61	5.71	5.80	5.88	5.95	6.02	6.09	6.15	6.21
13	3.06	3.73	4.15	4.45	4.69	4.88	5.05	5.19	5.32	5.43	5.53	5.63	5.71	5.79	5.86	5.93	5.99	6.05	6.11
14	3.03	3.70	4.11	4.41	4.64	4.83	4.99	5.13	5.25	5.36	5.46	5.55	5.64	5.71	5.79	5.85	5.91	5.97	6.03
15	3.01	3.67	4.08	4.37	4.59	4.78	4.94	5.08	5.20	5.31	5.40	5.49	5.57	5.65	5.72	5.78	5.85	5.90	5.96
16	3.00	3.65	4.05	4.33	4.56	4.74	4.90	5.03	5.15	5.26	5.35	5.44	5.52	5.59	5.66	5.73	5.79	5.84	5.90
17	2.98	3.63	4.02	4.30	4.52	4.70	4.86	4.95	5.11	5.21	5.31	5.39	5.47	5.54	5.61	5.67	5.73	5.79	5.84
18	2.97	3.61	4.00	4.28	4.49	4.67	4.82	4.96	5.07	5.17	5.27	5.35	5.43	5.50	5.57	5.63	5.69	5.74	5.79
19	2.96	3.59	3.98	4.25	4.47	4.65	4.79	4.92	5.04	5.14	5.23	5.31	5.39	5.46	5.53	5.59	5.65	5.70	5.75
20	2.95	3.58	3.96	4.23	4.45	4.62	4.77	4.90	5.01	5.11	5.20	5.28	5.36	5.43	5.49	5.55	5.61	5.66	5.71
24	2.92	3.53	3.90	4.17	4.37	4.54	4.68	4.81	4.92	5.01	5.10	5.18	5.25	5.32	5.38	5.44	5.49	5.55	5.59
30	2.89	3.49	3.85	4.10	4.30	4.46	4.60	4.72	4.82	4.92	5.00	5.08	5.15	5.21	5.27	5.33	5.38	5.43	5.47
40	2.86	3.44	3.79	4.04	4.23	4.39	4.52	4.63	4.73	4.82	4.90	4.98	5.04	5.11	5.16	5.22	5.27	5.31	5.36
60	2.83	3.40	3.74	3.98	4.16	4.31	4.44	4.55	4.65	4.73	4.81	4.88	4.94	5.00	5.06	5.11	5.15	5.20	5.24
120	2.80	3.36	3.68	3.92	4.10	4.24	4.36	4.47	4.56	4.64	4.71	4.78	4.84	4.90	4.95	5.00	5.04	5.09	5.13
∞	2.77	3.31	3.63	3.86	4.03	4.17	4.29	4.39	4.47	4.55	4.62	4.68	4.74	4.80	4.85	4.89	4.93	4.97	5.01

TABLE E.6   UPPER PERCENTAGE POINTS FOR STUDENTIZED RANGE DISTRIBUTIONS (CONT.)

$\alpha = 0.01$

Denom. df	Numerator df																		
	2	3	4	5	6	7	8	9	10	11	12	13	14	15	16	17	18	19	20
1	90.0	135	164	186	202	216	227	237	246	253	260	266	272	277	282	286	290	294	298
2	14.0	19.0	22.3	24.7	26.6	28.2	29.5	30.7	31.7	32.6	33.4	34.1	34.8	35.4	36.0	36.5	37.0	37.5	37.9
3	8.26	10.6	12.2	13.3	14.2	15.0	15.6	16.2	16.7	17.1	17.5	17.9	18.2	18.5	18.8	19.1	19.3	19.5	19.8
4	6.51	8.12	9.17	9.96	10.6	11.1	11.5	11.9	12.3	12.6	12.8	13.1	13.3	13.5	13.7	13.9	14.1	14.2	14.4
5	5.70	6.97	7.80	8.42	8.91	9.32	9.67	9.97	10.2	10.5	10.7	10.9	11.1	11.2	11.4	11.6	11.7	11.8	11.9
6	5.24	6.33	7.03	7.56	7.97	8.32	8.61	8.87	9.10	9.30	9.49	9.65	9.81	9.95	10.1	10.2	10.3	10.4	10.5
7	4.95	5.92	6.54	7.01	7.37	7.68	7.94	8.17	8.37	8.55	8.71	8.86	9.00	9.12	9.24	9.35	9.46	9.55	9.65
8	4.74	5.63	6.20	6.63	6.96	7.24	7.47	7.68	7.87	8.03	8.18	8.31	8.44	8.55	8.66	8.76	8.85	8.94	9.03
9	4.60	5.43	5.96	6.35	6.66	6.91	7.13	7.32	7.49	7.65	7.78	7.91	8.03	8.13	8.23	8.32	8.41	8.49	8.57
10	4.48	5.27	5.77	6.14	6.43	6.67	6.87	7.05	7.21	7.36	7.48	7.60	7.71	7.81	7.91	7.99	8.07	8.15	8.22
11	4.39	5.14	5.62	5.97	6.25	6.48	6.67	6.84	6.99	7.13	7.25	7.36	7.46	7.56	7.65	7.73	7.81	7.88	7.95
12	4.32	5.04	5.50	5.84	6.10	6.32	6.51	6.67	6.81	6.94	7.06	7.17	7.26	7.36	7.44	7.52	7.59	7.66	7.73
13	4.26	4.96	5.40	5.73	5.98	6.19	6.37	6.53	6.67	6.79	6.90	7.01	7.10	7.19	7.27	7.34	7.42	7.48	7.55
14	4.21	4.89	5.32	5.63	5.88	6.08	6.26	6.41	6.54	6.66	6.77	6.87	6.96	7.05	7.12	7.20	7.27	7.33	7.39
15	4.17	4.83	5.25	5.56	5.80	5.99	6.16	6.31	6.44	6.55	6.66	6.76	6.84	6.93	7.00	7.07	7.14	7.20	7.26
16	4.13	4.78	5.19	5.49	5.72	5.92	6.08	6.22	6.35	6.46	6.56	6.66	6.74	6.82	6.90	6.97	7.03	7.09	7.15
17	4.10	4.74	5.14	5.43	5.66	5.85	6.01	6.15	6.27	6.38	6.48	6.57	6.66	6.73	6.80	6.87	6.94	7.00	7.05
18	4.07	4.70	5.09	5.38	5.60	5.79	5.94	6.08	6.20	6.31	6.41	6.50	6.58	6.65	6.72	6.79	6.85	6.91	6.96
19	4.05	4.67	5.05	5.33	5.55	5.73	5.89	6.02	6.14	6.25	6.34	6.43	6.51	6.58	6.65	6.72	6.78	6.84	6.89
20	4.02	4.64	5.02	5.29	5.51	5.69	5.84	5.97	6.09	6.19	6.29	6.37	6.45	6.52	6.59	6.65	6.71	6.76	6.82
24	3.96	4.54	4.91	5.17	5.37	5.54	5.69	5.81	5.92	6.02	6.11	6.19	6.26	6.33	6.39	6.45	6.51	6.56	6.61
30	3.89	4.45	4.80	5.05	5.24	5.40	5.54	5.65	5.76	5.85	5.93	6.01	6.08	6.14	6.20	6.26	6.31	6.36	6.41
40	3.82	4.37	4.70	4.93	5.11	5.27	5.39	5.50	5.60	5.69	5.77	5.84	5.90	5.96	6.02	6.07	6.12	6.17	6.21
60	3.76	4.28	4.60	4.82	4.99	5.13	5.25	5.36	5.45	5.53	5.60	5.67	5.73	5.79	5.84	5.89	5.93	5.98	6.02
120	3.70	4.20	4.50	4.71	4.87	5.01	5.12	5.21	5.30	5.38	5.44	5.51	5.56	5.61	5.66	5.71	5.75	5.79	5.83
∞	3.64	4.12	4.40	4.60	4.76	4.88	4.99	5.08	5.16	5.23	5.29	5.35	5.40	5.45	5.49	5.54	5.57	5.61	5.65

*Copyright © 1959 by John Wiley and Sons, Inc. Reprinted by permission of John Wiley and Sons, Inc., from Henry Scheffé, *The Analysis of Variance* (New York, John Wiley and Sons, 1959), pp. 434–436.

TABLE E.7   UPPER PERCENTAGE POINTS FOR CHI-SQUARE DISTRIBUTIONS*

$\chi^2_{\alpha,\,\text{df}}$

Probability

df	0.9995	0.995	0.99	0.975	0.95	0.90	0.80	0.70	0.60
1	0.000000393	0.0000393	0.000157	0.000982	0.00393	0.0158	0.0642	0.148	0.275
2	0.00100	0.0100	0.0201	0.0506	0.103	0.211	0.446	0.713	1.022
3	0.0153	0.0717	0.115	0.216	0.352	0.584	1.005	1.424	1.869
4	0.0639	0.207	0.297	0.484	0.711	1.064	1.649	2.195	2.753
5	0.158	0.412	0.554	0.831	1.145	1.610	2.343	3.000	3.655
6	0.299	0.676	0.872	1.237	1.635	2.204	3.070	3.828	4.570
7	0.485	0.989	1.239	1.690	2.167	2.833	3.822	4.671	5.493
8	0.710	1.344	1.646	2.180	2.733	3.490	4.594	5.527	6.423
9	0.972	1.735	2.088	2.700	3.325	4.168	5.380	6.393	7.357
10	1.265	2.156	2.558	3.247	3.940	4.865	6.179	7.267	8.295
11	1.587	2.603	3.053	3.816	4.575	5.578	6.989	8.148	9.237
12	1.934	3.074	3.571	4.404	5.226	6.304	7.807	9.034	10.182
13	2.305	3.565	4.107	5.009	5.892	7.042	8.634	9.926	11.129
14	2.697	4.075	4.660	5.629	6.571	7.790	9.467	10.821	12.078
15	3.108	4.601	5.229	6.262	7.261	8.547	10.307	11.721	13.030
16	3.536	5.142	5.812	6.908	7.962	9.312	11.152	12.624	13.983
17	3.980	5.697	6.408	7.564	8.672	10.085	12.002	13.531	14.937
18	4.439	6.265	7.015	8.231	9.390	10.865	12.857	14.440	15.893
19	4.912	6.844	7.633	8.907	10.117	11.651	13.716	15.352	16.850
20	5.398	7.434	8.260	9.591	10.851	12.443	14.578	16.266	17.809
21	5.896	8.034	8.897	10.283	11.591	13.240	15.445	17.182	18.768
22	6.404	8.643	9.542	10.982	12.338	14.041	16.314	18.101	19.729
23	6.924	9.260	10.196	11.689	13.091	14.848	17.187	19.021	20.690
24	7.453	9.886	10.856	12.401	13.848	15.659	18.062	19.943	21.652
25	7.991	10.520	11.524	13.120	14.611	16.473	18.940	20.867	22.616
26	8.538	11.160	12.198	13.844	15.379	17.292	19.820	21.792	23.579
27	9.093	11.808	12.879	14.573	16.151	18.114	20.703	22.719	24.544
28	9.656	12.461	13.565	15.308	16.928	18.939	21.588	23.647	25.509
29	10.227	13.121	14.256	16.047	17.708	19.768	22.475	24.577	26.475
30	10.804	13.787	14.953	16.791	18.493	20.599	23.364	25.508	27.442
35	13.787	17.192	18.509	20.569	22.465	24.797	27.836	30.178	32.282
40	16.906	20.707	22.164	24.433	26.509	29.051	32.345	34.872	37.134
45	20.137	24.311	25.901	28.366	30.612	33.350	36.884	39.585	41.995
50	23.461	27.991	29.707	32.357	34.764	37.689	41.449	44.313	46.864
60	30.340	35.534	37.485	40.482	43.188	46.459	50.641	53.809	56.620
70	37.467	43.275	45.442	48.758	51.739	55.329	59.898	63.346	66.396
80	44.791	51.172	53.540	57.153	60.391	64.278	69.207	72.915	76.188
90	52.276	59.196	61.754	65.647	69.126	73.291	78.558	82.511	85.993
100	59.896	67.328	70.065	74.222	77.929	82.358	87.945	92.129	95.808
120	75.467	83.852	86.923	91.573	95.705	100.624	106.806	111.419	115.465
140	91.391	100.655	104.034	109.137	113.659	119.029	125.758	130.766	135.149
160	107.597	117.679	121.346	126.870	131.756	137.546	144.783	150.158	154.856
180	124.033	134.884	138.820	144.741	149.969	156.153	163.868	169.588	174.580
200	140.660	152.241	156.432	162.728	168.279	174.835	183.003	189.049	194.319

TABLE E.7   UPPER PERCENTAGE POINTS FOR CHI-SQUARE DISTRIBUTIONS (CONT.)

$$\chi^2_{\alpha,\,df}$$

df	Probability									
	0.50	0.40	0.30	0.20	0.10	0.05	0.025	0.01	0.005	0.0005
1	0.455	0.708	1.074	1.642	2.706	3.841	5.024	6.635	7.879	12.116
2	1.386	1.833	2.408	3.219	4.605	5.991	7.378	9.210	10.597	15.202
3	2.366	2.946	3.665	4.642	6.251	7.815	9.348	11.345	12.838	17.730
4	3.357	4.045	4.878	5.989	7.779	9.488	11.143	13.277	14.860	19.997
5	4.351	5.132	6.064	7.289	9.236	11.070	12.833	15.086	16.750	22.105
6	5.348	6.211	7.231	8.558	10.645	12.592	14.449	16.812	18.548	24.103
7	6.346	7.283	8.383	9.803	12.017	14.067	16.013	18.475	20.278	26.018
8	7.344	8.351	9.524	11.030	13.362	15.507	17.535	20.090	21.955	27.868
9	8.343	9.414	10.656	12.242	14.684	16.919	19.023	21.666	23.589	29.666
10	9.342	10.473	11.781	13.442	15.987	18.307	20.483	23.209	25.188	31.420
11	10.341	11.530	12.899	14.631	17.275	19.675	21.920	24.725	26.757	33.137
12	11.340	12.584	14.011	15.812	18.549	21.026	23.337	26.217	28.300	34.821
13	12.340	13.636	15.119	16.985	19.812	22.362	24.736	27.688	29.819	36.478
14	13.339	14.685	16.222	18.151	21.064	23.685	26.119	29.141	31.319	38.109
15	14.339	15.733	17.322	19.311	22.307	24.996	27.488	30.578	32.801	39.719
16	15.338	16.780	18.418	20.465	23.542	26.296	28.845	32.000	34.267	41.308
17	16.338	17.824	19.511	21.615	24.769	27.587	30.191	33.409	35.718	42.879
18	17.338	18.868	20.601	22.760	25.989	28.869	31.526	34.805	37.156	44.434
19	18.338	19.910	21.689	23.900	27.204	30.144	32.852	36.191	38.582	45.973
20	19.337	20.951	22.775	25.038	28.412	31.410	34.170	37.566	39.997	47.498
21	20.337	21.991	23.858	26.171	29.615	32.671	35.479	38.932	41.401	49.011
22	21.337	23.031	24.939	27.301	30.813	33.924	36.781	40.289	42.796	50.511
23	22.337	24.069	26.018	28.429	32.007	35.172	38.076	41.638	44.181	52.000
24	23.337	25.106	27.096	29.553	33.196	36.415	39.364	42.980	45.559	53.479
25	24.337	26.143	28.172	30.675	34.382	37.652	40.646	44.314	46.928	54.947
26	25.336	27.179	29.246	31.795	35.563	38.885	41.923	45.642	48.290	56.407
27	26.336	28.214	30.319	32.912	36.741	40.113	43.195	46.963	49.645	57.858
28	27.336	29.249	31.391	34.027	37.916	41.337	44.461	48.278	50.993	59.300
29	28.336	30.283	32.461	35.139	39.087	42.557	45.722	49.588	52.336	60.735
30	29.336	31.316	33.530	36.250	40.256	43.773	46.979	50.892	53.672	62.162
35	34.336	36.475	38.859	41.778	46.059	49.802	53.203	57.342	60.275	69.199
40	39.335	41.622	44.165	47.269	51.805	55.758	59.342	63.691	66.766	76.095
45	44.335	46.761	49.452	52.729	57.505	61.656	65.410	69.957	73.166	82.876
50	49.335	51.892	54.723	58.164	63.167	67.505	71.420	76.154	79.490	89.561
60	59.335	62.135	65.227	68.972	74.397	79.082	83.298	88.379	91.952	102.695
70	69.334	72.358	75.689	79.715	85.527	90.531	95.023	100.425	104.215	115.578
80	79.334	82.566	86.120	90.405	96.578	101.879	106.629	112.329	116.321	128.261
90	89.334	92.761	96.524	101.054	107.565	113.145	118.136	124.116	128.299	140.782
100	99.334	102.946	106.906	111.667	118.498	124.342	129.561	135.807	140.169	153.167
120	119.334	123.289	127.616	132.806	140.233	146.567	152.211	158.950	163.648	177.603
140	139.334	143.604	148.269	153.854	161.827	168.613	174.648	181.840	186.847	201.683
160	159.334	163.898	168.876	174.828	183.311	190.516	196.915	204.530	209.824	225.481
180	179.334	184.173	189.446	195.743	204.704	212.304	219.044	227.056	232.620	249.048
200	199.334	204.434	209.985	216.609	226.021	233.994	241.058	249.445	255.264	272.423

*Abstracted with permission from C. Lentner (Ed.), *Geigy Scientific Tables*, 8th ed., Volume 2, Ciba-Geigy, Basle, 1982, pp. 34–37.

TABLE E.8   CRITICAL VALUES FOR THE MCNEMAR M STATISTIC AND THE SIGN TEST S STATISTIC

n_D	Probability			
	0.10	0.05	0.02	0.01
1	none	none	none	none
2	none	none	none	none
3	none	none	none	none
4	none	none	none	none
5	0 or 5	none	none	none
6	0 or 6	0 or 6	none	none
7	0 or 7	0 or 7	0 or 7	none
8	≤ 1 or ≥ 7	0 or 8	0 or 8	0 or 8
9	≤ 1 or ≥ 8	≤ 1 or ≥ 8	0 or 9	0 or 9
10	≤ 1 or ≥ 9	≤ 1 or ≥ 9	0 or 10	0 or 10
11	≤ 2 or ≥ 9	≤ 1 or ≥ 10	≤ 1 or ≥ 10	0 or 11
12	≤ 2 or ≥ 10	≤ 2 or ≥ 10	≤ 1 or ≥ 11	≤ 1 or ≥ 11
13	≤ 3 or ≥ 10	≤ 2 or ≥ 11	≤ 1 or ≥ 12	≤ 1 or ≥ 12
14	≤ 3 or ≥ 11	≤ 2 or ≥ 12	≤ 2 or ≥ 12	≤ 1 or ≥ 13
15	≤ 3 or ≥ 12	≤ 3 or ≥ 12	≤ 2 or ≥ 13	≤ 2 or ≥ 13
16	≤ 4 or ≥ 12	≤ 3 or ≥ 13	≤ 2 or ≥ 14	≤ 2 or ≥ 14
17	≤ 4 or ≥ 13	≤ 4 or ≥ 13	≤ 3 or ≥ 14	≤ 2 or ≥ 15
18	≤ 5 or ≥ 13	≤ 4 or ≥ 14	≤ 3 or ≥ 15	≤ 3 or ≥ 15
19	≤ 5 or ≥ 14	≤ 4 or ≥ 15	≤ 4 or ≥ 15	≤ 3 or ≥ 16
20	≤ 5 or ≥ 15	≤ 5 or ≥ 15	≤ 4 or ≥ 16	≤ 3 or ≥ 17
21	≤ 6 or ≥ 15	≤ 5 or ≥ 16	≤ 4 or ≥ 17	≤ 4 or ≥ 17
22	≤ 6 or ≥ 16	≤ 5 or ≥ 17	≤ 5 or ≥ 17	≤ 4 or ≥ 18
23	≤ 7 or ≥ 16	≤ 6 or ≥ 17	≤ 5 or ≥ 18	≤ 4 or ≥ 19
24	≤ 7 or ≥ 17	≤ 6 or ≥ 18	≤ 5 or ≥ 19	≤ 5 or ≥ 19
25	≤ 7 or ≥ 18	≤ 7 or ≥ 18	≤ 6 or ≥ 19	≤ 5 or ≥ 20
26	≤ 8 or ≥ 18	≤ 7 or ≥ 19	≤ 6 or ≥ 20	≤ 6 or ≥ 20
27	≤ 8 or ≥ 19	≤ 7 or ≥ 20	≤ 7 or ≥ 20	≤ 6 or ≥ 21
28	≤ 9 or ≥ 19	≤ 8 or ≥ 20	≤ 7 or ≥ 21	≤ 6 or ≥ 22
29	≤ 9 or ≥ 20	≤ 8 or ≥ 21	≤ 7 or ≥ 22	≤ 7 or ≥ 22
30	≤ 10 or ≥ 20	≤ 9 or ≥ 21	≤ 8 or ≥ 22	≤ 7 or ≥ 23
31	≤ 10 or ≥ 21	≤ 9 or ≥ 22	≤ 8 or ≥ 23	≤ 7 or ≥ 24
32	≤ 10 or ≥ 22	≤ 9 or ≥ 23	≤ 8 or ≥ 24	≤ 8 or ≥ 24
33	≤ 11 or ≥ 22	≤ 10 or ≥ 23	≤ 9 or ≥ 24	≤ 8 or ≥ 25
34	≤ 11 or ≥ 23	≤ 10 or ≥ 24	≤ 9 or ≥ 25	≤ 9 or ≥ 25
35	≤ 12 or ≥ 23	≤ 11 or ≥ 24	≤ 10 or ≥ 25	≤ 9 or ≥ 26
36	≤ 12 or ≥ 24	≤ 11 or ≥ 25	≤ 10 or ≥ 26	≤ 9 or ≥ 27
37	≤ 13 or ≥ 24	≤ 12 or ≥ 25	≤ 10 or ≥ 27	≤ 10 or ≥ 27
38	≤ 13 or ≥ 25	≤ 12 or ≥ 26	≤ 11 or ≥ 27	≤ 10 or ≥ 28
39	≤ 13 or ≥ 26	≤ 12 or ≥ 27	≤ 11 or ≥ 28	≤ 11 or ≥ 28
40	≤ 14 or ≥ 26	≤ 13 or ≥ 27	≤ 12 or ≥ 28	≤ 11 or ≥ 29
41	≤ 14 or ≥ 27	≤ 13 or ≥ 28	≤ 12 or ≥ 29	≤ 11 or ≥ 30
42	≤ 15 or ≥ 27	≤ 14 or ≥ 28	≤ 13 or ≥ 29	≤ 12 or ≥ 30
43	≤ 15 or ≥ 28	≤ 14 or ≥ 29	≤ 13 or ≥ 30	≤ 12 or ≥ 31
44	≤ 16 or ≥ 28	≤ 15 or ≥ 29	≤ 13 or ≥ 31	≤ 13 or ≥ 31
45	≤ 16 or ≥ 29	≤ 15 or ≥ 30	≤ 14 or ≥ 31	≤ 13 or ≥ 32
46	≤ 16 or ≥ 30	≤ 15 or ≥ 31	≤ 14 or ≥ 32	≤ 13 or ≥ 33
47	≤ 17 or ≥ 30	≤ 16 or ≥ 31	≤ 15 or ≥ 32	≤ 14 or ≥ 33
48	≤ 17 or ≥ 31	≤ 16 or ≥ 32	≤ 15 or ≥ 33	≤ 14 or ≥ 34
49	≤ 18 or ≥ 31	≤ 17 or ≥ 32	≤ 15 or ≥ 34	≤ 15 or ≥ 34
50	≤ 18 or ≥ 32	≤ 17 or ≥ 33	≤ 16 or ≥ 34	≤ 15 or ≥ 35
51	≤ 19 or ≥ 32	≤ 18 or ≥ 33	≤ 16 or ≥ 35	≤ 15 or ≥ 36
52	≤ 19 or ≥ 33	≤ 18 or ≥ 34	≤ 17 or ≥ 35	≤ 16 or ≥ 36
53	≤ 20 or ≥ 33	≤ 18 or ≥ 35	≤ 17 or ≥ 36	≤ 16 or ≥ 37
54	≤ 20 or ≥ 34	≤ 19 or ≥ 35	≤ 18 or ≥ 36	≤ 17 or ≥ 37
55	≤ 20 or ≥ 35	≤ 19 or ≥ 36	≤ 18 or ≥ 37	≤ 17 or ≥ 38
56	≤ 21 or ≥ 35	≤ 20 or ≥ 36	≤ 18 or ≥ 38	≤ 17 or ≥ 39
57	≤ 21 or ≥ 36	≤ 20 or ≥ 37	≤ 19 or ≥ 38	≤ 18 or ≥ 39
58	≤ 22 or ≥ 36	≤ 21 or ≥ 37	≤ 19 or ≥ 39	≤ 18 or ≥ 40

TABLE E.8 CRITICAL VALUES FOR THE MCNEMAR *M* STATISTIC AND THE SIGN TEST *S* STATISTIC (CONT.)

	Probability			
n_D	0.10	0.05	0.02	0.01
59	≤ 22 or ≥ 37	≤ 21 or ≥ 38	≤ 20 or ≥ 39	≤ 19 or ≥ 40
60	≤ 23 or ≥ 37	≤ 21 or ≥ 39	≤ 20 or ≥ 40	≤ 19 or ≥ 41
61	≤ 23 or ≥ 38	≤ 22 or ≥ 39	≤ 20 or ≥ 41	≤ 20 or ≥ 41
62	≤ 24 or ≥ 38	≤ 22 or ≥ 40	≤ 21 or ≥ 41	≤ 20 or ≥ 42
63	≤ 24 or ≥ 39	≤ 23 or ≥ 40	≤ 21 or ≥ 42	≤ 20 or ≥ 43
64	≤ 24 or ≥ 40	≤ 23 or ≥ 41	≤ 22 or ≥ 42	≤ 21 or ≥ 43
65	≤ 25 or ≥ 40	≤ 24 or ≥ 41	≤ 22 or ≥ 43	≤ 21 or ≥ 44
66	≤ 25 or ≥ 41	≤ 24 or ≥ 42	≤ 23 or ≥ 43	≤ 22 or ≥ 44
67	≤ 26 or ≥ 41	≤ 25 or ≥ 42	≤ 23 or ≥ 44	≤ 22 or ≥ 45
68	≤ 26 or ≥ 42	≤ 25 or ≥ 43	≤ 23 or ≥ 45	≤ 22 or ≥ 46
69	≤ 27 or ≥ 42	≤ 25 or ≥ 44	≤ 24 or ≥ 45	≤ 23 or ≥ 46
70	≤ 27 or ≥ 43	≤ 26 or ≥ 44	≤ 24 or ≥ 46	≤ 23 or ≥ 47
71	≤ 28 or ≥ 43	≤ 26 or ≥ 45	≤ 25 or ≥ 46	≤ 24 or ≥ 47
72	≤ 28 or ≥ 44	≤ 27 or ≥ 45	≤ 25 or ≥ 47	≤ 24 or ≥ 48
73	≤ 28 or ≥ 45	≤ 27 or ≥ 46	≤ 26 or ≥ 47	≤ 25 or ≥ 48
74	≤ 29 or ≥ 45	≤ 28 or ≥ 46	≤ 26 or ≥ 48	≤ 25 or ≥ 49
75	≤ 29 or ≥ 46	≤ 28 or ≥ 47	≤ 26 or ≥ 49	≤ 25 or ≥ 50
76	≤ 30 or ≥ 46	≤ 28 or ≥ 48	≤ 27 or ≥ 49	≤ 26 or ≥ 50
77	≤ 30 or ≥ 47	≤ 29 or ≥ 48	≤ 27 or ≥ 50	≤ 26 or ≥ 51
78	≤ 31 or ≥ 47	≤ 29 or ≥ 49	≤ 28 or ≥ 50	≤ 27 or ≥ 51
79	≤ 31 or ≥ 48	≤ 30 or ≥ 49	≤ 28 or ≥ 51	≤ 27 or ≥ 52
80	≤ 32 or ≥ 48	≤ 30 or ≥ 50	≤ 29 or ≥ 51	≤ 28 or ≥ 52
81	≤ 32 or ≥ 49	≤ 31 or ≥ 50	≤ 29 or ≥ 52	≤ 28 or ≥ 53
82	≤ 33 or ≥ 49	≤ 31 or ≥ 51	≤ 30 or ≥ 52	≤ 28 or ≥ 54
83	≤ 33 or ≥ 50	≤ 32 or ≥ 51	≤ 30 or ≥ 53	≤ 29 or ≥ 54
84	≤ 33 or ≥ 51	≤ 32 or ≥ 52	≤ 30 or ≥ 54	≤ 29 or ≥ 55
85	≤ 34 or ≥ 51	≤ 32 or ≥ 53	≤ 31 or ≥ 54	≤ 30 or ≥ 55
86	≤ 34 or ≥ 52	≤ 33 or ≥ 53	≤ 31 or ≥ 55	≤ 30 or ≥ 56
87	≤ 35 or ≥ 52	≤ 33 or ≥ 54	≤ 32 or ≥ 55	≤ 31 or ≥ 56
88	≤ 35 or ≥ 53	≤ 34 or ≥ 54	< 32 or ≥ 56	≤ 31 or ≥ 57
89	≤ 36 or ≥ 53	≤ 34 or ≥ 55	≤ 33 or ≥ 56	≤ 31 or ≥ 58
90	≤ 36 or ≥ 54	≤ 35 or ≥ 55	≤ 33 or ≥ 57	≤ 32 or ≥ 58
91	≤ 37 or ≥ 54	≤ 35 or ≥ 56	≤ 33 or ≥ 58	≤ 32 or ≥ 59
92	≤ 37 or ≥ 55	≤ 36 or ≥ 56	≤ 34 or ≥ 58	≤ 33 or ≥ 59
93	≤ 38 or ≥ 55	≤ 36 or ≥ 57	≤ 34 or ≥ 59	≤ 33 or ≥ 60
94	≤ 38 or ≥ 56	≤ 37 or ≥ 57	≤ 35 or ≥ 59	≤ 34 or ≥ 60
95	≤ 38 or ≥ 57	≤ 37 or ≥ 58	≤ 35 or ≥ 60	≤ 34 or ≥ 61
96	≤ 39 or ≥ 57	≤ 37 or ≥ 59	≤ 36 or ≥ 60	≤ 34 or ≥ 62
97	≤ 39 or ≥ 58	≤ 38 or ≥ 59	≤ 36 or ≥ 61	≤ 35 or ≥ 62
98	≤ 40 or ≥ 58	≤ 38 or ≥ 60	≤ 37 or ≥ 61	≤ 35 or ≥ 63
99	≤ 40 or ≥ 59	≤ 39 or ≥ 60	≤ 37 or ≥ 62	≤ 36 or ≥ 63
100	≤ 41 or ≥ 59	≤ 39 or ≥ 61	≤ 37 or ≥ 63	≤ 36 or ≥ 64

TABLE E.9 CRITICAL VALUES FOR THE WILCOXON SIGNED RANK *W* STATISTIC*

	Probability			
n_D	0.10	0.05	0.02	0.01
1	none	none	none	none
2	none	none	none	none
3	none	none	none	none
4	none	none	none	none
5	0 or 15	none	none	none
6	≤ 2 or ≥ 19	0 or 21	none	none
7	≤ 3 or ≥ 25	≤ 2 or ≥ 26	0 or 28	none
8	≤ 5 or ≥ 31	≤ 3 or ≥ 33	≤ 1 or ≥ 35	0 or 36
9	≤ 8 or ≥ 37	≤ 5 or ≥ 40	≤ 3 or ≥ 42	≤ 1 or ≥ 44
10	≤ 10 or ≥ 45	≤ 8 or ≥ 47	≤ 5 or ≥ 50	≤ 3 or ≥ 52
11	≤ 13 or ≥ 53	≤ 10 or ≥ 56	≤ 7 or ≥ 59	≤ 5 or ≥ 61
12	≤ 17 or ≥ 61	≤ 13 or ≥ 65	≤ 9 or ≥ 69	≤ 7 or ≥ 71
13	≤ 21 or ≥ 70	≤ 17 or ≥ 74	≤ 12 or ≥ 79	≤ 9 or ≥ 82
14	≤ 25 or ≥ 80	≤ 21 or ≥ 84	≤ 15 or ≥ 90	≤ 12 or ≥ 93
15	≤ 30 or ≥ 90	≤ 25 or ≥ 95	≤ 19 or ≥ 101	≤ 15 or ≥ 105
16	≤ 35 or ≥ 101	≤ 29 or ≥ 107	≤ 23 or ≥ 113	≤ 19 or ≥ 117
17	≤ 41 or ≥ 112	≤ 34 or ≥ 119	≤ 27 or ≥ 126	≤ 23 or ≥ 130
18	≤ 47 or ≥ 124	≤ 40 or ≥ 131	≤ 32 or ≥ 139	≤ 27 or ≥ 144
19	≤ 53 or ≥ 137	≤ 46 or ≥ 144	≤ 37 or ≥ 153	≤ 32 or ≥ 158
20	≤ 60 or ≥ 150	≤ 52 or ≥ 158	≤ 43 or ≥ 167	≤ 37 or ≥ 173
21	≤ 67 or ≥ 164	≤ 58 or ≥ 173	≤ 49 or ≥ 182	≤ 43 or ≥ 188
22	≤ 75 or ≥ 178	≤ 66 or ≥ 187	≤ 55 or ≥ 198	≤ 48 or ≥ 205
23	≤ 83 or ≥ 193	≤ 73 or ≥ 203	≤ 62 or ≥ 214	≤ 54 or ≥ 222
24	≤ 91 or ≥ 209	≤ 81 or ≥ 210	≤ 69 or ≥ 231	≤ 61 or ≥ 239
25	≤ 100 or ≥ 225	≤ 89 or ≥ 236	≤ 76 or ≥ 249	≤ 68 or ≥ 257
26	≤ 110 or ≥ 241	≤ 98 or ≥ 253	≤ 84 or ≥ 267	≤ 75 or ≥ 276
27	≤ 119 or ≥ 259	≤ 107 or ≥ 271	≤ 93 or ≥ 285	≤ 83 or ≥ 295
28	≤ 130 or ≥ 276	≤ 116 or ≥ 290	≤ 101 or ≥ 305	≤ 91 or ≥ 315
29	≤ 140 or ≥ 295	≤ 126 or ≥ 309	≤ 110 or ≥ 325	≤ 100 or ≥ 335
30	≤ 151 or ≥ 314	≤ 137 or ≥ 328	≤ 120 or ≥ 345	≤ 109 or ≥ 356
31	≤ 163 or ≥ 333	≤ 147 or ≥ 349	≤ 130 or ≥ 366	≤ 118 or ≥ 378
32	≤ 175 or ≥ 353	≤ 159 or ≥ 369	≤ 140 or ≥ 388	≤ 128 or ≥ 400
33	≤ 187 or ≥ 374	≤ 170 or ≥ 391	≤ 151 or ≥ 410	≤ 138 or ≥ 423
34	≤ 200 or ≥ 395	≤ 182 or ≥ 413	≤ 162 or ≥ 433	≤ 148 or ≥ 447
35	≤ 213 or ≥ 417	≤ 195 or ≥ 435	≤ 174 or ≥ 456	≤ 159 or ≥ 471
36	≤ 227 or ≥ 439	≤ 208 or ≥ 458	≤ 186 or ≥ 480	≤ 171 or ≥ 495
37	≤ 241 or ≥ 462	≤ 221 or ≥ 482	≤ 198 or ≥ 505	≤ 183 or ≥ 520
38	≤ 256 or ≥ 485	≤ 235 or ≥ 506	≤ 211 or ≥ 530	≤ 195 or ≥ 546
39	≤ 271 or ≥ 509	≤ 249 or ≥ 531	≤ 224 or ≥ 556	≤ 207 or ≥ 573
40	≤ 286 or ≥ 534	≤ 264 or ≥ 556	≤ 238 or ≥ 582	≤ 220 or ≥ 600
41	≤ 302 or ≥ 559	≤ 279 or ≥ 582	≤ 252 or ≥ 609	≤ 234 or ≥ 627
42	≤ 319 or ≥ 584	≤ 294 or ≥ 609	≤ 266 or ≥ 637	≤ 247 or ≥ 656
43	≤ 336 or ≥ 610	≤ 310 or ≥ 636	≤ 281 or ≥ 665	≤ 262 or ≥ 684
44	≤ 353 or ≥ 637	≤ 327 or ≥ 663	≤ 296 or ≥ 694	≤ 276 or ≥ 714
45	≤ 371 or ≥ 664	≤ 343 or ≥ 692	≤ 312 or ≥ 723	≤ 291 or ≥ 744
46	≤ 389 or ≥ 692	≤ 361 or ≥ 720	≤ 328 or ≥ 753	≤ 307 or ≥ 774
47	≤ 407 or ≥ 721	≤ 378 or ≥ 750	≤ 345 or ≥ 783	≤ 323 or ≥ 805
48	≤ 427 or ≥ 749	≤ 396 or ≥ 780	≤ 362 or ≥ 814	≤ 339 or ≥ 837
49	≤ 446 or ≥ 779	≤ 415 or ≥ 810	≤ 380 or ≥ 845	≤ 356 or ≥ 869
50	≤ 466 or ≥ 809	≤ 434 or ≥ 841	≤ 397 or ≥ 878	≤ 373 or ≥ 902

*Adapted from "Table II. Probability Levels for the Wilcoxon Signed Rank Test," edited by the Institute of Mathematical Statistics, Coeditors; H. L. Harter and D. B. Owen, *Selected Tables in Mathematical Statistics*, (1973), Vol. 1, pp. 237–259, by permission of the American Mathematical Society.

TABLE E.10   CRITICAL VALUES FOR THE MANN-WHITNEY *MW* STATISTIC*

n_1	Two-tailed Prob.	n_2 1	2	3	4	5
1	0.10	none	none	none	none	none
	0.05	none	none	none	none	none
	0.02	none	none	none	none	none
	0.01	none	none	none	none	none
	0.002	none	none	none	none	none
2	0.10	none	none	none	none	≤ 3 or ≥ 13
	0.05	none	none	none	none	none
	0.02	none	none	none	none	none
	0.01	none	none	none	none	none
	0.002	none	none	none	none	none
3	0.10	none	none	≤ 6 or ≥ 15	≤ 6 or ≥ 18	≤ 7 or ≥ 20
	0.05	none	none	none	none	≤ 6 or ≥ 21
	0.02	none	none	none	none	none
	0.01	none	none	none	none	none
	0.002	none	none	none	none	none
4	0.10	none	none	≤ 10 or ≥ 22	≤ 11 or ≥ 25	≤ 12 or ≥ 28
	0.05	none	none	none	≤ 10 or ≥ 26	≤ 11 or ≥ 29
	0.02	none	none	none	none	≤ 10 or ≥ 30
	0.01	none	none	none	none	none
	0.002	none	none	none	none	none
5	0.10	none	≤ 15 or ≥ 25	≤ 16 or ≥ 29	≤ 17 or ≥ 33	≤ 19 or ≥ 36
	0.05	none	none	≤ 15 or ≥ 30	≤ 16 or ≥ 34	≤ 17 or ≥ 38
	0.02	none	none	none	≤ 15 or ≥ 35	≤ 16 or ≥ 39
	0.01	none	none	none	none	≤ 15 or ≥ 40
	0.002	none	none	none	none	none
6	0.10	none	≤ 21 or ≥ 33	≤ 23 or ≥ 37	≤ 24 or ≥ 42	≤ 26 or ≥ 46
	0.05	none	none	≤ 22 or ≥ 38	≤ 23 or ≥ 43	≤ 24 or ≥ 48
	0.02	none	none	none	≤ 22 or ≥ 44	≤ 23 or ≥ 49
	0.01	none	none	none	≤ 21 or ≥ 45	≤ 22 or ≥ 50
	0.002	none	none	none	none	none
7	0.10	none	≤ 28 or ≥ 42	≤ 30 or ≥ 47	≤ 32 or ≥ 52	≤ 34 or ≥ 57
	0.05	none	none	≤ 29 or ≥ 48	≤ 31 or ≥ 53	≤ 33 or ≥ 58
	0.02	none	none	≤ 28 or ≥ 49	≤ 29 or ≥ 55	≤ 31 or ≥ 60
	0.01	none	none	none	≤ 28 or ≥ 56	≤ 29 or ≥ 62
	0.002	none	none	none	none	none
8	0.10	none	≤ 37 or ≥ 51	≤ 39 or ≥ 57	≤ 41 or ≥ 63	≤ 44 or ≥ 68
	0.05	none	≤ 36 or ≥ 52	≤ 38 or ≥ 58	≤ 40 or ≥ 64	≤ 42 or ≥ 70
	0.02	none	none	≤ 36 or ≥ 60	≤ 38 or ≥ 66	≤ 40 or ≥ 72
	0.01	none	none	none	≤ 37 or ≥ 67	≤ 38 or ≥ 74
	0.002	none	none	none	none	≤ 36 or ≥ 76

TABLE E.10 CRITICAL VALUES FOR THE MANN-WHITNEY *MW* STATISTIC (CONT.)

n_1	Two-tailed Prob.	n_2 6	7	8	9
1	0.10	none	none	none	none
	0.05	none	none	none	none
	0.02	none	none	none	none
	0.01	none	none	none	none
	0.002	none	none	none	none
2	0.10	≤ 3 or ≥ 15	≤ 3 or ≥ 17	≤ 4 or ≥ 18	≤ 4 or ≥ 20
	0.05	none	none	≤ 3 or ≥ 19	≤ 3 or ≥ 21
	0.02	none	none	none	none
	0.01	none	none	none	none
	0.002	none	none	none	none
3	0.10	≤ 8 or ≥ 22	≤ 8 or ≥ 25	≤ 9 or ≥ 27	≤ 10 or ≥ 29
	0.05	≤ 7 or ≥ 23	≤ 7 or ≥ 26	≤ 8 or ≥ 28	≤ 8 or ≥ 31
	0.02	none	≤ 6 or ≥ 27	≤ 6 or ≥ 30	≤ 7 or ≥ 32
	0.01	none	none	none	≤ 6 or ≥ 33
	0.002	none	none	none	none
4	0.10	≤ 13 or ≥ 31	≤ 14 or ≥ 34	≤ 15 or ≥ 37	≤ 16 or ≥ 40
	0.05	≤ 12 or ≥ 32	≤ 13 or ≥ 35	≤ 14 or ≥ 38	≤ 14 or ≥ 42
	0.02	≤ 11 or ≥ 33	≤ 11 or ≥ 37	≤ 12 or ≥ 40	≤ 13 or ≥ 43
	0.01	≤ 10 or ≥ 34	≤ 10 or ≥ 38	≤ 11 or ≥ 41	≤ 11 or ≥ 45
	0.002	none	none	none	none
5	0.10	≤ 20 or ≥ 40	≤ 21 or ≥ 44	≤ 23 or ≥ 47	≤ 24 or ≥ 51
	0.05	≤ 18 or ≥ 42	≤ 20 or ≥ 45	≤ 21 or ≥ 49	≤ 22 or ≥ 53
	0.02	≤ 17 or ≥ 43	≤ 18 or ≥ 47	≤ 19 or ≥ 51	≤ 20 or ≥ 55
	0.01	≤ 16 or ≥ 44	≤ 16 or ≥ 49	< 17 or > 53	< 18 or ≥ 57
	0.002	none	none	≤ 15 or ≥ 55	≤ 16 or ≥ 59
6	0.10	≤ 28 or ≥ 50	≤ 29 or ≥ 55	≤ 31 or ≥ 59	≤ 33 or ≥ 63
	0.05	≤ 26 or ≥ 52	≤ 27 or ≥ 57	≤ 29 or ≥ 61	≤ 31 or ≥ 65
	0.02	≤ 24 or ≥ 54	≤ 25 or ≥ 59	≤ 27 or ≥ 63	≤ 28 or ≥ 68
	0.01	≤ 23 or ≥ 55	≤ 24 or ≥ 60	≤ 25 or ≥ 65	≤ 26 or ≥ 70
	0.002	none	≤ 21 or ≥ 63	≤ 22 or ≥ 68	≤ 23 or ≥ 73
7	0.10	≤ 36 or ≥ 62	≤ 39 or ≥ 66	≤ 41 or ≥ 71	≤ 43 or ≥ 76
	0.05	≤ 34 or ≥ 64	≤ 36 or ≥ 69	≤ 38 or ≥ 74	≤ 40 or ≥ 79
	0.02	≤ 32 or ≥ 66	≤ 34 or ≥ 71	≤ 35 or ≥ 77	≤ 37 or ≥ 82
	0.01	≤ 31 or ≥ 67	≤ 32 or ≥ 73	≤ 34 or ≥ 78	≤ 35 or ≥ 84
	0.002	≤ 28 or ≥ 70	≤ 29 or ≥ 76	≤ 30 or ≥ 82	≤ 31 or ≥ 88
8	0.10	≤ 46 or ≥ 74	≤ 49 or ≥ 79	≤ 51 or ≥ 85	≤ 54 or ≥ 90
	0.05	≤ 44 or ≥ 76	≤ 46 or ≥ 82	≤ 49 or ≥ 87	≤ 51 or ≥ 93
	0.02	≤ 42 or ≥ 78	≤ 43 or ≥ 85	≤ 45 or ≥ 91	≤ 47 or ≥ 97
	0.01	≤ 40 or ≥ 80	≤ 42 or ≥ 86	≤ 43 or ≥ 93	≤ 45 or ≥ 99
	0.002	≤ 37 or ≥ 83	≤ 38 or ≥ 90	≤ 40 or ≥ 96	≤ 41 or ≥ 103

TABLE E.10   CRITICAL VALUES FOR THE MANN-WHITNEY *MW* STATISTIC (CONT.)

n_1	Two-tailed Prob.	n_2			
		10	11	12	13
1	0.10	none	none	none	none
	0.05	none	none	none	none
	0.02	none	none	none	none
	0.01	none	none	none	none
	0.002	none	none	none	none
2	0.10	≤ 4 or ≥ 22	≤ 4 or ≥ 24	≤ 5 or ≥ 25	≤ 5 or ≥ 27
	0.05	≤ 3 or ≥ 23	≤ 3 or ≥ 25	≤ 4 or ≥ 26	≤ 4 or ≥ 28
	0.02	none	none	none	≤ 3 or ≥ 29
	0.01	none	none	none	none
	0.002	none	none	none	none
3	0.10	≤ 10 or ≥ 32	≤ 11 or ≥ 34	≤ 11 or ≥ 37	≤ 12 or ≥ 39
	0.05	≤ 9 or ≥ 33	≤ 9 or ≥ 36	≤ 10 or ≥ 38	≤ 10 or ≥ 41
	0.02	≤ 7 or ≥ 35	≤ 7 or ≥ 38	≤ 8 or ≥ 40	≤ 8 or ≥ 43
	0.01	≤ 6 or ≥ 36	≤ 6 or ≥ 39	≤ 7 or ≥ 41	≤ 7 or ≥ 44
	0.002	none	none	none	none
4	0.10	≤ 17 or ≥ 43	≤ 18 or ≥ 46	≤ 19 or ≥ 49	≤ 20 or ≥ 52
	0.05	≤ 15 or ≥ 45	≤ 16 or ≥ 48	≤ 17 or ≥ 51	≤ 18 or ≥ 54
	0.02	≤ 13 or ≥ 47	≤ 14 or ≥ 50	≤ 15 or ≥ 53	≤ 15 or ≥ 57
	0.01	≤ 12 or ≥ 48	≤ 12 or ≥ 52	≤ 13 or ≥ 55	≤ 13 or ≥ 59
	0.002	≤ 10 or ≥ 50	≤ 10 or ≥ 54	≤ 10 or ≥ 58	≤ 11 or ≥ 61
5	0.10	≤ 26 or ≥ 54	≤ 27 or ≥ 58	≤ 28 or ≥ 62	≤ 30 or ≥ 65
	0.05	≤ 23 or ≥ 57	≤ 24 or ≥ 61	≤ 26 or ≥ 64	≤ 27 or ≥ 68
	0.02	≤ 21 or ≥ 59	≤ 22 or ≥ 63	≤ 23 or ≥ 67	≤ 24 or ≥ 71
	0.01	≤ 19 or ≥ 61	≤ 20 or ≥ 65	≤ 21 or ≥ 69	≤ 22 or ≥ 73
	0.002	≤ 16 or ≥ 64	≤ 17 or ≥ 68	≤ 17 or ≥ 73	≤ 18 or ≥ 77
6	0.10	≤ 35 or ≥ 67	≤ 37 or ≥ 71	≤ 38 or ≥ 76	≤ 40 or ≥ 80
	0.05	≤ 32 or ≥ 70	≤ 34 or ≥ 74	≤ 35 or ≥ 79	≤ 37 or ≥ 83
	0.02	≤ 29 or ≥ 73	≤ 30 or ≥ 78	≤ 32 or ≥ 82	≤ 33 or ≥ 87
	0.01	≤ 27 or ≥ 75	≤ 28 or ≥ 80	≤ 30 or ≥ 84	≤ 31 or ≥ 89
	0.002	≤ 24 or ≥ 78	≤ 25 or ≥ 83	≤ 25 or ≥ 89	≤ 26 or ≥ 94
7	0.10	≤ 45 or ≥ 81	≤ 47 or ≥ 86	≤ 49 or ≥ 91	≤ 52 or ≥ 95
	0.05	≤ 42 or ≥ 84	≤ 44 or ≥ 89	≤ 46 or ≥ 94	≤ 48 or ≥ 99
	0.02	≤ 39 or ≥ 87	≤ 40 or ≥ 93	≤ 42 or ≥ 98	≤ 44 or ≥ 103
	0.01	≤ 37 or ≥ 89	≤ 38 or ≥ 95	≤ 40 or ≥ 100	≤ 41 or ≥ 106
	0.002	≤ 33 or ≥ 93	≤ 34 or ≥ 99	≤ 35 or ≥ 105	≤ 36 or ≥ 111
8	0.10	≤ 56 or ≥ 96	≤ 59 or ≥ 101	≤ 62 or ≥ 106	≤ 64 or ≥ 112
	0.05	≤ 53 or ≥ 99	≤ 55 or ≥ 105	≤ 58 or ≥ 110	≤ 60 or ≥ 116
	0.02	≤ 49 or ≥ 103	≤ 51 or ≥ 109	≤ 53 or ≥ 115	≤ 56 or ≥ 120
	0.01	≤ 47 or ≥ 105	≤ 49 or ≥ 111	≤ 51 or ≥ 117	≤ 53 or ≥ 123
	0.002	≤ 42 or ≥ 110	≤ 44 or ≥ 116	≤ 45 or ≥ 123	≤ 47 or ≥ 129

TABLE E.10   CRITICAL VALUES FOR THE MANN-WHITNEY _MW_ STATISTIC (CONT.)

n_1	Two-tailed Prob.	n_2 14	15	16	17
1	0.10	none	none	none	none
	0.05	none	none	none	none
	0.02	none	none	none	none
	0.01	none	none	none	none
	0.002	none	none	none	none
2	0.10	≤ 6 or ≥ 28	≤ 6 or ≥ 30	≤ 6 or ≥ 32	≤ 6 or ≥ 34
	0.05	≤ 4 or ≥ 30	≤ 4 or ≥ 32	≤ 4 or ≥ 34	≤ 5 or ≥ 35
	0.02	≤ 3 or ≥ 31	≤ 3 or ≥ 33	≤ 3 or > 35	≤ 3 or ≥ 37
	0.01	none	none	none	none
	0.002	none	none	none	none
3	0.10	≤ 13 or ≥ 41	≤ 13 or ≥ 44	≤ 14 or ≥ 46	≤ 15 or ≥ 48
	0.05	≤ 11 or ≥ 43	≤ 11 or ≥ 46	≤ 12 or ≥ 48	≤ 12 or ≥ 51
	0.02	≤ 8 or ≥ 46	≤ 9 or ≥ 48	≤ 9 or ≥ 51	≤ 10 or ≥ 53
	0.01	≤ 7 or ≥ 47	≤ 8 or ≥ 49	≤ 8 or ≥ 52	≤ 8 or ≥ 55
	0.002	none	none	none	≤ 6 or ≥ 57
4	0.10	≤ 21 or ≥ 55	≤ 22 or ≥ 58	≤ 24 or ≥ 60	≤ 25 or ≥ 63
	0.05	≤ 19 or ≥ 57	≤ 20 or ≥ 60	≤ 21 or ≥ 63	≤ 21 or ≥ 67
	0.02	≤ 16 or ≥ 60	≤ 17 or ≥ 63	≤ 17 or ≥ 67	≤ 18 or ≥ 70
	0.01	≤ 14 or ≥ 62	≤ 15 or ≥ 65	≤ 15 or ≥ 69	≤ 16 or ≥ 72
	0.002	< 11 or ≥ 65	≤ 11 or ≥ 69	≤ 12 or ≥ 72	≤ 12 or ≥ 76
5	0.10	≤ 31 or ≥ 69	≤ 33 or ≥ 72	≤ 34 or ≥ 76	≤ 35 or ≥ 80
	0.05	≤ 28 or ≥ 72	≤ 29 or ≥ 76	≤ 30 or ≥ 80	≤ 32 or ≥ 83
	0.02	≤ 25 or ≥ 75	≤ 26 or ≥ 79	≤ 27 or ≥ 83	≤ 28 or ≥ 87
	0.01	< 22 or ≥ 78	≤ 23 or ≥ 82	≤ 24 or ≥ 86	≤ 25 or ≥ 90
	0.002	≤ 18 or ≥ 82	≤ 19 or ≥ 86	≤ 20 or ≥ 90	≤ 20 or ≥ 95
6	0.10	≤ 42 or ≥ 84	≤ 44 or ≥ 88	≤ 46 or ≥ 92	≤ 47 or ≥ 97
	0.05	≤ 38 or ≥ 88	≤ 40 or ≥ 92	≤ 42 or ≥ 96	≤ 43 or ≥ 101
	0.02	≤ 34 or ≥ 92	≤ 36 or ≥ 96	≤ 37 or ≥ 101	≤ 39 or ≥ 105
	0.01	≤ 32 or ≥ 94	≤ 33 or ≥ 99	≤ 34 or ≥ 104	≤ 36 or ≥ 108
	0.002	≤ 27 or ≥ 99	≤ 28 or ≥ 104	≤ 29 or ≥ 109	≤ 30 or ≥ 114
7	0.10	≤ 54 or ≥ 100	≤ 56 or ≥ 105	≤ 58 or ≥ 110	≤ 61 or ≥ 114
	0.05	≤ 50 or ≥ 104	≤ 52 or ≥ 109	≤ 54 or ≥ 114	≤ 56 or ≥ 119
	0.02	≤ 45 or ≥ 109	≤ 47 or ≥ 114	≤ 49 or ≥ 119	≤ 51 or ≥ 124
	0.01	≤ 43 or ≥ 111	≤ 44 or ≥ 117	≤ 46 or ≥ 122	≤ 47 or ≥ 128
	0.002	≤ 37 or ≥ 117	≤ 38 or ≥ 123	≤ 39 or ≥ 129	≤ 41 or ≥ 134
8	0.10	≤ 67 or ≥ 117	≤ 69 or ≥ 123	≤ 72 or ≥ 128	≤ 75 or ≥ 133
	0.05	≤ 62 or ≥ 122	≤ 65 or ≥ 127	≤ 67 or ≥ 133	≤ 70 or ≥ 138
	0.02	≤ 58 or ≥ 126	≤ 60 or ≥ 132	≤ 62 or ≥ 138	≤ 64 or ≥ 144
	0.01	≤ 54 or ≥ 130	≤ 56 or ≥ 136	≤ 58 or ≥ 142	≤ 60 or ≥ 148
	0.002	≤ 48 or ≥ 136	≤ 50 or ≥ 142	≤ 51 or ≥ 149	≤ 53 or ≥ 155

TABLE E.10   CRITICAL VALUES FOR THE MANN-WHITNEY *MW* STATISTIC (CONT.)

n_1	Two-tailed Prob.	n_2		
		18	19	20
1	0.10	none	1 or 20	1 or 21
	0.05	none	none	none
	0.02	none	none	none
	0.01	none	none	none
	0.002	none	none	none
2	0.10	≤ 7 or ≥ 35	≤ 7 or ≥ 37	≤ 7 or ≥ 39
	0.05	≤ 5 or ≥ 37	≤ 5 or ≥ 39	≤ 5 or ≥ 41
	0.02	≤ 3 or ≥ 39	≤ 4 or ≥ 40	≤ 4 or ≥ 42
	0.01	none	≤ 3 or ≥ 41	≤ 3 or ≥ 43
	0.002	none	none	none
3	0.10	≤ 15 or ≥ 51	≤ 16 or ≥ 53	≤ 17 or ≥ 55
	0.05	≤ 13 or ≥ 53	≤ 13 or ≥ 56	≤ 14 or ≥ 58
	0.02	≤ 10 or ≥ 56	≤ 10 or ≥ 59	≤ 11 or ≥ 61
	0.01	≤ 8 or ≥ 58	≤ 9 or ≥ 60	≤ 9 or ≥ 63
	0.002	≤ 6 or ≥ 60	≤ 6 or ≥ 63	≤ 6 or ≥ 66
4	0.10	≤ 26 or ≥ 66	≤ 27 or ≥ 69	≤ 28 or ≥ 72
	0.05	≤ 22 or ≥ 70	≤ 23 or ≥ 73	≤ 24 or ≥ 76
	0.02	≤ 19 or ≥ 73	≤ 19 or ≥ 77	≤ 20 or ≥ 80
	0.01	≤ 16 or ≥ 76	≤ 17 or ≥ 79	≤ 18 or ≥ 82
	0.002	≤ 13 or ≥ 79	≤ 13 or ≥ 83	≤ 13 or ≥ 87
5	0.10	≤ 37 or ≥ 83	≤ 38 or ≥ 87	≤ 40 or ≥ 90
	0.05	≤ 33 or ≥ 87	≤ 34 or ≥ 91	≤ 35 or ≥ 95
	0.02	≤ 29 or ≥ 91	≤ 30 or ≥ 95	≤ 31 or ≥ 99
	0.01	≤ 26 or ≥ 94	≤ 27 or ≥ 98	≤ 28 or ≥ 102
	0.002	≤ 21 or ≥ 99	≤ 22 or ≥ 103	≤ 22 or ≥ 108
6	0.10	≤ 49 or ≥ 101	≤ 51 or ≥ 105	≤ 53 or ≥ 109
	0.05	≤ 45 or ≥ 105	≤ 46 or ≥ 110	≤ 48 or ≥ 114
	0.02	≤ 40 or ≥ 110	≤ 41 or ≥ 115	≤ 43 or ≥ 119
	0.01	≤ 37 or ≥ 113	≤ 38 or ≥ 118	≤ 39 or ≥ 123
	0.002	≤ 31 or ≥ 119	≤ 32 or ≥ 124	≤ 33 or ≥ 129
7	0.10	≤ 63 or ≥ 119	≤ 65 or ≥ 124	≤ 67 or > 129
	0.05	≤ 58 or ≥ 124	≤ 60 or ≥ 129	≤ 62 or ≥ 134
	0.02	≤ 52 or ≥ 130	≤ 54 or ≥ 135	≤ 56 or ≥ 140
	0.01	≤ 49 or ≥ 133	≤ 50 or ≥ 139	≤ 52 or ≥ 144
	0.002	≤ 42 or ≥ 140	≤ 43 or ≥ 146	≤ 44 or ≥ 152
8	0.10	≤ 77 or ≥ 139	≤ 80 or ≥ 144	≤ 83 or ≥ 149
	0.05	≤ 72 or ≥ 144	≤ 74 or ≥ 150	≤ 77 or ≥ 155
	0.02	≤ 66 or ≥ 150	≤ 68 or ≥ 156	≤ 70 or ≥ 162
	0.01	≤ 62 or ≥ 154	≤ 64 or ≥ 160	≤ 66 or ≥ 166
	0.002	≤ 54 or ≥ 162	≤ 56 or ≥ 168	≤ 57 or ≥ 175

TABLE E.10 CRITICAL VALUES FOR THE MANN-WHITNEY *MW* STATISTIC (CONT.)

n_1	Two-tailed Prob.	1	2	3	4	5
				n_2		
9	0.10	none	≤ 46 or ≥ 62	≤ 49 or ≥ 68	≤ 51 or ≥ 75	≤ 54 or ≥ 81
	0.05	none	≤ 45 or ≥ 63	≤ 47 or ≥ 70	≤ 49 or ≥ 77	≤ 52 or ≥ 83
	0.02	none	none	≤ 46 or ≥ 71	≤ 48 or ≥ 78	≤ 50 or ≥ 85
	0.01	none	none	≤ 45 or ≥ 72	≤ 46 or ≥ 80	≤ 48 or ≥ 87
	0.002	none	none	none	none	≤ 46 or ≥ 89
10	0.10	none	≤ 56 or ≥ 74	≤ 59 or ≥ 81	≤ 62 or ≥ 88	≤ 66 or ≥ 94
	0.05	none	≤ 55 or ≥ 75	≤ 58 or ≥ 82	≤ 60 or ≥ 90	≤ 63 or ≥ 97
	0.02	none	none	≤ 56 or ≥ 84	≤ 58 or ≥ 92	≤ 61 or ≥ 99
	0.01	none	none	≤ 55 or ≥ 85	≤ 57 or ≥ 93	≤ 59 or ≥ 101
	0.002	none	none	none	≤ 55 or ≥ 95	≤ 56 or ≥ 104
11	0.10	none	≤ 67 or ≥ 87	≤ 71 or ≥ 94	≤ 74 or ≥ 102	≤ 78 or ≥ 109
	0.05	none	≤ 66 or ≥ 88	≤ 69 or ≥ 96	≤ 72 or ≥ 104	≤ 75 or ≥ 112
	0.02	none	none	≤ 67 or ≥ 98	≤ 70 or ≥ 106	≤ 73 or ≥ 114
	0.01	none	none	≤ 66 or ≥ 99	≤ 68 or ≥ 108	≤ 71 or ≥ 116
	0.002	none	none	none	≤ 66 or ≥ 110	≤ 68 or ≥ 119
12	0.10	none	≤ 80 or ≥ 100	≤ 83 or ≥ 109	≤ 87 or ≥ 117	≤ 91 or ≥ 125
	0.05	none	≤ 79 or ≥ 101	≤ 82 or ≥ 110	≤ 85 or ≥ 119	≤ 89 or ≥ 127
	0.02	none	none	≤ 80 or ≥ 112	≤ 83 or ≥ 121	≤ 86 or ≥ 130
	0.01	none	none	≤ 79 or ≥ 113	≤ 81 or ≥ 123	≤ 84 or ≥ 132
	0.002	none	none	none	≤ 78 or ≥ 126	≤ 80 or ≥ 136
13	0.10	none	≤ 93 or ≥ 115	≤ 97 or ≥ 124	≤ 101 or ≥ 133	≤ 106 or ≥ 141
	0.05	none	≤ 92 or ≥ 116	≤ 95 or ≥ 126	≤ 99 or ≥ 135	≤ 103 or ≥ 144
	0.02	none	< 91 or > 117	≤ 93 or ≥ 128	≤ 96 or ≥ 138	≤ 100 or ≥ 147
	0.01	none	none	≤ 92 or ≥ 129	≤ 94 or ≥ 140	≤ 98 or ≥ 149
	0.002	none	none	none	≤ 92 or ≥ 142	≤ 94 or ≥ 153
14	0.10	none	≤ 108 or ≥ 130	≤ 112 or ≥ 140	≤ 116 or ≥ 150	≤ 121 or ≥ 159
	0.05	none	≤ 106 or ≥ 132	≤ 110 or ≥ 142	≤ 114 or ≥ 152	≤ 118 or ≥ 162
	0.02	none	≤ 105 or ≥ 133	≤ 107 or ≥ 145	≤ 111 or ≥ 155	≤ 115 or ≥ 165
	0.01	none	none	≤ 106 or ≥ 146	≤ 109 or ≥ 157	≤ 112 or ≥ 168
	0.002	none	none	none	≤ 106 or ≥ 160	≤ 108 or ≥ 172
15	0.10	none	≤ 123 or ≥ 147	≤ 127 or ≥ 158	≤ 132 or ≥ 168	≤ 138 or ≥ 177
	0.05	none	≤ 121 or ≥ 149	≤ 125 or ≥ 160	≤ 130 or ≥ 170	≤ 134 or ≥ 181
	0.02	none	≤ 120 or ≥ 150	≤ 123 or ≥ 162	≤ 127 or ≥ 173	≤ 131 or ≥ 184
	0.01	none	none	≤ 122 or ≥ 163	≤ 125 or ≥ 175	≤ 128 or ≥ 187
	0.002	none	none	none	≤ 121 or ≥ 179	≤ 124 or ≥ 191

TABLE E.10   CRITICAL VALUES FOR THE MANN-WHITNEY *MW* STATISTIC (CONT.)

n_1	Two-tailed Prob.	n_2 6	7	8	9
9	0.10	≤ 57 or ≥ 87	≤ 60 or ≥ 93	≤ 63 or ≥ 99	≤ 66 or ≥ 105
	0.05	≤ 55 or ≥ 89	≤ 57 or ≥ 96	≤ 60 or ≥ 102	≤ 62 or ≥ 109
	0.02	≤ 52 or ≥ 92	≤ 54 or ≥ 99	≤ 56 or ≥ 106	≤ 59 or ≥ 112
	0.01	≤ 50 or ≥ 94	≤ 52 or ≥ 101	≤ 54 or ≥ 108	≤ 56 or ≥ 115
	0.002	≤ 47 or ≥ 97	≤ 48 or ≥ 105	≤ 50 or ≥ 112	≤ 52 or ≥ 119
10	0.10	≤ 69 or ≥ 101	≤ 72 or ≥ 108	≤ 75 or ≥ 115	≤ 79 or ≥ 121
	0.05	≤ 66 or ≥ 104	≤ 69 or ≥ 111	≤ 72 or ≥ 118	≤ 75 or ≥ 125
	0.02	≤ 63 or ≥ 107	≤ 66 or ≥ 114	≤ 68 or ≥ 122	≤ 71 or ≥ 129
	0.01	≤ 61 or ≥ 109	≤ 64 or ≥ 116	≤ 66 or ≥ 124	≤ 68 or ≥ 132
	0.002	≤ 58 or ≥ 112	≤ 60 or ≥ 120	≤ 61 or ≥ 129	≤ 63 or ≥ 137
11	0.10	≤ 82 or ≥ 116	≤ 85 or ≥ 124	≤ 89 or ≥ 131	≤ 93 or ≥ 138
	0.05	≤ 79 or ≥ 119	≤ 82 or ≥ 127	≤ 85 or ≥ 135	≤ 89 or ≥ 142
	0.02	≤ 75 or ≥ 123	≤ 78 or ≥ 131	≤ 81 or ≥ 139	≤ 84 or ≥ 147
	0.01	≤ 73 or ≥ 125	≤ 76 or ≥ 133	≤ 79 or ≥ 141	≤ 82 or ≥ 149
	0.002	≤ 70 or ≥ 128	≤ 72 or ≥ 137	≤ 74 or ≥ 146	≤ 76 or ≥ 155
12	0.10	≤ 95 or ≥ 133	≤ 99 or ≥ 141	≤ 104 or ≥ 148	≤ 108 or ≥ 156
	0.05	≤ 92 or ≥ 136	≤ 96 or ≥ 144	≤ 100 or ≥ 152	≤ 104 or ≥ 160
	0.02	≤ 89 or ≥ 139	≤ 92 or ≥ 148	≤ 95 or ≥ 157	≤ 99 or ≥ 165
	0.01	≤ 87 or ≥ 141	≤ 90 or ≥ 150	≤ 93 or ≥ 159	≤ 96 or ≥ 168
	0.002	≤ 82 or ≥ 146	≤ 85 or ≥ 155	≤ 87 or ≥ 165	≤ 90 or ≥ 174
13	0.10	≤ 110 or ≥ 150	≤ 115 or ≥ 158	≤ 119 or ≥ 167	≤ 124 or ≥ 175
	0.05	≤ 107 or ≥ 153	≤ 111 or ≥ 162	≤ 115 or ≥ 171	≤ 119 or ≥ 180
	0.02	≤ 103 or ≥ 157	≤ 107 or ≥ 166	≤ 111 or ≥ 175	≤ 114 or ≥ 185
	0.01	≤ 101 or ≥ 159	≤ 104 or ≥ 169	≤ 108 or ≥ 178	≤ 111 or ≥ 188
	0.002	≤ 96 or ≥ 164	≤ 99 or ≥ 174	≤ 102 or ≥ 184	≤ 105 or ≥ 194
14	0.10	≤ 126 or ≥ 168	≤ 131 or ≥ 177	≤ 136 or ≥ 186	≤ 141 or ≥ 195
	0.05	≤ 122 or ≥ 172	≤ 127 or ≥ 181	≤ 131 or ≥ 191	≤ 136 or ≥ 200
	0.02	≤ 118 or ≥ 176	≤ 122 or ≥ 186	≤ 127 or ≥ 195	≤ 131 or ≥ 205
	0.01	≤ 116 or ≥ 178	≤ 120 or ≥ 188	≤ 123 or ≥ 199	≤ 127 or ≥ 209
	0.002	≤ 111 or ≥ 183	≤ 114 or ≥ 194	≤ 117 or ≥ 205	≤ 120 or ≥ 216
15	0.10	≤ 143 or ≥ 187	≤ 148 or ≥ 197	≤ 153 or ≥ 207	≤ 159 or ≥ 216
	0.05	≤ 139 or ≥ 191	≤ 144 or ≥ 201	≤ 149 or ≥ 211	≤ 154 or ≥ 221
	0.02	≤ 135 or ≥ 195	≤ 139 or ≥ 206	≤ 144 or ≥ 216	≤ 148 or ≥ 227
	0.01	≤ 132 or ≥ 198	≤ 136 or ≥ 209	≤ 140 or ≥ 220	≤ 144 or ≥ 231
	0.002	≤ 127 or ≥ 203	≤ 130 or ≥ 215	≤ 134 or ≥ 226	≤ 137 or ≥ 238

TABLE E.10 CRITICAL VALUES FOR THE MANN-WHITNEY *MW* STATISTIC (CONT.)

n_1	Two-tailed Prob.	n_2 10	11	12	13
9	0.10	≤ 69 or ≥ 111	≤ 72 or ≥ 117	≤ 75 or ≥ 123	≤ 78 or ≥ 129
	0.05	≤ 65 or ≥ 115	≤ 68 or ≥ 121	≤ 71 or ≥ 127	≤ 73 or ≥ 134
	0.02	≤ 61 or ≥ 119	≤ 63 or ≥ 126	≤ 66 or ≥ 132	≤ 68 or ≥ 139
	0.01	≤ 58 or ≥ 122	≤ 61 or ≥ 128	≤ 63 or ≥ 135	≤ 65 or ≥ 142
	0.002	≤ 53 or ≥ 127	≤ 55 or ≥ 134	≤ 57 or ≥ 141	≤ 59 or ≥ 148
10	0.10	≤ 82 or ≥ 128	≤ 86 or ≥ 134	≤ 89 or ≥ 141	≤ 92 or ≥ 148
	0.05	≤ 78 or ≥ 132	≤ 81 or ≥ 139	≤ 84 or ≥ 146	≤ 88 or ≥ 152
	0.02	≤ 74 or ≥ 136	≤ 77 or ≥ 143	≤ 79 or ≥ 151	≤ 82 or ≥ 158
	0.01	≤ 71 or ≥ 139	≤ 73 or ≥ 147	≤ 76 or ≥ 154	≤ 79 or ≥ 161
	0.002	≤ 65 or ≥ 145	≤ 67 or ≥ 153	≤ 69 or ≥ 161	≤ 72 or ≥ 168
11	0.10	≤ 97 or ≥ 145	≤ 100 or ≥ 153	≤ 104 or ≥ 160	≤ 108 or ≥ 167
	0.05	≤ 92 or ≥ 150	≤ 96 or ≥ 157	≤ 99 or ≥ 165	≤ 103 or ≥ 172
	0.02	≤ 88 or ≥ 154	≤ 91 or ≥ 162	≤ 94 or ≥ 170	≤ 97 or ≥ 178
	0.01	≤ 84 or ≥ 158	≤ 87 or ≥ 166	≤ 90 or ≥ 174	≤ 93 or ≥ 182
	0.002	≤ 78 or ≥ 164	≤ 81 or ≥ 172	≤ 83 or ≥ 181	≤ 86 or ≥ 189
12	0.10	≤ 112 or ≥ 164	≤ 116 or ≥ 172	≤ 120 or ≥ 180	≤ 125 or ≥ 187
	0.05	≤ 107 or ≥ 169	≤ 111 or ≥ 177	≤ 115 or ≥ 185	≤ 119 or ≥ 193
	0.02	≤ 102 or ≥ 174	≤ 106 or ≥ 182	≤ 109 or ≥ 191	≤ 113 or ≥ 199
	0.01	≤ 99 or ≥ 177	≤ 102 or ≥ 186	≤ 105 or ≥ 195	≤ 109 or ≥ 203
	0.002	≤ 92 or ≥ 184	≤ 95 or ≥ 193	≤ 98 or ≥ 202	≤ 101 or ≥ 211
13	0.10	≤ 128 or ≥ 184	≤ 133 or ≥ 192	≤ 138 or ≥ 200	≤ 142 or ≥ 209
	0.05	≤ 124 or ≥ 188	≤ 128 or ≥ 197	≤ 132 or ≥ 206	≤ 136 or ≥ 215
	0.02	≤ 118 or ≥ 194	≤ 122 or ≥ 203	≤ 126 or ≥ 212	≤ 130 or ≥ 221
	0.01	≤ 115 or ≥ 197	≤ 118 or ≥ 207	≤ 122 or ≥ 216	≤ 125 or ≥ 226
	0.002	≤ 108 or ≥ 204	≤ 111 or ≥ 214	≤ 114 or ≥ 224	≤ 117 or ≥ 234
14	0.10	≤ 146 or ≥ 204	≤ 151 or ≥ 213	≤ 156 or ≥ 222	≤ 161 or ≥ 231
	0.05	≤ 141 or ≥ 209	≤ 145 or ≥ 219	≤ 150 or ≥ 228	≤ 155 or ≥ 237
	0.02	≤ 135 or ≥ 215	≤ 139 or ≥ 225	≤ 143 or ≥ 235	≤ 148 or ≥ 244
	0.01	≤ 131 or ≥ 219	≤ 135 or ≥ 229	≤ 139 or ≥ 239	≤ 143 or ≥ 249
	0.002	≤ 124 or ≥ 226	≤ 127 or ≥ 237	≤ 130 or ≥ 248	≤ 134 or ≥ 258
15	0.10	≤ 164 or ≥ 226	≤ 170 or ≥ 235	≤ 175 or ≥ 245	≤ 181 or ≥ 254
	0.05	≤ 159 or ≥ 231	≤ 164 or ≥ 241	≤ 169 or ≥ 251	≤ 174 or ≥ 261
	0.02	≤ 153 or ≥ 237	≤ 157 or ≥ 248	≤ 162 or ≥ 258	≤ 167 or ≥ 268
	0.01	≤ 149 or ≥ 241	≤ 153 or ≥ 252	≤ 157 or ≥ 263	≤ 162 or ≥ 273
	0.002	≤ 141 or ≥ 249	≤ 144 or ≥ 261	≤ 148 or ≥ 272	≤ 152 or ≥ 283

TABLE E.10   CRITICAL VALUES FOR THE MANN-WHITNEY *MW* STATISTIC (CONT.)

n_1	Two-tailed Prob.	n_2 14	15	16	17
9	0.10	≤ 81 or ≥ 135	≤ 84 or ≥ 141	≤ 87 or ≥ 147	≤ 90 or ≥ 153
	0.05	≤ 76 or ≥ 140	≤ 79 or ≥ 146	≤ 82 or ≥ 152	≤ 84 or ≥ 159
	0.02	≤ 71 or ≥ 145	≤ 73 or ≥ 152	≤ 76 or ≥ 158	≤ 78 or ≥ 165
	0.01	≤ 67 or ≥ 149	≤ 68 or ≥ 156	≤ 72 or ≥ 162	≤ 74 or ≥ 169
	0.002	≤ 60 or ≥ 156	≤ 62 or ≥ 163	≤ 64 or ≥ 170	≤ 66 or ≥ 177
10	0.10	≤ 96 or ≥ 154	≤ 99 or ≥ 161	≤ 103 or ≥ 167	≤ 106 or ≥ 174
	0.05	≤ 91 or ≥ 159	≤ 94 or ≥ 166	≤ 97 or ≥ 173	≤ 100 or ≥ 180
	0.02	≤ 85 or ≥ 165	≤ 88 or ≥ 172	≤ 91 or ≥ 179	≤ 93 or ≥ 187
	0.01	≤ 81 or ≥ 169	≤ 84 or ≥ 176	≤ 86 or ≥ 184	≤ 89 or ≥ 191
	0.002	≤ 74 or ≥ 176	≤ 76 or ≥ 184	≤ 78 or ≥ 192	≤ 80 or ≥ 200
11	0.10	≤ 112 or ≥ 174	≤ 116 or ≥ 181	≤ 120 or ≥ 188	≤ 123 or ≥ 196
	0.05	≤ 106 or ≥ 180	≤ 110 or ≥ 187	≤ 113 or ≥ 195	≤ 117 or ≥ 202
	0.02	≤ 100 or ≥ 186	≤ 103 or ≥ 194	≤ 107 or ≥ 201	≤ 110 or ≥ 209
	0.01	≤ 96 or ≥ 190	≤ 99 or ≥ 198	≤ 102 or ≥ 206	≤ 105 or ≥ 214
	0.002	≤ 88 or ≥ 198	≤ 90 or ≥ 207	≤ 93 or ≥ 215	≤ 95 or ≥ 224
12	0.10	≤ 129 or ≥ 195	≤ 133 or ≥ 203	≤ 138 or ≥ 210	≤ 142 or ≥ 218
	0.05	≤ 123 or ≥ 201	≤ 127 or ≥ 209	≤ 131 or ≥ 217	≤ 135 or ≥ 225
	0.02	≤ 116 or ≥ 208	≤ 120 or ≥ 216	≤ 124 or ≥ 224	≤ 127 or ≥ 233
	0.01	≤ 112 or ≥ 212	≤ 115 or ≥ 221	≤ 119 or ≥ 229	≤ 122 or ≥ 238
	0.002	≤ 103 or ≥ 221	≤ 106 or ≥ 230	≤ 109 or ≥ 239	≤ 112 or ≥ 248
13	0.10	≤ 147 or ≥ 217	≤ 152 or ≥ 225	≤ 156 or ≥ 234	≤ 161 or ≥ 242
	0.05	≤ 141 or ≥ 223	≤ 145 or ≥ 232	≤ 150 or ≥ 240	≤ 154 or ≥ 249
	0.02	≤ 134 or ≥ 230	≤ 138 or ≥ 239	≤ 142 or ≥ 248	≤ 146 or ≥ 257
	0.01	≤ 129 or ≥ 235	≤ 133 or ≥ 244	≤ 136 or ≥ 254	≤ 140 or ≥ 263
	0.002	≤ 120 or ≥ 244	≤ 123 or ≥ 254	≤ 126 or ≥ 264	≤ 129 or ≥ 274
14	0.10	≤ 166 or ≥ 240	≤ 171 or ≥ 249	≤ 176 or ≥ 258	≤ 182 or ≥ 266
	0.05	≤ 160 or ≥ 246	≤ 164 or ≥ 256	≤ 169 or ≥ 265	≤ 174 or ≥ 274
	0.02	≤ 152 or ≥ 254	≤ 156 or ≥ 264	≤ 161 or ≥ 273	≤ 165 or ≥ 283
	0.01	≤ 147 or ≥ 259	≤ 151 or ≥ 269	≤ 155 or ≥ 279	≤ 159 or ≥ 289
	0.002	≤ 137 or ≥ 269	≤ 141 or ≥ 279	≤ 144 or ≥ 290	≤ 148 or ≥ 300
15	0.10	≤ 186 or ≥ 264	≤ 192 or ≥ 273	≤ 197 or ≥ 283	≤ 203 or ≥ 292
	0.05	≤ 179 or ≥ 271	≤ 184 or ≥ 281	≤ 190 or ≥ 290	≤ 195 or ≥ 300
	0.02	≤ 171 or ≥ 279	≤ 176 or ≥ 289	≤ 181 or ≥ 299	≤ 186 or ≥ 309
	0.01	≤ 166 or ≥ 284	≤ 171 or ≥ 294	≤ 175 or ≥ 305	≤ 180 or ≥ 315
	0.002	≤ 156 or ≥ 294	≤ 160 or ≥ 305	≤ 163 or ≥ 317	≤ 167 or ≥ 328

TABLE E.10   CRITICAL VALUES FOR THE MANN-WHITNEY *MW* STATISTIC (CONT.)

n_1	Two-tailed Prob.	n_2 18	19	20
9	0.10	≤ 93 or ≥ 159	≤ 96 or ≥ 165	≤ 99 or ≥ 171
	0.05	≤ 87 or ≥ 165	≤ 90 or ≥ 171	≤ 93 or ≥ 177
	0.02	≤ 81 or ≥ 171	≤ 83 or ≥ 178	≤ 85 or ≥ 185
	0.01	≤ 76 or ≥ 176	≤ 78 or ≥ 183	≤ 81 or ≥ 189
	0.002	≤ 68 or ≥ 184	≤ 70 or ≥ 191	≤ 71 or ≥ 199
10	0.10	≤ 110 or ≥ 180	≤ 113 or ≥ 187	≤ 117 or ≥ 193
	0.05	≤ 103 or ≥ 187	≤ 107 or ≥ 193	≤ 110 or ≥ 200
	0.02	≤ 96 or ≥ 194	≤ 99 or ≥ 201	≤ 102 or ≥ 208
	0.01	≤ 92 or ≥ 198	≤ 94 or ≥ 206	≤ 97 or ≥ 213
	0.002	≤ 82 or ≥ 208	≤ 84 or ≥ 216	≤ 87 or ≥ 223
11	0.10	≤ 127 or ≥ 203	≤ 131 or ≥ 210	≤ 135 or ≥ 217
	0.05	≤ 121 or ≥ 209	≤ 124 or ≥ 217	≤ 128 or ≥ 224
	0.02	≤ 113 or ≥ 217	≤ 116 or ≥ 225	≤ 119 or ≥ 233
	0.01	≤ 108 or ≥ 222	≤ 111 or ≥ 230	≤ 114 or ≥ 238
	0.002	≤ 98 or ≥ 232	≤ 100 or ≥ 241	≤ 103 or ≥ 249
12	0.10	≤ 146 or ≥ 226	≤ 150 or ≥ 234	≤ 155 or ≥ 241
	0.05	≤ 139 or ≥ 233	≤ 143 or ≥ 241	≤ 147 or ≥ 249
	0.02	≤ 131 or ≥ 241	≤ 134 or ≥ 250	≤ 138 or ≥ 258
	0.01	≤ 125 or ≥ 247	≤ 129 or ≥ 255	≤ 132 or ≥ 264
	0.002	≤ 115 or ≥ 257	≤ 118 or ≥ 266	≤ 120 or ≥ 276
13	0.10	≤ 166 or ≥ 250	≤ 171 or ≥ 258	≤ 175 or ≥ 267
	0.05	≤ 158 or ≥ 258	≤ 163 or ≥ 266	≤ 167 or ≥ 275
	0.02	≤ 150 or ≥ 266	≤ 154 or ≥ 275	≤ 158 or ≥ 284
	0.01	≤ 144 or ≥ 272	≤ 148 or ≥ 281	≤ 151 or ≥ 291
	0.002	≤ 133 or ≥ 283	≤ 136 or ≥ 293	≤ 139 or ≥ 303
14	0.10	≤ 187 or ≥ 275	≤ 192 or ≥ 284	≤ 197 or ≥ 293
	0.05	≤ 179 or ≥ 283	≤ 183 or ≥ 293	≤ 188 or ≥ 302
	0.02	≤ 170 or ≥ 292	≤ 174 or ≥ 302	≤ 178 or ≥ 312
	0.01	≤ 163 or ≥ 299	≤ 168 or ≥ 308	≤ 172 or ≥ 318
	0.002	≤ 151 or ≥ 311	≤ 155 or ≥ 321	≤ 159 or ≥ 331
15	0.10	≤ 208 or ≥ 302	≤ 214 or ≥ 311	≤ 220 or ≥ 320
	0.05	≤ 200 or ≥ 310	≤ 205 or ≥ 320	≤ 210 or ≥ 330
	0.02	≤ 190 or ≥ 320	≤ 195 or ≥ 330	≤ 200 or ≥ 340
	0.01	≤ 184 or ≥ 326	≤ 189 or ≥ 336	≤ 193 or ≥ 347
	0.002	≤ 171 or ≥ 339	≤ 175 or ≥ 350	≤ 179 or ≥ 361

TABLE E.10 CRITICAL VALUES FOR THE MANN-WHITNEY *MW* STATISTIC (CONT.)

n_1	Two-tailed Prob.	1	2	3	4	5
				n_2		
16	0.10	none	≤ 139 or ≥ 165	≤ 144 or ≥ 176	≤ 150 or ≥ 186	≤ 155 or ≥ 197
	0.05	none	≤ 137 or ≥ 167	≤ 142 or ≥ 178	≤ 147 or ≥ 189	≤ 151 or ≥ 201
	0.02	none	≤ 136 or ≥ 168	≤ 139 or ≥ 181	≤ 143 or ≥ 193	≤ 148 or ≥ 204
	0.01	none	none	≤ 138 or ≥ 182	≤ 141 or ≥ 195	≤ 145 or ≥ 207
	0.002	none	none	none	≤ 138 or ≥ 198	≤ 141 or ≥ 211
17	0.10	none	≤ 156 or ≥ 184	≤ 162 or ≥ 195	≤ 168 or ≥ 206	≤ 173 or ≥ 218
	0.05	none	≤ 155 or ≥ 185	≤ 159 or ≥ 198	≤ 164 or ≥ 210	≤ 170 or ≥ 221
	0.02	none	≤ 153 or ≥ 187	≤ 157 or ≥ 200	≤ 161 or ≥ 213	≤ 166 or ≥ 225
	0.01	none	none	≤ 155 or ≥ 202	≤ 159 or ≥ 215	≤ 163 or ≥ 228
	0.002	none	none	≤ 153 or ≥ 204	≤ 155 or ≥ 219	≤ 158 or ≥ 233
18	0.10	none	≤ 175 or ≥ 203	≤ 180 or ≥ 216	≤ 187 or ≥ 227	≤ 193 or ≥ 239
	0.05	none	≤ 173 or ≥ 205	≤ 178 or ≥ 218	≤ 183 or ≥ 231	≤ 189 or ≥ 243
	0.02	none	≤ 171 or ≥ 207	≤ 175 or ≥ 221	≤ 180 or ≥ 234	≤ 185 or ≥ 247
	0.01	none	none	≤ 173 or ≥ 223	≤ 177 or ≥ 237	≤ 182 or ≥ 250
	0.002	none	none	≤ 171 or ≥ 225	≤ 174 or ≥ 240	≤ 177 or ≥ 255
19	0.10	≤ 190 or ≥ 209	≤ 194 or ≥ 224	≤ 200 or ≥ 237	≤ 207 or ≥ 249	≤ 213 or ≥ 262
	0.05	none	≤ 192 or ≥ 226	≤ 197 or ≥ 240	≤ 203 or ≥ 253	≤ 209 or ≥ 266
	0.02	none	≤ 191 or ≥ 227	≤ 194 or ≥ 243	≤ 199 or ≥ 257	≤ 205 or ≥ 270
	0.01	none	≤ 190 or ≥ 228	≤ 193 or ≥ 244	≤ 197 or ≥ 259	≤ 202 or ≥ 273
	0.002	none	none	≤ 190 or ≥ 247	≤ 193 or ≥ 263	≤ 197 or ≥ 278
20	0.10	≤ 210 or ≥ 230	≤ 214 or ≥ 246	≤ 221 or ≥ 259	≤ 228 or ≥ 272	≤ 235 or ≥ 285
	0.05	none	≤ 212 or ≥ 248	≤ 218 or ≥ 262	≤ 224 or ≥ 276	≤ 230 or ≥ 290
	0.02	none	≤ 211 or ≥ 249	≤ 215 or ≥ 265	≤ 220 or ≥ 280	≤ 226 or ≥ 294
	0.01	none	≤ 210 or ≥ 250	≤ 213 or ≥ 267	≤ 218 or ≥ 282	≤ 223 or ≥ 297
	0.002	none	none	≤ 210 or ≥ 270	≤ 213 or ≥ 287	≤ 217 or ≥ 303

TABLE E.10   CRITICAL VALUES FOR THE MANN-WHITNEY _MW_ STATISTIC (CONT.)

n_1	Two-tailed Prob.	n_2 6	7	8	9
16	0.10	≤ 161 or ≥ 207	≤ 166 or ≥ 218	≤ 172 or ≥ 228	≤ 178 or ≥ 238
	0.05	≤ 157 or ≥ 211	≤ 162 or ≥ 222	≤ 167 or ≥ 233	≤ 173 or ≥ 243
	0.02	≤ 152 or ≥ 216	≤ 157 or ≥ 227	≤ 162 or ≥ 238	≤ 167 or ≥ 249
	0.01	≤ 149 or ≥ 219	≤ 154 or ≥ 230	≤ 158 or ≥ 242	≤ 163 or ≥ 253
	0.002	≤ 144 or ≥ 224	≤ 147 or ≥ 237	≤ 151 or ≥ 249	≤ 155 or ≥ 261
17	0.10	≤ 179 or ≥ 229	≤ 186 or ≥ 239	≤ 192 or ≥ 250	≤ 198 or ≥ 261
	0.05	< 175 or > 233	≤ 181 or ≥ 244	≤ 187 or ≥ 255	≤ 192 or ≥ 267
	0.02	≤ 171 or ≥ 237	≤ 176 or ≥ 249	≤ 181 or ≥ 261	≤ 186 or ≥ 273
	0.01	≤ 168 or ≥ 240	≤ 172 or ≥ 253	≤ 177 or ≥ 265	≤ 182 or ≥ 277
	0.002	≤ 162 or ≥ 246	≤ 166 or ≥ 259	≤ 170 or ≥ 272	≤ 174 or ≥ 285
18	0.10	≤ 199 or ≥ 251	≤ 206 or ≥ 262	≤ 212 or ≥ 274	≤ 219 or ≥ 285
	0.05	≤ 195 or ≥ 255	≤ 201 or ≥ 267	≤ 207 or ≥ 279	≤ 213 or ≥ 291
	0.02	≤ 190 or ≥ 260	≤ 195 or ≥ 273	≤ 201 or ≥ 285	≤ 207 or ≥ 297
	0.01	≤ 187 or ≥ 263	≤ 192 or ≥ 276	≤ 197 or ≥ 289	≤ 202 or ≥ 302
	0.002	≤ 181 or ≥ 269	≤ 185 or ≥ 283	≤ 189 or ≥ 297	≤ 194 or ≥ 310
19	0.10	≤ 220 or ≥ 274	≤ 227 or ≥ 286	≤ 234 or ≥ 298	≤ 241 or ≥ 310
	0.05	≤ 215 or ≥ 279	≤ 222 or ≥ 291	≤ 228 or ≥ 304	≤ 235 or ≥ 316
	0.02	≤ 210 or ≥ 284	≤ 216 or ≥ 297	≤ 222 or ≥ 310	≤ 228 or ≥ 323
	0.01	≤ 207 or ≥ 287	≤ 212 or ≥ 301	≤ 218 or ≥ 314	≤ 223 or ≥ 328
	0.002	≤ 201 or ≥ 293	≤ 205 or ≥ 308	≤ 210 or ≥ 322	≤ 215 or ≥ 336
20	0.10	≤ 242 or ≥ 298	≤ 249 or ≥ 311	≤ 257 or ≥ 323	≤ 264 or ≥ 336
	0.05	≤ 237 or ≥ 303	≤ 244 or ≥ 316	≤ 251 or ≥ 329	≤ 258 or ≥ 342
	0.02	≤ 232 or ≥ 308	≤ 238 or ≥ 322	≤ 244 or ≥ 336	≤ 250 or ≥ 350
	0.01	≤ 228 or ≥ 312	≤ 234 or ≥ 326	≤ 240 or ≥ 340	≤ 246 or ≥ 354
	0.002	≤ 222 or ≥ 318	≤ 226 or ≥ 334	≤ 231 or ≥ 349	≤ 236 or ≥ 364

TABLE E.10   CRITICAL VALUES FOR THE MANN-WHITNEY *MW* STATISTIC (CONT.)

n_1	Two-tailed Prob.	10	11	12	13
16	0.10	≤ 184 or ≥ 248	≤ 190 or ≥ 258	≤ 196 or ≥ 268	≤ 201 or ≥ 279
	0.05	≤ 178 or ≥ 254	≤ 183 or ≥ 265	≤ 189 or ≥ 275	≤ 195 or ≥ 285
	0.02	≤ 172 or ≥ 260	≤ 177 or ≥ 271	≤ 182 or ≥ 282	≤ 187 or ≥ 293
	0.01	≤ 167 or ≥ 265	≤ 172 or ≥ 276	≤ 177 or ≥ 287	≤ 181 or ≥ 299
	0.002	≤ 159 or ≥ 273	≤ 163 or ≥ 285	≤ 167 or ≥ 297	≤ 171 or ≥ 309
17	0.10	≤ 204 or ≥ 272	≤ 210 or ≥ 283	≤ 217 or ≥ 293	≤ 223 or ≥ 304
	0.05	≤ 198 or ≥ 278	≤ 204 or ≥ 289	≤ 210 or ≥ 300	≤ 216 or ≥ 311
	0.02	≤ 191 or ≥ 285	≤ 197 or ≥ 296	≤ 202 or ≥ 308	≤ 208 or ≥ 319
	0.01	≤ 187 or ≥ 289	≤ 192 or ≥ 301	≤ 197 or ≥ 313	≤ 202 or ≥ 325
	0.002	≤ 178 or ≥ 298	≤ 182 or ≥ 311	≤ 187 or ≥ 323	≤ 191 or ≥ 336
18	0.10	≤ 226 or ≥ 296	≤ 232 or ≥ 308	≤ 239 or ≥ 319	≤ 246 or ≥ 330
	0.05	≤ 219 or ≥ 303	≤ 226 or ≥ 314	≤ 232 or ≥ 326	≤ 238 or ≥ 338
	0.02	≤ 212 or ≥ 310	≤ 218 or ≥ 322	≤ 224 or ≥ 334	≤ 230 or ≥ 346
	0.01	≤ 208 or ≥ 314	≤ 213 or ≥ 327	≤ 218 or ≥ 340	≤ 224 or ≥ 352
	0.002	≤ 198 or ≥ 324	≤ 203 or ≥ 337	≤ 208 or ≥ 350	≤ 213 or ≥ 363
19	0.10	≤ 248 or ≥ 322	≤ 255 or ≥ 334	≤ 262 or ≥ 346	≤ 270 or ≥ 357
	0.05	≤ 242 or ≥ 328	≤ 248 or ≥ 341	≤ 255 or ≥ 353	≤ 262 or ≥ 365
	0.02	≤ 234 or ≥ 336	≤ 240 or ≥ 349	≤ 246 or ≥ 362	≤ 253 or ≥ 374
	0.01	≤ 229 or ≥ 341	≤ 235 or ≥ 354	≤ 241 or ≥ 367	≤ 247 or ≥ 380
	0.002	≤ 219 or ≥ 351	≤ 224 or ≥ 365	≤ 230 or ≥ 378	≤ 235 or ≥ 392
20	0.10	≤ 272 or ≥ 348	≤ 279 or ≥ 361	≤ 287 or ≥ 373	≤ 294 or ≥ 386
	0.05	≤ 265 or ≥ 355	≤ 272 or ≥ 368	≤ 279 or ≥ 381	≤ 286 or ≥ 394
	0.02	≤ 257 or ≥ 363	≤ 263 or ≥ 377	≤ 270 or ≥ 390	≤ 277 or ≥ 403
	0.01	≤ 252 or ≥ 368	≤ 258 or ≥ 382	≤ 264 or ≥ 396	≤ 270 or ≥ 410
	0.002	≤ 242 or ≥ 378	≤ 247 or ≥ 393	≤ 252 or ≥ 408	≤ 258 or ≥ 422

TABLE E.10   CRITICAL VALUES FOR THE MANN-WHITNEY _MW_ STATISTIC (CONT.)

n_1	Two-tailed Prob.	n_2 14	15	16	17
16	0.10	≤ 207 or ≥ 289	≤ 213 or ≥ 299	≤ 219 or ≥ 309	≤ 225 or ≥ 319
	0.05	≤ 200 or ≥ 296	≤ 206 or ≥ 306	≤ 211 or ≥ 317	≤ 217 or ≥ 327
	0.02	≤ 192 or ≥ 304	≤ 197 or ≥ 315	≤ 202 or ≥ 326	≤ 207 or ≥ 337
	0.01	≤ 186 or ≥ 310	≤ 191 or ≥ 321	≤ 196 or ≥ 332	≤ 201 or ≥ 343
	0.002	≤ 175 or ≥ 321	≤ 179 or ≥ 333	≤ 184 or ≥ 344	≤ 188 or ≥ 356
17	0.10	≤ 230 or ≥ 314	≤ 236 or ≥ 325	≤ 242 or ≥ 336	≤ 249 or ≥ 346
	0.05	≤ 222 or ≥ 322	≤ 228 or ≥ 333	≤ 234 or ≥ 344	≤ 240 or ≥ 355
	0.02	≤ 213 or ≥ 331	≤ 219 or ≥ 342	≤ 224 or ≥ 354	≤ 230 or ≥ 365
	0.01	≤ 207 or ≥ 337	≤ 213 or ≥ 348	≤ 218 or ≥ 360	≤ 223 or ≥ 372
	0.002	≤ 196 or ≥ 348	≤ 200 or ≥ 361	≤ 205 or ≥ 373	≤ 210 or ≥ 385
18	0.10	≤ 253 or ≥ 341	≤ 259 or ≥ 353	≤ 266 or ≥ 364	≤ 273 or ≥ 375
	0.05	≤ 245 or ≥ 349	≤ 251 or ≥ 361	≤ 257 or ≥ 373	≤ 264 or ≥ 384
	0.02	≤ 236 or ≥ 358	≤ 241 or ≥ 371	≤ 247 or ≥ 383	≤ 253 or ≥ 395
	0.01	≤ 229 or ≥ 365	≤ 235 or ≥ 377	≤ 241 or ≥ 389	≤ 246 or ≥ 402
	0.002	≤ 217 or ≥ 377	≤ 222 or ≥ 390	≤ 227 or ≥ 403	≤ 232 or ≥ 416
19	0.10	≤ 277 or ≥ 369	≤ 284 or ≥ 381	≤ 291 or ≥ 393	≤ 299 or ≥ 404
	0.05	≤ 268 or ≥ 378	≤ 275 or ≥ 390	≤ 282 or ≥ 402	≤ 289 or ≥ 414
	0.02	≤ 259 or ≥ 387	≤ 265 or ≥ 400	≤ 272 or ≥ 412	≤ 278 or ≥ 425
	0.01	≤ 253 or ≥ 393	≤ 259 or ≥ 406	≤ 264 or ≥ 420	≤ 271 or ≥ 432
	0.002	≤ 240 or ≥ 406	≤ 245 or ≥ 420	≤ 250 or ≥ 434	≤ 256 or ≥ 447
20	0.10	≤ 302 or ≥ 398	≤ 310 or ≥ 410	≤ 317 or ≥ 423	≤ 325 or ≥ 435
	0.05	≤ 293 or ≥ 407	≤ 300 or ≥ 420	≤ 308 or ≥ 432	≤ 315 or ≥ 445
	0.02	≤ 283 or ≥ 417	≤ 290 or ≥ 430	≤ 297 or ≥ 443	≤ 303 or ≥ 457
	0.01	≤ 277 or ≥ 423	≤ 283 or ≥ 437	≤ 289 or ≥ 451	≤ 296 or ≥ 464
	0.002	≤ 264 or ≥ 436	≤ 269 or ≥ 451	≤ 275 or ≥ 465	≤ 280 or ≥ 480

TABLE E.10 CRITICAL VALUES FOR THE MANN-WHITNEY *MW* STATISTIC (CONT.)

n_1	Two-tail Prob.	n_2 18	n_2 19	n_2 20
16	0.10	≤ 231 or ≥ 329	≤ 237 or ≥ 339	≤ 243 or ≥ 349
	0.05	≤ 222 or ≥ 338	≤ 228 or ≥ 348	≤ 234 or ≥ 358
	0.02	≤ 212 or ≥ 348	≤ 218 or ≥ 358	≤ 223 or ≥ 369
	0.01	≤ 206 or ≥ 354	≤ 210 or ≥ 366	≤ 215 or ≥ 377
	0.002	≤ 192 or ≥ 368	≤ 196 or ≥ 380	≤ 201 or ≥ 391
17	0.10	≤ 255 or ≥ 357	≤ 262 or ≥ 367	≤ 268 or ≥ 378
	0.05	≤ 246 or ≥ 366	≤ 252 or ≥ 377	≤ 258 or ≥ 388
	0.02	≤ 235 or ≥ 377	≤ 241 or ≥ 388	≤ 246 or ≥ 400
	0.01	≤ 228 or ≥ 384	≤ 234 or ≥ 395	≤ 239 or ≥ 407
	0.002	≤ 214 or ≥ 398	≤ 219 or ≥ 410	≤ 223 or ≥ 423
18	0.10	≤ 280 or ≥ 386	≤ 287 or ≥ 397	≤ 294 or ≥ 408
	0.05	≤ 270 or ≥ 396	≤ 277 or ≥ 407	≤ 283 or ≥ 419
	0.02	≤ 259 or ≥ 407	≤ 265 or ≥ 419	≤ 271 or ≥ 431
	0.01	≤ 252 or ≥ 414	≤ 258 or ≥ 426	≤ 263 or ≥ 439
	0.002	≤ 237 or ≥ 429	≤ 242 or ≥ 442	≤ 247 or ≥ 455
19	0.10	≤ 306 or ≥ 416	≤ 313 or ≥ 428	≤ 320 or ≥ 440
	0.05	≤ 296 or ≥ 426	≤ 303 or ≥ 438	≤ 309 or ≥ 451
	0.02	≤ 284 or ≥ 438	≤ 291 or ≥ 450	≤ 297 or ≥ 463
	0.01	≤ 277 or ≥ 445	≤ 283 or ≥ 458	≤ 289 or ≥ 471
	0.002	≤ 261 or ≥ 461	≤ 267 or ≥ 474	≤ 272 or ≥ 488
20	0.10	≤ 333 or ≥ 447	≤ 340 or ≥ 460	≤ 348 or ≥ 472
	0.05	≤ 322 or ≥ 458	≤ 329 or ≥ 471	≤ 337 or ≥ 483
	0.02	≤ 310 or ≥ 470	≤ 317 or ≥ 483	≤ 324 or ≥ 496
	0.01	≤ 302 or ≥ 478	≤ 309 or ≥ 491	≤ 315 or ≥ 505
	0.002	≤ 286 or ≥ 494	≤ 292 or ≥ 508	≤ 298 or ≥ 522

*Adapted with permission from C. Lentner (Ed.), *Geigy Scientific Tables*, 8th ed., Volume 2, Ciba-Geigy, Basle, 1982, pp. 156–162.

INDEX

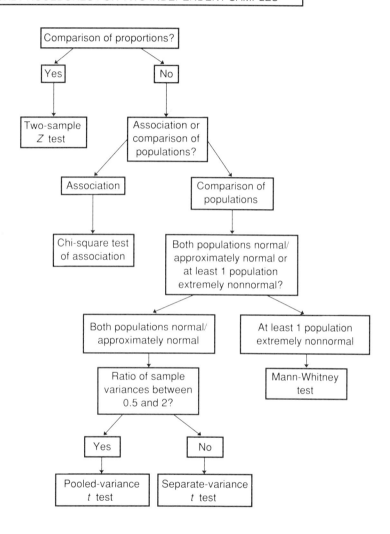

STATISTICAL PROCEDURES FOR TWO INDEPENDENT SAMPLES

Comparison of proportions?

Yes

No

Two-sample
Z test

Association or
comparison of
populations?

Association

Comparison of
populations

Chi-square test
of association

Both populations normal/
approximately normal or
at least 1 population
extremely nonnormal?

Both populations normal/
approximately normal

At least 1 population
extremely nonnormal

Ratio of sample
variances between
0.5 and 2?

Mann-Whitney
test

Yes

No

Pooled-variance
t test

Separate-variance
t test

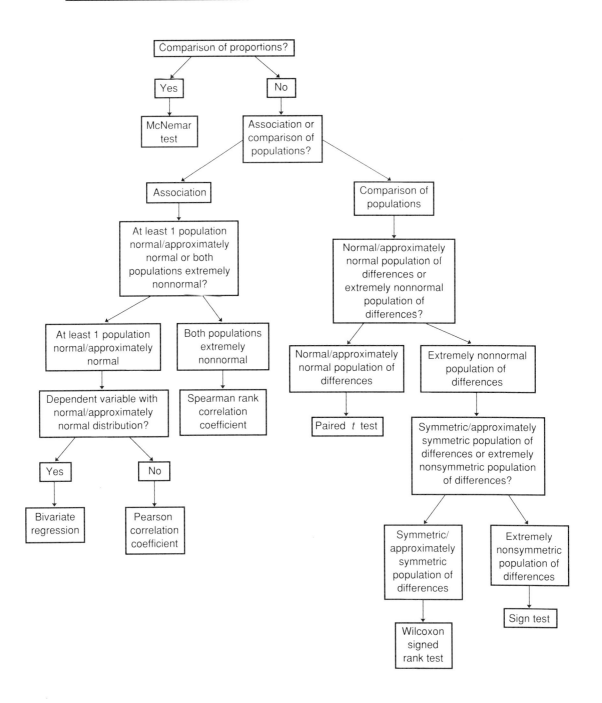

STATISTICAL PROCEDURES FOR TWO PAIRED SAMPLES

Comparison of proportions?

Yes → McNemar test

No → Association or comparison of populations?

Association

At least 1 population normal/approximately normal or both populations extremely nonnormal?

At least 1 population normal/approximately normal

Dependent variable with normal/approximately normal distribution?

Yes → Bivariate regression

No → Pearson correlation coefficient

Both populations extremely nonnormal

Spearman rank correlation coefficient

Comparison of populations

Normal/approximately normal population of differences or extremely nonnormal population of differences?

Normal/approximately normal population of differences

Paired *t* test

Extremely nonnormal population of differences

Symmetric/approximately symmetric population of differences or extremely nonsymmetric population of differences?

Symmetric/ approximately symmetric population of differences

Wilcoxon signed rank test

Extremely nonsymmetric population of differences

Sign test